HANDBOOK OF NONPRESCRIPTION DRUGS *fifth edition*

Health professionals and government officials alike expend vast amounts of energy and taxpayer dollars to constantly refine the distinction between prescription and nonprescription drug products. Unfortunately, the human body makes no such distinction. And so while the lay public often believes that nonprescription drugs may be used *ad infinitum* without concern or risk, the fact remains that some nonprescription medications are potentially more hazardous than some prescription drugs. Conversely, some prescription drugs are less effective than certain nonprescription drugs are for their respective indicated uses.

These facts, of course, contradict popular notions about drugs, and are among the principal reasons why the American Pharmaceutical Association, the national professional society of pharmacists, published the First Edition of this *Handbook* in 1967. Prior to its appearance, such information was rarely available to even the medical and pharmacy professions. This newest edition, a totally revised publication, is now a reflection of consumers' demands for increasingly sophisticated and comprehensive information on the drugs they self-prescribe and self-administer—and an increasing public awareness that pharmacists can provide the information and professional advice they seek.

Because Americans are the world's most liberal utilizers of self-medication, the American Pharmaceutical Association continues to devote its efforts to the rational, intelligent use of nonprescription drugs as well as prescription drugs. With the professional knowledge, judgment, and guidance of the nation's pharmacists, the consuming public can be assured that the nonprescription drugs it uses each day will both protect and advance good health.

William S. Apple, Ph.D.
Executive Director
American Pharmaceutical Association

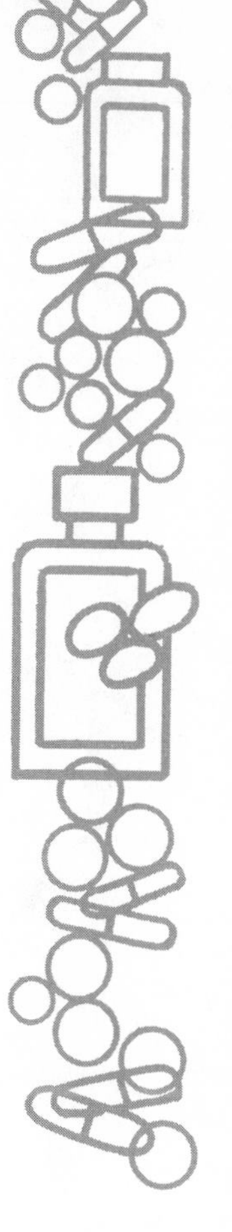

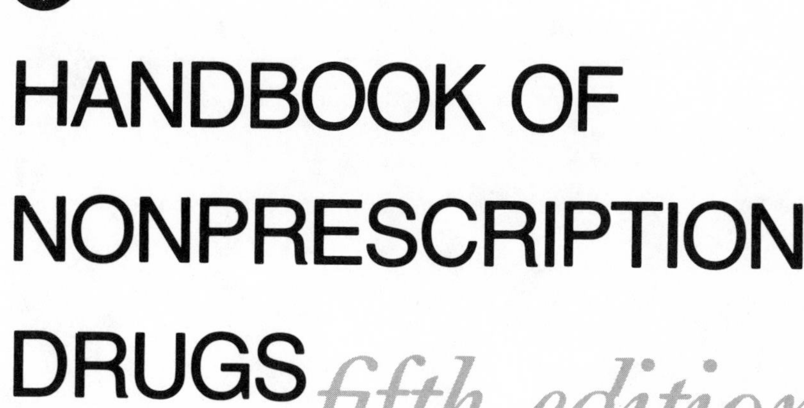

HANDBOOK OF NONPRESCRIPTION DRUGS *fifth edition*

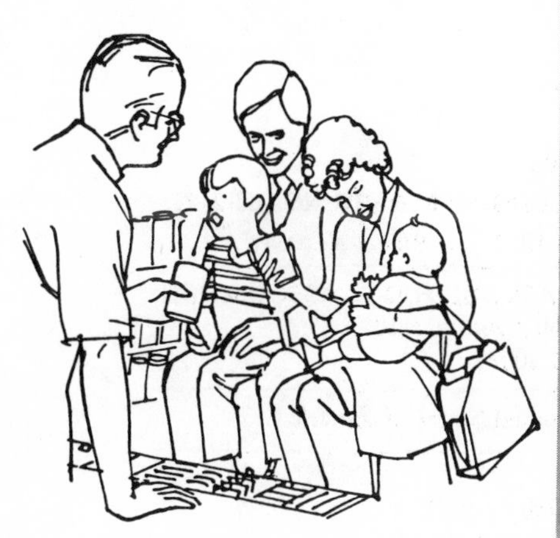

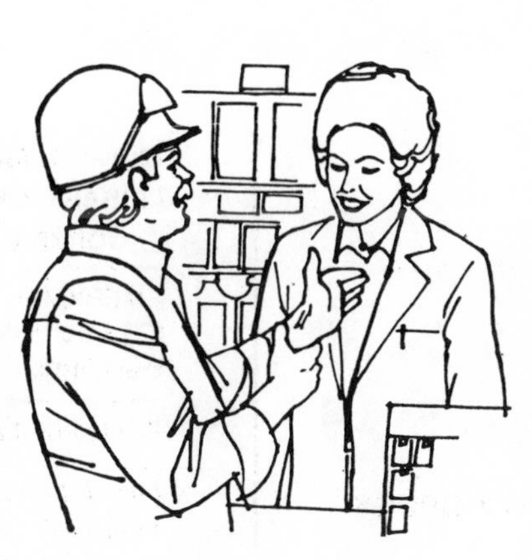

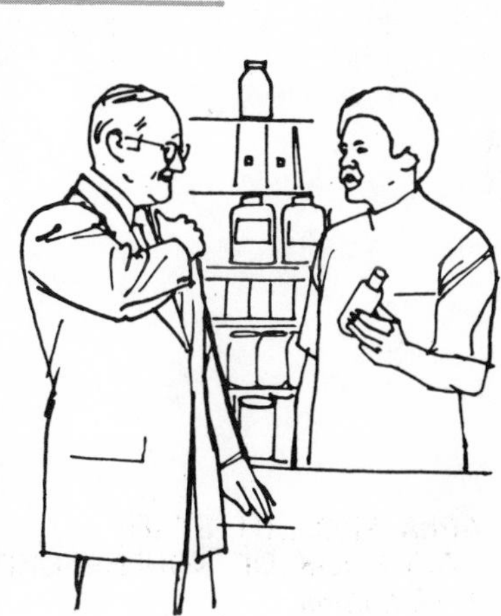

Published by
AMERICAN PHARMACEUTICAL ASSOCIATION
2215 Constitution Avenue, N.W.
Washington, DC 20037
(202) 628-4410

THE NATIONAL PROFESSIONAL SOCIETY OF PHARMACISTS

APhA PROJECT STAFF
HANDBOOK OF NONPRESCRIPTION DRUGS
Fifth Edition

Richard P. Penna, Pharm. D., *Project Director*
Cynthia Kleinfeld, *Project Editor*
David R. Bohardt, *Acting Director of Publications*
Margaret F. Rose

Consultants
James P. Caro, R. Ph.
Gene Anne Sandbach, R.Ph., *Product Tables*
John Sandbach, M.D., *Anatomical Drawings*

BOOK DESIGN: *Henry J. Bausili*
ANATOMICAL DRAWINGS: *Walter Hilmers*

ISBN 0-917330-08-0
LIBRARY OF CONGRESS CARD NO. 68-2177

AMERICAN PHARMACEUTICAL ASSOCIATION
2215 Constitution Avenue, N.W.
Washington, DC 20037

Printed in the United States of America

First Edition
Published September, 1967

Second Edition
Published January, 1969

Third Edition
Published January, 1971

Fourth Edition
Published March, 1973

Fifth Edition
Published January, 1977
Second Printing February, 1977
Third Printing June, 1977
Fourth Printing December, 1977

TABLE OF CONTENTS

PREFACE

"It is always rewarding to see the fruits of one's labors ripen and mature. The APhA proposal on drug reclassification and a steady flow of articles and editorials concerning it have placed the need for professional guidance of the public in self-medication into sharper focus."

This prophetic observation introduced the editorial in the November, 1965, issue of the *Journal of the American Pharmaceutical Association* which noted that APhA had been receiving an ever-increasing number of inquiries and suggestions on upgrading the type of information needed by pharmacists to serve the public better in this area of competence. It was reported that a California pharmaceutical educator called for better "courses in over-the-counter medication" while a Massachusetts community pharmacist asked if there was a guidebook on self-medication for the practitioner. But a review of existing published literature on nonprescription drugs revealed a decided inadequacy. The 1965 editorial put it this way:

"More and more literature today is concerned with the evaluation of prescription drugs and seemingly less and less literature is being devoted to reviews of OTC's. It is unfortunate that *all* currently available standard drug information sources either completely ignore, or include only a very limited number of examples of formulas and evaluations on use, toxicity and contraindications of home medication. . . . For these reasons, this month's [*APhA*] *Journal* is devoted to home medication. Admittedly, it is only a beginning but, hopefully, in 1966 we will be able to publish a series of comprehensive articles on various widely used classes of home remedies."

A total of 22 articles on various classes of nonprescription drugs were published in the *APhA Journal* between September 1966 and August 1967. The series met with such overwhelming acclaim that the articles were published in September 1967 as a separate 108-page soft cover handbook complete with an alphabetical product index of more than 1,000 different OTC's. Book reviews praised the *Handbook of Non-Prescription Drugs* as "a first" and "a valuable guide." *Drug Intelligence* noted in particular that "for the first time, there is now available in one handbook a wealth of information about drug products which the patient may obtain without a prescription."

The unprecedented and continuing demand for facts on nonprescription drugs resulted in the publication of the 1969 edition of the *Handbook* with a hard cover, expanded to 160 pages with 29 chapters, and both a product and manufacturers' index. Medical, dental, and other health professional journals added their accolades via book reviews.

By the time the 1971 edition of the *Handbook* was published—expanded to 202 pages with 31 chapters—it had become a universally accepted reference. It is not surprising, therefore, that the 1971 edition went through 9 printings before the 1973 edition was published containing 32 chapters and 232 pages. Linda L. Hawkins joined as co-editor of the 1971 and 1973 editions.

The profession of pharmacy has witnessed the evolution of many continuing standard references over the years. These include the *United States Pharmacopeia* in 1820; the *United States Dispensatory* in 1833; *Remington's Practice of Pharmacy* in 1885 (now *Remington's Pharmaceutical Sciences*); and the *National Formulary* in 1888. But no publication on home remedies designed for the health professions has achieved similar continuity. As pharmacists and physicians were attempting to determine the composition of the secret remedies at the turn of the century, pharmacist A. Emil Hiss published in 1898 a *Thesaurus of Proprietary Preparations* with the admonition that "the editor holds it to be the bounden duty of every physician and pharmacist to know everything possible concerning the constituents of everything he may prescribe or dispense. In this way only can he discharge his obligations to the physical welfare of his patrons." The Hiss *Thesaurus* was patterned after Charles W. Oleson's *Secret Nostrums* first published in 1889.

With the passage of the 1906 Federal Food and Drug Act, there was a decided decline in literature for the health professions on nonprescription drugs. Instead, the interest in OTC's shifted from the professions to lay groups. There was Arthur Kallet and F. J. Schlink's fiery best-seller entitled *100,000,000 Guinea Pigs* published in 1933, but the enactment of the 1938 Federal Food, Drug, and Cosmetic Act appeared to quiet the muckrakers for a time. As the public grew exceedingly interested in knowing more about all drugs, Consumer's Union published in 1955 the first edition of *The Medicine Show*, subtitled "Some Plain Truths about Popular Remedies for Common Ailments." The early editions based evaluations more often on price alone than on actual evaluation of product composition. However, the 1974 Revised Edition of *The Medicine Show* is much more sophisticated in its approach, noting that among the "respected Books" consulted was APhA's *Handbook of Non-Prescription Drugs*, fourth edition. In fact, Consumer's Union borrowed much of the quantitative data of actual constituents for leading OTC products from APhA's *Handbook*.

It will be for impartial historians to place the *Handbook* into proper perspective, but we already have a preliminary analysis in James Harvey Young's *American Self-Dosage Medicines: An Historical Perspective* (Coronado Press, 1974). This noted historian records that "pharmacists, physicians, and other professionals, the compilers hoped, might use the *Handbook* to counsel patients about non-prescription drugs. To judge by the number of copies sold, the work filled a most pressing need." More importantly, Dr. Young's history suggests that APhA's efforts were an important factor in stimulating FDA to launch in 1972 its OTC Drug Products Evaluation Program. Originally estimated to take 3 years, the FDA/OTC panel process is necessarily slow. In the meanwhile, the American Pharmaceutical Association offers in this Fifth Edition of the *Handbook of Nonprescription Drugs* the only definitive compilation of facts on home remedies. As we stated in the introduction of previous editions, we feel confident that this *Handbook* will make the reader a little wiser, the self-medicating public a little safer, and nonprescription drugs a little more useful. —*George B. Griffenhagen*

ACKNOWLEDGMENTS

HANDBOOK OF NONPRESCRIPTION DRUGS REVISION PROJECT

ADVISORY COMMITTEE

Linwood F. Tice, D.Sc., *Chairman*
Dean Emeritus
The Philadelphia College of Pharmacy and Science
Philadelphia, Pennsylvania

George B. Griffenhagen
Associate Executive Director for Communications
American Pharmaceutical Association
Washington, DC

Richard P. Penna, Pharm.D.
Assistant Executive Director for Professional Affairs
Director, Handbook Revision Project
American Pharmaceutical Association
Washington, DC

Cynthia Kleinfeld
Editor, Handbook Revision Project
American Pharmaceutical Association
Washington, DC

Howard C. Ansel, Ph.D.
University of Georgia
Athens, Georgia

David S. Roffman
University of Maryland
Baltimore, Maryland

Leland J. Arney
Director of Publications
American Pharmaceutical Association
Washington, DC

Ivan R. Sanzel, R.Ph.
Community Pharmacist
Rochester, New York

Robert K. Chalmers, Ph.D.
Purdue University
West Lafayette, Indiana

Armond M. Welch, R.Ph.
Food and Drug Administration/Bureau of Drugs
Rockville, Maryland

Pierre S. Del Prato, Pharm.D.
Director of Clinical Practices
American Pharmaceutical Association
Washington, DC

Sara J. White, R.Ph.
University of Kansas Medical Center
Kansas City, Kansas

Neil E. Esterson, R.Ph.
Community Pharmacist
Seaford, Delaware

AUTHORS

Howard C. Ansel, Ph.D.
University of Georgia
Athens, Georgia

Glenn D. Appelt, Ph.D.
University of Colorado
Boulder, Colorado

Kenneth J. Bender, Pharm.D.
University of Illinois at the Medical Center
Chicago, Illinois

Bobby G. Bryant, Pharm.D.
Purdue University
West Lafayette, Indiana

Nancy Burdock, R.Ph.
University of Mississippi
University, Mississippi

James P. Caro, R.Ph.
American Pharmaceutical Association
Washington, DC

John F. Cormier, M.S.
Medical University of South Carolina
Charleston, South Carolina

Roy C. Darlington, Ph.D.
Howard University
Washington, DC

Robert L. Day, Pharm.D.
University of California
San Francisco, California

William R. Garnett, Pharm.D.
Virginia Commonwealth University
Richmond, Virginia

Lawrence J. Hak, Pharm.D.
University of North Carolina
Chapel Hill, North Carolina

Nathan A. Hall, Ph.D.
University of Washington
Seattle, Washington

Luis Hernandez, M.Sc.
Strong Memorial Hospital
Rochester, New York

Stephen G. Hoag, Ph.D.
North Dakota State University
Fargo, North Dakota

Raymond E. Hopponen, Ph.D.
South Dakota State University
Brookings, South Dakota

James Huff, Ph.D.
Oak Ridge National Laboratories
Oak Ridge, Tennessee

Marianne Ivey, B.S.
University of Washington
Seattle, Washington

Michael L. Kleinberg, M.S.
The Ohio State University
Columbus, Ohio

K. Richard Knoll, M.S.
University of Arkansas
Little Rock, Arkansas

Peter P. Lamy, Ph.D.
University of Maryland
Baltimore, Maryland

Max A. Lemberger, M.S.
University of Florida
Gainesville, Florida

Paul W. Lofholm, Pharm.D.
Ross Valley Medical Clinic
Greenbrae, California

R. Leon Longe, Pharm.D.
Medical College of Georgia
Augusta, Georgia

James W. McFadden, M.S.
Overlake Memorial Hospital
Bellevue, Washington

Michael W. McKenzie, M.S.
University of Florida
Gainesville, Florida

Keith O. Miller, M.S.
Medical University of South Carolina
Charleston, South Carolina

Gary M. Oderda, Pharm.D.
University of Maryland
Baltimore, Maryland

Frank A. Pettinato, Ph.D.
University of Montana
Missoula, Montana

Nicholas G. Popovich, Ph.D.
Purdue University
West Lafayette, Indiana

Keith W. Reichmann, Ph.D.
Southwestern Oklahoma State University
Weatherford, Oklahoma

Joseph R. Robinson, Ph.D.
University of Wisconsin
Madison, Wisconsin

Farid Sadik, Ph.D.
University of South Carolina
Columbia, South Carolina

A. Jeanece Seals
Tennessee Department of Public Health
Nashville, Tennessee

Ralph F. Shangraw, Ph.D.
University of Maryland
Baltimore, Maryland

Paul Skierkowski, Ph.D.
University of Mississippi
University, Mississippi

Gary H. Smith, Pharm.D.
University of Washington
Seattle, Washington

George Torosian, Ph.D.
University of Florida
Gainesville, Florida

W. Kent Van Tyle, Ph.D.
Butler University
Indianapolis, Indiana

Charles A. Walker, Ph.D.
The Florida A&M University
Tallahassee, Florida

Sheila West, Pharm.D.
Johns Hopkins Medical Institution
Baltimore, Maryland

Henry Wormser, Ph.D.
Wayne State University
Detroit, Michigan

Paul Zanowiak, Ph.D.
Temple University
Philadelphia, Pennsylvania

REVIEW PANEL MEMBERS

Kenneth Bachmann, Ph.D.
Paul Bass, Ph.D.
Robert L. Beamer, Ph.D.
Hyland A. Bickerman, M.D.
Norman F. Billups, Ph.D.
Billy Jim Blankenship, D.D.S., M.D.
Eddie L. Boyd, Pharm.D.
George B. Browning, R.Ph., F.A.C.A.
W. Ray Burns, Pharm.D.
F. David Butler, M.S.
Bruce C. Carlstedt, Ph.D.
Kenneth Crahan, M.S.
D. Stephen Crawford, B.S.
Gregory R. D'Angelo, R.Ph.
Alexander F. Demetro, Pharm.D.
Robert E. Duncan, B.S.
Thomas W. Dunphy, Pharm.D.
S. Albert Edwards, Pharm.D.
Carl F. Emswiller, Jr., B.S.
James C. Eoff III, Pharm.D.
Donald O. Fedder, B.S.
Stuart Feldman, Ph.D.
Earl L. Giacolini, B.S.
James H. Harelik, Pharm.D.
Charles I. Hicks, M.S.
George M. Hocking, Ph.D.
Benjamin Hodes, Ph.D.

J. Heyward Hull, M.S.
James O. Inashima, Ph.D.
Arthur I. Jacknowitz, Pharm.D.
Raymond W. Jurgens, Jr., Ph.D.
Ronald B. Kluza, Ph.D.
Charma A. Konnor, Pharm.B.S., R.Ph.
Wayne A. Kradjan, Pharm.D.
Kermit E. Krantz, M.D., Litt.D.
Ruth Kroeger, Ph.D.
William S. Lackey, B.S.
Lawrence A. Lemchen, R.Ph.
Lawrence J. Lesko, Ph.D.
Mary M. Losey, M.S.
Irwin I. Lubowe, M.D., F.A.C.A.
Gregory A. Maggini, Pharm.D.
Shabir Z. Masih, Ph.D.
Jeremy A. Matchett, R.Ph., M.S.
John W. Mauger, Ph.D.
Arthur J. McBay, Ph.D.
Richard Y. Miller, R.Ph., F.A.C.A.
Roger B. Miller, B.S.
William A. Miller, M.Sc., Pharm.D.
Larry D. Milne, Ph.D.
Donald W. Moore, F.A.C.A.
Timothy Moore, B.S.
Robert S. Mosser, M.D.

George Narinian, M.S.
Edward G. Nold, M.S.
Thomas W. O'Connor, Pharm.D.
James O'Donnell, Ph.D.
Kenneth B. Paiva, Pharm.D.
Hugh T. Polson, B.S.
Arnold J. Repta, Ph.D.
Charles R. Rettig, D.P.M.
Joseph A. Romano, Pharm.D.
E. William Rosenberg, M.D.
Brandt Rowles, Ph.D.
Charles F. Ryan, Ph.D.
Roger H. Scholle, D.D.S.
Anthony J. Silvagni, Pharm.D.
Harold I. Silverman, D.Sc.
Stewart B. Siskin, Pharm.D.
Valentino J. Stella, Ph.D.
Curtis A. Taber, Ph.D.
C. Larry Thomasson, Ph.D.
Ralph W. Trottier, Jr., Ph.D.
C. Wayne Weart, Pharm.D.
Matthew B. Wiener, Pharm.D.
Byron B. Williams, Jr., Ph.D.
Dennis D. Williams, Pharm.D.
Phillip I. Wizwer, M.S.
Colin R. Woolf, M.D.
Thom J. Zimmerman, M.D.

Introduction

A Pharmacist should always strive to perfect and enlarge his professional knowledge. He should utilize and make available this knowledge as may be required in accordance with his best professional judgment.

Section 3 *Code of Ethics*
American Pharmaceutical Association

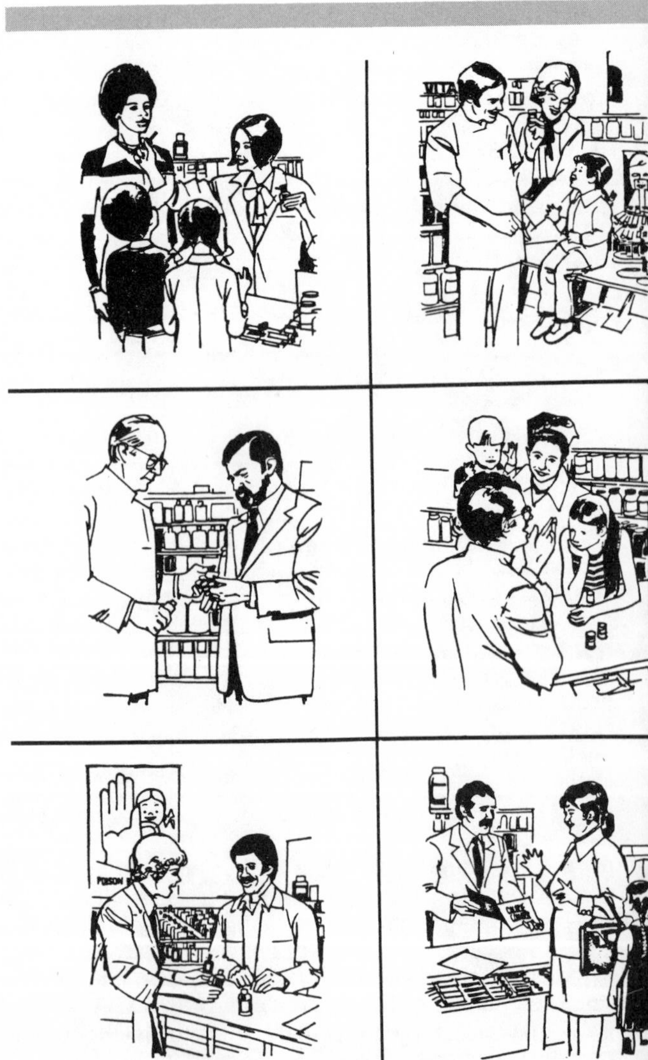

Health care can be divided into two general categories: medical care—that provided by physicians, nurses, dentists, pharmacists, hospitals, etc.—and self-care—patients caring for themselves. The American public spends about 8 percent of its gross national product (approximately $118 billion) on medical care. This same public spends between $4 and $8 billion per year on self-prescribed and self-administered drugs for self-diagnosed illnesses.

While self-care (at least viewed from the money spent for OTC drugs) may rank low on a monetary basis with medical care, it maintains if not exceeds this ratio when analyzed according to other statistics. It has been estimated that between 65 and 85 percent of illness episodes in the U.S.—including life-endangering situations—are cared for by the individual or the family. Some studies estimate that more than 70 percent of illnesses are treated with self-prescribed medication, indicating that self-diagnosis and self-medication constitute a significant and important component of self-care.

The relative contributions of self-care to the overall health status of the American people and the economics of health care are now being recognized. It stands to reason that the degree to which the American people engage in self-care, safely and effectively, directly affects the pressures which are placed on America's health care system. The economic impact is obvious. Victor Fuchs put it this way:

> "By changing institutions and creating new programs, we can make medical care more accessible and deliver it more efficiently, but the greatest potential for improving health lies in what we do and do not do for and to ourselves. The choice is ours."

Professor Lowell Levin defined self-care as "the self-initiated and self-controlled application of skills necessary to the promotion of health, reduction of undesired risks, diagnosis and treatment of disease, and the *effective use of professional health resources.*" This definition clearly establishes the interface between the self-diagnosing public and pharmacists—the intelligent use of available and knowledgeable resources—as a key to effective self-care.

Decisions by pharmacists based on knowledge of illnesses, patients, and drugs comprises the essence of professional services which pharmacists offer the self-caring public. This is what the American Pharmaceutical Association's *Handbook of Nonprescription Drugs* is all about.

The self-medicating person is a day-to-day reality for most pharmacists. In certain respects, the self-medicating patient can represent the most challenging and demanding part of a pharmacist's professional responsibilities. The self-medicating patient is most frequently a self-diagnosing patient. Such patients enter the pharmacy having already determined (a) the nature of their problem, (b) its probable resolution with nonprescription [over-the-counter (OTC)] drugs, and (c) perhaps the product or product type they intend to use. The pharmacist then must not only answer specific patient questions but also must help the patient retrace the steps taken to arrive at the "self-diagnosis," and, if appropriate, recommend a product and provide adequate instructions and warnings.

The pharmacist's responsibilities

The first responsibility of the pharmacist in counseling the self-medicating patient is to help the patient determine if the problem requires professional medical attention. The pharmacist's general knowledge of disease and specific knowledge of the patient are important in fulfilling this responsibility.

The second responsibility of the pharmacist is assisting the self-medicating patient who does not require medical assistance in choosing the most suitable course of action, e.g., let the condition run its course, recommend an OTC product, or suggest methods to reduce or eliminate the problem. Third, if the pharmacist decides that a product is indicated, the best available OTC product must be recommended from among the many that may be claimed to be effective.

Such recommendations necessarily must consider other drugs (prescription and OTC) that the person is taking, and the general condition of the person, i.e., age, weight, activity, etc.

The fourth area of responsibility involves being sure that the patient has all the essential information needed for safe and effective utilization of the products, e.g., instructions for use, possible side effects, when to discontinue, how long to wait before seeking medical attention, or when to check back with the pharmacist.

There was a time when organized pharmacy and pharmaceutical education generally frowned upon the practice of the pharmacist talking with patients about self-diagnosis and self-medication. Indeed, such "counter prescribing" was considered taboo, and even an early version of the APhA Code of Ethics contained a prohibition against such a practice. As late as the mid-1950's, schools of pharmacy were teaching students to "refer all questions about self-medication to the physician."

In the past 20 years, however, changes have occurred in the attitude of pharmacists toward their practice, and in pharmaceutical education toward the role of the pharmacist in self-medication. Many schools of pharmacy now include either required or elective courses on self-medication, and self-medication is considered an indispensable component of a pharmacy student's practical experience or internship requirement. APhA supports and encourages pharmacists to become more fully involved in advising self-medicating patients, despite the cries from certain medical associations that pharmacists are invading areas previously considered as the physicians' domain.

The elaboration of clinical pharmacy concepts over the last decade has emphasized the clinical functions of pharmaceutical service, particularly regarding the pharmacist's understanding minor illnesses, the OTC drugs available to treat them, and the reactions of patients to these drugs.

As the public becomes more involved in self-care, it more frequently will look to the pharmacist for advice in this area. Hence, the clinical aspects of self-care will grow as a challenge to pharmacy practice. The decision (professional judgment) is the key factor in the pharmacist/patient interaction relating to advice for self-medicating patients.

The entire range of functions relating to a pharmacist's clinical role in serving the self-medicating patient revolves around the recommendations that pharmacists make to the patient. The pharmacist's continuing education, experience, knowledge of specific products and individual patients all affect the pharmacist's final decision as to the course of action to advise for the patient. But pharmacists' recommendations are not made in isolation. The manufacturers and distributors of OTC drugs spend about $1.2 billion annually to advertise and promote the use of OTC medication. Advertising and promotion not only stimulate utilization but also perpetuate misinformation about the treatment of minor illnesses. How much these promotional efforts contribute to overuse and misuse has been, and continues to be, hotly debated.

Regardless of the precise extent to which promotion contributes to overuse and misuse of OTC drugs, the fact remains that the overuse and misuse of these drugs constitute a public health problem.

Nonprescription drugs

The Food, Drug, and Cosmetics Act defines a nonprescription drug as a drug for which directions for safe use by the public can be written. It does not necessarily follow that these drugs are without danger. A degree of hazard is involved in the use of all nonprescription drugs. For example, in a 3-year study of adverse drug reactions as a cause of hospitalization in one hospital, 18 percent of the admissions involved nonprescription drugs. Nonprescription drugs can interact with both nonprescription and prescription drugs. APhA's *Evaluations of Drug Interactions*, Second Edition, discusses more than 50 potential interactions involving aspirin.

Approaching the situation logically, if nonprescription drugs are effective, that is, if a function of the body is altered, then nonprescription drugs possess an element of danger to those who use them. That danger might arise from:

☐ The use of the agent according to instructions (adverse drug reaction).

☐ The use of the drug in combination with other drugs (adverse drug-drug interaction).

☐ The overuse or excessive use of the drug (toxicity).

☐ The use of the drug according to instructions, but for inappropriate purposes, such as conditions which have been misdiagnosed by patients.

The APhA *Handbook of Nonprescription Drugs*

In 1966, the American Pharmaceutical Association published articles in the *Journal of the American Pharmaceutical Association* dealing with specific classes of drugs. In 1967, many of these articles were compiled and became the first edition of the APhA *Handbook of Nonprescription Drugs*. Among pharmacists, interest in the *Handbook* was so encouraging that APhA revised the *Handbook* in 1969, 1971, and 1973. More chapters were added to each revision, and the existing chapters were expanded.

The objectives of the *Handbook* are to provide pharmacists and other health professionals with up-to-date information on commonly self-diagnosed conditions and the drugs used to treat them. In order to help meet these objectives, product tables are included in each chapter listing quantitative amounts of active ingredients (supplied by the manufacturer) of the more popular OTC products. As the *Handbook* has grown, so too have the product tables—it is estimated that the products responsible for approximately 90 percent of the dollar volume of OTC products sold in the U.S. are now represented in these tables. Further, the listing of quantitative amounts of active ingredients (where available) has provided a unique resource. The *Handbook* is the only compilation of quantitative amounts of active ingredients for OTC drugs.

In revising the *Handbook* for the Fifth Edition, the APhA Board of Trustees decided to add new chapters, combine some existing ones, and to delete others. In order to provide for effective practitioner input into the project design and implementation, the Board appointed an Advisory Committee to help design the publication. The Advisory Committee prepared a chapter outline for authors to follow as a guide to ensure design consistency. Each author was requested to approach the chapter by discussing the etiology of the condition; the anatomy, physiology, and pathophysiology of the affected systems; the signs and symptoms; the treatment and adjunctive measures; an evaluation of ingredients in OTC products; and important patient and product considerations.

Each chapter went through an in-depth review. Ten Review Panels were chosen, each responsible for reviewing an average of three chapters. Each Panel was composed of pharmacists, physicians, and other health professionals, in order that each chapter reflect a consensus of scientific thought. After initial editing, chapters were reviewed by APhA staff, then sent to the appropriate Panel. The Panel members were asked to comment on the accuracy and appropriateness of the material presented. The Panel's comments were referred back to the authors for revision of the chapters. These steps were repeated after the chapters were set in type. In addition to review by APhA staff and Review Panels, all chapters (at each stage) were sent to the Advisory Committee and to a member of the Food and Drug Administration's Division of OTC Drug Evaluation.

Interpreting product table data

Information contained in the product tables of this *Handbook* was obtained directly from the manufacturers of the more than 1,500 included products.

Product ingredients are classified either by pharmacologic class (e.g., analgesic) or by drug entity (e.g., aspirin). In columns which specify pharmacologic class, entries are either the name of the drug entity and the quantitative amount (when supplied) or a dash. A dash indicates that the product contains no ingredients in that class.

In columns which specify drug entity, entries are identified by: a) Quantitative data—the amount of the drug entity in the product; b) NS—the product contains the drug entity, but the amount was not supplied; or c) A dash —the product does not contain the drug entity.

Many of the tables include a column headed "other." This column is used to designate additional active and/or inactive ingredients. A dash in this column signifies that the manufacturer did not supply additional information; it should *not* be interpreted to mean that no other ingredients are contained in the product. For example, even though tablets contain fillers, binders, and color, dashes may appear in the "other" column for tablet preparations.

The FDA review program

The Food and Drug Administration (FDA) established an OTC Drug Review Program in 1972 to establish standards of safety, efficacy, and labeling for all OTC drug products on the market. The goals for the program are:

- ☐ To identify safe and effective ingredients for OTC drug products.
- ☐ To establish acceptable combinations of ingredients and their rationale for inclusion.
- ☐ To define safe and effective dose ranges for these ingredients in OTC products.
- ☐ To determine indications for self-medication use that are acceptable as manufacturer claims.
- ☐ To determine information to appear on OTC product labels including indications, directions for use, and appropriate warnings and cautions.
- ☐ To develop acceptable testing methods for each pharmacologic category of ingredients to determine safety and effectiveness for use.

To reach these objectives, FDA has formed 17 Panels of physicians, pharmacists, pharmacologists, and other health professionals to review specific classes of OTC drugs assigned to them. The Panels are to report their findings to the FDA Commissioner. The Panels' final reports are submitted to the FDA Commissioner and appear in the Federal Register.

APhA staff has maintained a close liaison with Panel activities and has arranged for *Handbook* authors to receive minutes and reports of all Panel meetings. The minutes are tentative, however, and recommendations made therein are subject to change.

The Panels' final reports may necessitate a revision of a particular chapter in this *Handbook,* in order that pharmacists be kept up-to-date with the FDA Panel reports as they affect *Handbook* chapters. APhA will review Panel reports and, where deemed necessary, request chapter authors to prepare clarifying language which will be published in the *Journal of the American Pharmaceutical Association*. Future *Handbook* revisions will reflect FDA OTC Panel reports as they become available.

This edition of the *Handbook of Nonprescription Drugs* culminates 3 years of intensive research and review by the Advisory Committee, authors, Review Panel members, and APhA staff. Each chapter, illustration, and table reflects their best professional and scientific judgments on what information will prove most valuable to pharmacists and their self-medicating patients.

If the pharmacist's involvement with patients is essential to safe and effective self-medication, reliable and practical reference information is the key to initiating their interaction. This Fifth Edition of the *Handbook* fulfills the APhA commitment to provide practitioners with that key. It is the most comprehensive publication of its kind and, in our opinion, no book better helps pharmacists live up to their professional responsibilities and earn the trust and confidence of the self-medicating public.

—Richard P. Penna, Director
Handbook Revision Project
January 1977

Antacid Products

William R. Garnett

Questions to ask the patient

How long has the pain been present?

When does the pain occur? Immediately after meals or several hours after meals?

Is the pain relieved by food?

Have you vomited blood or black "coffee ground" material?

Have you noticed blood in the stool or have the stools been black?

What medicines are you currently taking?

Have you used antacids before? Which ones?

Did they relieve the pain?

Are you on any dietary restrictions such as a low salt diet?

Are you under the care of a physician?

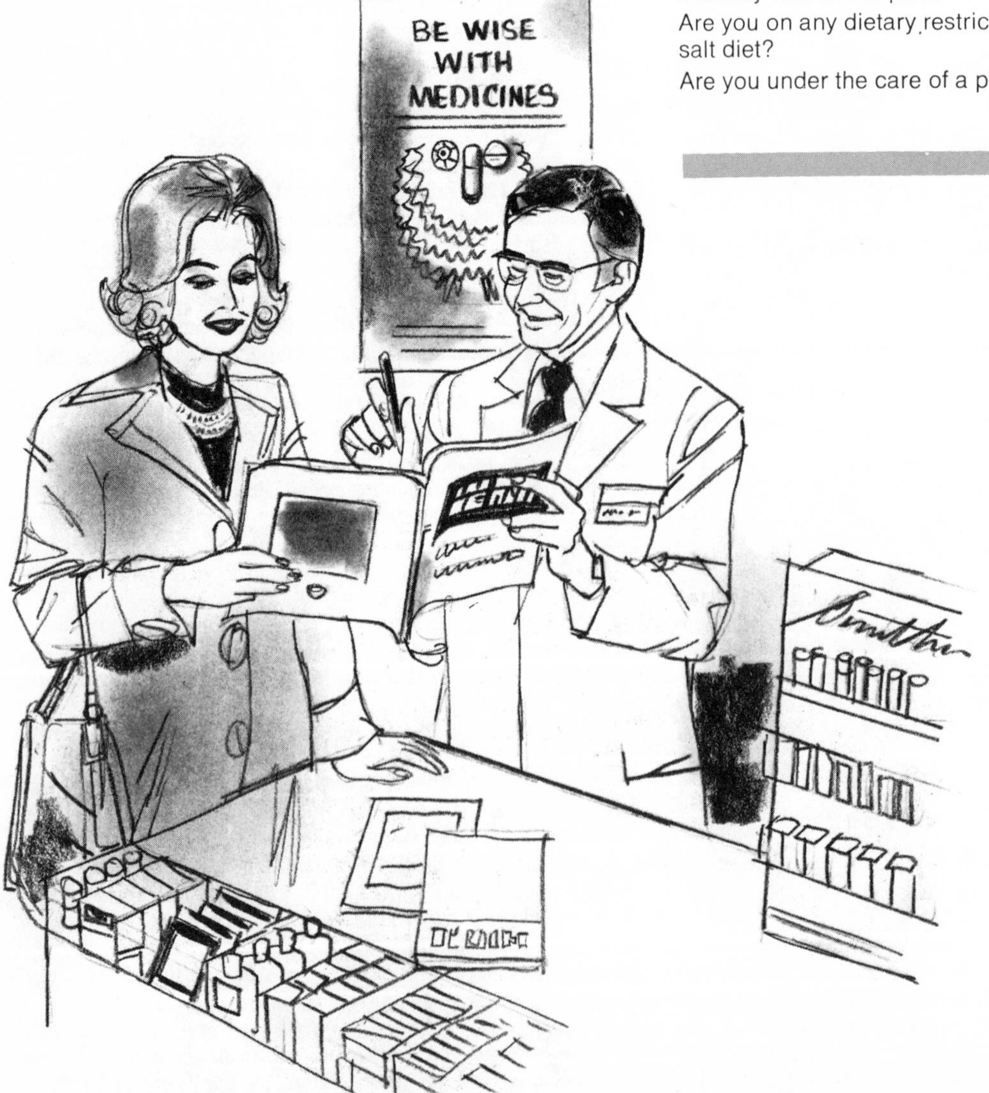

CHAPTER 1

The American public currently spends more than $140 million per year for the treatment of "sour stomach," "acid indigestion," "upset stomach," "heartburn," and other symptoms of gastrointestinal (GI) distress. These terms are used by the public and by antacid advertisers as synonyms for indigestion or discomfort located almost anywhere in the chest or abdomen. Pharmaceutical manufacturers have released more than 8,000 gels, suspensions, tablets, powders, and gums in an attempt to capture a part of this lucrative market. They devote millions of dollars to advertising the instant relief provided by their products. The pharmacist can provide an essential service by knowing when an antacid is indicated, when more extensive medical evaluation is needed, and how to select a product for an individual patient.

Physiology of the GI system

The upper GI system (Fig. 1) is made up of the esophagus, the stomach, the duodenum, the jejunum, and the ileum.[1-3] Peptic ulcer disease may occur at any site of the GI tract which is exposed to the digestive action of acid and pepsin. However, ulcers requiring antacid therapy occur most often in the stomach or duodenum.[4]

After food is ingested and masticated by the teeth, voluntary swallowing is initiated. Following the initiation of swallowing, an involuntary reflex, peristaltic movement, occurs in the pharynx and esophagus, which carries the food into the stomach. Gravity exerts an additional effect to pull food downward.

Anatomy of the stomach

The stomach consists of the cardia, fundus, body, and antrum. The cardia is a narrow strip (0.5 to 3.0 cm wide) that starts at the esophagogastric sphincter. It is lined with cardiac mucosa.

Gastric mucosa lines the fundus and the body (the largest part) of the stomach. This lining contains surface mucous cells, mucous neck cells, argentaffin cells, parietal cells, and chief cells. The gastric juice is a mixture of the various secretions of these cells. The parietal cells of the fundus secrete mainly hydrochloric acid; the chief cells of the glands, mainly pepsinogen; and the mucosal cells of the covering epithelium and the other cells of the glands secrete an alkaline, mucous juice for protection and lubrication. The hydrochloric acid reacts with the pepsinogen to form the active proteolytic enzyme, pepsin.[1,5] Intrinsic factor is also secreted by the parietal cells. It enables the absorption of extrinsic cyanocobalamin (vitamin B_{12}).

The antrum (which extends from the notch in the lesser curvature), the prepyloric canal (which is the narrow, last 2 to 5 cm of the antrum), and the pyloric sphincter (which opens into the duodenum) make up the distal portion of the stomach. Pyloric mucosa and surface mucosal cells line the distal portion of the stomach and are responsible for the release of gastrin and a protective mucus.[1,5]

Gastric secretion

The three phases of gastric secretion are cephalic, gastric, and intestinal.[6] They proceed simultaneously, initiated by the introduction of food, and continue for several hours.[7] The cephalic and gastric phases are synergistic.

Cephalic phase. The cephalic phase, which is a parasympathetic response transmitted by the vagus nerve, is stimulated by the sight, smell, or thought of food. Vagotomy or large doses of anticholinergics prevent this phase. Vagal stimulation causes the release of hydrochloric acid, pepsinogen, and gastrin.[6,8]

Gastric phase. The presence of food in the stomach initiates the gastric phase of secretion by physical and chemical actions. The physical stretching of fundic mucosa mediates the release of hydrochloric acid. In addition, gastrin, also released by food, chemically stimulates the release of hydrochloric acid.[9] Gas also distends the stomach, stretching the fundic mucosa and increasing gastric secretions. The physical and chemical stimulation of gastric secretion are synergistic.[6]

Gastrin plays an important role as a neurohumoral stimulus to gastric secretion. There are several kinds of gastrin which vary in their molecular weight and site of release. "Little" gastrin is a major component of antral gastrin and is more potent than "big" gastrin, which has a longer half-life and is released mainly in the small intestine.[10] "Big big" gastrin is secreted from the jejunum.[11] The gastric mucosa makes no distinction between the gastrins and responds to all of them by secreting hydrochloric acid and pepsinogen.[12]

Gastrin release may be stimulated by ingested material and neural and blood-borne stimulants.[13] Peptides and amino acids are potent stimuli for the release of gastrin. Gastric distention initiates reflexes to release gastrin. The blood-borne stimuli—epinephrine and calcium—do not normally reach levels high enough to initiate release. Gastrin release is inhibited by acid and by circulating secretin, glucagon, and calcitonin.[14]

Gastrin is significant in other physiologic gastric functions.[7] It may help prevent peptic ulcers by stimulating gastric mucosal cell proliferation and by tightening the gastric mucosal cell barrier.[15,16] It also increases lower esophageal sphincter tone which helps prevent peptic esophagitis.[17] The chemical structural relationship of gastrin to pancreozymin and cholecystokinin explains why gastrin increases pancreatic secretions, increases the flow of peptic bile, and increases gastric and intestinal motility.[8]

Intestinal phase. The third phase of gastric secretion, called the intestinal phase, is controlled by the intestine and involves stimulation and inhibition. As long as chyme, or partly digested food, is in the intestine, there is continued gastric secretion, probably mediated by "big" gastrin.[6] Other intestinal secretions, such as cholecystokinin and pancreozymin, stimulate gastric secretion of acid and pepsinogen but inhibit the action of gastrin.[18,19] This inhibition is believed to be caused by the release of enterogastrone.[8] Enterogastrone is any substance secreted from the small intestine that inhibits gastric secretion.[7] An enterogastrone may inhibit gastric secretion and motility by direct inhibition of acid-pepsinogen release, by inhibiting gastrin activity, or both. Cholecystokinin, pancreozymin, and glucagon inhibit the action of gastrin.[19, 20] Secretin blocks acid secretion and inhibits the release of gastrin.[21, 22]

The stomach secretes acid and proteolytic enzymes to help digest food. Autodigestion of the stomach and intestine is prevented by the mucus barriers, the intestinal inhibition of gastric secretion, cellular regeneration, rapid blood flow, and an epithelial cell barrier.[1] Normally, these defense mechanisms are sufficient. However, the balance may be altered so that the acid-pepsin complex predominates and an ulcer forms.

Ulcers: acute and chronic

An ulcer is an open sore or lesion of the skin or mucous membrane of the body with loss of substance, sometimes accompanied by pus.[23] In the GI tract, ulcers can be acute or chronic.

Acute ulcers are single or multiple lesions mainly in the stomach and, rarely, in the duodenum. They are shallow and usually are associated with an identifiable cause: surgery and trauma (Cushing's ulcer), burns (Curling's ulcer), infection, uremia, cerebrovascular accidents, endogenous steroids, alcohol, and drugs.[4, 24, 25] Drugs that have acute ulcerogenic potential include aspirin, phenylbutazone, indomethacin, reserpine, caffeine, and corticosteroids.[26] Acute ulcers may be caused by the digestive action of acid and pepsin, erosion of the gastric mucosa, or change in the production of mucosa.[27] They can occur in the course of daily activity and may be asymptomatic or may cause acute GI hemorrhage and pain, necessitating hospitalization. This kind of ulcer heals rapidly and rarely requires chronic antacid therapy. Prevention of acute ulcers has involved antacids and the avoidance of ulcerogenic drugs in high-risk patients.[8] There are no controlled studies as to the effectiveness of this therapy.

Peptic ulcers are chronic but may have sudden flareups. They are most often solitary and occur at all levels of the GI tract that are exposed to the digestive action of acid and pepsin. In decreasing order of frequency, they occur in the duodenum, stomach (gastric), esophagus, stoma of a gastroenterostomy, Meckel's diverticulum, and the jejunum.[10] However, the only significant sites of peptic ulcers are the duodenum and the stomach. It is unlikely that there is one etiology for peptic ulcer disease. The actual formation of an ulcer may require an interrelationship of several of the proposed etiologies.[28] It is usually agreed, however, that in order for an ulcer to occur, there must be acid and pepsin.[29]

Prior to World War I, gastric ulcers were more common than duodenal ulcers, but the incidence has shifted so that duodenal ulcers now occur about 10 times more frequently than gastric ulcers. Both types occur more frequently in males—4:1 for duodenal and 2:1 for gastric. Both types have a low mortality but may cause morbidity.[29] Neither occurs in primitive tribes or lower primates until they live in conditions of "civilization."

Gastric ulcer

Gastric ulcers occur most often along the lesser curvature and the adjacent posterior wall of the antrum to within 4 to 5 cm of the pyloric sphincter. They may occur occasionally in the cardia, pyloric canal, and the greater curvature of the body and fundus. Hyperacidity is a less frequent cause of gastric ulcers than of duodenal ulcers. Individuals with gastric ulcers may have low or normal acid secretion, but the ulcers occur next to the acid-secreting mucosa. Patients with normal acid secretion who develop gastric ulcers also tend to have duodenal ulcers; those with increased acid production have prepyloric gastric ulcers. Thus, acid seems to be more important in determining where, rather than when, a gastric ulcer originates.[29]

Etiology. Damaged or abnormal gastric mucosa may cause an ulcer.[30] Increased permeability to hydrogen ion, decreased mucus formation, decreased cell proliferation, and decreased mucosal blood flow have been postulated as causes of damaged mucosa.[30-33] However, none of these factors has been documented or takes into account other known factors of ulcer formation.

The major theories of gastric ulcer formation involve pyloric dysfunction. A slow gastric emptying time caused by an abnormality or stenosis of the pyloris leads to distention of the antrum and gastric stasis. This serves as a stimulus for gastrin release and increased gastric secretion.[34]

The second theory involves a dysfunction in motility of the pyloric sphincter which causes a reflux of duodenal fluid concentrated with bile salts into the stomach.[35] Normally, the pyloric sphincter prevents reflux of duodenal contents into the stomach, but when gastric ulcer is present, the sphincter allows this reflux.[36-38] Gastric analysis reveals more frequent and higher concentrations of bile in individuals with gastric ulcers than in those with no ulcers or with duodenal ulcers.[39] Once they are in the stomach, bile salts damage the gastric mucosa by changing the nature of the epithelial cells, by removing and depleting mucus, and by altering gastric permeability to acid, salt, and water. Bile salts also stimulate the release of gastrin and histamine, causing increased gastric secretion.[40] Pyloric dysfunction may be the result rather than the cause of the disease.

Several predisposing factors are associated with ulcer formation. There is a higher incidence of ulcers where there is a family history of ulcers or blood type O, suggesting a genetic influence.[29] A higher incidence is found in people who smoke tobacco or take ulcerogenic drugs.[41, 42] Causative factors may exist in the diet or environment that have not yet been elucidated. Currently, it is believed that ulcer formation is a result of several factors working in an unknown relationship in a predisposed individual.

Symptoms. Although the erosion of gastric mucosa may be asymptomatic, the most common complaints are pain and GI bleeding. The pain of gastric ulcers occurs within 30 to 60 minutes after meals and lasts between 60 and 90 minutes. This pain may be described by the patient as "heartburn," "acid indigestion," "sour stomach," etc. Its relationship to food intake results from the distention of inflamed areas and the release of acid. Rhythm or chronicity associated with the pain is rare, and the pain covers a wide area of the midepigastrium. Somatic pain that may radiate into the back indicates penetration, perforation, or obstruction. Nausea, bloating, anorexia, vomiting, and weight loss are also reported. The vomitus or stool may contain blood.

The pharmacist should obtain a history of the type, site, and duration of pain and the presence of bleeding. A small percentage (1 to 4 percent) of gastric ulcers are actually carcinomas of the stomach; therefore, definitive diagnosis is needed for chronic or recurring symptoms.

Bleeding, either acute or chronic, requires a medical evaluation. Although a patient history is helpful, it is not as useful a diagnostic aid for gastric ulcers as it is for duodenal ulcers. Definitive diagnosis of gastric ulcer is accomplished by examination of the stomach by X-ray, gastroscopy, gastric analysis for acid production and cytogenic cells, and testing for occult blood in the feces.

The mortality rate from gastric ulcers is low, but morbidity is high. Gastric ulcers are less responsive to medical management than duodenal ulcers and require surgery more often. They also have a higher incidence of recurrence than duodenal ulcers.

Duodenal ulcer

Duodenal ulcers are mucosal lesions that occur most often in the anterior wall of the proximal end of the duodenum.[4] The "typical" duodenal ulcer patient is male, between 30 and 50 years old, and has an aggressive personality. Based on current incidence, it is predicted that 1 out of 10 American males will develop a duodenal ulcer.[8]

Etiology. Hypersecretion of acid and pepsin is a causative factor of ulcer formation. The small intestine regulates acid production and protects itself from digestion by secreting a thick, viscous, alkaline fluid from the glands of Brunner.[1] However, in people with duodenal ulcers, there is an increase in the acidity and erosion of the duodenal mucosa. The increase in acid and pepsin may occur through abnormal vagal stimulation and gastrin concentration; it may also occur through impaired intestinal inhibition of gastric secretion because of decreased release of enterogastrones.[27 43 44] The increased acid secretion increases the conversion of pepsinogen to pepsin and prolongs the duration of proteolytic activity. It is the acid-pepsin complex that is responsible for the destruction of mucous membranes.[27]

Factors may predispose an individual to duodenal ulcers or may interact with the acid-pepsin to increase the potential for ulcers. The increased incidence of duodenal ulcers in individuals with a positive family history or blood type O suggests a genetic influence. The blood type association occurs in both gastric and duodenal ulcers but is more significant in duodenal ulcer patients. Many people can relate the onset of ulcer symptoms to a particularly stressful event, but the role played by emotional and psychological factors is still undefined.[8] Endocrine abnormalities resulting from elevated calcium or gastrin, e.g., the Zollinger-Ellison syndrome, may cause ulcers.[4] People who suffer from cirrhosis of the liver, chronic pancreatitis, chronic pulmonary disease, and arthritis have an increased incidence of duodenal ulcers.[8 27]

A medical workup should be performed to document the existence of the intestinal lesion. The definitive diagnostic tests for the presence of a duodenal ulcer are an X-ray following the barium swallow procedure and duodenoscopy.

Symptoms. Obtaining a good history of symptoms is important in the diagnosis of duodenal ulcers. The pain

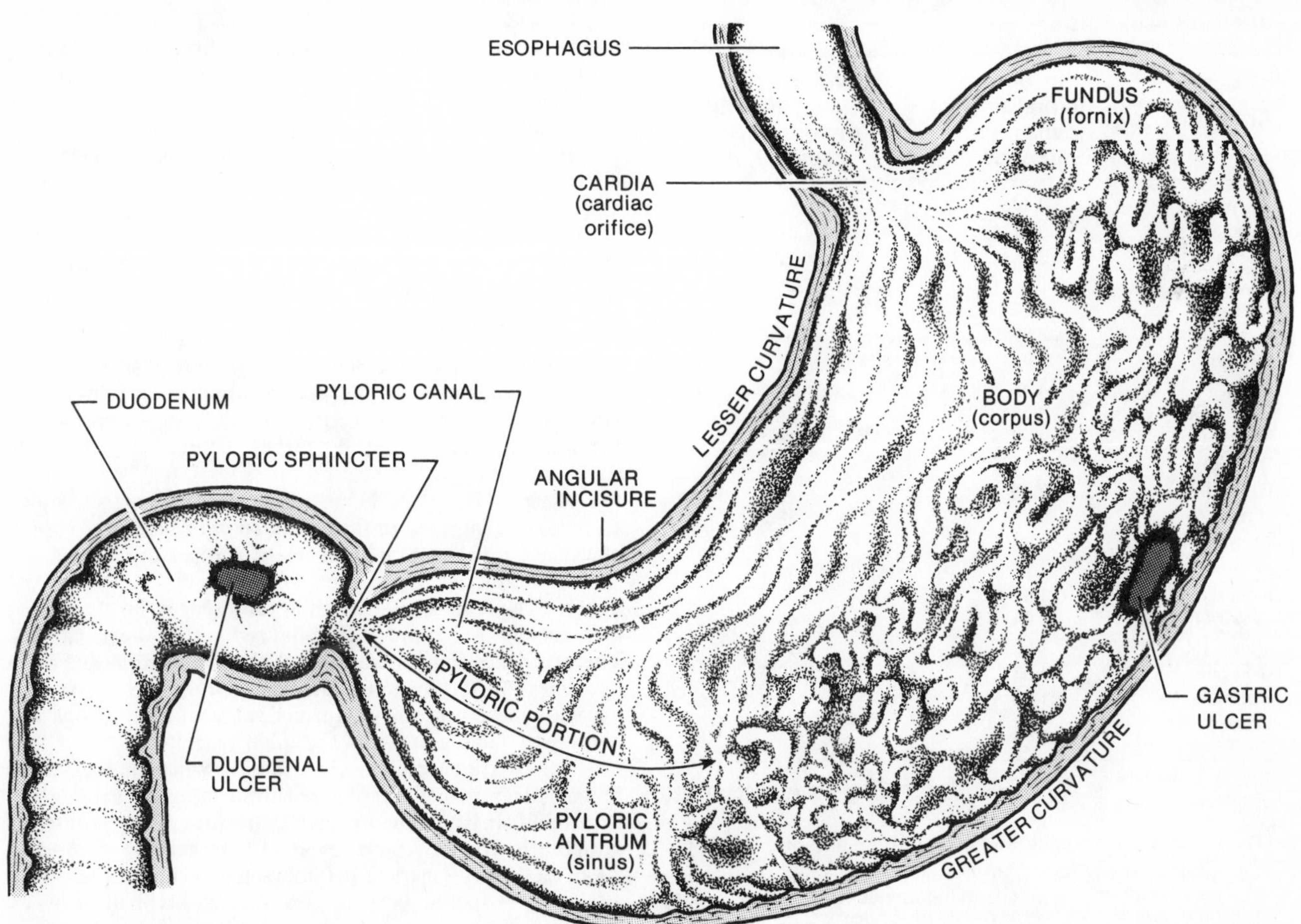

Figure 1. Sites of duodenal and gastric ulcers. Adapted from "The Ciba Collection of Medical Illustrations" by Frank H. Netter, M.D.

is rhythmical, periodic, and chronic. Its rhythmical nature corresponds to the release of gastric acid and usually begins 2 to 3 hours after meals and may continue until the next meal. The pain occurs when the stomach is empty and is relieved by food. The sensation is described as gnawing, burning, pressing, aching, or resembling hunger pain and often wakes the person at night. It is usually located in an area in the midepigastrium between the xiphoid and the umbilicus. The pain is prone to exacerbation and remission with or without therapy.[4 8] Exacerbations are most common in the spring and fall and may last for days to months.

Other GI symptoms include retrosternal burning, alteration in bowel habits, and, rarely, nausea and vomiting. The individual's appetite is good and frequently there is weight gain resulting from increased food intake to allay pain. Bleeding and/or perforation are frequent complications and may be the initial manifestation, especially in children. If there is bleeding, there is a change in color and consistency of the stool.[4] Duodenal bleeding is suspected when the patient complains of black, tarry stools. When the site of bleeding is high in the GI tract, the blood mixes with the feces giving it the black, tarry appearance. Red or red-streaked stools indicate lower GI bleeding.

Stenosis, or gastric outlet obstruction, is also a complication of peptic ulcer disease. It occurs more frequently with duodenal ulcers than with gastric ulcers. It results in vomiting, pain, and anorexia.

Table 1. Neutralizing Capacity of Various Antacids[a]

Antacid[b]	*In vitro* neutralizing capacity, mEq/ml	Volume[c] to equal 80 mEq of neutralizing capacity, ml
Mylanta-II	4.14	19.3
Titralac	3.87	20.7
Camalox	3.59	22.3
Aludrox	2.81	28.5
Maalox	2.58	31.0
Creamalin	2.57	31.1
Di-Gel	2.45	32.7
Mylanta	2.38	33.6
Silain-Gel	2.31	34.6
Marblen	2.28	35.1
WinGel	2.25	35.6
Gelusil M	2.23	35.9
Riopan	2.21	36.2
Amphojel	1.93	41.5
A.M.T.	1.79	44.7
Kolantyl Gel	1.69	47.3
Trisogel	1.65	48.5
Malcogel	1.59	50.3
Gelusil	1.33	60.2
Robalate	1.13	70.8
Phosphaljel	0.42	190.5

[a] Adapted from J. S. Fordtran *et al.*, *N. Engl. J. Med.*, **288(18)**, 923 (1973).

[b] For antacid components, see listing at the end of this chapter.

[c] To determine volume, divide the milliequivalents per milliliter capacity into the desired milliequivalent of antacid. For example, the neutralizing capacity of Maalox is 2.58 mEq/ml. To achieve 156 mEq of antacid activity, 60 ml of Maalox must be given; to achieve the same antacid potency using Gelusil, 117 ml must be given.

Treatment of ulcers

Because the main therapy for ulcers is OTC antacids, it is often difficult for the pharmacist to convince a patient who may have an ulcer to seek a more extensive medical examination. If the pharmacist believes that the GI distress is related to overeating, dietary indiscretion, or tension, antacids can be recommended. However, if the problem seems chronic, if there is an increase in the frequency of the distress, or if there are any other symptoms, medical help is indicated. Bleeding, vomiting, or obstruction may endanger a person's life. Bleeding may be suspected by the patient complaining of black, tarry stools or "coffee ground" vomitus. A loss of 50 to 100 ml of blood will result in black, tarry stools, whereas the loss of 500 ml of blood will result in systemic symptoms of anemia. The pharmacist should obtain a history from all patients returning frequently or trying different antacids. If the history is positive for signs of bleeding or suggestive of ulcer pain, the patient should be referred to a physician.

More serious diseases—gastritis, hiatal hernia, ulcerating gastric carcinoma, duodenal neoplasms, pancreatitis, insufficiency of the coronary arteries, pancreatic carcinoma, and radiating pleuretic chest pains—may mimic ulcer pain and require further diagnostic techniques.[45] If the complaint is limited and an antacid is recommended, the pharmacist should check to see if relief is obtained, how long the relief lasts, and if discomfort returns. If relief is not obtained after 2 weeks and is not sustained, the pharmacist should refer the patient to a physician.

Even without therapy, an ulcer may become quiescent, but it always has the potential to reactivate. During the period of active disease, therapy is directed at reducing pain. Ulcer treatment is unique in that nonprescription medications are also the initial medical management. An individual frequently initiates therapy with antacids, and a physician alters it only by changing the dose or the dosage interval. If antacids fail after an "adequate therapeutic trial," anticholinergics may be initiated by the physician. If rest, diet, antacids, and anticholinergics fail to control the disease, surgery to remove the lesion may be necessary.

Antacids and relief of pain

The rationale for antacid therapy has been to control the pain and to promote the healing of peptic ulcers. However, there are few controlled trials to support either hypothesis. Hollander and Harlan[46] found a statistically significant increase in healing rate ($P=0.04$) and in control of pain ($P=0.03$) in gastric ulcer patients treated with an antacid compared to those treated with placebo. A high placebo response rate prevented statistically significant results in duodenal ulcer patients. However, Butler and Gersh[47] were not able to show differences in healing or pain control in a group of hospitalized gastric ulcer patients. There are no controlled trials that test the differences in potencies of the various antacids. Until such time that many of these tests are performed, clinical impressions will continue to make antacids the main ulcer therapy.

There are several mechanisms by which antacids can reduce ulcer pain. Although neutralization of acid brings pain relief, it is not the only mechanism; epigastric distress of achlorhydria may be relieved with antacids.[48 49] Adding alkali elevates the gastric pH above the optimum for pepsin activity. Pepsin activity is completely inhibited between pH 4.0 and 5.0; partial pepsin inhibition occurs at a lower pH by progressive proteolytic neutralization.[50] This decrease in pepsin activity depends on alteration of pH and does not reflect intrinsic antipeptic activity of the antacids.[51] Other proposed mechanisms of antacid activity include tightening of the mucosal barrier and increasing lower esophageal sphincter tone.[52,53] The increase is believed to be responsible for the effectiveness of antacids in esophageal reflux (heartburn).[54] Antacids do not seem to have a coating effect on ulcers.[55] Thus, the primary effect of antacids is to neutralize acid, elevating gastric pH.

Ingredients in OTC products

Sodium bicarbonate. Sodium bicarbonate is a potent, effective antacid. However, because it is completely soluble in gastric and intestinal secretions, it should not be used in chronic therapy. Large doses or prolonged therapy may lead to systemic alkalosis.[56] Chronic administration with milk or calcium leads to an increase in calcium absorption and may precipitate the milk-alkali syndrome.[57,58] The syndrome is characterized by hypercalcemia, renal insufficiency, and metabolic alkalosis; it improves with the discontinuance of the antacid and calcium.[59,60] The symptoms include nausea, vomiting, headache, mental confusion, and anorexia.

Sodium bicarbonate may elevate the gastric pH above the desired 4.0 to 5.0. The stomach responds to this excess alkalinization by increasing acid output which results in an acid rebound phenomenon. Acid may also be released by the gastric distention that results from the carbon dioxide released during the reaction of sodium bicarbonate and hydrochloric acid. Thus, although sodium bicarbonate is a potent antacid, it may stimulate further acid secretion.

Each gram of sodium bicarbonate contains 12 mEq of sodium. Sodium retention becomes a problem when sodium-containing antacids are used in large doses or in individuals with decreased renal function.[61] The suggested daily maximum intake is 200 mEq bicarbonate in patients under 60 and 100 mEq in those over 60.[62] Gastric distention and flatulence may occur with effervescent sodium bicarbonate. Therefore, effervescent sodium bicarbonate (e.g., Alka-Seltzer) should be used only occasionally, for relief from overeating or indigestion. It is contraindicated for use in chronic therapy.

Calcium carbonate. Calcium carbonate exerts rapid, prolonged, and potent neutralization of gastric acid. Although there has been much enthusiasm for the use of calcium carbonate, the recognition of its systemic side effects has prompted a reevaluation of the agent.[63,64]

Calcium carbonate reacts with hydrochloric acid to form calcium chloride. Calcium chloride is highly soluble and available for absorption while in the stomach. The absorption is limited because about 90 percent of the calcium chloride is converted back to insoluble calcium salts, mainly calcium carbonate, in the small intestine.[65] However, enough calcium may be absorbed after several days of frequent use to induce hypercalcemia. In one study 30 percent of the patients developed hypercalcemia after 3 days of intensive antacid therapy.[66] The hypercalcemia may induce neurologic symptoms, renal calculi, and decreased renal function.[60,66]

Although most renal failure patients have hypocalcemia secondary to impaired vitamin D metabolism, hypercalcemia has been reported in patients undergoing dialysis.[67]

The milk-alkali syndrome is more common with sodium bicarbonate but may occur with calcium carbonate.[58] Increased absorption of calcium promotes alkalosis. If there is less calcium present in the small intestine secondary to absorption, there is also more bicarbonate absorbed. Thus, the hypercalcemia and the alkalosis of the milk-alkali syndrome occur.[65]

Calcium carbonate has been shown to induce gastric hypersecretion[68,69] as first reported by Breuhaus *et al.*,[70] who found that gastric secretory volume and acidity were greater the night after a day of calcium carbonate ingestion than after aluminum hydroxide or food ingestion. Fordtran[71] observed 24 patients with chronic duodenal ulcers and found that 4 or 8 g of calcium carbonate induced gastric hypersecretion 3 to 5.5 hours after ingestion, whereas 30 to 60 ml of aluminum and magnesium hydroxides or 4 or 8 g of sodium bicarbonate did not. He observed one subject closely and suggested that the mechanism is mediated by the action of calcium ions in the GI tract. Barreras[72] administered four equivalent neutralizing doses of calcium carbonate, sodium bicarbonate, and magnesium hydroxide at random to 20 duodenal ulcer patients. The mean gastric output in the 60-minute period beginning 2 hours after the last dose of antacid and 30 minutes after the insertion of a nasogastric tube was twice as great with calcium carbonate as it was in the basal state or with the other antacids. He concluded that it was the calcium carbonate itself rather than a nonspecific action of antacids that produced these effects. Reeder *et al.*,[73] after observing increased gastric secretion after calcium infusion, concluded that calcium increases serum gastrin and that it is the hypergastrinemia that is responsible for the hypersecretion. As little as 0.5 g of calcium carbonate (the amount found in most antacids) can increase the acid secretion in men with and without duodenal ulcers.[74] Although several theories have been presented to explain this acid rebound, it seems most likely that the mechanism is a local effect of calcium on the gastrin-producing cells.[68]

Constipation is another limiting factor for the chronic use of calcium carbonate. Calcium carbonate may be safely used in low doses for occasional relief of intermittent hyperacidity. It causes too many severe and frequent side effects to be recommended for chronic therapy.

Aluminum. Aluminum is administered most often as the hydroxide but also may be given as the carbonate, phosphate, or aminoacetate. The main side effect of aluminum antacids is constipation. Intestinal obstruction may occur in the elderly and in patients with decreased bowel motilities, dehydration, or fluid restriction.[56] Impaction may be increased by agents such as sodium polystyrene sulfonate resin (Kayexalate).[75] Constipation is usually managed by combining aluminum with magnesium compounds and by administering laxatives and stool softeners.

It was thought that aluminum did not cause systemic toxicity. However, several studies now report elevated serum or bone levels of aluminum in patients on chronic aluminum hydroxide therapy.[76-78] Alfrey *et al.*[79] have reported the first possible systemic toxicity of aluminum. They found elevated aluminum levels in brain gray matter of uremic patients who died of neurologic syndrome of unknown causes. The encephalopathy syndrome has been reported elsewhere, but this group was the first to monitor aluminum levels.[80-82] The patients developing the dementia all took aluminum hydroxide as a phosphate binder for 3 years or longer. It was concluded that patients with little or no renal function who chronically ingest aluminum may accumulate aluminum in the brain, inducing a neurological syndrome.

Aluminum binds with and decreases absorption of phosphate in the gut. It is useful for individuals with renal failure who have hyperphosphatemia, but it can cause phosphate depletion in others. In the restoration of renal function after a renal transplant, phosphate excretion and the hypophosphatemia produced by aluminum antacids may be enhanced.[83] Hypophosphatemia is manifested by anorexia, malaise, and muscle weakness.[56] Phosphate depletion can cause bone resorption of calcium and demineralization of the bone with resulting osteomalacia.[84] It has been suggested that serum phosphate levels be monitored bimonthly during therapy with aluminum.[85] The syndrome may occur as early as the third week of therapy and is complicated by a low phosphate diet and/or diarrhea.[86] Aluminum phosphate may reverse this process.

Aluminum hydroxide has the greatest neutralizing capacity of the aluminum salts but has less neutralizing capacity than magnesium hydroxide. Products that contain large quantities of anhydrous aluminum oxide react too slowly to be useful as antacids. Aluminum hydroxide gel loses much of its neutralizing capacity in the process of drying to a tablet or powder form. Once the gel dries, reconstitution with water cannot restore the neutralizing capacity.[56]

Magnesium. The salts of magnesium that have antacid properties are the oxide, hydroxide, and trisilicate. Of these, magnesium hydroxide is the most potent. The major side effect of magnesium is osmotic diarrhea, which can have systemic manifestations of fluid and electrolyte depletion.[65] This side effect may be a main cause of patient noncompliance.

After the neutralization of hydrochloric acid by magnesium salts, magnesium chloride is formed. It is partly absorbed and is rapidly eliminated by the kidney, but in the presence of renal disease, magnesium may accumulate causing hypermagnesemia.[56] Hypermagnesemia is manifested by hypotension, nausea, vomiting, depressed reflexes, respiratory depression, and coma.[87] It may be complicated by the administration of other magnesium-containing products and can occur after a renal transplant.[88] The author has seen hypermagnesemia develop in two patients with renal dysfunction after they ingested 300 ml of magnesium citrate and followed this with the ingestion of 30 ml of magaldrate for 3 to 5 days. Caution should be used if more than 50 mEq of magnesium is given daily to a patient with renal disease.[62]

An infrequent side effect of magnesium trisilicate is the development of renal stones. When this antacid is taken daily for long periods, silica renal stones may develop.[89-91] The stones formed after the ingestion of 15 g of magnesium trisilicate daily for 3 to 4 years.

Magnesium and aluminum hydroxides. Magnesium and aluminum ions have been mixed as hydroxide gels to balance the alterations of bowel habit caused by either alone. Because both ions are present, there may be normal bowel function, diarrhea, or constipation; diarrhea seems to be the more common alteration. Magaldrate is a chemical entity of aluminum and magnesium hydroxides, not a physical mixture. Its commercial form has the unique advantage of having the lowest sodium content of all antacids on the market.

Dosage recommendations

Dosage recommendations for antacids depend on which antacid is used and its neutralizing capacity, frequency of meals, dosage intervals, and palatability of the antacid.[92 93]

It has been recognized that not all antacids have the same neutralizing capacity *in vitro. In vitro* neutralization has been correlated with *in vivo* potency.[93] Following a standard test meal, it was found that the gastric acidity increased slowly for the first 1.5 hours while the food provided a buffer; then, acidity increased rapidly to an average maximum of 65 mEq/liter. The ingestion of an antacid containing 156 mEq of aluminum and magnesium hydroxides, 1 hour after eating, prevented acidity from increasing above 3 mEq/liter at the end of 3 hours. Although the *in vivo* potency of equal volumes of antacids varied widely, an *in vitro* test predicted the *in vivo* potency. Using this test, a 17-fold difference was found in commercial products. Antacids that contain calcium carbonate and concentrated antacids are the most potent. However, as previously discussed, calcium carbonate should be avoided for chronic, intensive therapy. Therapy is best instituted with an aluminum-magnesium preparation.

The buffer capacity of the antacid must also be considered; a dose of 15 to 30 ml of an antacid may not be sufficient. The dose should be calculated in terms of milliequivalents (mEq) of antacid and converted to volume. A milliequivalent of antacid is defined by the milliequivalents of hydrochloric acid that are required to keep an antacid suspension at pH 3.0 for 2 hours *in vitro.*[93] Table 1 lists the neutralizing capacity (in milliequivalents per milliliter) for various antacids.

For initial treatment of gastric ulcers, intensive antacid therapy initiated with 40 mEq of antacid is recommended every hour while the person is awake. Treatment for duodenal ulcers starts with 80 mEq of antacid every hour.[65] Although Fordtran [65] recommends "that doses should be as large as reasonably tolerable," Morrissey and Barreras [56] are concerned about toxicity. They feel that smaller doses should be used, e.g., four to eight doses of 10 to 15 ml of aluminum and magnesium hydroxides and four to eight doses of aluminum hydroxide. They state that 90 percent of the acid is neutralized at pH 2.3 and 99 percent at pH 3.3; additional neutralization is considered inconsequential. The actual amount given depends on the person's response—a low dose is used initially with gradual increases if the patient does not respond. Intensive antacid therapy should be reserved for institutionalized patients and should be closely monitored for side effects. For occasional use, 20 to 40 mEq of liquid antacid or 2 to 4 g of sodium bicarbonate or calcium carbonate is effective.

The dose of antacid can be altered by the temporal relationship to meals. Food acts as a buffer even though it triggers the release of acid and the formation of pepsin.[94] Taken 1 hour after meals, antacids can reduce acidity for as long as 3 hours; antacids that are ingested when there is no food in the stomach have a much shorter duration of action (20 to 40 minutes).[93 95] Information about the duration of action can be used when there is no pain on which to base the dosage interval. For gastric ulcers, 80 mEq of antacid 1 hour after meals and at bedtime is suggested for chronic therapy.[65] A Veterans Administration study suggests that this dosage should be continued for 6 weeks, the period needed to heal 80 percent of gastric ulcers; the actual healing rate depends on the size of the ulcer.[96] Dosage for duodenal ulcers is 80 to 160 mEq of antacid 1 hour after meals and at bedtime for about 6 to 8 weeks.

Palatability may determine the dose. In some individuals, larger doses taken less frequently may be better tolerated, although small frequent amounts are less likely to stimulate gastric secretion.[97] Unpalatability may be a major cause of noncompliance in outpatients. Side effects may require converting to another antacid. When selecting an alternative, the relative buffering capacity should be considered and the volume of antacid adjusted accordingly.

Formulations of antacids

Antacids are available as chewing gums, tablets, lozenges, powders, and liquids.[98] Insoluble antacids depend on particle size for neutralization of acid. A smaller particle size increases the surface area of the antacid; the greater surface area increases the wettability and the ease of mixing with gastric contents. Therefore, an increased surface area means an increased antacid effect. Many solid dosage forms must be thoroughly masticated before they will disintegrate and react with acid in the stomach. Liquid suspensions of antacids are milled to a fine particle size and provide a greater surface area.[99] It has been shown that tablet antacids are not equal to liquid antacids on a milligram for milligram basis.[65] This may be due to the desiccation process used in the manufacturing procedure. Tablets that do not disintegrate may lodge in the bowel and cause obstruction.[100] Powders must be suspended in water before ingestion. Liquids (suspensions) generally are easier to ingest and have a greater neutralizing capacity. Tablets may be reserved for people who find liquids awkward or inconvenient.

Drug interactions

Antacids may interfere with other drugs by forming insoluble complexes, by altering absorption, and by altering the pH of the urine. They contain polyvalent cations which are capable of forming insoluble chelates with other drugs given concurrently.

Absorption of tetracycline is decreased with the concurrent administration of antacids.[101] The decreased serum levels are clinically significant, and antacids containing polyvalent cations should not be given within 1 to 2 hours of tetracycline.[102] The American Pharmaceutical Association has advised practitioners to warn people against the concurrent use of tetracycline and antacids or milk.[103]

Although they are not well documented, the therapeutic effects of iron and chlorpromazine may be inhibited by antacids. The absorption of ferrous sulfate was measured in patients without antacid and with the administration of magnesium trisilicate. In all subjects the absorption of iron was inhibited.[104] The adsorption of chlorpromazine to antacids resulted in a decreased clinical response.[105,106] Concomitant administration of iron and chlorpromazine with antacids is not contraindicated but does indicate closer monitoring.

In vitro adsorption to antacids has been reported with anticholinergic drugs, alkaloids (only with magnesium trisilicate), and digoxin.[107-109] There are no clinical studies to suggest a significant *in vivo* interaction, and these drugs are not contraindicated. The antacids with the highest potential for adsorption contain magnesium trisilicate or magnesium hydroxide; calcium carbonate and aluminum hydroxide have an intermediate potential; and kaolin and bismuth subcarbonate have the lowest potential.[110]

By making the gastric contents more alkaline, antacids may alter the absorbability of weak acids and bases by altering the degree of ionization. An increase in gastric pH increases the un-ionized concentration of basic drugs and decreases the un-ionized concentration of acidic drugs. Thus, absorption is increased for basic drugs and decreased for acidic drugs. Absorption of pseudoephedrine, morphine, and quinine—all weak bases—is increased by antacids.[111] Decreased absorption is reported with the following acidic drugs: isoniazid, pentobarbital, nalidixic acid, nitrofurantoin, penicillin, sulfonamides, and salicylates; the clinical significance has not been established.[60,102,112,113] The most clinically significant decrease of absorption occurs with tetracycline.[114] The dissolution rate and absorption of tetracycline are inhibited as much as 50 percent by 2 g of sodium bicarbonate, which has no chelation activity. Antacids may alter the effect of enteric-coated products by causing an increased release of the drug in the stomach.[115] This may increase or decrease absorption or increase GI irritation.

Patients taking an antacid and requiring an anticoagulant should be placed on warfarin. The absorption of dicumarol has been shown to be increased 50 percent by 15 ml of magnesium hydroxide and 30 ml of aluminum hydroxide gel.[81] The absorption or the effect of warfarin is not altered by antacids.[81,82] Patients with a history of ulcers who require anticoagulants should be monitored for signs of GI bleeding, e.g., coffee ground vomitus or black, tarry stools.

Alteration of urine pH affects the renal excretion of drugs.[116] The effect of sodium bicarbonate on alkalinizing the urine is well known. However, Gibaldi *et al.*[117] have shown that "nonabsorbable" antacids may also affect urine pH. They administered the following doses of antacids four times a day: 10 ml of aluminum hydroxide (Amphojel), 15 ml of magnesium and aluminum hydroxides gel (Maalox), 5 ml of magnesium hydroxide (Phillips' Milk of Magnesia), 5 ml of dihydroxyaluminum aminoacetate (Robalate), and 5 ml of calcium carbonate and glycine (Titralac). On the average, suspensions of aluminum hydroxide and dihydroxyaluminum aminoacetate had no effect on the urine pH. The magnesium hydroxide and calcium carbonate suspensions raised the urine pH by 0.4 to 0.5 unit, and magnesium and aluminum hydroxides gel raised the urine pH by 0.9 unit. With regular administration, these changes are sufficient to affect the kinetics of elimination of certain acidic and basic drugs.

Levy *et al.*[118] showed that 20 ml of aluminum and magnesium hydroxides gel suspended in 50 ml of water given with two 300 mg aspirin tablets raised the urinary pH. The increased urinary pH increased the renal elimination of the salicylate and lowered the serum concentration by 30 to 70 percent. One case of quinidine intoxication resulting from antacid- and diet-induced alkaline urine has been reported.[119] Alkalinization of the urine to pH 8.5 with sodium bicarbonate has been shown to increase the activity of gentamicin against most gram-negative bacteria by 100 times or more.[80] This may allow a reduced dose in selected patients.

Systemic alkalosis has been reported following the administration of nonsystemic antacids and cation exchange resins, e.g., sodium polystyrene sulfonate.[120,121] The resin binds polyvalent cations, preventing them from forming an insoluble complex with bicarbonate. The bicarbonate is absorbed, resulting in systemic alkalosis.

Secondary formulation ingredients

Alginic acid. After the tablet is chewed, alginic acid reacts with the sodium bicarbonate in the tablet (in the presence of saliva in the oral cavity) to form a highly viscous solution of sodium alginate; there is not enough antacid to alter gastric pH. The sodium alginate is swallowed with a glass of water and is supposed to float on the surface of the gastric contents. If there is esophageal reflux, the mucosa comes in contact with the alginate rather than with the acidic contents.[122] The effectiveness of the sodium alginate depends on the individual remaining in a vertical position.[123] To ensure effectiveness, the patient should sleep propped up on pillows or elevate the head of the bed. Although there are reports in the literature attesting to the effectiveness of sodium alginate, the studies are poorly controlled, and the Food and Drug Administration (FDA) has withheld classification of effectiveness.[62 124] Large doses of alginate have been reported to deplete divalent cations.[125] If alginic acid is used, it should be restricted to reflux esophagitis.

Anticholinergics. Anticholinergics frequently are administered to prolong the duration of action of antacids. If they are used, the dose of both the antacid and anticholinergic should be individualized; side effects from the anticholinergic may occur if it is administered in fixed combinations. The FDA considers the combinations unsafe.[62]

Simethicone. Simethicone is an antifoaming agent. It causes small gas bubbles to coalesce and form larger ones. Simethicone is safe and effective as an antiflatulent, but its clinical benefit has not been established. It has no activity as an antacid.[62]

Additives. Additives such as analgesics and anticholinergics can cause side effects. Therefore, antacids which are given chronically should not contain analgesics, local anesthetics, sedatives, or anticholinergics. Additives such as bismuth and kaolin are of little therapeutic value.

Guidelines for product selection

The FDA OTC Panel on Antacids has set minimum criteria for a drug to be called an antacid. These data must accompany the professional literature and advertising. The test is based on *in vitro* neutralization, and the Panel does not provide comparative data nor does it make specific dosage recommendations. Thus, product selection and dosage must be based on the current literature and the individual.

Antacid therapy should be initiated with aluminum and magnesium hydroxides gel, unless other medical problems contraindicate it. Congestive heart failure, edema, hypertension, and renal failure should be included on a patient's medication profile. The sodium content of antacids is important to patients who must restrict their salt intake. It must be printed on the label of antacids if the content is more than 0.2 mEq per dosage unit.[62] Antacids should be selected carefully for patients with renal failure. Although magnesium is minimally absorbed, hypermagnesemia may develop in uremic patients or patients undergoing dialysis.[126 127]

Antacids that contain aluminum may cause constipation. The bowel habits of the patient should be reviewed. Antacids that may cause constipation or diarrhea should not be given to patients who already have these complaints.

The medical history should include antacids which have been tried. If self-medication with therapeutic doses of an acceptable antacid has been used without relief for at least 2 weeks, medical attention is indicated. It may be necessary to increase the volume and frequency of dosage.

Other drugs taken concurrently with an antacid should be checked for possible interactions. Although the effectiveness of an antacid is not likely to be diminished by other drugs, antacids may alter the effect of those drugs.

Although cost is not a main consideration in product selection, it should be taken into account; a considerable sum can be involved in the chronic use of antacids. The cheapest, most effective agent should be used, but a superior drug should not be avoided because of cost. Added ingredients, such an antiflatulents, which do not offer therapeutic benefit, add to the cost. Cost should be computed for equipotent not equivolume quantities.

Ulcer diets are ineffective in treating ulcers, regardless of patient compliance.[128-130] Alcohol and caffeine should be avoided because they directly stimulate gastric secretion. The prevailing philosophy is: "If a food causes ulcer pain, avoid it." Anticholinergics can be used after an unsuccessful response to an adequate trial of antacids or when antacids are contraindicated.[49 65] Research continues for alternatives to alkali and anticholinergic management of peptic ulcers. Bank and Marks[131] provide a review of the newer drugs for peptic ulcer disease.

Antacids are mainly used to reduce gastric acidity; they are occasionally used for other purposes. Sodium bicarbonate and Shol's solution (sodium citrate-citric acid) can be used to prevent the acidosis of chronic renal failure. Sodium bicarbonate is also used to increase the renal excretion of barbiturates and salicylates in cases of intoxication. In renal failure, calcium is absorbed poorly, and calcium carbonate helps replace the decreased serum calcium. Low calcium concentration leads to an elevated phosphorus concentration. Aluminum hydroxide or aluminum carbonate may be used as phosphate binders in the gut.

Antacids are administered prophylactically when ulcerogenic drugs, e.g., corticosteroids, are used for a long period. The clinical efficacy of prophylactic use is not proven.

The Pharmacist's Advice to the Patient

Compliance. The antacid should be taken on schedule—1 hour after meals, unless otherwise directed—to provide maximum duration of activity.

Change in bowel habits. To prevent self-medication for an iatrogenic condition, the patient should understand that the antacid may cause diarrhea or constipation. Control is usually provided by giving an alternative antacid.

Sodium content. Patients with restricted salt intake should be informed of the amount of sodium in the medications and advised of those products with a low sodium content.

Tablets. The lesser effectiveness of tablets should be made clear. If liquid antacids are unacceptable, tablets should be chewed thoroughly and followed with a full glass of water to help dissolution and dispersion in the stomach. Effervescent tablets should be dissolved in water and the bubbles should subside before swallowing.

Other medications. Additional medication should be identified to enable the pharmacist to monitor for drug interactions.

Changing antacids. The taste or side effects of the antacid may be intolerable. If another antacid is tried, the change should be supervised by the pharmacist to ensure than an equipotent, not necessarily equivolume, dose is administered.

Side effects of antacids. Several antacids (e.g., sodium bicarbonate) are absorbed and produce alterations in systemic pH. Others may induce nonsystemic changes such as changes in bowel function. For example, aluminum and calcium may cause constipation, but magnesium may cause diarrhea. Some cations (e.g., magnesium) are absorbed minimally, producing toxicity only if they cannot be excreted. This should be considered in patients with renal failure. The type and severity of side effects must be considered when antacids are used chronically and are major considerations in choosing an antacid for a particular patient. No antacid is devoid of side effects.

Summary

Before recommending an antacid, the pharmacist should ascertain the reason for the antacid. Obtaining a good medical history about the type of pain experienced can help determine if the problem is secondary to peptic ulceration.

If the problem is heartburn, indigestion, or upset stomach, an antacid may be suggested for self-medication—20 to 40 mEq of liquid antacid or 2 to 4 g of sodium bicarbonate or calcium carbonate is effective. The pharmacist should caution against frequent use. If the discomfort is not relieved after 2 weeks of therapeutic doses, medical help is indicated.

If the pain is consistent with peptic ulcer disease, the patient should be referred to a physician. The pharmacist may be asked to recommend an antacid for physician-supervised management of peptic ulcer disease. In the absence of other complications, an aluminum and magnesium hydroxides gel may be used as initial therapy. Individuals with renal failure, those on low sodium diets, and those with abnormal bowel function may require other agents. Therapy should continue for 6 to 8 weeks after the pain is controlled.

Subjectively, antacids are employed to control the pain of a peptic ulcer.[132] Failure may be the result of a poor selection of antacids, an infrequent dosage schedule, or an inadequate dose. Caution should be used if side effects necessitate switching an effective treatment regimen for another antacid.

New FDA standards for antacids require that ingredients be safe and effective, that the indications be limited to conditions related to excess stomach acid, that the patient instructions be clear and concise, that combination products have a reason for the combination, and that drug interactions be listed on the label.[133]

Whether prescribed or used as self-medication, antacids are the main treatment for peptic ulcer disease. There should be an adequate trial period with antacids before other drugs or surgery are considered.

References

1. "Peptic Ulcer," H. M. Spiro, Ed., Medcom for William H. Rorer, Inc., Fort Washington, Pa., 1971.
2. H. M. Spiro, "Clinical Gastroenterology," Collier-Macmillan, London, England, 1970.
3. "Gray's Anatomy of the Human Body," 28th ed., C. M. Goss, Ed., Lea and Febiger, Philadelphia, Pa., 1974.
4. S. L. Robbins, "Pathologic Basis of Disease," 4th ed., Saunders, Philadelphia, Pa., 1974.
5. S. Ito, in "Handbook of Physiology," C. F. Code, Ed., American Physiological Society, Washington, D. C., 1967.
6. A. C. Guyton, "Textbook of Medical Physiology," 4th ed., Saunders, Philadelphia, Pa., 1971.
7. K. J. Ivey, *Am. J. Med.*, **58,** 389(1975).
8. "Harrison's Principles of Internal Medicine," 7th ed., M. M. Wintrobe *et al.*, Eds., McGraw-Hill, New York, N.Y., 1974.
9. T. Scratcherd, *Clin. Gastroenterol.*, **2(2),** 259(1973).
10. J. E. McGuigan, *Gastroenterology*, **64(3),** 497(1973).
11. D. H. Stern and J. H. Walsh, *Gastroenterology*, **64(3),** 363(1973).
12. G. M. Makhlouf, *Fed. Proc.*, **27(6),** 1322(1968).
13. J. H. Walsh and M. I. Grossman, *N. Engl. J. Med.*, **292(25),** 1324(1975).
14. J. H. Walsh and M. I. Grossman, *N. Engl. J. Med.*, **292(26),** 1377(1975).
15. S. Cohen and W. Lipshutz, *J. Clin. Invest.*, **50(2),** 449(1971).
16. M. L. Chapman *et al.*, *Gastroenterology*, **63(6),** 962(1972).
17. M. G. Moshal *et al.*, *Am. J. Clin. Nutr.*, **23(3),** 336(1970).
18. K. G. Wormsley, *Scand. J. Gastroenterol.*, **3(6),** 632(1968).
19. A. M. Brooks and M. I. Grossman, *Gastroenterology*, **59(1),** 114(1970).
20. D. E. Wilson *et al.*, *Gastroenterology*, **63(1),** 45(1972).
21. K. G. Wormsley, *Gastroenterology*, **62(1),** 156(1972).
22. J. Hansky *et al.*, *Gastroenterology*, **61(1),** 62(1971).
23. C. W. Taber, "Taber's Cyclopedic Medical Dictionary," Davis, Philadelphia, Pa., 1969.
24. E. David *et al.*, *Mayo Clin. Proc.*, **46,** 15(1971).
25. F. P. Brooks, *Med. Clin. North Am.*, **50(5),** 1447(1966).
26. H. S. Murray *et al.*, *Br. Med. J.*, **1(5896),** 19(1974).
27. Rene Menguy, *Am. J. Surg.*, **120,** 282(1970).
28. L. Wise, *Ann. R. Coll. Surg. Engl.*, **50(3),** 145(1972).
29. M. J. S. Langman, *Clin. Gastroenterol.*, **2(2),** 219(1973).
30. P. H. Guth, *Gastroenterology*, **64(6),** 1187(1973).
31. H. W. Davenport, *Gastroenterology*, **46(3),** 254(1964).
32. W. M. Ludwig and M. Lipkin, *Gastroenterology*, **56(5),** 895(1969).
33. W. A. Mersereau and E. J. Hinchey, *Gastroenterology*, **64(6),** 1130(1973).
34. L. R. Dragstedt and E. R. Woodward, *Scand. J. Gastroenterol.*, **5(6),** 243(1970).
35. *Ann. Gastroenterol.*, **9,** 327(1973).
36. R. S. Fisher and S. Cohen, *Gastroenterology*, **64(1),** 67(1973).
37. R. S. Fischer and S. Cohen, *N. Engl. J. Med.*, **288(6),** 273(1973).
38. J. B. Cochina and P. Grech, *Gut*, **14(7),** 555(1973).
39. J. Rhodes *et al.*, *Gastroenterology*, **57(3),** 241(1969).
40. J. Rhodes and B. Calcraft, *Clin. Gastroenterol.*, **2(2),** 227(1973).
41. G. D. Friedman *et al.*, *N. Engl. J. Med.*, **290(9),** 469(1974).
42. W. C. MacDonald, *Gastroenterology*, **65(3),** 381(1973).
43. J. S. Fordtran and J. H. Walsh, *J. Clin. Invest.*, **52(3),** 645(1973).
44. J. E. McGuigan and W. L. Trudeau, *N. Engl. J. Med.*, **288(2),** 64(1973).
45. "Cecil and Loeb Textbook of Medicine," 13th ed., P. B. Beeson and W. McDermott, Eds., Saunders, Philadelphia, Pa., 1971.
46. D. Hollander and J. Harlan, *J. Am. Med. Assoc.*, **226(10),** 1181(1973).
47. M. L. Butler and H. Gersh, *Am. J. Dig. Dis.*, **20(9),** 803(1975).
48. D. W. Piper and T. R. Heap, *Drugs*, **3(5-6),** 366(1972).
49. A. Littman and B. H. Pine, *Ann. Intern. Med.*, **82(4),** 544(1975).
50. D. W. Piper and B. H. Fenton, *Gut*, **5(6),** 585(1964).
51. J. T. Kuruvilla, *Gut*, **12,** 897(1971).
52. J. E. Dill, *Gastroenterology*, **62(4),** 697(1972).
53. D. O. Castell and S. M. Levine, *Ann. Intern. Med.*, **74(2),** 223(1971).
54. R. H. Higgs *et al.*, *N. Engl. J. Med.*, **291(10),** 486(1974).
55. J. F. Morrissey *et al.*, *Arch. Intern. Med.*, **119(5),** 510(1967).
56. J. F. Morrissey and R. F. Barreras, *N. Engl. J. Med.*, **290(10),** 550(1974).
57. C. H. Burnett *et al.*, *N. Engl. J. Med.*, **240(20),** 787(1949).
58. C. J. Riley, *Practitioner*, **205(1229),** 657(1970).
59. F. W. Green *et al.*, *Am. J. Hosp. Pharm.*, **32(4),** 425(1975).
60. D. W. Piper, *Clin. Gastroenterol.*, **2(2),** 361(1973).
61. R. K. Maudlin, "Applied Therapeutics for Clinical Pharmacists," Y. Young and M. A. Kimble, Eds., Applied Therapeutics, 1975.
62. A. M. Schmidt, *Fed. Regist.*, **39(108),** 19862(1974).
63. D. E. McMillan and R. B. Freeman, *Medicine*, **44(6),** 485(1965).
64. J. B. Kirsner, *Gastroenterology*, **54(5),** 945(1968).
65. "Gastrointestinal Disease," M. H. Sleisenger and J. S. Fordtran, Eds., Saunders, Philadelphia, Pa., 1973.
66. J. Stiel *et al.*, *Gastroenterology*, **53(6),** 900(1967).
67. D. A. Ginzburg *et al.*, *Lancet*, **1,** 1271(1973).
68. R. F. Barreras, *Gastroenterology*, **64(6),** 1168(1973).
69. R. M. Case, *Digestion*, **8(3),** 269(1973).
70. H. Breuhaus *et al.*, *Gastroenterology*, **16,** 172(1950).
71. J. S. Fordtran, *N. Engl. J. Med.*, **279(17),** 900(1968).
72. R. F. Barreras, *N. Engl. J. Med.*, **282(25),** 1402(1970).
73. D. D. Reeder *et al.*, *Ann. Surg.*, **172(4),** 540(1970).
74. J. A. Levant *et al.*, *N. Engl. J. Med.*, **289(11),** 555(1973).
75. C. M. Townsend *et al.*, *N. Engl. J. Med.*, **288(20),** 1058(1973).
76. E. M. Clarkson *et al.*, *Clin. Sci.*, **43(4),** 519(1972).
77. G. M. Berlyne *et al.*, *Lancet*, **2,** 494(1970).
78. V. Parsons *et al.*, *Br. Med. J.*, **4,** 273(1971).
79. A. C. Alfrey *et al.*, *N. Engl. J. Med.*, **294(4),** 184(1976).
80. L. D. Sabath *et al.*, *Clin. Pharm. Ther.*, **11(2),** 161(1970).
81. J. J. Ambre and L. J. Fischer, *Clin. Pharm. Ther.*, **14(2),** 231(1973).
82. D. S. Robinson *et al.*, *Clin. Pharm. Ther.*, **12(3),** 491(1971).
83. R. E. Chojnacki, *Ann. Intern. Med.*, **74(2),** 297(1971).
84. C. E. Dent and C. S. Winter, *Br. Med. J.*, **1(5907),** 551(1974).
85. D. E. Abrams *et al.*, *West. J. Med.*, **120(2),** 157(1974).

86. M. Lotz *et al.*, *N. Engl. J. Med.*, **278(8)**, 409(1968).
87. R. E. Randall *et al.*, *Ann. Intern. Med.*, **61(1)**, 73(1964).
88. A. C. Alfrey *et al.*, *Ann. Intern. Med.*, **73(3)**, 367(1970).
89. J. R. Herman and A. S. Goldberg, *J. Am. Med. Assoc.*, **174(9)**, 1206(1960).
90. A. M. Joekes *et al.*, *Br. Med. J.*, **1(5846)**, 146(1973).
91. C. Lagergren, *J. Urol.*, **87(6)**, 994(1962).
92. D. W. Piper and B. H. Fenton, *Gut*, **5(6)**, 585(1964).
93. J. S. Fordtran *et al.*, *N. Engl. J. Med.*, **288(18)**, 923(1973).
94. J. S. Fordtran and J. H. Walsh, *J. Clin. Invest.*, **52**, 645(1973).
95. J. S. Fordtran and J. A. H. Collyns, *N. Engl. J. Med.*, **274(17)**, 921(1966).
96. A. Littman, Ed., *Gastroenterology*, **61(4)**, 567(1971).
97. E. S. Alday and H. S. Goldsmith, *Surg. Gynecol. Obstet.*, **139(3)**, 333(1974).
98. G. C. Cupit *et al.*, *Am. J. Nurs.*, **72(12)**, 2210(1972).
99. R. P. Penna in "Handbook of Non-Prescription Drugs," American Pharmaceutical Association, Washington, D. C., 1973, p. 7.
100. D. Patyk, *N. Engl. J. Med.*, **283(3)**, 134(1970).
101. S. A. Kabins, *J. Am. Med. Assoc.*, **219(2)**, 206(1972).
102. "Evaluations of Drug Interactions," 2d ed., American Pharmaceutical Association, Washington, DC 20037, 1976, p. 227.
103. *Apharmacy Weekly*, **14(25)**, 2(1975).
104. G. J. L. Hall and A. E. David, *Med. J. Aust.*, **2(2)**, 95(1969).
105. F. M. Forrest *et al.*, *Biol. Psychiatry*, **2(1)**, 53(1970).
106. W. E. Fann *et al.*, *J. Clin. Pharmacol.*, **13**, 388(1973).
107. S. M. Blaug and M. R. Gross, *J. Pharm. Sci.*, **54(2)**, 289(1965).
108. V. D. Gupta and K. L. Euler, *J. Pharm. Sci.*, **61(9)**, 1458(1972).
109. S. A. H. Khalil, *J. Pharm. Sci.*, **63(10)**, 1641(1974).
110. S. Khalil and M. Moustafa, *Die Pharmazie*, **28(2)**, 116(1973).
111. R. Lucarotti *et al.*, *J. Pharm. Sci.*, **61(6)**, 903(1972).
112. A. Hurwitz and D. L. Schlozman, *Am. Rev. Respir. Dis.*, **109(1)**, 41(1974).
113. A. Hurwitz and M. B. Sheehan, *J. Pharm. Exp. Ther.*, **179(1)**, 124(1971).
114. W. H. Barr *et al.*, *Clin. Pharm. Ther.*, **12(5)**, 779(1971).
115. S. Feldman and B. C. Carlstedt, *J. Am. Med. Assoc.*, **227(6)**, 660(1974).
116. "Evaluations of Drug Interactions," 2d ed., American Pharmaceutical Association, Washington, DC 20037, 1976, p. 320.
117. M. Gibaldi *et al.*, *Clin. Pharm. Ther.*, **16(3)**, 520(1974).
118. G. Levy *et al.*, *N. Engl. J. Med.*, **293(7)**, 323(1975).
119. M. D. Zinn, *Tex. Med.*, **66**, 64(1970).
120. E. T. Schroeder, *Gastroenterology*, **56(5)**, 868(1969).
121. P. C. Fernandez and P. J. Kovnat, *N. Engl. J. Med.*, **286(1)**, 23(1972).
122. C. Stanciu and J. R. Bennett, *Lancet*, **1(7848)**, 109(1974).
123. G. L. Beckloff *et al.*, *J. Clin. Pharm.*, **12(1)**, 11(1972).
124. M. Beeley and J. O. Warner, *Curr. Med. Res. Opin.*, **1**, 63(1972).
125. A. Littman, "Nutrients in Processed Foods," vol. 3, Boston Publishing Science Group, 1974.
126. S. Jameson, *Scand. J. Urol. Nephrol.*, **6(3)**, 260(1972).
127. F. J. Goodwin and F. P. Vince, *Br. J. Urol.*, **42(5)**, 586(1970).
128. R. Doll *et al.*, *Lancet*, **1**, 5(1956).
129. E. Buchman *et al.*, *Gastroenterology*, **56(6)**, 1016(1969).
130. H. S. Caron and H. P. Roth, *Am. J. Med. Sci.*, **261(1)**, 61(1971).
131. S. Bank and I. N. Marks, *Clin. Gastroenterol.*, **2(2)**, 379(1973).
132. G. L. W. Bonney and G. W. Pickering, *Clin. Sci.*, **6(1,2)**, 63(1946).
133. *FDA Consumer*, **8(6)**, 25(1974).

Product (manufacturer)	Dosage form	Calcium carbonate	Aluminum hydroxide	Magnesium oxide or hydroxide	Magnesium trisilicate	Other	Sodium content [b]
Alka-2 Chewable Antacid (Miles)	chewable tablet	500 mg	—	—	—	—	—
Alka-Seltzer Effervescent Antacid (Miles)	tablet	—	—	—	—	sodium bicarbonate, 1.008 g citric acid, 800 mg potassium bicarbonate, 300 mg	276 mg/tablet
Alkets (Upjohn)	tablet	780 mg	—	65 mg	—	magnesium carbonate, 130 mg	—
Aludrox (Wyeth)	tablet suspension	—	233 mg/tablet 307 mg/5 ml	84 mg/tablet 103 mg/5 ml	—	—	1.6 mg/tablet 1.5 mg/5 ml
Alurex (Rexall)	tablet suspension	—	NS [a]	NS [a] (hydroxide)	—	—	—
Aluscop (O'Neal, Jones & Feldman)	capsule suspension	—	gel, 150 mg (suspension)	180 mg/capsule 150 mg/5 ml (hydroxide)	—	dihydroxyaluminum acetate, 325 mg/capsule, 200 mg/5 ml methylparaben, 0.15% (suspension)	—
Amitone (Norcliff-Thayer)	tablet	350 mg	—	—	—	mint flavor	—
Amphojel (Wyeth)	tablet suspension	—	300 or 600 mg/tablet 320 mg/5 ml	—	—	—	1.4 or 1.8 mg/tablet 6.9 mg/5 ml
A.M.T. (Wyeth)	tablet suspension	—	164 mg/tablet 305 mg/5 ml	—	250 mg/tablet 625 mg/5 ml	—	3.5 mg/tablet 7.2 mg/5 ml
Antacid Powder (DeWitt)	powder	—	dried gel, 15%	—	31%	sodium bicarbonate, 25% magnesium carbonate (heavy), 10%	—
Anti-Acid No. 1 (North American)	tablet	227.5 mg	—	—	—	magnesium carbonate, 130 mg bismuth subnitrate, 32.5 mg aromatics	—
Banacid (Buffington)	tablet	—	NS [a]	NS [a] (hydroxide)	NS [a]	—	—
Basaljel (Wyeth)	suspension capsule tablet	—	400 mg/5 ml 500 mg/capsule or tablet	—	—	—	1.8 mg/5 ml 2.8 mg/capsule 2.1 mg/tablet
Basaljel Extra Strength (Wyeth)	suspension	—	1.0 g/5 ml	—	—	—	17 mg/5 ml
Bell-Ans (Dent)	tablet	—	—	—	—	sodium bicarbonate, 264 or 527 mg wintergreen ginger	—
BiSoDol (Whitehall)	tablet powder	195 mg (tablet)	—	180 mg (tablet)	—	sodium bicarbonate (powder) magnesium carbonate (powder) peppermint oil (tablet, powder)	0.036 mg/tablet 157 mg/tsp of powder

Product (manufacturer)	Dosage form	Calcium carbonate	Aluminum hydroxide	Magnesium oxide or hydroxide	Magnesium trisilicate	Other	Sodium content [b]
Camalox (Rorer)	suspension tablet	250 mg/5 ml or tablet	225 mg/5 ml or tablet	200 mg/5 ml or tablet (hydroxide)	—	—	2.5 mg/5 ml 1.5 mg/tablet
Chooz (Plough)	gum tablet	360 mg	—	—	268 mg	—	3.15 mg/tablet
Citrocarbonate (Upjohn)	suspension powder	—	—	—	—	sodium bicarbonate, 780 mg/3.9 g (suspension), 1.06 g/5.1 g (powder) sodium citrate, anhydrous, 1.82 g/3.9 g (suspension), 1.33 g/5.1 g (powder)	—
Creamalin (Winthrop)	tablet	—	248 mg	75 mg	—	mint flavor	41 mg
Delcid (Merrell-National)	suspension	—	600 mg/5 ml	665 mg/5 ml (hydroxide)	—	—	—
Dialume (Armour)	tablet	—	dried gel, 500 mg	—	—	—	—
Diatrol (Otis Clapp)	tablet	NS [a]	—	—	—	pectin sodium bicarbonate	—
Dicarbosil (Arch)	tablet	500 mg	—	—	—	peppermint oil	2.7 mg
Di-Gel (Plough)	tablet liquid	—	codried with magnesium carbonate, 282 mg/ tablet 282 mg/5 ml (liquid)	85 mg/tablet 87 mg/5 ml	—	simethicone, 25 mg/tablet or 5 ml	10.6 mg/tablet 8.5 mg/5 ml
Dimacid (Otis Clapp)	tablet	NS [a]	—	—	—	magnesium carbonate	—
Eno (Beecham Products)	powder	—	—	—	—	sodium bicar-bonate, 7.6% sodium tartrate, 65.2% sodium citrate, 27.2%	—
Estomul-M (Riker)	tablet liquid	—	codried with magnesium carbonate, 500 mg/ tablet 918 mg/5 ml	45 mg (tablet) (oxide)	—	—	—
Fizrin (Glenbrook)	powder	—	—	—	—	sodium bicarbonate, 1825 mg/ packet aspirin, 325 mg/ packet sodium carbonate, 400 mg/packet citric acid, 1448.5 mg/ packet	—

Product (manufacturer)	Dosage form	Calcium carbonate	Aluminum hydroxide	Magnesium oxide or hydroxide	Magnesium trisilicate	Other	Sodium content [b]
Flacid (Amfre-Grant)	tablet	—	NS [a]	85 mg (hydroxide)	—	simethicone, 25 mg magnesium carbonate, 282 mg	—
Gelumina (Amer. Pharm.)	tablet	—	250 mg	—	500 mg	sorbitol, 18.8 mg lactose saccharin sodium	0.3 mg
Gelusil (Warner-Chilcott)	tablet liquid	—	250 mg/tablet or 5 ml	—	500 mg/tablet or 5 ml	mint flavor	9 mg/tablet 8 mg/5 ml
Gelusil Flavor-Pack (Warner-Chilcott)	liquid	—	250 mg/5 ml	—	500 mg/5 ml	raspberry, spearmint, and pineapple flavors	—
Gelusil-Lac (Warner-Chilcott)	powder	—	1 g/packet	—	2 g/packet	high protein, low fat milk solids	7.5 mg/packet
Gelusil M (Warner-Chilcott)	tablet liquid	—	250 mg/tablet or 5 ml	100 mg/tablet or 5 ml	500 mg/tablet or 5 ml	mint flavor mannitol (tablet)	10 mg/tablet 9 mg/5 ml
Glycate (O'Neal, Jones & Feldman)	tablet	300 mg	—	—	—	glycine, 150 mg	—
Glycogel (Central Pharmacal)	tablet	325 mg	codried with magnesium carbonate, 175 mg	—	—	—	—
Gustalac (Geriatric Pharmaceutical)	tablet	300 mg	—	—	—	defatted skim milk powder, 200 mg	—
Kessadrox (McKesson)	suspension	—	1.0 g/15 ml	165 mg/15 ml (hydroxide)	—	peppermint oil sorbitol	—
Kolantyl (Merrell-National)	gel tablet wafer	—	150 mg/5 ml 300 mg/tablet (dried gel) 180 mg/wafer (dried gel)	150 mg/5 ml (hydroxide) 185 mg/tablet (oxide) 170 mg/wafer (hydroxide)	—	—	—
Krem (Mallinckrodt)	tablet	400 mg	—	—	—	magnesium carbonate, 200 mg milk base mint or cherry flavor	—
Kudrox (Kremers-Urban)	tablet liquid	—	codried with magnesium carbonate, 400 mg/tablet 565 mg/5 ml	180 mg/5 ml (only in suspension)	—	sorbitol solution, 1 ml/5 ml (only in suspension)	16 mg/tablet 15 mg/5 ml
Liquid Antacid (McKesson)	liquid	—	1.0 g/15 ml	165 mg/15 ml (hydroxide)	—	peppermint oil sorbitol	—
Maalox (Rorer)	suspension	—	225 mg/5 ml	200 mg/5 ml	—	—	2.5 mg/5 ml
Maalox #1 (Rorer)	tablet	—	200 mg	200 mg	—	—	0.84 mg
Maalox #2 (Rorer)	tablet	—	400 mg	400 mg	—	—	1.95 mg
Maalox Plus (Rorer)	tablet suspension	—	dried gel, 200 mg/tablet 225 mg/5 ml	200 mg/tablet or 5 ml (hydroxide)	—	simethicone, 25 mg/tablet or 5 ml	0.84 mg/tablet 2.5 mg/5 ml

Products 1 ANTACID

Product (manufacturer)	Dosage form	Calcium carbonate	Aluminum hydroxide	Magnesium oxide or hydroxide	Magnesium trisilicate	Other	Sodium content [b]
Magna Gel (North American)	suspension	—	NS [a]	NS [a] (hydroxide)	—	peppermint flavor	—
Magnatril (Lannett)	tablet suspension	—	260 mg/tablet or 5 ml	130 mg/tablet or 5 ml	454 mg/tablet 260 mg/5 ml	—	—
Magnesia and Alumina Oral Suspension (Philips Roxane)	suspension	—	—	1.24 g/30 ml	—	aluminum oxide, 720 mg/30 ml sorbitol saccharin sodium peppermint	50.4 mg/30 ml
Malcogel (Upjohn)	suspension	—	330 mg/5 ml	—	660 mg/5 ml	—	—
Marblen (Fleming)	tablet suspension	NS [a]	NS [a]	—	NS [a]	magnesium carbonate peach or apricot flavor	NS [a]
Maxamag Suspension (Vitarine)	suspension	—	gel, NS [a]	NS [a]	—	—	—
Mylanta (Stuart)	tablet suspension	—	200 mg/tablet or 5 ml	200 mg/tablet or 5 ml (hydroxide)	—	simethicone, 20 mg/tablet or 5 ml	0.79 mg/tablet 11.7 mg/15 ml
Mylanta-II (Stuart)	tablet suspension	—	400 mg/tablet or 5 ml	400 mg/tablet or 5 ml (hydroxide)	—	simethicone, 30 mg/tablet or 5 ml	1.5 mg/tablet 4–10 mg/5 ml
Noralac (North American)	tablet	—	codried with magnesium carbonate, 300 mg	—	magnesium trisilicate, 100 mg	bismuth aluminate, 100 mg alginic acid, 50 mg	—
Nutrajel (Cenci)	suspension	—	300 mg/5 ml	—	—	—	—
Nutramag (Cenci)	suspension	—	—	NS [a] (hydroxide)	—	aluminum oxide	—
Pama (North American)	tablet	—	dried gel, 260 mg	—	260 mg	—	—
Phillips' Milk of Magnesia (Glenbrook)	suspension tablet	—	—	2.27–2.62 g/30 ml 311 mg/tablet	—	peppermint oil, 1.166 mg/30 ml or tablet	—
Phosphaljel (Wyeth)	suspension	—	—	—	—	aluminum phosphate, 233 mg	12.5 mg/5 ml
Ratio (Warren-Teed)	tablet	400 mg	—	—	—	magnesium carbonate, 50 mg	0.6–0.8 mg
Riopan (Ayerst)	tablet chewable tablet suspension	—	—	—	—	magaldrate, 400 mg/tablet or 5 ml	0.7 mg/tablet or 5 ml
Robalate (Robins)	tablet	—	—	—	—	dihydroxyaluminum aminoacetate, 500 mg	0.14 mg
Rolaids (Warner-Lambert)	tablet	—	—	—	—	dihydroxyaluminum sodium carbonate, 334 mg	53 mg
Salcedrox (Beecham Labs)	tablet	—	dried gel, 120 mg	—	—	sodium salicylate, 300 mg calcium ascorbate, 60 mg calcium carbonate, 60 mg	—

Product (manufacturer)	Dosage form	Calcium carbonate	Aluminum hydroxide	Magnesium oxide or hydroxide	Magnesium trisilicate	Other	Sodium content [b]
Silain-Gel (Robins)	suspension tablet	—	gel, 282 mg/ 5 ml codried with magnesium carbonate, 282 mg/ tablet	85 mg/5 ml or tablet	—	simethicone, 25 mg/5 ml or tablet	4.78 mg/5 ml 7.68 mg/tablet
Soda Mint (Lilly)	tablet	—	—	—	—	sodium bicarbonate, 324 mg peppermint oil	87.4 mg
Spastosed (North American)	tablet	precipitated, 226 mg	—	—	—	magnesium carbonate, 162 mg	—
Syntrogel (Block)	tablet	—	codried with magnesium carbonate, 38%	14% (hydroxide)	—	—	—
Titralac (Riker)	tablet suspension	420 mg/ tablet 1 g/5 ml	—	—	—	glycine, 180 mg/tablet 300 mg/5 ml	11 mg/5 ml
Trimagel (Columbia Medical)	tablet	—	dried gel, 250 mg	—	500 mg	—	—
Trisogel (Lilly)	capsule suspension	—	100 mg/ capsule 150 mg/5 ml	300 mg/ capsule 583 mg/5 ml	—	—	48 mg/15 ml
Tums (Lewis-Howe)	tablet	500 mg	—	—	—	peppermint oil	2.7 mg
WinGel (Winthrop)	tablet suspension	—	180 mg/tablet or 5 ml	160 mg/tablet or 5 ml	—	—	2.5 mg/tablet or 5 ml

[a] Quantity not specified.
[b] If no amount is given, it should not be assumed that the product contains no sodium.

Anthelmintic Products

Frank A. Pettinato

Questions to ask the patient

Have you had nausea, diarrhea, or abdominal pain?
Have you been bothered by itching in the anal area?
Have you lost weight or do you become fatigued easily?
How long have the symptoms been present?
If the patient is not an adult, what is the age and approximate weight of the patient?
Have worms appeared in your stool?
Are other members of your family also affected?

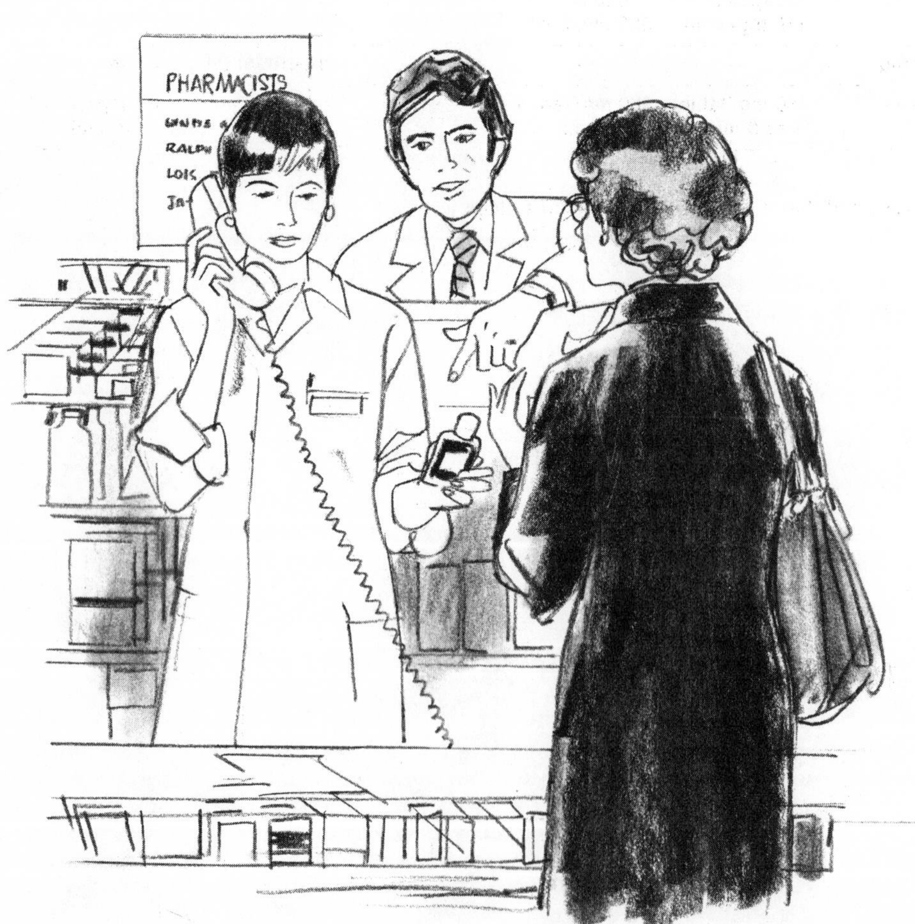

CHAPTER 2

Anthelmintics are used to treat worm (helminth) infections. It has been estimated that 800 million to 1.1 billion humans, or more than one-third of the world's population, harbor helminths.[1] The incidence of helminth infection exceeds 90 percent in primitive areas where sanitation is neglected, economic conditions are poor, and preventive medicine practices are inadequate. Helminthiasis is a serious health problem, particularly in the tropics, that results in a general debilitation of large populations. Efficiency, resistance to disease, physical development in children, and productivity are reduced by these infections. In the U.S. and other temperate-zone countries, these infections are probably more of an annoyance than a major health problem.

Helminth infections that are commonly encountered in the U.S. are trichinosis, enterobiasis (pinworm infections), ascariasis (roundworm infections), and hookworm infections. In the U.S., the incidence of death caused by helminth infestation is low. So few effective nonprescription drugs are available for helminth infections that self-medication should be discouraged. Common helminth infections of humans and their symptoms are listed in Table 1.

The parasitic worms that infect humans include the nematodes (roundworms), the cestodes (tapeworms), and the trematodes (flukes). Roundworms are the most frequently encountered human helminthic parasites in the U.S.

Trichinosis

Trichinosis is caused by a small nematode (*Trichinella spiralis*). When pork that contains the larvae is eaten, the action of the gastric juices frees the larvae which then penetrate the wall of the small intestine. The larvae develop into sexually mature adults, the males and females mate, and the female deposits larvae in the intestinal mucosa. These larvae enter the bloodstream and are carried throughout the body and enter striated muscle fibers, where they complete their development. Most often affected are the muscles of the diaphragm, tongue, eye, and the deltoid pectoral and intercostal muscles. Larvae that reach other tissues, such as the heart and the brain, disintegrate and are absorbed.

The incidence of trichinosis in the U.S., as determined by autopsy, was about 15 percent from 1931 to 1950; from 1951 to 1968, only 4 percent of autopsied bodies were infected.[2] This decline is attributed to laws that require the cooking of garbage fed to hogs, storage of meat at low temperatures, and public education programs concerning the need to thoroughly cook pork.

Symptoms

Symptoms of trichinosis are extremely variable and depend on the severity of the infection. If the meat is heavily infected, the invasion into the intestinal mucosa 1 to 4 days after ingestion may cause local irritation leading to nausea, vomiting, and diarrhea. In some cases, no symptoms are evident. After the seventh day, the migration of the larvae may produce muscle weakness, stiffness or pain, and irregular, persistent fever from 100° to 105° F (37.7° to 40.5° C). These symptoms may be accompanied by an urticarial rash and respiratory symptoms such as cough and bronchospasm. Invasion of skeletal muscle produces muscular pain, tenderness, and often, severe weakness. There may be pain on chewing, swallowing, breathing, or moving the eyes or limbs. Another common symptom is edema which usually appears as puffiness around the eyes involving the upper eyelids. When the larvae have become encysted, the only symptom may be vague aching in the muscles.

The clinical diagnosis of trichinosis is difficult because of the asymptomatic nature of most mild infections and because of the protean nature of the symptoms. A combination of irregular fever, periorbital edema, GI disturbances, muscle soreness, hypereosinophilia, and hemorrhages under fingernails and toenails may be suggestive of trichinosis. Attempting self-diagnosis is foolish because similar symptoms are characteristic of many other ailments. The pharmacist should refer patients with these symptoms to a physician for diagnosis and to a laboratory for evaluation.

Treatment of trichinosis

Treatment is mostly symptomatic. Mild analgesics for relief of pain, sedatives, adequate diet, and anti-inflammatory steroids are recommended. Thiabendazole (prescription only) has been shown to kill the larvae in experimental animals; results in humans have varied. Thiabendazole has also been effective in reducing the fever and relieving the muscle pain, tenderness, and edema of trichinosis.[3]

There are no nonprescription drugs available for the mitigation of the disease.

Enterobiasis

Enterobiasis is commonly called pinworm, seatworm, threadworm, or oxyuriasis. The intestinal infection in humans is caused by *Enterobius vermicularis*. Unlike many helminth infections, enterobiasis is not limited to the rural and the poor but occurs in urban communities of every economic status. *E. vermicularis* is common in temperate climates and is especially prevalent among school children. The female adult is about 10 mm long, and the adult male, about 3 mm. The adult worms inhabit the first portion of the large intestine. The mature female usually does not pass her eggs into the intestinal lumen but stores them in her body until several thousand accumulate, at which time she migrates down the colon, out the anus, and deposits the eggs in the perianal region. Within a few hours each egg develops into an infective larva. Ingestion of the larvae releases them in the small intestine. Within 1 month from the time of ingestion, newly developed, gravid females migrate to the anal area and discharge eggs, and the cycle continues.

Table 1. Helminth Infections (human) and their Symptoms

	Common name	Source of infestation	Symptoms
Roundworm			
Ancylostoma duodenale and Necator americanus	Hookworm	Spreading by contact with contaminated soil; larvae are ingested or penetrate the skin on contact.	Anemia caused by blood loss (0.5 ml/worm/day); indigestion, anorexia, headache, cough, vomiting, diarrhea, weakness; urticaria at the site of entry into the skin.
Ascaris lumbricoides	Roundworm	Ingesting eggs through contact with fecally contaminated soil.	Mild cases may be asymptomatic; GI discomfort, pain, and diarrhea; intestinal obstruction in severe cases; occasionally, bile or pancreatic duct may be obstructed; allergic reactions.
Enterobius (Oxyuris) vermicularis	Pinworm, seatworm, threadworm	Ingesting eggs by fecal contamination of hands, food, clothing, and bedding; reinfection is common; the most common worm infestation in the U.S., especially in school children.	Indigestion, intense perianal itching, especially at night, resulting in loss of sleep; scratching may cause infection; irritability and fatigue in children.
Strongyloides stercoralis	None	Most frequently by larvae penetrating the skin; rarely by ingestion.	Similar to hookworm infestation.
Trichinella spiralis	None	Ingesting infected, "rare" pork; particularly prevalent in the U.S.	Adult worms in intestinal tract cause vomiting, nausea, and diarrhea; migrating larvae cause malaise, weakness, fever, sweating, dermatitis, and cardiac and respiratory distress; can be fatal.
Trichuris trichiura	Whipworm	Ingesting eggs through contact with fecally contaminated soil.	Heavy infestation causes indigestion, mild anemia, insomnia, diarrhea, and urticaria.
Tapeworm			
Diphyllobothrium latum	Fish tapeworm	Eating raw or inadequately cooked fish.	Similar to beef tapeworm infestation.
Hymenolepis nana	Dwarf tapeworm	Eating food contaminated with human feces.	Similar to beef tapeworm infestation.
Taenia saginata	Beef tapeworm	Eating "rare," infected beef.	No characteristic symptoms; digestive upset, diarrhea, anemia, and dizziness vary with the degree of infestation.
Taenia solium	Pork tapeworm	Eating inadequately cooked, infected pork.	Similar to beef tapeworm infestation.

The most common way of transmitting pinworm infection in children is probably by direct anus-to-mouth transfer of eggs by contaminated fingers and by eating food which has been handled by soiled hands. Reinfection may readily occur—eggs are frequently found under the fingernails of infected children. The eggs may be dislodged from the perianal region of the host into the environment and may enter the mouth via hands or food or by swallowing airborne eggs.

Symptoms

The first apparent symptom of pinworm infection is usually severe and irritating itching in the perianal and perineal regions. If the area is scratched, a bacterial infection of the area may result. Children may lose sleep and become tired during the day. Because the worms in various stages of development are frequently seen in the appendix, they are sometimes suspected of causing appendicitis. Worms occasionally may enter the female genital tract and become encapsulated within the uterus or fallopian tubes, or migrate into the peritoneal cavity, resulting in the formation of granulomas in these areas. The cycle of a pinworm infestation is illustrated in Figure 1.

Treatment of enterobiasis

Prescription-only drugs (e.g., piperazine salts, pyrvinium pamoate, pyrantel pamoate, thiabendazole, and mebendazole) can cure 80 to 95 percent of pinworm infections. Pyrantel pamoate and mebendazole are the drugs of choice because of ease of administration and patient

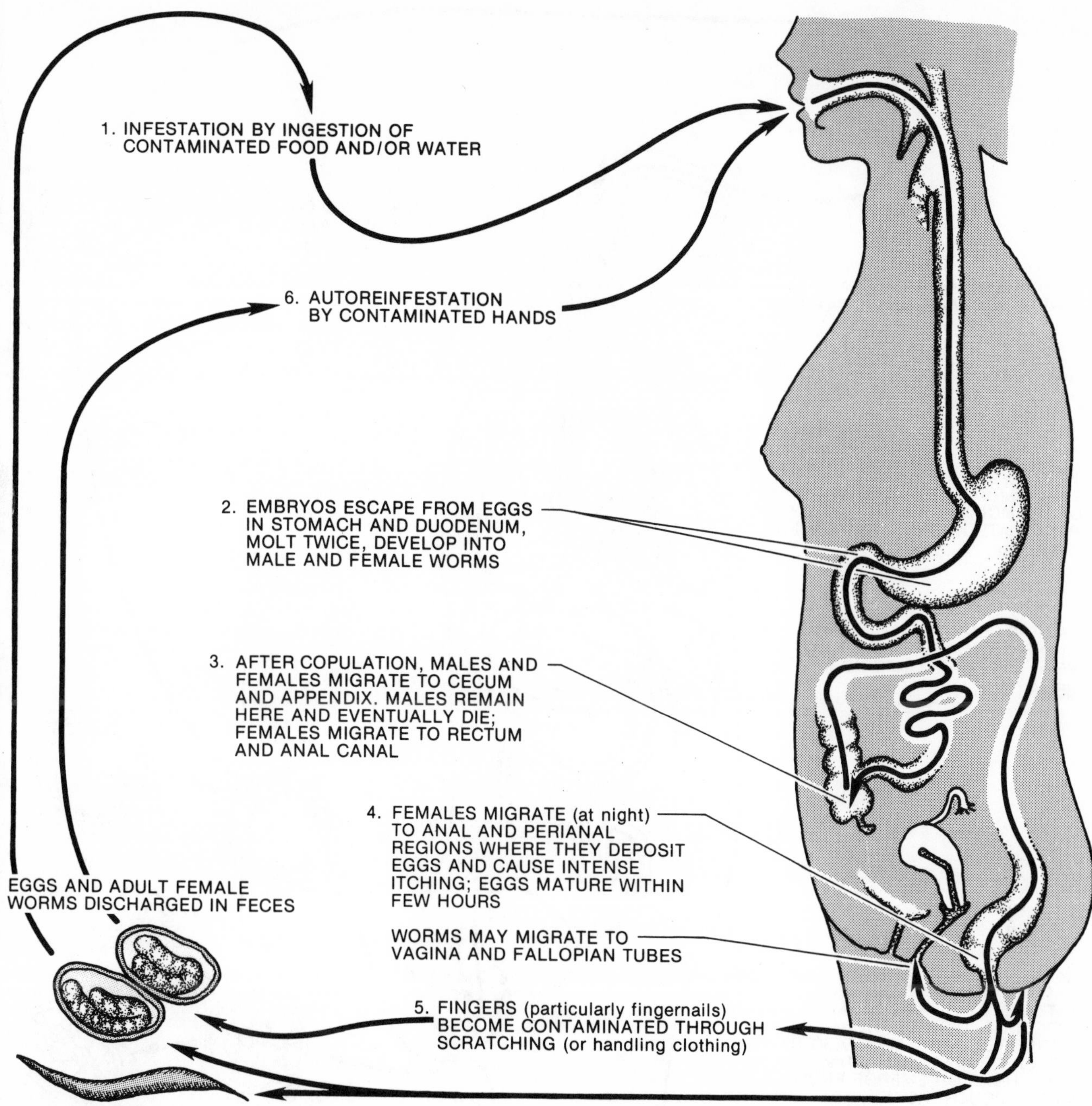

Figure 1. Cycle of pinworm infestation. Adapted from "The Ciba Collection of Medical Illustrations" by Frank H. Netter, M.D.

tolerance.[4] Gentian violet (methylrosaniline chloride) is the only OTC drug available for treatment of pinworm infections. It is questionable whether this drug should be recommended in view of the efficient, easily administered, and well-tolerated prescription drugs available.

Simultaneous treatment of every member of the family is advised for best results. Measures that are recommended to prevent reinfection include: [4]

☐ A daily morning shower to remove eggs deposited in the perianal region during the night.

☐ Regular application of an antipruritic ointment over the perianal region at bedtime. (Avoid contaminating the ointment.)

☐ The use of close-fitting shorts under one-piece pajamas.

☐ Regular trimming of an infected child's nails and scrubbing of the fingers with a brush after going to the bathroom.

☐ Daily use of disinfectants on the toilet seat.

☐ Frequent washing of the hands, especially before meals.

Gentian violet. The oral use of gentian violet may produce nausea, vomiting, diarrhea, and mild abdominal pain. The drug should be used with caution in patients with cardiac, hepatic, or renal disease or intestinal disorders. It should not be used in treating pinworm infection complicated by roundworm infection until the roundworms have been expelled. The reason for this precaution is to avoid possible intestinal obstruction from clumping of the roundworms.[5] However, it has been reported that the drug has been used safely in the presence of roundworms.[6]

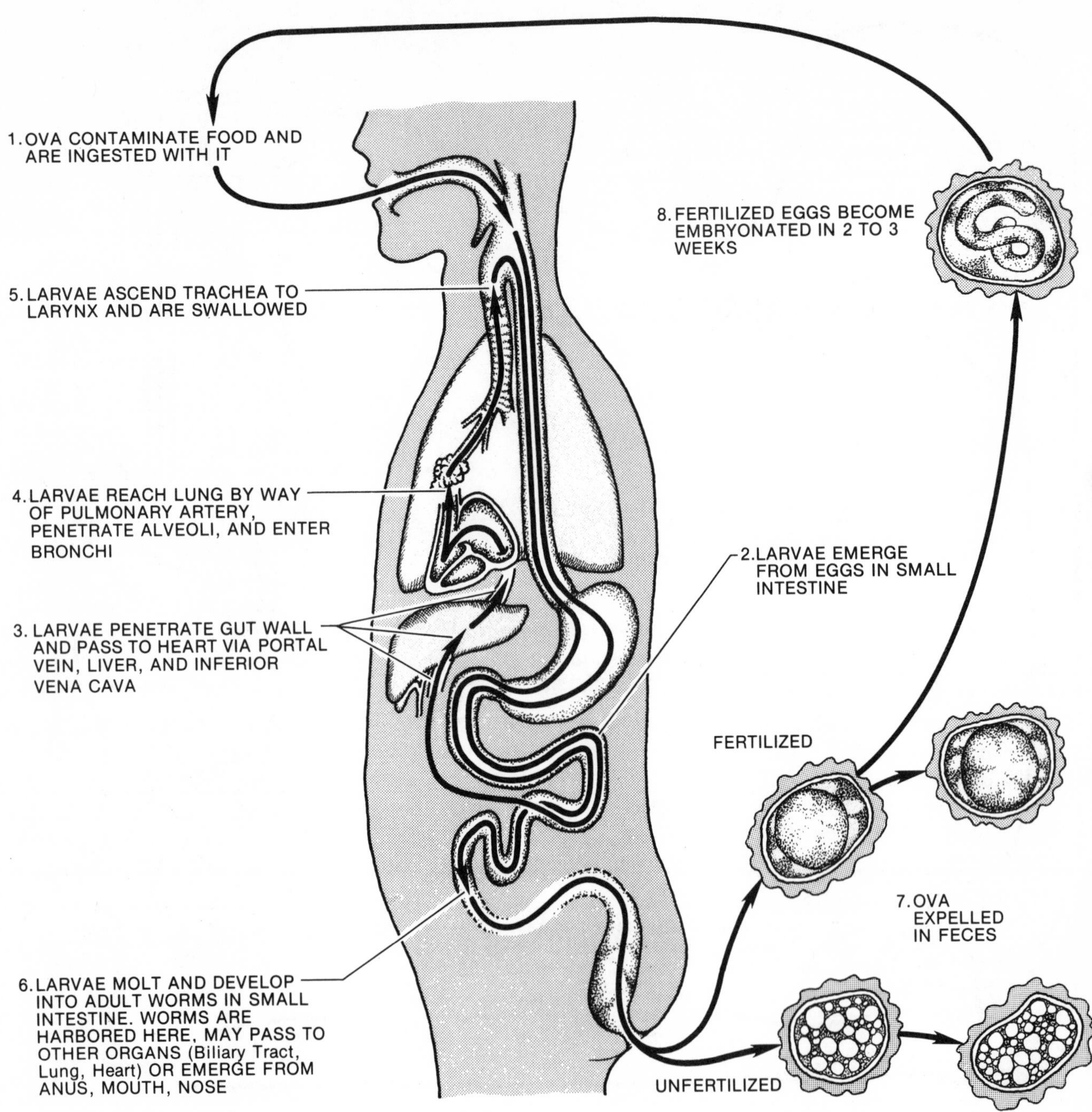

Figure 2. Cycle of roundworm infestation. Adapted from "The Ciba Collection of Medical Illustrations" by Frank H. Netter, M.D.

The usual adult dose is 60 mg three times a day; for children, 3 mg three times a day for each year of age up to a maximum of 90 mg/day is recommended. Jayne's P.W. (Glenbrook) is available as 9.6-mg, red-coated tablets for children and 25-mg, black-coated tablets for adults.

Although gentian violet is a dye and can discolor tissue and clothing, staining is not a problem with the coated tablets if they are swallowed whole, not chewed.

Ascariasis

Ascariasis is caused by *Ascaris lumbricoides* (roundworm) (Fig. 2). Adult ascarides, 15 to 35 cm long, live in the small intestine, where they get their nourishment. The female lays eggs which are passed in the feces and develop into infective larvae in the soil. Although the mature larvae in the shell remain viable in the soil for many months, the eggs do not hatch until ingested by humans. Upon ingestion, the larvae are released in the small intestine. They penetrate the intestinal wall and migrate via the bloodstream to the lungs, up the respiratory tree to the epiglottis where they are swallowed, and develop into male and female adults in the small intestine.

Symptoms

Light infections usually are not noticed until an adult worm is discovered in the stool. The most frequent complaint is colic or vague abdominal pain. The larvae may cause irritation and inflammation of the lung tissue and may sensitize the host, who then develops allergic reactions. Edema, weight loss, anorexia, and nervousness may occur in the sensitized individual. Children may fail to grow normally. More serious complications and death may results if the adult worms migrate into the bile duct, gallbladder, liver, or appendix. Adult worms may penetrate the intestinal wall, migrate to the peritoneal cavity, and cause peritonitis.

Treatment of ascariasis

There are no nonprescription drugs available for treating ascariasis. Cure rates of more than 90 percent are achieved with piperazine salts, pyrantel, and thiabendazole, which are available only by prescription.

Hookworm disease

Hookworm infection in humans is caused by *Ancylostoma duodenale* or *Necator americanus.* The adult worms, which are about 1 cm long, attach themselves to the small intestine. Their eggs are excreted in the feces, hatch in warm, moist soil, and develop into an active filariform larvae. Upon contact with humans, the larvae rapidly penetrate the skin, enter the bloodstream, and are carried to the lungs. They then enter the alveoli, ascend the trachea to the throat, are swallowed, and pass into the small intestine where they develop into mature adults.

Symptoms

When the larvae penetrate the skin they produce a dermatitis called "ground itch." An eruption may develop at the site, usually between the toes. Heavy infection may produce a cough and fever as the larvae pass through the lungs. Mild intestinal infection may be asymptomatic; moderately severe infection may result in indigestion, dizziness, headache, weakness, fatigue, nausea, and vomiting. In advanced cases there is epigastric pain, abdominal tenderness, chronic fatigue, and alternating constipation and diarrhea. While in the intestine, each adult extracts about 0.5 ml of blood per day, resulting in anemia.

Treatment of hookworm disease

Tetrachloroethylene. This drug is effective in treating hookworm disease. It has been demonstrated that a single dose of 5 ml for adults and 0.05 to 0.06 ml per pound of body weight up to 5 ml maximum for children is safe, produces few side effects, and will remove approximately 92 percent of the worms.[7] A light meal is eaten the night before treatment, no breakfast is given in the morning, and the tetrachloroethylene is given between 7 and 8 a.m. A relatively fat-free noon meal may be eaten. Purgation is not necessary. Another dose may be needed in 4 to 7 days to assure complete removal of the worms.

Tetrachloroethylene has replaced carbon tetrachloride as an anthelmintic for the treatment of hookworm disease because it is much less toxic. Although it is claimed that this drug is not absorbed to any extent from the intestine in the absence of alcohol, some absorption must occur because CNS depression has frequently been reported following the use of this drug.[8] This depression is manifested as giddiness and inebriation. A burning sensation in the stomach, cramps, nausea, and vomiting often occur when taking tetrachloroethylene.

Summary

The pharmacist should be familiar with the common helminth infections and their effects in order to discourage self-diagnosis and treatment. The clinical manifestations of these parasitic diseases are so general and so characteristic of other illnesses that attempts at self-diagnosis of helminthiasis are not only difficult but could lead to the neglect of a more serious condition. Diagnosis should be made on the basis of clinical and laboratory evidence.

Self-medication should be discouraged at every opportunity. The availability of effective, relatively safe, easy-to-take prescription-only drugs which can eradicate many infections in one or two doses should be reason enough to avoid self-medication. A pharmacist is the person most available and capable to encourage the patient to consult a physician for treatment.

References

1. E. Bueding, in "Drill's Pharmacology in Medicine," 4th ed., J. R. DiPalma, Ed., McGraw-Hill, New York, N.Y., 1971, p. 1822
2. W. J. Zimmerman *et al., Health Service Report,* **88,** 606-623; through E. C. Faust *et al.,* "Animal Agents and Vectors in Human Disease," Lea and Febiger, Philadelphia, Pa., 1975, p. 227.
3. W. C. Campbell and A. C. Cuckler, *Tex. Rep. Biol. Med.,* **27(Supp. 2),** 665-692(1969); through B. H. Keane and D. W. Hoskins, in "Drugs of Choice 1976-1977," W. Modell, Ed., Mosby, St. Louis, Mo., 1976, p. 362.
4. B. H. Keane and D. W. Hoskins, in "Drugs of Choice 1976-1977," W. Modell, Ed., Mosby, St. Louis, Mo., 1976, p. 362.
5. W. H. Wright and F. J. Brady, *J. Am. Med. Assoc.,* **114,** 862-863(1940).
6. H. W. Brown, *J. Pediatr.,* **28,** 160(1946); through "The United States Dispensatory," 25th ed., A. Osol and G. Farrar, Eds., 1955, p. 859.
7. H. P. Carr *et al., J. Trop. Med.,* **3,** 495-503(1954).
8. W. O. Negherbon, "Handbook of Toxicology," vol. III, Saunders, Philadelphia, Pa., 1959, p. 736.

Additional References

I. L. Bennett, Jr., "Principles of Internal Medicine," 5th ed., McGraw-Hill, New York, N.Y., 1966, pp. 1778-1785.

E. C. Faust *et al.,* "Animal Agents and Vectors in Human Disease," Lea and Febiger, Philadelphia, Pa., 1975, pp. 217-284.

P. D. Mardsen, "Textbook of Medicine," 13th ed., Saunders, Philadelphia, Pa., 1971, pp. 756-776.

I. M. Rollo, in "The Pharmacological Basis of Therapeutics," 5th ed., L. S. Goodman and A. Gilman, Eds., Macmillan, New York, N.Y., 1975, pp. 1018-1044.

Antidiarrheal and Other Gastrointestinal Products

R. Leon Longe
Howard C. Ansel

Questions to ask the patient

Is the diarrhea associated with other symptoms such as fever, vomiting, or pain?

How long has the problem existed? Was it sudden in onset?

Can you relate the onset of diarrhea to a specific cause such as a particular food or drug?

Is the patient an infant or small child?

Is there blood or mucus present in the stool?

What medicines are you currently taking?

Do you have diabetes or other chronic disease?

Have you tried any antidiarrheal products? Which ones? How effective were they?

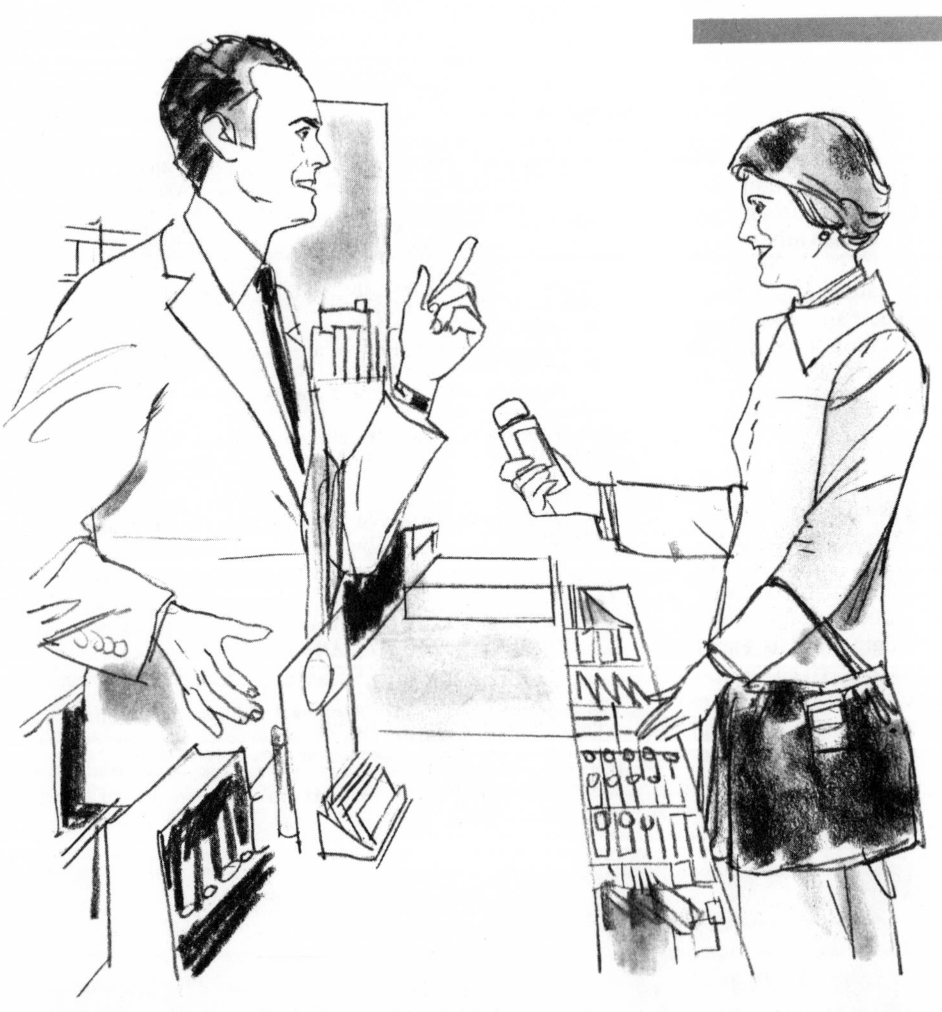

CHAPTER 3

Diarrhea is the abnormally frequent passage of watery stools. The frequency of bowel movements varies with the individual. Some healthy adults may have as many as three stools a day; others may defecate once in 2 or more days. The mean daily fecal weight is 100 to 150 g. A change from 150 to 300 g would be interpreted as diarrhea. The major factor contributing to diarrhea is excess water. Normally, about ". . . 7 liters of digestive fluid are secreted into the GI tract each day. This is made up of about 1 liter of saliva, 2 liters of gastric juice, 2 liters of pancreatic juice, about 1 liter of fluid from the liver, and 1 liter from the small bowel. In addition, another 2 liters enter the GI tract with food and drinks. Of these 9 liters all but one are reabsorbed in the small intestine. The large bowel reabsorbs about 850 milliliters of the remaining 1 liter, leaving about 150 milliliters to be excreted in the stool each day." [1] A disruption in the water absorption process that results in the accumulation of even a few hundred milliliters of water may cause diarrhea.[1,2]

Diarrhea is usually viewed and treated as a symptom of an undiagnosed and presumed minor and transient GI disorder. More than 50 medical conditions, including diseases of the kidneys, heart, liver, thyroid, and lungs are associated with diarrhea illness. However, diarrhea is not usually the only symptom when it is part of the clinical picture of a major illness.[3-5]

If differential diagnosis and management of diarrhea are desired, a distinction must be made between acute and chronic diarrhea. Acute diarrhea is characterized by sudden onset of frequent, liquid stools accompanied by weakness, gas urgency, pain, and often fever and vomiting. Chronic diarrheal illness is the persistent or recurrent passage of unformed stools and is usually the result of multiple etiologic factors. Englert[1] has classified the possible causes of acute and chronic diarrhea (Table 1). The great variability in etiologies of diarrhea may make a proper identification of the responsible pathophysiologic mechanism difficult and may make a complete physical examination necessary, including supportive clinical laboratory tests. The causes of diarrhea can be psychogenic, neurogenic, surgical, endocrine, irritative, osmotic, dietary, allergenic, malabsorptive, and inflammatory.

Physiology of the digestive system

The small intestine originates at the pylorus and terminates at the cecum of the ascending colon (Fig. 1). It is a convoluted tube, 6.4 m long, made up of the duodenum, jejunum, and ileum. The small intestine is the site of digestion, absorption of nutrients, and retention of waste material; these activities depend on normal musculature, nerve tone, and digestive enzymes.

The alimentary tract is basically a long, hollow tube surrounded by layers of smooth muscle—a thick, circular layer on the mucosal side of the intestine, a thinner, longitudinal one on the serosal side, and a third layer of both circular and longitudinal muscle fibers. The active contractions of the various muscles control the tone, or tension, of the intestinal wall. Normally, this tone is maintained with little expenditure of energy so that the muscles remain generally free from fatigue and capable of continued performance. Lining the walls of the intestine is a mucous layer which protects and lubricates the walls. The mucus, composed of glycoproteins and sulfurated aminopolysaccharides, is released from goblet cells interspersed among the columnar epithelial cells in the intestine. Secretion of mucus is increased by colonic irritation, purgation, or psychic trauma, suggesting control by the autonomic nervous system. The mucus is more viscous in the upper part of the small intestine than in the colon and forms a protective physical barrier to the intestinal lining, reducing contact with irritating substances and bacteria. The alkalinity of the mucus further contributes to the protection of the intestinal lining by neutralizing acidic bacterial products.

Normal intestinal motility and peristalsis are maintained by the smooth muscles and the intrinsic nerves (Auerbach's and Meissner's plexuses). The vagus and parasympathetic pelvic nerves stimulate intestinal motility, whereas sympathetic innervation provides inhibitory stimuli to intestinal motility and secretion. Extrinsic autonomic innervation influences the strength and frequency of these movements and mediates reflexes by which activity in one part of the intestine influences another.

Following a meal, the lumen of the intestine is distended, causing the smooth muscle layers to contract. Normally, the segmental contractions of the circular muscles are accompanied by a decrease in the propulsive activity of the gut. This retains the food in the lumen and increases the duration of its exposure to the digestive elements, enhancing digestion and absorption.

Approximately 3 liters of fluid containing electrolytes and nutrients enters the small intestine every 24 hours.[4] Reabsorption reduces the quantity that reaches the large intestine to 500 ml of an isotonic semiliquid substance (chyme).

The large intestine (about 1.5 m long) extends from the cecum to the rectum. It is composed of the cecum, ascending colon, transverse colon, descending colon, sigmoid colon, and rectum. The colon has primarily two functions: absorption and storage. The first two-thirds handles absorption; the rest functions as storage. Chyme has an average electrolyte content of 85 mEq of sodium, 20 mEq of bicarbonate, 6 mEq of potassium, and 60 mEq of chloride.[6] The proximal half (ascending and transverse parts) of the colon reduces chyme to a semisolid substance called feces, or stool. Feces is made up of three-fourths water and one-fourth solid material, which consists of nonabsorbed food residue, bacteria, desquamated epithelial cells, unabsorbed minerals, and a small amount of electrolytes (Table 2). The stool is stored in the descending colon until voiding.

The colon is structured similarly to the intestine with both circular and longitudinal muscles. The longitudinal muscles are shorter than the underlying colon and tend to draw the colon into sacs. The segmental contractions of

Table 1. Etiologies of Diarrhea[a]

Acute		Chronic	
Amebic dysentery	Addison's disease	Intracranial disease	Surgery
Antibiotics	Bacterial overgrowth	Irritable colon	(a) Subtotal gastrectomy and vagotomy
Carcinoma	Blind loops	Lactase deficiency	(b) Gastroenterostomy and vagotomy
Cholera	Carcinoid syndrome	Malabsorption syndrome	(c) Vagotomy and pyloroplasty
Diverticulitis	Carcinoma	Parasitosis	(d) Afferent loop syndrome from gastrojejunostomy or subtotal gastrectomy and Bilroth II anastomosis
Escherichia coli toxin	Diabetic neuropathy	Prostaglandins	(e) Ileal resection
Food poisoning	Dihydroxy bile acids	Protein-losing enteropathy	(f) Short-bowel syndrome
Giardiasis	Diverticulitis	Regional enteritis	Tuberculosis
Medication	GI hormones	Scleroderma	Ulcerative colitis
Radiation	Gluten enteropathy	Stricture	Uremia
Regional enteritis	Hydroxy fatty acids		Villus tumor
Salmonellosis	Hyperthyroidism		Zollinger-Ellison syndrome
Shigellosis			
Staphylococcal infection			
Ulcerative colitis			
Viral gastroenteritis			

[a]Adapted from E. Englert, in "Dealing with Diarrhea," G. D. Searle and Co., Jan., 1974.

the circular musculature further cause the division of the colon into sausagelike units which facilitate the churning of the colonic contents and the absorption of water. A decrease in the occurrence or intensity of the segmental contractions and the predominance of the propulsive force of the longitudinal muscles may lead to the diarrheal state. In the absence of circular muscle contractions, mass colonic movements may occur, during which the colon may contract to half its length and may resemble a smooth, hollow tube devoid of segmented units.

Colonic activity is increased by parasympathetic stimulation or by the administration of parasympathomimetic drugs. Sympathetic stimulation inhibits colonic motor activity.

The normal bowel movement, or defecation, begins with the stimulation of stretch receptors in the rectum by feces. Peristaltic waves propel the feces to the anal canal where the voluntarily controlled external anal sphincter controls defecation.[7]

In the colon, nonpathogenic bacterial flora produce enzymes necessary for degradation of waste products, synthesize certain vitamins, and generate ammonia. Bacteroides and anaerobic lactobacilli make up the majority of the colonic flora; Enterobacteriaceae (e.g., *Escherichia coli*), hemolytic streptococci, Clostridia, and yeasts are also found. Many factors such as diet, pH, GI disease, and drugs (e.g., antibiotics) influence their population control. If they are uncontrolled, these minority pathogens can present serious complications.[8]

Table 2. Electrolyte and Water Content of Normal and Diarrheal Feces

Component	Normal[a]	Diarrheal[b]
Bicarbonate, mEq/24 hr	30	135–450
Chloride, mEq/24 hr	60	120–400
Potassium, mEq/24 hr	11.3	105–350
Sodium, mEq/24 hr	6.5	130–500
Water, ml/24 hr	111	3,000–10,000

[a]Adapted from "Documenta Geigy: Scientific Tables," K. Diem and C. Lentner, Eds., Ciba-Geigy Limited, Basel, Switzerland, 1970, pp. 657-658.

[b]Adapted from "Manual of Medical Therapeutics," M. G. Rosenfeld, Ed., Little Brown, Boston, Mass., 1971, p. 38.

Etiology of diarrhea

Acute diarrhea

Acute diarrhea may be of infectious, toxic, drug-induced, or dietary origin or the result of another acute or chronic illness. Of the infectious diarrhea class, most diarrhea in adults is bacterial; viral diarrhea is more frequent in pediatric patients.

Infectious diarrhea. In the U.S., the bacterial pathogens most commonly responsible for acute diarrhea are Salmonella, Shigella, and enteropathic *E. coli.*[9] Enteroviruses and adenoviruses are also suspected causative agents in acute diarrheal illness. In the majority of cases of acute diarrheal illness of suspected infectious origin, the causative agents are not identified. However, when a patient is first seen, the history often leads to identifying the source of the problem. For example, diarrhea developing in a number of patients within 12 to 24 hours after a common meal may be caused by a Salmonella infection. Fever, malaise, muscle aching, and profound epigastric or periumbilical discomfort with severe anorexia suggest an infectious, inflammatory disease of the small intestine. Severe periumbilical pain and vomiting is commonly experienced with

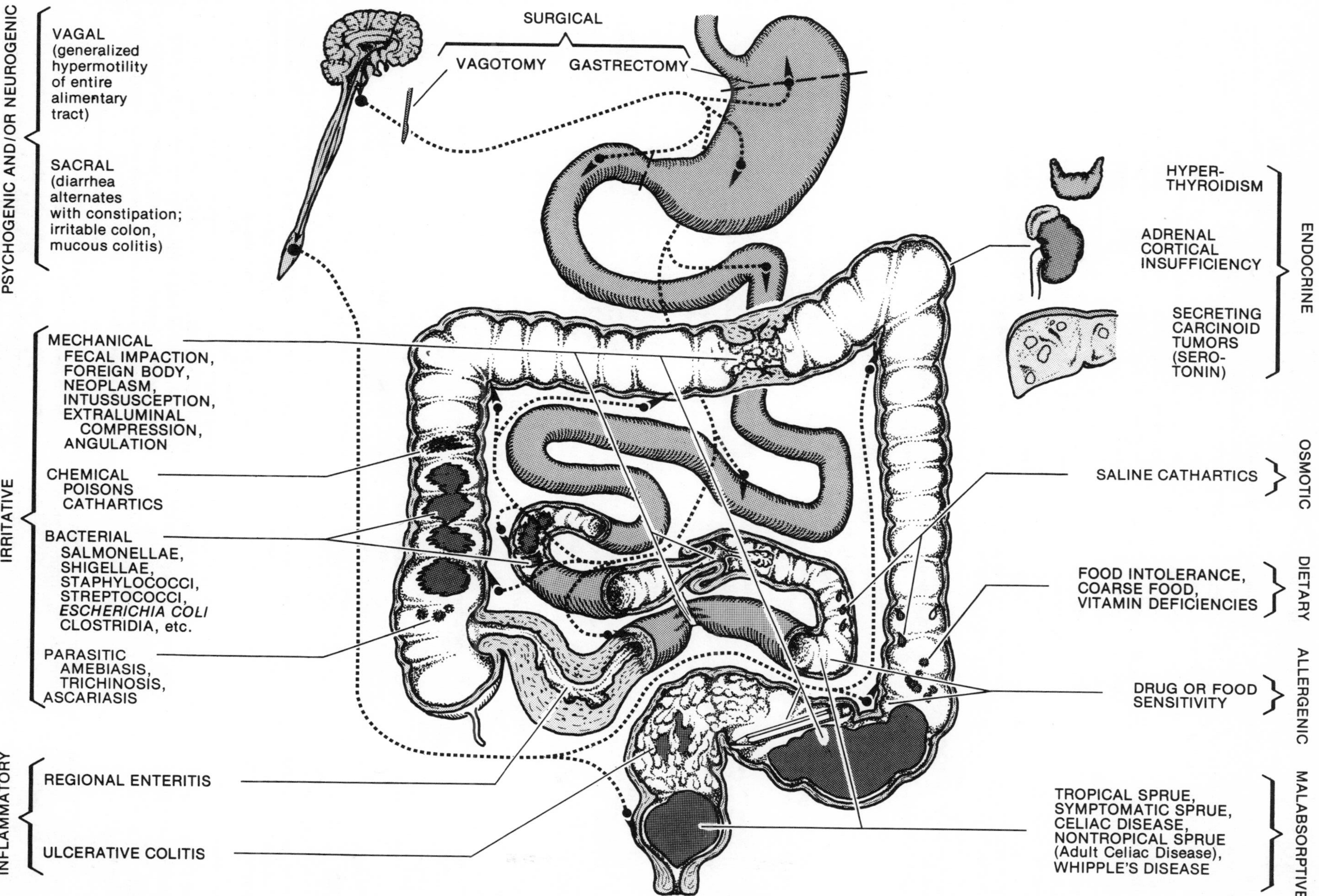

Figure 1. The lower digestive tract showing the induction of diarrhea by various causes. Adapted from "The Ciba Collection of Medical Illustrations" by Frank H. Netter, M.D.

viral gastroenteritis and is acute for 2 to 3 days, then gradually subsides.[10]

The treatment of diarrhea of infectious origin is based on combating the proliferation of the pathogen, generally with a prescribed antibiotic or other anti-infective agent. In many instances the illness is self-limiting, and normalcy of the alimentary tract is restored, with or without treatment, in 24 to 48 hours.

Infantile diarrhea. Diarrhea in infants and young children is common. The etiology usually cannot be identified. It is often attributed to a viral infection of the intestinal tract; however, diet and systemic and local infections are other known causes of acute diarrheal episodes in children. Viral diarrhea has an abrupt onset, lasts 1 to 21 days, and produces a low-grade fever. The child frequently complains of upper respiratory symptoms. The disease usually is self-limiting and requires only symptomatic treatment.

Severe acute diarrhea, where water and electrolytes are lost in a short period, causes severe dehydration in children, especially infants. In the newborn, water may make up 75 percent of the total body weight; water loss in severe diarrhea may be 10 percent or more of body weight. After 8 to 10 bowel movements in 24 hours, a 2-month-old infant could lose enough fluid to cause circulatory collapse and renal failure. The pharmacist must be cautious in recommending treatment for pediatric patients.[11 12]

Travelers' diarrhea. The acute diarrhea that frequently develops among tourists visiting foreign countries with warm climates and relatively poor sanitation cannot usually be ascribed to known pathogens. However, in a recent study conducted during the Fifth World Congress of Gastroenterology, Merson [13] reports enterotoxigenic *E. coli* was the most common cause of travelers' diarrhea in Mexico. It probably results from an extensive alteration in the bacterial flora of the gut caused by exposure, through food and drink, to a markedly different microbial population. Travelers' diarrhea is characterized by a sudden onset of loose stools, nausea, occasional vomiting, and abdominal cramping. Children seem particularly susceptible, and most cases develop during the first week of exposure to the new location.

In many parts of the world, iodochlorhydroxyquin (Entero-Vioform) has been given prophylactically to travelers to protect them against travelers' diarrhea. The FDA has recommended that the drug not be used for this purpose.[14] Its conclusion is based on findings from Japan, Australia, and Sweden, implicating iodochlorhydroxyquin as the cause of a severe, subacute, myelo-optic neuropathy (SMON).[15] As a result, oral iodochlorhydroxyquin and diiodohydroxyquin were removed from the U.S. market. There is no acceptable evidence that iodochlorhydroxyquin or other halogenated oxyquinolines, e.g., chiniofon, are effective in the treatment or prevention of travelers' diarrhea.[16]

The FDA suggests that travelers to areas where hygiene and sanitation are poor may possibly prevent diarrhea by eating only recently peeled or thoroughly cooked foods and by drinking only boiled or bottled water, bottled carbonated soft drinks, beer, or wine. Tapwater used for brushing teeth or for ice in drinks may be a source of infection.

Drug-induced diarrhea. Drug-induced diarrhea is a side effect that frequently accompanies the administration of drugs. All antibiotics can produce adverse GI symptoms including diarrhea, but the severity of the diarrhea depends largely on the specific antibiotic used. Antibiotics that have a broad spectrum of activity against aerobic and anaerobic organisms are most frequently found to be the cause of drug-induced diarrhea. They include the tetracyclines, erythromycin, ampicillin, lincomycin, clindamycin, and neomycin. Severe and persistent diarrhea has been reported by patients receiving lincomycin and clindamycin.[17] Deaths have been associated with colitis induced by these drugs. Sigmoidoscopic examination reveals an erythematous, purulent, ulcerative mucosa consistent with pseudomembranous colitis. These antibiotic agents should be used only in serious infections when other less toxic antibiotics have not been effective. A recent report questions the advisability of treating lincomycin-induced diarrhea with atropine–diphenoxylate or codeine because GI irritation was more prominent with these treatments.[18]

Two processes can account for antibiotic-induced diarrhea. Diarrhea associated with the first few doses is attributed to mild irritant properties of the drug. Diarrhea beginning within a few days of the initial antibiotic therapy is most likely due to a disruption in the normal intestinal flora.

In general, orally administered antibiotics are not completely absorbed. The unabsorbed parts may be irritating to the intestinal mucosa and cause alterations in intestinal motility and induce diarrhea. Even the soluble antibiotics may cause irritation if they form strongly acid solutions as does tetracycline hydrochloride. Some antibiotics, e.g., neomycin and kanamycin, affect intestinal absorption of nutrients, even at usual dosage levels.[3]

Antibiotic-induced diarrhea most likely is caused by a disruption in the normal intestinal flora. It may also be caused by an overgrowth of an antibiotic-resistant bacterial or fungal strain. Intestinal micro-organisms that tend to proliferate in the presence of antibiotic therapy include *Staphylococcus aureus, Pseudomonas aeruginosa, Streptococcus faecalis, Candida albicans,* and species of Salmonella and Proteus. Except for severe staphylococcal enterocolitis, a reduction in the dose of the drug, a change to the parenteral route of administration, or the withdrawal of the antibiotic agent relieves the problem. (Oral vancomycin and fecal enemas to restore competitive bacterial flora are indicated in staphylococcal enterocolitis.)

Other drugs, such as cathartics, which are irritating to the intestinal mucosa may precipitate diarrhea as might drugs that cause the retention of salts and water in the intestinal lumen. Certain antacid preparations contain magnesium to prevent the constipating effects of aluminum and calcium. Depending on the dose taken and the individual, these types of antacid preparations may induce diarrhea. Drugs that alter autonomic control of intestinal motility may cause diarrhea. For example, it is not uncommon for the antiadrenergic, antihypertensive agents such as reserpine, guanethidine, and methyldopa to produce diarrhea. Generalized cramping and diarrhea may follow the use of a parasympathomimetic drug.

Food intolerance, caused by allergy or by the ingestion of foods that are excessively fatty or spicy or that contain a high degree of roughage or a large number of seeds can also provoke diarrhea. If diarrhea occurs in more than one person, within 24 hours of ingestion of the same food, it is likely that a preformed toxin (food poison) has been ingested.

Chronic diarrhea

Usually, chronic diarrhea is the result of multiple etiologic factors and, therefore, can be difficult to diagnose. The pharmacist should refer patients with persistent or

Table 3. Diarrhea and Its Treatment[a]

Type	History	Symptoms	Usual duration	Treatment	Prognosis
Acute					
Salmonella (infectious)	Recent ingestion of contaminated food, affects all age groups.	Sudden onset of abdominal cramps, watery diarrhea, nausea, vomiting, fever; onset of symptoms usually within 12-24 hours after ingestion.	1-5 days	Symptomatic, bed rest, fluid and electrolyte replacement.	Usually self-limiting.
Shigella (infectious)	Affects all age groups.	Sudden onset of abdominal cramps, diarrhea containing shreds of mucus and specks of blood, tenesmus (frequently), fever.	4-7 days	Symptomatic, bed rest, fluid and electrolyte replacement.	Usually self-limiting.
Escherichia coli (infectious)	Affects children under 2 and the elderly in an overcrowded environment (e.g., hospital nursery or nursing home).	Abdominal cramps, fever, tenesmus.	7-21 days	Antibiotics, fluid and electrolyte replacement.	Severe if not treated.
Viral, infantile (infectious)	Predilection for children and infants, usually occurs in summer and autumn, very contagious.	Abrupt onset, profuse, watery diarrhea, slight fever; frequent vomiting; upper respiratory symptoms.	1-21 days	Symptomatic and supportive.	Usually self-limiting.
Travelers'	Travel outside of normal locus.	Sudden onset, nausea, abdominal cramps.	1-14 days	Symptomatic and supportive.	Usually self-limiting.
Drug induced	Broad-spectrum antibiotics, autonomic drugs, laxatives, nitrofurantoin, antacids, antineoplastics, antituberculins, ferrous sulfate, colchicine.	Sudden onset, rectal urgency, abdominal cramps.	Variable	Reduce dosage or discontinue drug.	Usually self-limiting.
Chronic	History of repeated episodes, poor health history.	Weight loss, anorexia, mucus and/or blood in feces.	Weeks to years	Depends on etiology.	Severe if not treated.

[a]From "Gastroenterology," A. Bogoch, Ed., McGraw-Hill, New York, N.Y., 1973, pp. 33-38, 602-721; A. I. Mendeloff, in "Harrison's Principles of Internal Medicine," 7th ed., McGraw-Hill, New York, N.Y., 1974, pp. 213-217; and S. M. Mellinkoff, "The Differential Diagnosis of Diarrhea," McGraw-Hill, New York, N.Y., 1964, pp. 310-325.

recurrent diarrhea to a physician. Correct causative diagnosis usually can be made only after a physician carefully studies the patient's history and performs a physical examination and appropriate laboratory tests. Chronic diarrheal illness may be caused by many conditions but generally may be related to diseases of the stomach, small and large intestines, or to factors resulting in disturbed GI motility.

One of the most frequent causes of chronic diarrhea is psychogenic in origin. Psychogenic diarrhea is usually characterized by small, frequent stools and abdominal pain. The stool may be watery and may follow a normal bowel movement or may appear shortly after eating. Psychogenic diarrhea is related to emotional stress which may lead to a periodic increase in parasympathetic nervous system impulses to the GI tract. It may alternate with constipation.

Some people who suffer from persistent diarrhea are aware of the cause and can manage the condition. For example, about 2.5 percent of adult diabetics and 22 percent of diabetics with evident neuropathy have chronic diarrhea. Individuals who have persistent or recurrent diarrhea and are unaware of its cause should seek prompt medical attention because conditions such as cancer of the stomach or colon or an endocrine tumor may be the cause of the diarrhea. One of the seven "warning signals of cancer" is a change in bowel habits. In both sexes, cancer of the colon and rectum is the most frequently reported type of cancer. The American Cancer Society estimates that almost three out of four patients might be saved by early diagnosis and proper treatment.[19] A follow-up study of patients who had been suffering from "unexplained" diarrhea revealed the risk of missing a diagnosis such as neoplasm.[20]

Common complaints and history

The most common complaints voiced by patients with acute diarrhea are abrupt onset of frequent, watery, loose stools and abdominal cramping, fever, muscle ache, vomiting, and malaise. In chronic diarrhea, the most significant finding usually is a history of previous bouts of diarrhea and complaints of anorexia, weight loss, and chronic weakness. These patients generally have histories of poor health.

The pharmacist should obtain a history of present illness before recommending self-treatment. Four groups of patients with either type of diarrhea should, as a rule, be referred to a physician for a complete diagnostic evaluation: children under 3 or patients over 60 who have a poor medical history; patients with a medical history of chronic illness (e.g., asthma, peptic ulcer, heart disease); and pregnant patients. Clinical judgment must be used in evaluating these patients. For example, access to medical treatment may not be readily available, and temporary self-treatment may be needed until a medical appointment can be arranged.

The medication history helps rule out drug-induced diarrhea. With this background, the pharmacist should find out about self-treatments already tried, age of the patient, symptoms, date of onset, and characteristics of stools (e.g., number, consistency, odor, and appearance). Stool character gives valuable information about diarrhea. For example, undigested food particles in the stool indicate small bowel irritation; black, tarry stool can mean GI bleeding; and red stool suggests possible lower bowel bleeding or simply the recent ingestion of red-colored food (e.g., beets).

Treatment of diarrhea

Diarrhea is a symptom, and symptomatic relief must not be interpreted as a cure for the underlying cause. Symptomatic relief generally suffices in simple functional diarrhea which is only temporary and relatively uncomplicated. More than 100 OTC products are readily available; however, the pharmacist should exercise propriety in recommending their use in self-medication. Certain diseases which cause diarrhea might be serious or more effectively treated with specific agents. The following statement is required by the FDA on all OTC antidiarrheal preparations:

> "WARNING—Do not use for more than 2 days or in the presence of high fever or in infants or children under 3 years of age unless directed by a physician."

Some antidiarrheal drugs are directed against the symptom, diarrhea; others act against the cause; and others against the effect of the disease such as loss of nutrients or electrolytes. The categories of drugs generally used are opiates, adsorbents, astringents, electrolytes, nutrients, bulk laxatives, anti-infectives, digestive enzymes, intestinal flora modifiers, sedatives and tranquilizers, smooth muscle relaxants, and anticholinergic drugs. In some of these categories, the drug of choice may require a prescription. They include opiates, anti-infectives, the tranquilizers and sedatives used to combat emotional and nervous diarrhea, and anticholinergic drugs.

In 1975, the FDA OTC Panel on Laxatives, Antidiarrheals, Antiemetic and Emetic Drugs published its report on antidiarrheal agents.[21] According to the Panel, only opiates and polycarbophil were recognized as safe and effective and not misbranded. The Panel concluded that "adequate and reliable scientific evidence is not available at this time to permit final classification" of other ingredients submitted, including attapulgite, charcoal, kaolin, pectin, belladonna alkaloids, alumina powder, bismuth salts, calcium hydroxide, salol, zinc phenolsulfonate, lactobacilli species, calcium carbonate, and sodium carboxymethylcellulose. Generally, the Panel agreed that the agents are safe in recommended doses but believed there was a lack of acceptable clinical evidence to establish their effectiveness as antidiarrheal agents.

Opiates

The opiates (opium powder, tincture of opium, and paregoric) are safe and effective in doses of 15 to 20 mg of opium or 1.5 to 2.0 mg of morphine.[21] Most opiate-containing OTC antidiarrheals contain paregoric or its equivalent in the usual dose; 1 tsp of paregoric contains 20 mg of powdered opium (2 mg of morphine). Several products incorporate paregoric or its equivalent. However, the usual dose may not provide enough to reach the recognized effective dose.

Because of their morphine content, paregoric-containing products inhibit effective propulsive movements in the small intestine and colon. Thus, hyperperistaltic movements decrease, and the passage of intestinal contents slows, resulting in absorption of water and electrolytes. In the usual oral antidiarrheal doses, addiction liability is low for acute diarrheal episodes because the morphine is not well absorbed orally and thus, the low dose is not large enough to produce analgesia or euphoria. However, chronic use, as in ulcerative colitis, increases the risk of physical addiction.[22] Paregoric per se is a schedule III prescription-only item, but it is a schedule V item available for OTC purchase in combination with antidiarrheals that contain not more than 100 mg of opium (5 tsp paregoric/ 100 ml of mixture). Opium derivatives are CNS depressants, and excessive sedation may be a problem in patients taking other CNS depressants concomitantly with the diarrhea remedy.

Polycarbophil

Polycarbophil is an absorbent which has a marked capacity to bind free fecal water. Paradoxically, it is recommended both in the treatment of diarrhea and constipation. In diarrhea, polycarbophil absorbs about 60 times its weight in water, producing formed stools; in constipation, this same action prevents desiccation of fecal material and allows passage of soft stools.[21] According to the FDA, polycarbophil has been shown to be nontoxic and nonabsorbed, to have no effect on digestive enzymes and nutritional status, and to be metabolically inactive.[21] For adults, the effective oral dose is 4 to 6 g divided in four doses a day. The dose is 0.5 to 1.0 g for infants under 2; 1.0 to 1.5 g from 2 to 5 years; and 1.5 to 3.0 g for children over 5.[21]

Adsorbents

The adsorbents are the most frequently used type of drug in OTC antidiarrheal preparations. Because of the large doses generally used and because they improve palatability properties, most of the commercially available products are in liquid-suspension form. Adsorbents generally are used in the treatment of mild functional diarrhea.

Adsorption is not a specific action, and materials possessing this capability, when given orally, adsorb nutrients and digestive enzymes as well as toxins, bacteria, and various noxious materials. They may also have the effect of adsorbing drugs (e.g., lincomycin) from the GI tract. Although the systemic absorption of a drug might be expected to be poor from the GI tract during a diarrheal episode, its absorption may be further hampered by the concomitant administration of an antidiarrheal adsorbent. Thus, a judgment must be made when drugs other than the antidiarrheal preparation are taken by the patient, perhaps for an unrelated condition. Depending on the medication involved, its usual rate and site of adsorption, and the absolute necessity of attaining specific and consistent blood levels of the drug, an alteration of the dose or the dosage regimen may be required. In some cases, it might be better to administer the drug parenterally until the diarrheal illness is over and the adsorbent drugs are discontinued.

Following the initial treatment, most antidiarrheal preparations containing adsorbents are taken after each loose bowel movement until the diarrhea is controlled. In instances in which the diarrheal episodes occur in rapid succession and for several hours, the total amount of adsorbent taken may be quite large. Because there is no systemic absorption of the adsorbent drug, the usual consequence is constipation.

The main GI adsorbents used are kaolin, attapulgite, aluminum hydroxide, magnesium trisilicate, bismuth subsalts, pectin, and activated charcoal. Adsorbents used with ion exchange resins combine their individual activities in relieving gastric distress and diarrhea. These agents are relatively inert and nontoxic except for possible interference with drugs and nutrient absorption. Kaolin, which has long been used in the Orient against diarrhea and dysentery, is a native hydrated aluminum silicate. Attapulgite is a hydrous magnesium aluminum silicate. It is activated by thermal treatment and used in a finely powdered form. Although it is seldom used as an antidiarrheal today, activated charcoal, which in a single gram has a surface area of about 100 m^2, possesses excellent adsorption properties and has been used for conditions of various origin, including cholera and infantile and nervous diarrhea.[23]

Pectin, a purified carbohydrate extracted from the rind of citrus fruit or from apple pomace, is widely used in the treatment of diarrhea, although its exact mechanism of action is not known. Pectin generally is found in combination with other adsorbents; however, it may be used alone as an intestinal adsorbent, absorbent, and protective.

The bismuth subsalts as the subnitrate and subsalicylate are used in antidiarrheal preparations as adsorbents, astringents, and protectives. However, subnitrate may form nitrite ion in the bowel which, upon absorption, may cause hypotension and methemoglobinemia. Bismuth subnitrate is contraindicated in infants under 2. Stools may become dark with use of a bismuth compound. The FDA Panel concludes that bismuth salts are safe in amounts taken orally (0.6 to 2.0 g of bismuth subsalicylate every 6 to 8 hours), but data establishing the effectiveness of bismuth in diarrhea are questionable.[21]

In summary, the adsorbents [attapulgite (activated), charcoal (activated), kaolin, pectin] are safe in the usual doses; however, there is insufficient evidence to classify these agents as effective antidiarrheals.[21]

Anticholinergics

The formulations of adsorbents are frequently fortified by the addition of agents such as belladonna alkaloids (anticholinergics), making them prescription drugs. When the diarrhea is due to an increase in intestinal tone and peristalsis, belladonna alkaloids are effective "when given in doses which are equivalent to 0.6 to 1.0 milligram of atropine sulfate." [21] As a therapeutic rule, decreased intestinal motility is evidenced by a dry feeling in the mouth. However, in some available combination OTC antidiarrheal products, the usual dose of belladonna alkaloids is less than the recognized effective dose. Hence, the FDA Antidiarrheal Panel recommends that "antidiarrheal products containing anticholinergics when given in doses which are equivalent to 0.6 to 1.0 milligram of atropine sulfate be available only by prescription." [21]

Anticholinergics have a narrow margin of safety, especially in young children. Their containers carry the following warning statement which should be reviewed before dispensing:

> WARNING—Not to be used by persons having glaucoma or excessive pressure within the eye, or by elderly persons (when undiagnosed glaucoma or excessive pressure within the eye occurs most frequently), or by children under 6 years of age, unless directed by a physician. Discontinue use if blurring of vision, rapid pulse or dizziness occurs. Do not exceed recommended dosage. Not for frequent or prolonged use. If dryness of the mouth occurs, decrease dosage. If eye pain occurs, discontinue use and see your physician immediately as this may indicate undiagnosed glaucoma.

Lactobacillus preparations

One of the most controversial forms of diarrhea treatment is the use of preparations of lactobacillus organisms.

The bacteriology of the intestinal tract is extremely complex, and it is difficult to explain many changes in the numbers and types of micro-organisms found. The flora of the GI tract plays a significant role in the maintenance of bowel function, in nutrition, and in the overall well-being of the individual. Antibiotic therapy often disrupts the balance of intestinal micro-organisms, resulting in abnormal intestinal and bowel function. Seeding the bowel with viable *Lactobacillus acidophilus* and *L. bulgaricus* micro-organisms has been suggested as an effective treatment for functional intestinal disturbances, including diarrhea. These micro-organisms are believed to be effective in suppressing the growth of pathogenic micro-organisms and in reestablishing the normal intestinal flora. However, the FDA Panel states that a diet (e.g., milk) containing 240 to 400 g of lactose or dextrin is as effective in colonizing the intestine without supplemental lactobacilli.[21]

Guidelines for product selection

The information obtained during the patient interview and from the family medication record must be assessed prior to product selection. The treatment alternatives are: an adsorbent such as kaolin-pectin mixture; an opiate-containing antidiarrheal product; or physician referral.

It is better to undertreat than to overtreat. No product should be recommended that has been tried and found unsatisfactory. A kaolin-pectin mixture should be recommended unless clear indications warrant a more potent pharmacologic agent such as an anticholinergic or opiate-containing antidiarrheal product. OTC antidiarrheal products can usually manage mild to moderate acute diarrhea; severe acute diarrhea probably requires a prescription drug such as diphenoxylate or paregoric.

Patient consultation

The pharmacist should be contacted if control of diarrhea is not achieved in 24 hours. After this period, a reassessment can be made and another treatment chosen, i.e., continue treatment for another 24 hours with the same or more potent product or advise the patient to consult a physician. If control of the symptoms is not achieved after the second 24-hour period, a physician should be consulted.

The pharmacist should review the label contents as to appropriate dosage schedule based on age of the patient, maximum number of doses per 24 hours, proper storage, and auxiliary dispensing advice (e.g., shake well before using). The patient must be questioned about special precautions on the label such as contraindications to use. Adjunctive therapy includes rest, drinking fluids, and appropriate diet. Physical and GI rest should be encouraged by advising bed rest and discontinuation of all solid foods.

Fluid and electrolyte losses are a primary problem, especially in infants and young children. Commercial electrolyte formulas (e.g., Pedialyte, Lytren) might be helpful but must be used with caution because of possible electrolyte overload.[24] The diet should consist primarily of clear liquids (e.g., broth, gelatin, fruit juices) for the first 24 hours and progress to more solid foods as the diarrhea subsides.

Other GI disorders

The agents found in products recommended as GI "protectives" and antidiarrheal mixtures sometimes overlap. GI protectives are intended to soothe acutely irritated or inflamed gastric mucosa or intestinal linings, resulting from the ingestion of an irritant or the contraction of an illness affecting the digestive tract.

Acute gastritis. Inflammation of the gastric mucosa is called gastritis. Acute gastritis occurs suddenly, occasionally violently, lasts for short periods, and involves the inflammation and erosion of the mucosa of the stomach.

Acute erosive gastritis. This is a common disorder caused by acute alcoholism; drugs (especially aspirin); hot, spicy foods; allergenic foods in hypersensitive individuals (especially milk, eggs, fish); bacteria or toxins in food poisoning; or an acute illness, such as a viral infection.

Acute corrosive gastritis. This is a much more serious disorder caused by swallowing corrosive materials such as strong acids or alkalis, iodine, potassium permanganate, or salts of heavy metals. It requires hospitalization and immediate emergency treatment directed toward removing or neutralizing the offending agent and providing supportive measures.[25]

Acute gastroenteritis. This is the acute inflammation of the lining of the stomach and intestine. It may be precipitated by excessive use of harsh cathartics, salicylates, and other irritant drugs.

The OTC products for relief of acute GI irritation and inflammation contain adsorbents, bulk formers, astringents (especially the bismuth subsalts), antacids, and GI analgesics. The commercial claims for some of the products refer to their ability to coat the stomach, reducing irritation and inflammation. The report of the FDA Panel on OTC Antacids states that "the evidence currently available is inadequate to support the claim that such properties as . . . 'coating' . . . and . . . 'demulcent' . . . contribute to the relief of gastrointestinal symptoms."[26]

Chronic gastritis. Chronic gastritis is an inflammatory reaction of the gastric mucosa which may be associated with serious underlying diseases such as gastric carcinoma, pernicious anemia, diabetes mellitus, and thyroid disease or may be the result of chronic drug ingestion, e.g., aspirin.

Colitis. Colitis is inflammation and pain of the colon. It is classified as ulcerative, amoebic, or bacillary.

Irritable colon. Irritable colon ("spastic colon" or "mucous colitis") is a motor disorder of the colon, resulting in abdominal discomfort and pain, usually with alternating episodes of diarrhea and constipation.[25]

Patients with chronic conditions should be under the care of a physician. Treatment is based on managing the underlying cause and avoiding the ingestion of agents that contribute to the condition. The medications prescribed may include prescription-only drugs such as antispasmodics and anti-inflammatory agents and OTC products such as intestinal bulk formers or mucilaginous products.

Many of the commercial products sold as "protectives" are thick, viscous suspensions which probably physically protect the mucous membranes from the irritating agent. The adsorbent drugs can bind certain offending agents. The drug substances that form bulk or thick mucilaginous fluids within the GI tract can dilute the concentration of the irritant, act as a physical barrier between it and the GI walls, and hasten the passage of the irritant toward the bowel.

Summary

Diarrhea, frequent passage of unformed stools, is often treated as a simple disorder, but it can be a symptom of a more serious underlying disease. Diarrhea is either acute or chronic. Acute diarrhea is characterized by a sudden onset of loose stools in a previously healthy patient. Chronic diarrhea is characterized by persistent or recurrent episodes with anorexia, weight loss, and chronic weakness. Simple functional diarrhea can usually be treated without sequela with an OTC product.

The debilitating effect of persistent diarrhea is caused, to a large extent, by loss of water and electrolytes through excretion. The replacement of these vital fluids and electrolytes has become a part of diarrhea therapy, particularly in infants and children. This can be accomplished by the ingestion of the appropriate foodstuffs or by the use of proprietary oral electrolyte formulations which provide, in powdered form for reconstitution, a balanced formulation of important electrolytes and carbohydrates.

Complaints of GI irritation should be evaluated for their severity and nature (acute or chronic). For the relatively minor acute problems, e.g., food or drink intolerance, relief may be provided by OTC protectives containing adsorbent, bulk-forming, or mucilaginous ingredients. All severely acute, uncontrolled, or chronic GI complaints should be referred promptly to a physician. The pharmacist can contribute to better patient care by being familiar with the disease processes involved in diarrhea and other GI illnesses and by appropriate selection and use of pharmacologic agents.

References

1. E. Englert, "Dealing with Diarrhea," Science and Medical Publishing Co., 1974.
2. S. F. Phillips, "Diarrhea—Pathogenesis and Diagnosis Techniques," *Postgrad. Med.*, **57,** 65-71(1974).
3. H. L. DuPont and R. B. Hornick, in "Disease a Month," Year Book Medical Publishers, Chicago, Ill., July, 1969, pp. 1-40.
4. "The Macmillan Medical Cyclopedia," W. A. R. Thomas, Ed., Macmillan, New York, N.Y., 1955, p. 244.
5. W. C. Matousek, "Manual of Differential Diagnosis," Year Book Medical Publishers, Chicago, Ill., 1959, p. 84.
6. "Documenta Geigy: Scientific Tables," 7th ed., K. Diem and C. Lentner, Eds., Ciba-Geigy Limited, Basel, Switzerland, 1970, pp. 657-658.
7. A. C. Guyton, in "Textbook of Medical Physiology," 5th ed., Saunders, Philadelphia, Pa., 1976, pp. 850-866.
8. "Gastroenterology," A. Bogoch, Ed., McGraw-Hill, New York, N.Y., 1973, pp. 33-38, 602-721.
9. G. F. Grady and G. T. Keusch, *N. Engl. J. Med.*, **285,** 831-841, 891-901(1971).
10. A. I. Mendeloff, in "Harrison's Principles of Internal Medicine," 7th ed., M. M. Wintrobe *et al.*, Eds., McGraw-Hill, New York, N.Y., 1974, pp. 213-217.
11. S. M. Mellinkoff, "The Differential Diagnosis of Diarrhea," McGraw-Hill, New York, N.Y., 1964, pp. 310-325.
12. "Pediatric Therapy," 5th ed., H. C. Shirkey, Ed., Mosby, St. Louis, Mo., 1975, pp. 505-509.
13. M. H. Merson *et al.*, *N. Engl. J. Med.*, **294,** 1299-1305(1976).
14. *FDA Drug Bulletin,* (May, 1972).
15. G. P. Oakley, *J. Am. Med. Assoc.*, **225,** 395(1973).
16. M. H. Merson and E. J. Gangarosa, *J. Am. Med. Assoc.*, **234,** 200-201(1975).
17. *FDA Drug Bulletin,* (January-March, 1975).
18. Ervin Novak *et al.*, *J. Am. Med. Assoc.*, **235,** 1451-1454(1976).
19. *Cancer Facts and Figures,* American Cancer Society, New York, N.Y., 1975.
20. C. F. Hawkins and R. Cockel, *Gut,* **12,** 208(1971).
21. *Fed. Regist.*, **40,** 12924-12933(1975).
22. *Opium Preparations,* American Hospital Formulary Service, American Society of Hospital Pharmacists, Washington, D. C., Section 28:08.
23. J. A. Riese and F. Damrau, *J. Am. Geriatr. Soc.*, **12,** 500(1964).
24. H. F. Eichenwald and G. H. McCracken, *Med. Clin. North Am.*, **54,** 443-453(1970).
25. "The Merck Manual of Diagnosis and Therapy," 12th ed., D. N. Holvey, Ed., Merck, Sharp, and Dohme Research Laboratories, Rahway, N.J., 1972, pp. 673-731.
26. *Fed. Regist.*, **39,** No. 108, 19874(1974).

Products **3** DIARRHEA

Product (manufacturer)	**Dosage form**	**Opiates** [a]	**Adsorbents**	**Other active ingredients**	**Inactive ingredients**
Amogel (North American)	tablet	powdered opium, 1.2 mg	bismuth subgallate, 120 mg kaolin, 120 mg pectin, 15 mg	zinc phenolsulfonate, 15 mg	—
Bacid (Fisons)	tablet	—	—	carboxymethylcellulose sodium, 100 mg *Lactobacillus acidophilus*	—
Bisilad (Central)	suspension	—	kaolin, 5.5 g/15 ml bismuth subgallate, 150 mg/15 ml	—	thymol, menthol, eucalyptus oil, methyl salicylate, preservatives
Corrective Mixture (Beecham Labs)	liquid	—	bismuth subsalicylate, 80 mg/5 ml	pepsin, 40 mg/5 ml phenyl salicylate, 20 mg/5 ml zinc phenolsulfonate, 10 mg/5 ml	alcohol, 1.5%; carminatives; demulcents; flavoring
Corrective Mixture with Paregoric (Beecham Labs)	liquid	paregoric, 0.6 ml/ 5 ml	bismuth subsalicylate, 80 mg/5 ml	pepsin, 40 mg/5 ml phenyl salicylate, 20 mg/5 ml zinc phenolsulfonate, 10 mg/5 ml	alcohol, 2%; carminatives; demulcents; flavoring
Diabismul (O'Neal, Jones & Feldman)	suspension	opium, 7 mg/15 ml	kaolin, 2.5 g/15 ml pectin, 80 mg/15 ml	—	methylparaben, propylparaben
DIA-quel (International Pharmaceutical)	liquid	paregoric, 0.75 ml/ 5 ml	pectin, 24 mg/5 ml	homatropine methylbromide, 0.15 mg/5 ml	alcohol, 10%

Product (manufacturer)	Dosage form	Opiates[a]	Adsorbents	Other active ingredients	Inactive ingredients
Digestalin (North American)	tablet	—	activated charcoal, 5.30 mg bismuth subgallate, 3.80 mg	pepsin, 2.00 mg berberis, 1.20 mg papain, 1.20 mg pancreatin, 0.40 mg hydrastis, 0.08 mg animal diastate, 0.06 mg	—
Donnagel (Robins)	suspension	—	kaolin, 6 g/30 ml pectin, 142.8 mg/30 ml	sodium benzoate, 60 mg/30 ml hyoscyamine sulfate, 0.1037 mg/30 ml atropine sulfate, 0.0194 mg/30 ml hyoscine hydrobromide, 0.0065 mg/30 ml	alcohol, 3.8%
Donnagel-PG (Robins)	suspension	powdered opium, 24 mg/30 ml	kaolin, 6 g/30 ml pectin, 142.8 mg/30 ml	sodium benzoate, 60 mg/30 ml hyoscyamine sulfate, 0.1037 mg/30 ml atropine sulfate, 0.0194 mg/30 ml hyoscine hydrobromide, 0.0065 mg/30 ml	alcohol, 5%
Infantol Pink (First Texas)	liquid	opium camphorated fluid, 0.078 ml/5 ml	bismuth subsalicylate, 65.78 mg/5 ml pectin powder, 37.27 mg/5 ml	calcium carrageenan, 18.0 mg/5 ml zinc phenolsulfonate, 17.57 mg/5 ml	saccharin sodium, 1.37 mg/5 ml glycerin, 0.25 ml/5 ml alcohol, 0.068 ml/5 ml peppermint oil, 0.00078 ml/5 ml
Kaolin Pectin Suspension (Philips Roxane)	suspension	—	kaolin, 5.83 g/30 ml pectin, 130 mg/30 ml	saccharin sodium glycerin carboxymethylcellulose sodium	lime mint flavor
Kaomagma (Wyeth)	suspension	—	kaolin, 6 g/30 ml alumina gel	—	—
Kaopectate (Upjohn)	suspension	—	kaolin, 5.83 g/30 ml pectin, 130 mg/30 ml	—	—
Kaopectate Concentrate (Upjohn)	suspension	—	kaolin, 8.75 g/30 ml pectin, 194 mg/30 ml	—	—
Lactinex (Hynson, Westcott & Dunning)	tablet granules	—	—	*Lactobacillus acidophilus* *Lactobacillus bulgaricus*	—
Pabizol with Paregoric (Rexall)	suspension	paregoric, 3.69 mg/30 ml	bismuth subsalicylate, 517 mg/30 ml	aluminum magnesium silicate, 265 mg/30 ml phenyl salicylate, 97.4 mg/30 ml zinc phenolsulfonate, 51.8 mg/30 ml	alcohol, 8% carminatives
Parelixir (Purdue Frederick)	liquid	tincture of opium, 0.2 ml/30 ml	pectin, 145 mg/30 ml	—	alcohol, 18%
Parepectolin (Rorer)	suspension	paregoric, 3.7 ml/30 ml	kaolin, 5.5 g/30 ml pectin, 162 mg/30 ml	—	alcohol, 0.69%
Pargel (Parke-Davis)	suspension	—	kaolin, 6 g/30 ml pectin, 130 mg/30 ml	—	—
Pektamalt (Warren-Teed)	liquid	—	kaolin, 6.5 g/30 ml pectin, 600 mg/30 ml	—	—

Product (manufacturer)	Dosage form	Opiates [a]	Adsorbents	Other active ingredients	Inactive ingredients
Pepto-Bismol (Norwich)	tablet suspension	—	bismuth subsalicylate	—	calcium carbonate, 350 mg/tablet
Polymagma Plain (Wyeth)	suspension	—	activated attapulgite, 3 g/30 ml pectin, 270 mg/30 ml alumina gel	—	—
Quintess (Lilly)	suspension	—	activated attapulgite, 3 g/30 ml colloidal attapulgite, 900 mg/30 ml	—	—

[a] Schedule V drug: OTC sale forbidden in some states.

Laxative Products

Roy C. Darlington

Questions to ask the patient

What is the normal frequency of your bowel movements? How has it changed?

How long has constipation been a problem?

Have you experienced symptoms such as abdominal pain, bloating, or weight loss?

Are you under the care of a physician for any illness? Did the physician recommend a particular laxative?

What medicines are you currently taking?

Have you attempted to alleviate constipation by dietary measures such as increasing fruit consumption?

Which laxative products have you used previously? Were they effective?

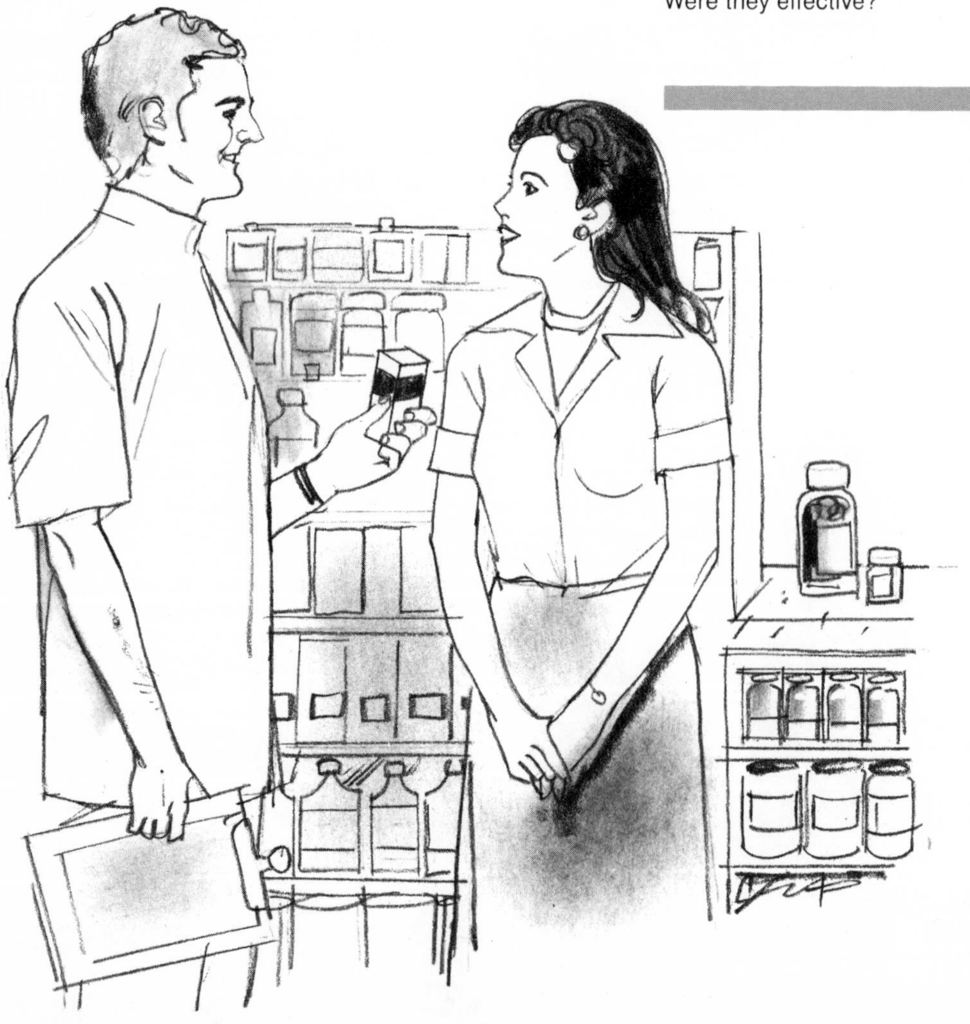

CHAPTER 4

Laxative products facilitate the passage and elimination of feces from the colon and rectum.[1] Because there are few valid indications for their use, these products are misused by many people to alleviate what they consider to be constipation. Constipation is "infrequent or difficult evacuation."[2] It usually results from the abnormally slow movement of feces through the colon; dry and hard feces accumulate in the descending colon.

Physiology of the lower GI tract

The mechanisms that are responsible for the digestive and absorptive functions of the GI system depend on the intrinsic properties of intestinal smooth muscle, visceral reflexes, and GI hormones (Fig. 1). (See Chapter 3 for a discussion of GI tract anatomy.) Little absorption occurs in the stomach or duodenum. About 94 percent of the absorption takes place in the small intestine. Of approximately 6 liters of fluids that are ingested and supplied by secretions of the GI tract, about 1.5 percent, or 100 ml, is excreted with the feces.[3]

Tonic contractions of the stomach churn and knead food, and large peristaltic waves start at the fundus and move food toward the duodenum. The rate at which the stomach empties into the duodenum is regulated by mechanisms operating through autonomic reflexes or a hormonal link between the duodenum and stomach. Carbohydrates leave the stomach most rapidly, proteins leave more slowly, and fats have the slowest emptying time. Vagotomy and fear slow emptying time; excitement hastens it. Most of the mechanisms that slow emptying time of the stomach also inhibit secretion of hydrochloric acid and pepsin. When the osmotic pressure of the stomach contents is higher or lower than that of the plasma, gastric emptying time is slowed until isotonicity is achieved.

The movement of the contents of the small and large intestines is a result of four movements. Pendular movements result from contractions of the longitudinal muscles of the intestine. The contractions pass up and down small segments of the gut at the rate of about 10 per minute. They mix, rather than propel, the contents. Segmental movements result from contractions of the circular muscles and occur at about the same rate as pendular movements. These movements are also primarily for mixing. Pendular and segmental movements are caused by the intrinsic contractility of smooth muscle, and they occur in the absence of innervation of intestinal tissue.

Peristaltic movements propel intestinal contents. They are caused by circular contractions that form behind a point of stimulation and pass along the GI tract toward the rectum. The rate of contraction ranges from 2 to 20 cm/second. These contractions require an intact myenteric (Auerbach's) nerve plexus which apparently is located in the intestinal mucosa. Peristaltic waves move the intestinal contents through the small intestine about 6 to 7 meters in about 3.5 hours. Vermiform (wormlike) movements occur mainly in the large intestine (colon) and are caused by the contraction of several centimeters of the colonic tissue at one time. In the cecum and ascending colon the contents are fluid, and peristaltic and antiperistaltic waves occur quite frequently. However, the activity of the transverse, descending, and sigmoid segments of the colon is very irregular, and here the contents are semisolid.

Three or four times a day a strong peristaltic wave (mass movement) propels the contents about one-third (38 cm) the length of the colon. This activity seems to be associated with the entrance of food into the stomach. The sigmoid colon serves as a storage place for fecal matter until defecation occurs. Except for the fauces and anus, the entire alimentary canal normally functions involuntarily as a coordinated whole.[4]

The presence of fecal material in the rectum is not in itself sufficient to initiate the defecation reflex; it must be large enough to exceed the individual threshold of the distention stimulus. The internal anal sphincter is relaxed when the rectum is distended. The nerve supply to the striated muscle of the external anal sphincter maintains it in a state of tonic contraction which, when relaxed by voluntary action, permits the reflex contraction of the distended colon to expel the feces. Defecation is a spinal reflex which is voluntarily inhibited by keeping the external sphincter contracted or is facilitated by relaxing the sphincter and contracting the abdominal muscles.

Distention of the stomach by food initiates contractions of the rectum (gastrocolic reflex) and, frequently, a desire to defecate. Children usually defecate after meals; in adults, however, habits and cultural factors play a significant role in determining the time of defecation.

Pathophysiology of the lower GI tract

Alteration in motor activities is responsible for symptoms of disorders in the small intestine. Distention or irritation of the small intestine can cause nausea and vomiting; the duodenum is the most sensitive part. The motility in the small intestine is intensified when the mucosa is irritated by bacterial toxins, chemical agents, and mechanical obstruction.

Pain caused by functional disturbances of the jejunoileum is "referred" to the periumbilical region; pain in the midabdomen is suggestive of a lesion of the small intestine. One of the most common disorders of the small intestine is the formation of gallstones in the gallbladder and bile ducts. The stones do not alter the function of the small intestine unless the flow of bile into the intestine is blocked, in which case, fat digestion and absorption are impaired.[5] Diminished pancreatic secretion affects the digestion and absorption of fats, carbohydrates, and proteins.

The pain associated with regional ileitis is similar to that caused by appendicitis. The enterointestinal reflexes elicited from the pain cause inhibition of intestinal motility. As a result, functional obstruction often occurs in the small intestine, causing all the symptoms of acute intestinal obstruction.

Disorders of the colon may cause constipation or diarrhea. The main causes of the disorder are ulcerative colitis, excessive parasympathetic stimulation of the colon, and the chronic misuse of irritant laxative drugs. Some clinicians believe that ulcerative colitis is an infectious disease; others believe that it is caused by the digestive action of the contents of the large intestine on the mucosa. The irritation of the inflamed mucosa can initiate enough propulsive contractions to cause complete evacuation of the colon. A watery diarrhea may result.

The diarrhea caused by excessive parasympathetic stimulation is called neurogenic diarrhea. It can occur during periods of nervous tension, when there is an increase in the motility and the mucus secretion of the colon. This type of diarrhea can cause the loss of large amounts of water and electrolytes.

The prolonged misuse of laxative drugs can cause morbid, anatomical changes in the colon. In a study of 12 chronic laxative users, the main anatomical changes were loss of intrinsic innervation, atrophy of smooth muscle coats, and pigmentation of the colon. Most of the users had been taking laxatives regularly for 30 to 40 years; two were less than 30 years old when they had the colon removed and, therefore, had a much shorter history. In these cases the myenteric plexus showed many swollen, but otherwise normal, neurones. This suggests that the initial action of an irritant laxative is to stimulate neurones and that prolonged and continuous stimulation causes the death of the cell. Surgery in such cases shows that the transverse colon is often pendulous, the sigmoid section is highly dilated, and the muscle coats are thin and contain excess adipose tissue, indicating some tissue loss.

Melanosis coli suggests prolonged use of anthraquinone laxatives. Pigment-containing macrophages appear in the mucosa, but staining reactions indicate that the pigment is not melanin but has many of the characteristics of lipofuscin. It has been suggested that it is a combination of a pigment of this type and either anthraquinone or one of its breakdown products.[6]

In some cases, especially in older people, large masses of fecal material can accumulate in a greatly dilated rectum. The loss of tonicity in the rectal musculature may be caused by ignoring or suppressing the urge to defecate. It may also be caused by the degeneration of nerve pathways concerned with defecation reflexes. Sometimes, enemas or fecal-softening laxatives may be necessary for defecation.

Painful lesions of the anal canal, such as ulcers, fissures, and thrombosed hemorrhoidal veins, impede defecation by causing a spasm of the sphincters and by promoting voluntary suppression of defecation to avoid pain.

Table 1. Clinical Features of Laxative Abuse[a]

Cathartic colon
Electrolyte imbalance:
hypermagnesemia
hypocalcemia
hypokalemia
Factitious diarrhea
Liver disease
Osteomalacia
Protein losing enteropathy
Steatorrhea

[a]Adapted from R. R. Babb, *West. J. Med.*, **122**, 93 (January, 1975).

The normal rectal mucosa is relatively insensitive to cutting or burning. However, when it is inflamed, it becomes highly sensitive to all stimuli, including those acting on the receptors mediating the stretch reflex. A constant urge to defecate in the absence of appreciable material in the rectum may occur with inflamed rectal mucosa.[7]

The normal symptoms of constipation are slight anorexia and mild, abdominal discomfort and distention even in children with congenital aganglionic megacolon of Hirschsprung's disease; these children may defecate as infrequently as once every 3 weeks. Thus, the symptoms which many unwittingly attribute to the absorption of toxic substances because of infrequency of bowel evacuation are due to other causes.[8]

The main symptoms of constipation are the result of chronic abuse or misuse of stimulating laxatives. Abdominal discomfort and inadequate response to increasing varieties and doses of irritant laxatives are frequent complaints. Responses to questions may disclose that a person produces loose stools and has misconceptions concerning normal bowel movement.[9]

The pharmacist cannot effectively counsel on the proper use of laxatives without a knowledge of an individual's habits. Counseling requires not only a comprehensive knowledge of properties of the laxative product but also an appreciation of significant physiological and psychological factors.

Excessive use of laxatives can cause diarrhea and vomiting, leading to fluid and electrolyte losses and hypokalemia, where there is a general loss of tone of smooth and striated muscle (Table 1).[10] In a study of seven hospitalized female patients, 26 to 65 years old, the main complaints were abdominal pain and diarrhea, the number of hospital admissions ranged from 2 to 11, and the number of days spent in the hospital ranged from 58 to 202.[10] Diagnosis was difficult because all the women denied taking laxatives, and none of the colonic tissue characteristics usually associated with excessive laxative use was observed on sigmoidoscopy or radiological examination. However, additional tests revealed excessive laxative use.

Causes of constipation

Constipation is a functional impairment of the colon in producing properly formed stools at regular intervals. The main causes include:

- ☐ Neglecting to respond to the defecation urge
- ☐ Failure to acquire the habit of regular defecation
- ☐ Faulty eating habits
- ☐ Environmental changes
- ☐ Atony or hypertonicity of the colon
- ☐ Hypertonicity of the ileocecal valve
- ☐ Insensitivity of the defecation reflex initiated by fecal mass in the rectum
- ☐ Mental stress
- ☐ Excessive ingestion of foods that harden stools, such as processed cheese
- ☐ Prolonged use of drugs such as aluminum hydroxide, calcium carbonate, opiates, liquid petrolatum, and anticholinergic drugs.[11]

A frequent cause of constipation is irregular bowel habits which have developed over a long period of inhibition of the normal defecation reflexes. Clinical experience has shown that if defecation is not allowed to occur when the defecation reflexes are excited, the reflexes become progressively weaker. Constipation can also result from atony of the colon or from spasm of a small segment of the sigmoid part of the colon. Motility in the colon normally is weak, and a slight spasm in any part of the descending or sigmoid colon can often block the movement of feces.

Stress-producing situations or emotions can cause constipation, and many drugs may induce or aggravate it. These drugs include antacids, antihistamines, anticholinergics, muscle relaxants, narcotics, diuretics, tranquilizers, adrenergic agents, and rauwolfia preparations.

Faulty information, undue apprehension concerning the normal frequency of bowel evacuation, and prolonged use of irritating or mineral oil laxatives are the main causes of chronic constipation in the absence of organic origin and inadequate roughage in the diet. Constipation of organic origin may be due to hypothyroidism, megacolon, stricture, or lesions (benign or malignant). Laxatives are contraindicated in such cases; proper diagnosis and medical treatment should be used.

In many cases of chronic constipation, not of organic origin, there is a misunderstanding as to what constitutes normal frequency of bowel movement. Although limited quantitative data are available, the results of one study indicate that the range of bowel movement frequency in humans is from three times a day to three times a week.[12] Therefore, constipation cannot be defined in terms of the number of bowel movements in any given period.

Treatment of constipation

If drug therapy for constipation is chosen, the recommendations of the FDA OTC Panel on Laxatives, Antidiarrheals, Emetic and Anti-Emetic Products should be followed.[13] Stimulant laxatives should be limited to short-term use—no longer than one week. The dose of the

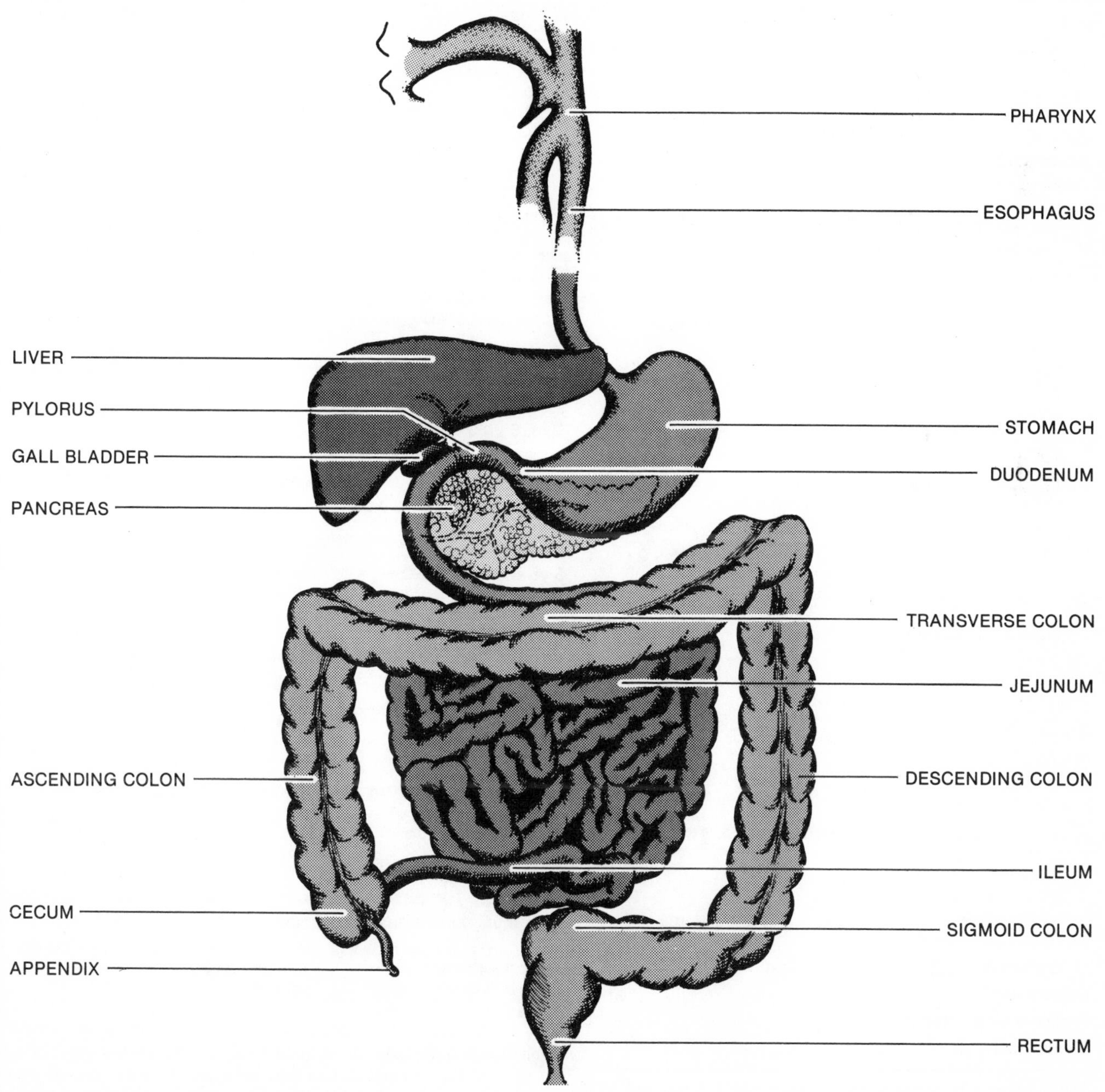

Figure 1. Anatomy of the digestive system.

Table 2. Classification and Properties of Laxatives

Class and drug	Dosage form	Daily dosage range: Adult	Daily dosage range: Pediatric	Site of action	Approximate hours required for action
Stimulants					
Anthraquinones					
Aloe	Solid	0.12–0.25 g	Under 6 yr: not recommended 6-8 yr: 0.04-0.08 g	Colon	8–12
Cascara sagrada	Fluidextract	0.5–1.5 ml		Colon	6–8
	Aromatic fluidextract	2–6 ml	Under 2 yr: ¼ adult dose		
	Bark	0.3–1.0 g			
	Extract	0.2–0.4 ml	2–12 yr: ½ adult dose		
	Casanthranol	0.03–0.09 ml			
Danthron	Solid	0.075–0.15 g	Under 12 yr: not recommended	Colon	8
Senna	Powder	0.5–2.0 g	Under 2 yr: ⅛ adult dose	Colon	6–10
	Fluidextract	2.0 ml			
	Syrup	8.0 ml	1–6 yr: ¼ adult dose		
	Fruit extract	3.4–4.0 ml	6–12 yr: ½ adult dose		
Sennosides A and B	Solid	0.012–0.036 g	0.0015-0.018 g	Colon	6–10
Diphenylmethanes					
Bisacodyl	Tablet	0.005–0.015 g	Over 3 yr: 0.005 g	Colon	6-10
	Suppository	0.010 g	Under 2 yr: 0.005 g		0.25-1
Phenolphthalein	Solid	0.03–0.27 g	Under 2 yr: not recommended 2-6 yr: 0.015-0.020 g Over 6 yr: 0.03-0.06 g	Colon	6–8
Saline					
Magnesium citrate	Solid	11–18 g	2-5 yr: 2.5-5.0 g 6 yr and over: 5.0-10.0 g	Small and large intestines	0.5-3
Magnesium hydroxide	Solid	2.4–4.8 g	2-5 yr: 0.4-1.2 g 6 yr and over: 1.2-2.4 g	Small and large intestines	0.5-3
Magnesium sulfate	Solid	10–30 g	2-5 yr: 2.5-5.0 g 6 yr and over: 5.0-10.0 g	Small and large intestines	0.5-3
Dibasic sodium phosphate	Solid (oral)	1.9–3.8 g	5–10 yr: ¼ adult dose 10 yr and over: ½ adult dose	Small and large intestines	0.5-3
	Solid (rectal)	3.8 g	Over 2 yr: ½ adult dose	Colon	2-15 min
Monobasic sodium phosphate	Solid (oral)	8.3–16.6 g	5–10 yr: ¼ adult dose 10 yr and over: ½ adult dose	Small and large intestines	0.5-3
	Solid (rectal)	16.6 g	Over 2 yr: ½ adult dose	Colon	2-15 min
Sodium biphosphate	Solid (oral)	9.6–19.2 g	5–10 yr: ¼ adult dose 10 yr and over: ½ adult dose	Small and large intestines	0.5-3
	Solid (rectal)	19.2 g	Over 2 yr: ½ adult dose	Colon	2-15 min

Table 2. Continued

Class and drug	Dosage form	Daily dosage range		Site of action	Approximate hours required for action
		Adult	*Pediatric*		
Bulk-forming					
Methylcellulose	Solid	4-6 g	Over 6 yr: 1-1.5 g	Small and large intestines	12-72
Carboxymethyl-cellulose sodium	Solid	4-6 g	Over 6 yr: 1-1.5 g	Small and large intestines	12-72
Polycarbophil	Solid	4-6 g	Under 2 yr: 0.5-1.0 g 2-5 yr: 1-1.5 g 6-12 yr: 1.5-3.0 g	Small and large intestines	12-72
Psyllium seeds	Solid	2.5-30 g	Over 6 yr: 1.25-15 g	Small and large intestines	12-72
Emollient					
Dioctyl calcium sulfosuccinate	Solid	0.05-0.36 g	Under 2 yr: 0.025 g 2 yr and over: 0.05-0.150 g	Small and large intestines	12-72
Dioctyl sodium sulfosuccinate	Solid	0.05-0.36 g	Under 2 yr: 0.02-0.05 g 2 yr and over: 0.05-0.15 g	Small and large intestines	12-72
Dioctyl potassium sulfosuccinate	Solid (rectal)	0.05-0.25 g	Children: 0.1 g	Colon	2-15 min
Lubricant					
Mineral oil	Liquid (oral)	15-45 ml	Over 6 yr: 10-15 ml	Colon	6-8
Hyperosmotic					
Glycerin	Suppository	3 g	Under 6 yr: 1.15 g	Colon	0.25 - 1
Miscellaneous					
Castor oil	Liquid	15-60 ml	Under 2 yr: 1-5 ml 2-12 yr: 5-15 ml	Small intestine	2-6

laxative should be within the dosage range indicated as safe and effective.

An ideal laxative should be nonirritating, nontoxic, and should act only on the descending and sigmoid colon. Within a few hours it should produce a normally formed stool. Its action should then cease and permit the resumption of normal bowel activity. Such a laxative is not now available.

Cathartics, or laxatives, are not used to treat constipation associated with intestinal pathology. They are also not a cure for functional constipation and, therefore, are only of secondary importance in its treatment. The case history often reveals that the use of laxatives is unnecessary. A diet with adequate roughage and fluid intake, exercise (if necessary), and the establishment of proper stool habits are often all that is required. Sedation and psychotherapy are often needed to combat responsible emotional factors.

Stimulant laxatives, such as castor oil or bisacodyl, are frequently used prior to radiological examination of the GI tract and prior to bowel surgery. Bisacodyl is also used orally or rectally instead of an enema for emptying the colon before proctological examination.

In cases of food or drug poisoning, the saline laxatives are used in purging doses. Magnesium sulfate is recommended except in cases of a depressed CNS or renal dysfunction.[11]

People with hernia, severe hypertension, or cardiovascular disease should not strain to defecate; neither should those who are about to undergo or have undergone surgery for hemorrhoids or other anorectal disorders. An emollient or fecal-softening laxative is indicated in such cases.

Laxative drugs have been classified according to site of action, severity of action, chemical structure, or mechanism of action. The most meaningful method is the mechanism of action, under which laxatives are classified as stimulant, bulk forming, emollient, lubricant, saline, and hyperosmotic (see Table 2).

Stimulant laxatives

A comprehensive review of stimulant laxatives has been reported, and several investigators have related the structure-activity significance of the anthraquinone or emodin-bearing laxatives.[14-17] Stimulant laxatives increase the propulsive peristaltic activity of the intestine by local irritation of the mucosa or by a more selective action on the intramural nerve plexus of intestinal smooth muscle, thus increasing motility. Their site of action ranges from the small intestine (with castor oil) or colon (with anthracene derivatives) to the small and large intestines (with jalap). Intensity of action is proportional to dosage, but individually effective doses vary. All stimulant laxatives produce griping, increased mucus secretion, and in some people, excessive evacuation of fluid. Listed doses and dosage ranges are only guides to the correct individual dose. Stimulating laxatives are contraindicated with abdominal pain, nausea, or vomiting, which are some of the symptoms of appendicitis.

Anthraquinones. The drugs of choice in this group are the cascara and senna compounds. Rhubarb, which contains an astringent (tannin), and aloe, which is too irritating, are not recommended. The properties of each of the anthraquinone laxatives vary, depending on the anthraquinone content and the speed of liberation of the active principles from their glycosidic combinations. Crude drug formulations may also contain active constituents not found in extractive preparations or more highly purified compounds.

The precise mechanism by which peristalsis is increased has not been determined. The cathartic activity of anthraquinones is limited primarily to the colon. The drugs reach the colon by direct passage. Bacterial enzymes are partly responsible for hydrolysis of the glycosides in the intestinal tract. Anthraquinones usually produce their action in 8 to 12 hours after administration but may require up to 24 hours.

The active principles of anthraquinones appear in body secretions, including human breast milk. The practical significance of this in nursing infants is controversial. After taking a senna laxative, postpartum women reported a brown discoloration of breast milk and subsequent catharsis of their nursing infants. The result of a study initiated by this report indicated that the amount of senna laxative principles in breast milk was inadequate to cause defecation.[18] In another study with constipated, postpartum, breast-feeding women, it was reported that 17 percent of their infants experienced diarrhea.[19]

Chrysophanic acid, a component of rhubarb excreted in the urine, colors acidic urine yellowish brown and alkaline urine reddish violet after ingesting rhubarb and senna. The prolonged use of anthraquinone laxatives, especially cascara sagrada, can result in a melanotic pigmentation of the colonic mucosa. The pigmentation is usually reversible in 4 to 12 months after the drug is discontinued.

The liquid preparations of cascara sagrada (fluidextracts) are more reliable than the solid dosage forms (extract and tablet). Aromatic cascara fluidextract USP is less active and less bitter than cascara sagrada fluidextract NF. Magnesium oxide, which is used in the preparation of the former, removes some of the bitter and irritating principles from the crude drug.

Preparations of senna are more potent than those of cascara and produce considerably more griping. Those that contain the crystalline glycosides of senna are more stable, more reliable, and cause less griping than those made from the crude drug.[20]

Danthron (1,8-dihydroxyanthraquinone) is a free anthraquinone rather than a glycoside. Its action, use, properties, and limitations are similar to those of the natural anthraquinone drugs. Its site of action is the colon. It is partly absorbed from the small intestine, and a large part is metabolized by the liver; the metabolites are excreted by the kidneys, sometimes causing a harmless discoloration of the urine.

Diphenylmethane laxatives. The most common diphenylmethane laxatives are phenolphthalein and bisacodyl.

Phenolphthalein. This drug exerts its stimulating effect mainly on the colon, but the activity of the small intestine may also be increased. Its exact mechanism of action is not known, and it is usually active in 6 to 8 hours after administration.

A therapeutic dose of phenolphthalein passes through the stomach unchanged and is dissolved by the bile salts and the alkaline intestinal secretions. As much as 15 percent of the dose is absorbed, and the rest is excreted unchanged in the feces. Some of the drug that is absorbed appears in the urine, which if sufficiently alkaline, is colored pink to red. Similarly, the drug excreted in the feces causes a red coloration if the feces are alkaline enough (soap enemas). This may cause alarm to people who are unaware of this property.

Part of the absorbed phenolphthalein is excreted back into the intestinal tract with the bile. Reports show that the resulting enterohepatic cycle has prolonged the action of a dose of phenolphthalein for 3 or 4 days. It has also been reported that phenolphthalein is ineffective in people with obstructive jaundice. It functions as a laxative when administered intravenously and is excreted into the intestine with the bile.

Phenolphthalein is usually nontoxic. The main hazard of phenolphthalein overdosage is usually electrolyte and fluid deficit resulting from excessive catharsis. The danger of hypokalemia which may result cannot be overemphasized.

At least two types of allergic toxicity may follow the use of phenolphthalein. In susceptible individuals, a large dose may cause diarrhea, colic, cardiac and respiratory distress, or collapse. The other reaction is a polychromatic rash that ranges from pink to deep purple. The eruptions may be pinhead sized or as large as the palm of the hand. Itching and burning may be moderate or severe. If the rash is severe, it may lead to vesication and erosion, especially around the mouth and genitalia.

Osteomalacia has been attributed to the excessive ingestion of phenolphthalein.[21] A female patient in an orthopedic clinic had been suffering for 6 months with back and hip pain. The dietary history indicated a balanced and adequate diet, but the clinical symptoms and laboratory findings were typical of osteomalacia. The cause of the osteomalacia was not apparent until investigation disclosed a 20-year history of ingestion of 15 to 20 phenolphthalein tablets daily. Discontinuance of the laxative quickly led to normal bowel habits and the resolution of the osteomalacia.

Bisacodyl. Bisacodyl was introduced as a cathartic as a result of structure-activity studies of compounds related to phenolphthalein. It is practically insoluble in water or in alkaline media. Bisacodyl exerts its action in the colon upon contact with the mucosal nerve plexus. Stimulation is segmented and axonal, producing contractions of the entire colon. Its action is independent of intestinal tone, and the drug is not systemically absorbed. Action on the small intestine is negligible. A soft, formed stool is usually produced 6 to 10 hours after oral administration and in 15 to 60 minutes when given rectally.

Bisacodyl is recommended for cleaning the colon before and after surgery and prior to X-ray examinations. It is effective in colostomies and reducing or eliminating the need for irrigations. No systemic effects or adverse effects on the liver, kidney, or hematopoietic system have been observed following its administration. Bisacodyl has not been detected in the milk of nursing women. The suppository form may produce a burning sensation in the rectum.

Bulk-forming laxatives

These laxatives are natural and semisynthetic, polysaccharides and cellulose derivatives that dissolve or swell in the intestinal fluid. They form emollient gels which facilitate the passage of the intestinal contents and stimulate peristalsis. The bulk-forming drugs usually exert a laxative effect in 12 to 24 hours but may require as much as 3 days. This type of laxative may be indicated for people on low-residue diets that cannot be corrected.

The hydrophilic colloid laxatives do not seem to interfere with the absorption of nutrients. They should be mixed with water just before ingestion and administered with a large amount of fluid. When they are administered properly, these agents are essentially free from systemic side effects because they are not absorbed. Esophageal obstruction has occurred in patients with strictures of the esophagus when these drugs are chewed or taken in dry form. Because of the danger of fecal impaction or intestinal obstruction, the bulk-forming laxatives should not be taken by individuals with intestinal ulcerations, stenosis, disabling adhesions, or difficulty in swallowing.

The bulk-forming drugs are derived from agar, plantago (psyllium) seed, kelp (alginates), and plant gums (tragacanth, chondrus, sterculia, karaya, and others). The synthetic cellulose derivatives—methylcellulose and carboxymethylcellulose sodium—are being used more frequently, and many preparations that contain these drugs also contain stimulant and/or fecal-softening laxative drugs.

Each dose of the laxative should be taken with a full glass of water. These drugs may interact and combine with other drugs, including salicylates and digitalis glycosides. They should not be taken if prescription drugs or drugs that contain a salicylate are also used.[13]

Emollient laxatives

Dioctyl sodium sulfosuccinate (DSS) is a surface active agent (detergent) which, when administered orally, increases the wetting efficiency of intestinal water and promotes the formation of oil-in-water emulsions. It facilitates admixture of aqueous and fatty substances with the fecal mass to soften it.

DSS does not retard absorption of nutrients from the intestinal tract. It is useful in alleviating spastic constipation, but its value in atonic constipation is dubious. It prevents the development of constipation, but does not improve existing constipation.[22]

This drug is recommended for the treatment of constipation associated with hard, dry stools. It is also considered valuable in conditions that require the avoidance of straining at the stool; combinations of DSS and peristaltic stimulants, bulk-forming laxatives, and choleretic agents are also used. A solution of DSS is added to the enema fluid in cases of fecal impaction. DSS and its congeners are claimed to be nonabsorbable, nontoxic, and pharmacologically inert.

Other fecal-softener laxatives are dioctyl calcium sulfosuccinate (anionic surfactant) and poloxamer 188 (nonionic surfactant). The latter has no irritant properties and is compatible with electrolytes. Both can be used when the sodium ion is contraindicated.

Lubricant laxatives

Liquid petrolatum and certain digestible plant oils (e.g., olive oil) soften fecal contents by coating them and thus preventing colonic absorption of fecal water. There is little difference in their cathartic efficacy, although emulsions of mineral oil penetrate and soften fecal matter more effectively than nonemulsified preparations. Liquid petrolatum is useful when it is used judiciously in cases that require the maintenance of a soft stool to avoid straining, e.g., after a hemorrhoidectomy or abdominal surgery, hernias, aneurysms, hypertension, and cerebrovascular accidents.

The side effects and toxicity of mineral oil are associated with repeated and prolonged use. The results of several studies indicate that significant absorption of mineral oil may occur. The oil is readily apparent in the mesenteric lymph nodes, but may also be present in the intestinal mucosa, liver, and spleen, where liquid petrolatum elicits a typical foreign-body reaction characterized by cells of chronic inflammation, including giant cells.

Lipid pneumonia caused by the use of oily nose drops may also result from the oral ingestion and subsequent aspiration of mineral oil. The pharynx becomes coated with the oil, and droplets gain access to the trachea and the posterior part of the lower lobes of the lungs. The effect of mineral oil on the absorption of fat-soluble nutrients is controversial, but there is sufficient evidence to make this property significant. The absorption of calcium, phosphates, and vitamins A and D may be affected. It has been reported that the mineral oil affects the absorption of the carotenes to a greater extent; the plasma level of carotene may be reduced as much as 50 percent.

Mineral oil should not be taken with meals because it may delay gastric emptying. If large doses are taken, the oil may leak through the anal sphincter. This leakage may produce anal pruritus, hemorrhoids, cryptitis, and other perianal disease and can be avoided by reducing the dose, dividing the dose, or using a stable emulsion of mineral oil. Prolonged use should be avoided, and mineral oil should not be taken with surface active fecal softeners.

Saline laxatives

The active constituents of saline laxatives are nonabsorbable anions and cations such as the magnesium and sulfate ions. The intestinal wall, acting as a semipermeable membrane to the magnesium, sulfate, tartrate, phosphate, and citrate ions, osmotically causes the retention of water in the intestinal lumen. The increased intraluminal pressure exerts a mechanical stimulus which increases intestinal motility. However, reports indicate that different mechanisms, independent of osmotic effect, are responsible for the laxative properties of the salts. Saline laxatives have a complex series of actions, both secretory and motor, on the GI tract.

It has been shown that the action of magnesium sulfate on the GI tract is similar to that of cholecystokinin-pancreozymin (C.C.K.-P.Z.). There is evidence that this hormone is released from the intestinal mucosa when saline laxatives are administered.[23]

The choice of a saline laxative should be dictated mainly by cost and palatability. However, there are cases where the injudicious choice of a saline laxative results in serious effects. As much as 20 percent of the administered magnesium ion may be absorbed from magnesium salts. If renal function is normal, the absorbed ion is excreted so rapidly that no change in the blood level of the ion can be detected. If, however, the renal function is impaired, toxic concentrations of the magnesium ion can accumulate in the extracellular body fluids. Magnesium can exert a depressant effect on the CNS and the neuromuscular mechanism. Cathartics that contain sodium may be toxic to individuals with edema and congestive heart disease. Dehydration may occur from the repeated use of hypertonic solutions of saline cathartics and should not be used by those who cannot afford fluid loss.

Miscellaneous

Castor Oil. The laxative action of castor oil USP is due to ricinoleic acid which is produced when castor oil is hydrolyzed in the small intestine by pancreatic lipase; its mechanism of action is unknown. The assumption that laxation results from increased peristalsis due to the irritant effect of ricinoleic acid is not supported by experimental evidence.

Castor oil, a glyceride, may be absorbed from the GI tract and is probably metabolized like other fatty acids. Because the main site of action is the small intestine, its prolonged use may result in excessive loss of fluid, electrolytes, and nutrients. Castor oil is not recommended for the treatment of constipation.

Enemas

Enemas are used routinely in hospitals to prepare patients for surgery, child delivery, and radiological examination. They are also used in certain cases of constipation. The enema fluid (warmed or at room temperature) determines the mechanism by which evacuation is produced. Tapwater, normal saline, and milk add bulk by osmotic effects; vegetable oils lubricate, soften, and facilitate the passage of hardened fecal matter; and soapsuds and hydrogen peroxide produce defecation by their irritant action.

According to Modell,[24] a properly administered enema cleans only the distal colon, most nearly approximating a normal bowel movement. He concludes, therefore, that a properly administered enema is the "nearest substitute" available for an ideal laxative. "Properly administered" means that the diagnosis, the enema fluid, and the technique of administration must be correct. Improperly administered, an enema can produce fluid and electrolyte imbalances and colonic perforation. A misdirected nozzle or the use of an inadequately lubricated nozzle may cause abrasion of the anal canal and rectal wall.

Enema fluids that contain substances foreign to the bowel have caused mucosal changes or spasm of the intestinal wall. Hydrogen peroxide enemas can cause proctitis and gross hemorrhaging, and mucosal irritation has been severe enough to resemble the early changes of ulcerative colitis. Water intoxication has resulted from the use of tapwater or soapsuds enemas in the presence of megacolon.[25]

The proper administration of an enema requires that the person be in a horizontal position and reclining on the side; the use of an enema while sitting on a stool clears only the rectum of fecal material. The container holding the fluid should be 1 or 2 inches above the hips to allow free but not forcible flow of the fluid from the tube. A pint of fluid, properly introduced, usually causes adequate evacuation, if it is retained until definite lower abdominal cramping is felt. Two or three pints of a nonirritating fluid usually produce a clean bowel and a nonirritated mucosa.

Suppositories

Glycerin suppositories are used as a laxative to relieve constipation. They are available for infants and adults and, until recently, were the main suppositories for lower bowel evacuation. However, several other effective laxatives in suppository form have been developed: bisacodyl, DSS, senna concentrate, and chemical combinations that release carbon dioxide after insertion. They are used for constipation of the lower bowel, but other uses for the newer suppositories have been proposed.

The bisacodyl, senna, and carbon dioxide releasing suppositories are being promoted as replacements for enemas in cases where cleaning the distal colon is required. The suppositories that contain senna concentrate are advertised as effective in postsurgical and postpartum care; those that contain bisacodyl are promoted for postoperative, antepartum, and postpartum care and are adequate in the preparation for proctosigmoidoscopy. A suppository that exerts its action by the pressure of the released carbon dioxide is recommended for the same uses "or whenever the last 25 cm of the lower bowel must be emptied."[26]

Although bisacodyl suppositories are prescribed and used more frequently than others, reports from pharmacies and hospitals indicate that, as yet, the laxative suppository has not replaced the enema as an agent for cleaning the lower bowel.

It has been suggested that the carbon dioxide releasing suppository might serve as a beneficial replacement for some of the uses of the enema. Shirkey[25] reported that it was used successfully in institutionalized, spastic, and mentally retarded pediatric patients to replace enemas. It also replaced enemas in preparing these patients for intravenous pyelograms and for the installation of basal or rectal anesthetics.

Oxyphenisatin and oxyphenisatin acetate. Oxyphenisatin (phenolisatin) acts directly on the colonic mucosa and is administered rectally only as a solution. It is promoted as a cleaning enema preoperatively or prior to radiological examination of the colon or proctosigmoidoscopy. It may be used in severe constipation, but frequent or repeated use should be avoided. Extreme caution is indicated in the case of an irritated and inflamed colon.

Oxyphenisatin acetate (acetphenolisatin) is used orally and functions like oxyphenisatin in the colon; its pharmacological properties resemble those of phenolphthalein. Investigations have indicated that oxyphenisatin acetate was not absorbed from the GI tract. However, reports now support the opinion that, in combination with DSS, absorption does occur; they indicate that the daily use of oxyphenisatin acetate for 8 months or longer may produce chronic active liver disease with the attendant symptoms, including jaundice.[27-30]

As a result of these reports and recommendations of the medical profession, laxatives that contain oxyphenisatin acetate have been removed from the market.[31]

Diet and exercise

Chronic constipation, not of organic origin, may be treated without the use of drugs. This is especially true for cases involving a low fiber diet and the habitual use of laxatives. A low fiber diet produces a low-bulk stool, and the habitual use of laxatives weakens the bowel muscle tone.

Dietary fiber is that part of whole grain, vegetables, fruits, and nuts that resists digestion in the GI tract. It is composed of the carbohydrates cellulose, hemicelluloses, polysaccharides, and pectin and a noncarbohydrate, lignin.

The fiber content of food is expressed in terms of crude fiber residue after treatment with dilute acid and alkali. The fiber has a significant effect on bowel habits. Because fiber holds water, stools tend to be softer, bulkier, and heavier in persons with a higher fiber intake and probably pass through the colon more rapidly.

It has been reported that diverticula and diverticulitis are rare in countries with high fiber content diets. In industrialized countries, where diets are usually low in fiber content, diverticulitis and constipation occur frequently. It is believed that an increase in dietary fiber can lessen the incidence of constipation and provide symptomatic relief in cases of colonic diverticulitis.[32]

Intestinal transit times and stool weights have been related to fiber content of food in different countries of the world. In addition, the bowel behavior has been related to the prevalence of many of the diseases which are common in the industrialized western world.

Studies have shown that people in less developed countries living on minimally refined plant food diets have intestinal transit times of 30 to 35 hours. People consuming this high fiber content diet usually pass 250 to 400 g of soft stool each day. Those who live on a mixed diet, with some highly refined carbohydrates added to less processed foods, have intestinal transit times of about 48 hours and average daily stool weights of approximately 200 g. People in highly developed countries who live on diets containing highly refined foods and a low fiber content have intestinal transit times exceeding 3 days. They usually pass about 110 g of firm stool each day.

In addition to these changes in transit time and stool weight and consistency, the fiber content of food alters the rate of absorption of energy-yielding foodstuff, bile acid metabolism, and intraluminal pressures within the bowel.

Foods with a high fiber content take longer to eat than refined foods. Increased production of saliva and gastric juices, together with the fiber content of the food, leave less space in the stomach to be filled with high energy food before a sense of satiety is achieved. It is the foods which have a high energy satiety ratio that encourage overconsumption of calories. Not only does more energy tend to be consumed with highly refined foods, but also the energy is utilized more quickly from foods in which the sugars and starches have been, in part, liberated from the encasing cell walls prior to ingestion. Increased consumption of highly refined foods and their subsequent rapid utilization have been implicated in the development of obesity and diabetes.

In high fiber diets, more of the cholesterol and bile acids are believed to be excreted in the feces. In low fiber diets, more cholesterol is absorbed. In addition, the lithocholate is only absorbed in low fiber diets, and this appears to depress the synthesis of bile acids from cholesterol. This may be one of the reasons for elevated serum cholesterol levels. This effect on cholesterol and bile acid metabolism may influence gallstone formation.[33]

It has been shown that as little as 2 g of cereal fiber (bran) added to the usual daily diet will significantly lessen intestinal transit time and increase stool volume.

Exercise in any form improves muscle tone, but that which involves abdominal muscles is the most useful in improvement of intestinal muscle tone.[34] Daily exercise, an increase in the crude fiber content of the diet, and the elimination of laxative use should be effective in the relief of constipation.

Summary

The widespread abuse of OTC laxatives is evidence of a greater need for professional consultation. Pharmacists are qualified and professionally responsible for providing this service. Their main determination should be whether referral to a physician or self-therapy is indicated, which requires a knowledge of the case history and current symptoms. This information is also needed for the selection of the correct laxative. Proper consultation includes education concerning the importance of restoring normal bowel function—the significance of a proper diet and the establishment of correct stool habits must be emphasized.

If the case history discloses a sudden change in bowel habits that has persisted for 2 weeks, the pharmacist should refer the patient to a physician. Abdominal pain, nausea, and vomiting also contraindicate the use of stimulating laxatives.

Advice to patients concerning laxative products should include:

- ☐ Laxatives are not designed for long-term use, and if they are not effective after 1 week, a physician should be consulted.
- ☐ Laxative products that contain more than 15 mEq (345 mg) of sodium, more than 25 mEq (975 mg) of potassium, or more than 50 mEq (600 mg) of magnesium in the maximum daily dose should not be used if kidney disease or its symptoms are present.
- ☐ If a skin rash appears after taking a laxative containing phenolphthalein, it should be discontinued.
- ☐ Saline laxatives should not be used daily and should not be administered orally to children under 6 or rectally to infants under 2. (Mineral oil should not be given to children under 6, and castor oil should not be used to treat constipation.)
- ☐ Enemas and suppositories must be administered properly to be effective.

References

1. "New and Nonofficial Drugs," Lippincott, Philadelphia, Pa., 1965, p. 615.
2. "Dorland's Illustrated Medical Dictionary," 25th ed., Saunders, Philadelphia, Pa., 1974, p. 354.
3. J. R. DiPalma, "Drill's Pharmacology in Medicine," 4th ed., McGraw-Hill, New York, N.Y., 1971, p. 747.
4. W. F. Ganong, "Review of Medical Physiology," 6th ed., Lange Medical Publications, Los Altos, Calif., 1971, p. 357.
5. A. C. Guyton, "Textbook of Medical Physiology," 3d ed., Saunders, Philadelphia, Pa., 1971, p. 738.
6. B. Smith, *Dis. Colon Rectum,* **16(6),** 455(1973).
7. F. H. Netter, "The Ciba Collection of Medical Illustrations," vol. 3, part II, Ciba Pharmaceutical Products, 1962, p. 98.
8. A. Grollman and E. F. Grollman, "Pharmacology and Therapeutics," 6th ed., Lea and Febiger, Philadelphia, Pa., 1965, p. 615.
9. G. E. Sladen, *Proc. R. Soc. Med.,* **65,** 289(1972).
10. J. H. Cummings, *Br. Med. J.,* **1(907),** 537(1974).
11. "The Pharmacological Basis of Therapeutics," 5th ed., L. S. Goodman and A. Gilman, Eds. Macmillan, New York, N.Y., 1975, p. 976.
12. A. M. C. Connell *et al., Br. Med. J.,* **2,** 1095(1965).
13. *Fed. Regist.,* **40,** 12907(1975).
14. J. Travel, *Ann. N.Y. Acad. Sci.,* **58,** 416(1954).
15. S. J. Loewe, *J. Pharmacol. Exp. Ther.,* **94,** 288(1948).
16. L. Schmidt and E. Seeger, *Arzneim.-Forsche.,* **b,** 22(1965).
17. M. H. Hubacher and S. Doernberg, *J. Pharm. Sci.,* **53,** 1067(1964).
18. M. W. Werthmann and S. V. Krees, *Med. Ann. D.C.,* **42,** 4(1973).
19. M. B. Greenhalf and H. S. D. Leonard, *Practitioner,* **210(256),** 259(1973).
20. M. Browne *et al., Br. Med. J.,* **1,** 436(1957).
21. B. Frame *et al., Arch. Intern. Med.,* **128,** 794(1971).
22. B. B. Weybrew *et al., U.S. Armed Forces Med. J.,* **11,** 567(1960).
23. R. F. Harvey and A. E. Read, *Lancet,* **2,** 185(1973).
24. "Drugs of Choice," W. Modell, Ed., Mosby, St. Louis, Mo., 1960, p. 370.
25. H. C. Shirkey, *Nebr. State Med. J.,* **50,** 67(1965).
26. "Physicians' Desk Reference," Medical Economics, Oradell, N.J., 1966.
27. T. B. Reynolds *et al., N. Engl. J. Med.,* **285,** 813(1971).
28. E. Gjone *et al., Scand. J. Gastroenterol.,* **7(4),** 395(1972).
29. O. Dietrichson *et al., Scand. J. Gastroenterol.,* **9(5),** 473(1974).
30. R. L. Willing and R. Hecker, *Med. J. Aus.,* **1,** 1179(1971).
31. Editorial, *J. Am. Med. Assoc.,* **211,** 114(1970).
32. *Med. Lett. Drugs Ther.,* **17(23),** 93(1975).
33. D. P. Burkitt, *Community Health,* **6,** 190(1975).
34. *Drug Therapy,* "Combating Constipation Without Laxatives," March 1975.

Products 4 LAXATIVE

Product (manufacturer)	Dosage form	Stimulant	Bulk forming	Emollient/ Lubricant	Other laxatives	Other ingredients
Afko-Lube (Amer. Pharm.)	capsule	—	—	dioctyl sodium sulfosuccinate, 100 mg	—	—
Afko-Lube Lax (Amer. Pharm.)	capsule	casanthranol, 30 mg	—	dioctyl sodium sulfosuccinate, 100 mg	—	—
Agoral (Warner-Chilcott)	emulsion	phenolphthalein, 1.3 mg/100 ml	agar gel tragacanth acacia	mineral oil	—	egg albumen glycerin
Alophen (Parke-Davis)	tablet	phenolphthalein, 32.4 mg aloin, 16.2 mg	—	—	—	—
Amlax (North American)	tablet	cascara sagrada extract, 32.5 mg phenolphthalein, 32.5 mg aloin, 8 mg	—	—	bile salts, 65 mg	—
Black Draught (Chattem)	tablet syrup granules	senna, 180 mg/tablet 100 mg/ml syrup 660 mg/g granules	—	—	—	anise peppermint cinnamon clove nutmeg (spices only in syrup)
Caroid and Bile Salts with Phenolphthalein (Breon)	tablet	cascara sagrada extract, 48.6 mg phenolphthalein, 32.4 mg	—	—	capsicum, 6 mg bile salts, 70 mg	papaya extract, 75 mg
Carter's Little Pills (Carter)	tablet	aloe, 16 mg podophyllum, 4.0 mg	—	—	—	—
Casakol (Upjohn)	capsule	casanthranol, 30 mg	—	poloxamer 188, 250 mg	—	—

Product (manufacturer)	Dosage form	Stimulant	Bulk forming	Emollient/ Lubricant	Other laxatives	Other ingredients
Casa-Laud (Amfre-Grant)	tablet	casanthranol, 30 mg	—	dioctyl sodium sulfosuccinate, 100 mg	—	—
Cas-Evac (Parke-Davis)	liquid	cascara sagrada, 200 mg/100 ml	—	—	—	alcohol, 18%
Casyllium (Upjohn)	powder	cascara fluidextract, 15 ml/30 g	psyllium husk, 20.5 g/30 g prune powder, 6 g/30 g	—	—	—
Colace (Mead Johnson)	capsule liquid syrup	—	—	dioctyl sodium sulfosuccinate, 50 and 100 mg/ capsule 1% (liquid) 20 mg/5 ml syrup	—	—
Coloctyl (Vitarine)	capsule	—	—	dioctyl sodium sulfosuccinate, 100 mg	—	—
Comfolax (Searle)	capsule	—	—	dioctyl sodium sulfosuccinate, 100 mg	—	—
Comfolax Plus (Searle)	capsule	casanthranol, 30 mg	—	dioctyl sodium sulfosuccinate, 100 mg	—	—
Constiban (Columbia Medical)	capsule	casanthranol, 30 mg	—	dioctyl sodium sulfosuccinate, 100 mg	—	—
Correctol (Plough)	tablet	yellow phenol-phthalein, 64.8 mg	—	dioctyl sodium sulfosuccinate, 100 mg	—	—
Dialose (Stuart)	capsule	—	carboxymethyl-cellulose sodium, 400 mg	dioctyl sodium sulfosuccinate, 100 mg	—	—
Dialose Plus (Stuart)	capsule	casanthranol, 30 mg	carboxymethyl-cellulose sodium, 400 mg	dioctyl sodium sulfosuccinate, 100 mg	—	—
Dio Medicone (Medicone)	tablet	—	—	dioctyl sodium sulfosuccinate, 50 mg	—	—
Dio-Sul (North American)	capsule	—	—	dioctyl sodium sulfosuccinate, 100 mg	—	—
Diothron (North American)	capsule	casanthranol, 30 mg	—	dioctyl sodium sulfosuccinate, 100 mg	—	—
Disanthrol (Lannett)	capsule	casanthranol, 30 mg	—	dioctyl sodium sulfosuccinate, 100 mg	—	—
Disolan (Lannett)	capsule	casanthranol, 30 mg	—	dioctyl sodium sulfosuccinate, 100 mg	—	—

Product (manufacturer)	Dosage form	Stimulant	Bulk forming	Emollient/ Lubricant	Other laxatives	Other ingredients
Disolan Forte (Lannett)	capsule	casanthranol, 30 mg	carboxymethyl-cellulose sodium, 400 mg	dioctyl sodium sulfosuccinate, 100 mg	—	—
Disonate (Lannett)	capsule liquid syrup	—	—	dioctyl sodium sulfosuccinate, 60, 100, and 240 mg/ capsule 10 mg/ml liquid 20 mg/5 ml syrup	—	—
Disoplex (Lannett)	capsule	—	carboxymethyl-cellulose sodium, 400 mg	dioctyl sodium sulfosuccinate, 100 mg	—	—
Doctate (Meyer)	capsule	—	—	dioctyl sodium sulfosuccinate, 100 and 300 mg	—	—
Doctate-P (Meyer)	capsule	danthron, 40 mg	—	dioctyl sodium sulfosuccinate, 60 mg	—	—
Dorbane (Riker)	tablet	danthron, 75 mg	—	—	—	—
Dorbantyl (Riker)	capsule	danthron, 25 mg	—	dioctyl sodium sulfosuccinate, 50 mg	—	—
Dorbantyl Forte (Riker)	capsule	danthron, 50 mg	—	dioctyl sodium sulfosuccinate, 100 mg	—	—
Doxan (Hoechst-Roussel)	tablet	danthron, 50 mg	—	dioctyl sodium sulfosuccinate, 60 mg	—	—
Doxidan (Hoechst-Roussel)	capsule	danthron, 50 mg	—	dioctyl calcium sulfosuccinate, 60 mg	—	—
Doxinate (Hoechst-Roussel)	capsule 5% solution	—	—	dioctyl sodium sulfosuccinate, 60 and 240 mg	—	—
Dr. Caldwell's Senna Laxative (Glenbrook)	liquid	senna, 412.05 mg/ 5 ml	—	—	—	alcohol, 4.5% peppermint oil, 0.95 mg/ 5 ml
Dual Formula Feen-A-Mint (Plough)	tablet	yellow phenolphthalein, 64.8 mg	—	dioctyl sodium sulfosuccinate, 100 mg	—	—
Dulcolax (Boehringer-Ingelheim)	tablet suppository	bisacodyl, 5 mg/ tablet 10 mg/suppository	—	—	—	—
Effersyllium (Stuart)	powder	—	psyllium hydrocolloid, 3 g/7 g	—	—	—

Product (manufacturer)	Dosage form	Stimulant	Bulk forming	Emollient/ Lubricant	Other laxatives	Other ingredients
Enemeez (Armour)	enema	—	—	—	sodium biphosphate, 16 g/100 ml sodium phosphate, 6 g/100 ml	methylparaben, 100 mg/ 100 ml propylparaben, 100 mg/ 100 ml
Espotabs (Combe)	tablet	yellow phenolphthalein	—	—	—	—
Evac-Q-Kit (Warren-Teed)	liquid tablet suppository	phenolphthalein, 2 tablets (Evac-Q-Tabs), 130 mg each	—	—	magnesium citrate (Evac-Q-Mag), 300 ml carbon dioxide-releasing suppository (Evac-Q-Sert)	—
Evac-U-Gen (Walker Corp)	tablet	yellow phenolphthalein, 97.2 mg	—	—	—	—
Ex-Lax (Ex-Lax)	tablet (regular, chocolate)	yellow phenolphthalein, 90 mg	—	—	—	—
Feen-A-Mint (Plough)	gum tablet mint	yellow phenolphthalein, 97.2 mg	—	—	—	—
Fleet Bagenema (Fleet)	enema	—	—	—	liquid castile soap, 19.7 ml	—
Fleet Enema (Fleet)	enema	—	—	—	sodium biphosphate, 19 g/118 ml sodium phosphate, 7 g/118 ml	—
Fleet Enema Oil Retention (Fleet)	enema	—	—	mineral oil, 118 ml	—	—
Fleet Pediatric Enema (Fleet)	enema	—	—	—	sodium biphosphate, 9.5 g/59 ml sodium phosphate, 3.5 g/59 ml	—
Fletcher's Castoria (Glenbrook)	liquid	senna, 6.5%	—	—	—	—
Gentlax (Blair)	tablet granules	senna concentrate, 326 mg/tablet or tsp granules	guar gum, 1 g/tablet or tsp granules	—	—	polygalacturonic acid, 100 mg/ tablet or tsp granules
Gentlax B (Blair)	tablet granules	senna concentrate, 108.7 mg/tablet 326.1 mg/tsp granules	guar gum, 333 mg/tablet 1 g/tsp granules	—	—	—
Gentlax S (Blair)	tablet	senna concentrate, 187 mg	—	dioctyl sodium sulfosuccinate, 50 mg	—	—

Product (manufacturer)	Dosage form	Stimulant	Bulk forming	Emollient/ Lubricant	Other laxatives	Other ingredients
Glysennid (Sandoz)	tablet	sennosides A and B (as calcium salt), 12 mg	—	—	—	—
G-W Emulsoil (Canfield)	instant-mix liquid	—	—	—	castor oil, 30 and 60 ml	—
Haley's M-O (Glenbrook)	emulsion	—	—	mineral oil, 25%	magnesium hydroxide, 75%	—
Hydrocil (Fuller)	powder	—	psyllium, 40% karaya gum, 10%	—	—	dextrose, 50%
Hydrocil Fortified (Fuller)	powder	casanthranol, 30 mg/6 g	psyllium, 40% karaya gum, 10%	—	—	dextrose, 50%
Hydrolose (Upjohn)	syrup	—	methylcellulose, 5.91 g/30 ml	—	—	—
Imbicoll (Upjohn)	granules	(in Imbicoll with cascara sagrada fluidextract), 1.27 ml/7 g	karaya gum, 86%	—	—	(in Imbicoll with vitamin B_1), 1.75 mg/7 g
Instant Mix Metamucil (Searle)	powder in single dose packets	—	psyllium mucilloid, 3.7 g/packet	—	citric acid sodium bicarbonate (equiv. to 250 mg sodium)	—
Kondremul (Fisons)	micro-emulsion	—	chondrus	heavy mineral oil, 55%	—	—
Laxsil (Reed & Carnrick)	liquid	—	—	—	magnesium hydroxide, 1.25 g/15 ml	simethicone, 100 mg/ 15 ml
Magcyl (Elder)	capsule	danthron, 25 mg	—	dioctyl sodium sulfosuccinate, 100 mg	—	—
Maltsupex (Wallace)	tablet	—	malt soup extract, 750 mg	—	—	—
Metamucil (Searle)	powder	—	psyllium mucilloid, 50%	—	—	dextrose, 50%
Milkinol (Kremers-Urban)	liquid	—	—	dioctyl sodium sulfosuccinate, 3.3 mg/5 ml mineral oil, 4.75 ml/5 ml	—	—
Modane (Warren-Teed)	tablet liquid	danthron, 75 mg/ tablet or 10 ml	—	—	—	—
Modane Mild (Warren-Teed)	tablet	danthron, 37.5 mg	—	—	—	—
Mucilose (Winthrop)	flakes granules	—	psyllium, 50%	—	—	dextrose, 50% (granules)
Nature's Remedy Juniors (Lewis-Howe)	tablet	aloe, 48 mg cascara sagrada, 42 mg	—	—	—	—

Product (manufacturer)	Dosage form	Stimulant	Bulk forming	Emollient/ Lubricant	Other laxatives	Other ingredients
Nature's Remedy Regular and Candy Coated (Lewis-Howe)	tablet	aloe, 143 mg cascara sagrada, 127 mg	—	—	—	—
Neo-Cultol (Fisons)	suspension	—	—	refined mineral oil jelly	—	chocolate flavor
Neoloid (Lederle)	emulsion	—	—	—	castor oil, 36.4%	—
Nujol (Plough)	liquid	—	—	mineral oil	—	—
Oxothalein (O'Neal, Jones & Feldman)	tablet	phenolphthalein, 32 mg cascara sagrada extract, 32 mg aloin, 8 mg	—	—	—	—
Peri-Colace (Mead Johnson)	capsule syrup	casanthranol, 30 mg/capsule 10 mg/5 ml	—	dioctyl sodium sulfosuccinate, 100 mg/ capsule 20 mg/5 ml	—	—
Peristim Forte (Mead Johnson)	capsule	casanthranol, 90 mg	—	—	—	—
Petrogalar (Wyeth)	emulsion	phenolphthalein, 0.3% or cascara aqueous extract, 13.2%	agar sodium alginate	mineral oil, 65%	—	acacia glycerin
Petro-Syllium No. 1 Plain (Whitehall)	liquid	—	psyllium seed	mineral oil	—	—
Petro-Syllium No. 2 with Phenolphthalein (Whitehall)	liquid	phenolphthalein, 243.8 mg/30 ml	psyllium seed	mineral oil	—	—
Phenolax (Upjohn)	wafer	phenolphthalein, 64.8 mg	—	—	—	sugar aromatics
Phillips Milk of Magnesia (Glenbrook)	suspension tablet	—	—	—	magnesium hydroxide, 2.27-2.62 g/30 ml 311 mg/tablet	peppermint oil, 1.166 mg/ 30 ml or tablet
Phospho-Soda (Fleet)	liquid	—	—	—	sodium biphosphate, 48 g/100 ml sodium phosphate, 18 g/100 ml	artificial sweeteners flavors
Plova (Washington Ethical)	powder	—	psyllium, 100% (plain) 50% (flavored)	—	—	dextrose, 50% (cocoa flavored)
Polykol (Upjohn)	capsule	—	—	poloxamer 188, 25 mg	—	—
Rectalad (Wallace)	enema	—	—	dioctyl potassium sulfosuccinate, 5%	glycerin, 76% soft soap, 10%	—

Product (manufacturer)	Dosage form	Stimulant	Bulk forming	Emollient/ Lubricant	Other laxatives	Other ingredients
Regul-Aid (Columbia Medical)	capsule syrup	—	—	dioctyl sodium sulfosuccinate, 100 mg/ capsule 20 mg/5 ml	—	—
Regutol (Plough)	tablet	—	—	dioctyl sodium sulfosuccinate, 100 mg	—	—
Sal Hepatica (Bristol-Meyers)	granules	—	—	—	sodium phosphate sodium bicarbonate citric acid, anhydrous sodium citrate, tribasic sodium citrate, dibasic	—
Saraka (Plough)	granules	frangula	karaya gum	—	—	—
Senokap DSS (Purdue Frederick)	capsule	senna concentrate, 163 mg	—	dioctyl sodium sulfosuccinate, 50 mg	—	—
Senokot (Purdue Frederick)	granules tablet suppository syrup	senna concentrate, 326 mg/tsp granules 187 mg/tablet 652 mg/suppository 218 mg extract/5 ml syrup	—	—	—	—
Senokot-S (Purdue Frederick)	tablet	senna concentrate, 187 mg	—	dioctyl sodium sulfosuccinate, 50 mg	—	—
Senokot with Psyllium (Purdue Frederick)	powder	senna concentrate, 326 mg/5 ml	psyllium, 1 g/5 ml	—	—	—
Serutan (J. B. Williams)	powder granules	—	psyllium, 100%	—	—	—
Siblin (Parke-Davis)	granules	—	psyllium seed husks, 62.4%	—	—	sugar caramel sodium chloride
Stimulax (Geriatric Pharmaceutical)	capsule	cascara, 30 mg	—	dioctyl sodium sulfosuccinate, 250 mg	—	—
Surfak (Hoechst-Roussel)	capsule	—	—	dioctyl calcium sulfosuccinate, 50 and 240 mg	—	—
Swiss Kriss (Modern Products)	powder	senna	—	—	—	herbs
Syllact (Wallace)	powder	—	psyllium seed husks, 50%	—	—	dextrose, 50%
Syllamalt (Wallace)	powder	—	malt soup extract, 50% psyllium seed husks, 50%	—	—	—

Product (manufacturer)	Dosage form	Stimulant	Bulk forming	Emollient/ Lubricant	Other laxatives	Other ingredients
Syllamalt Effervescent (Wallace)	powder	—	malt soup extract, 25% psyllium seed husks, 25%	—	sodium bicarbonate citric acid	dextrose
Theralax (Beecham Labs)	tablet suppository	bisacodyl, 5 mg/ tablet 10 mg/suppository	—	—	—	triglyceride base (suppository)
Tonelax (A.V.P.)	tablet	danthron, 75 mg	—	—	—	calcium panto-thenate, 25 mg
Tucks Saf-Tip Oil Retention Enema (Fuller)	enema	—	—	light mineral oil	—	—
Tucks Saf-Tip Phosphate Enema (Fuller)	enema	—	—	—	sodium biphosphate, 16 g/100 ml sodium phosphate, 6 g/100 ml	—
Vacuetts Adult (Dorsey)	suppository	—	—	—	sodium biphosphate sodium acid pyrophosphate sodium bicarbonate	polyethylene glycols
X-Prep (Gray)	liquid powder	senna extract (liquid) senna concentrate (powder)	—	—	—	—

Emetic and Antiemetic Products

Gary M. Oderda
Sheila West

Questions to ask the patient

Will you be using the product for nausea of motion sickness?

Are you requesting an emetic for immediate emergency use or for possible future use?

What is the age of the patient for whom the antiemetic is intended?

Is the patient pregnant?

How long has nausea and/or vomiting been a problem?

Have you noted blood in the vomitus?

Have you noted other symptoms such as abdominal pain, headache, or diarrhea?

What medicines are you currently taking?

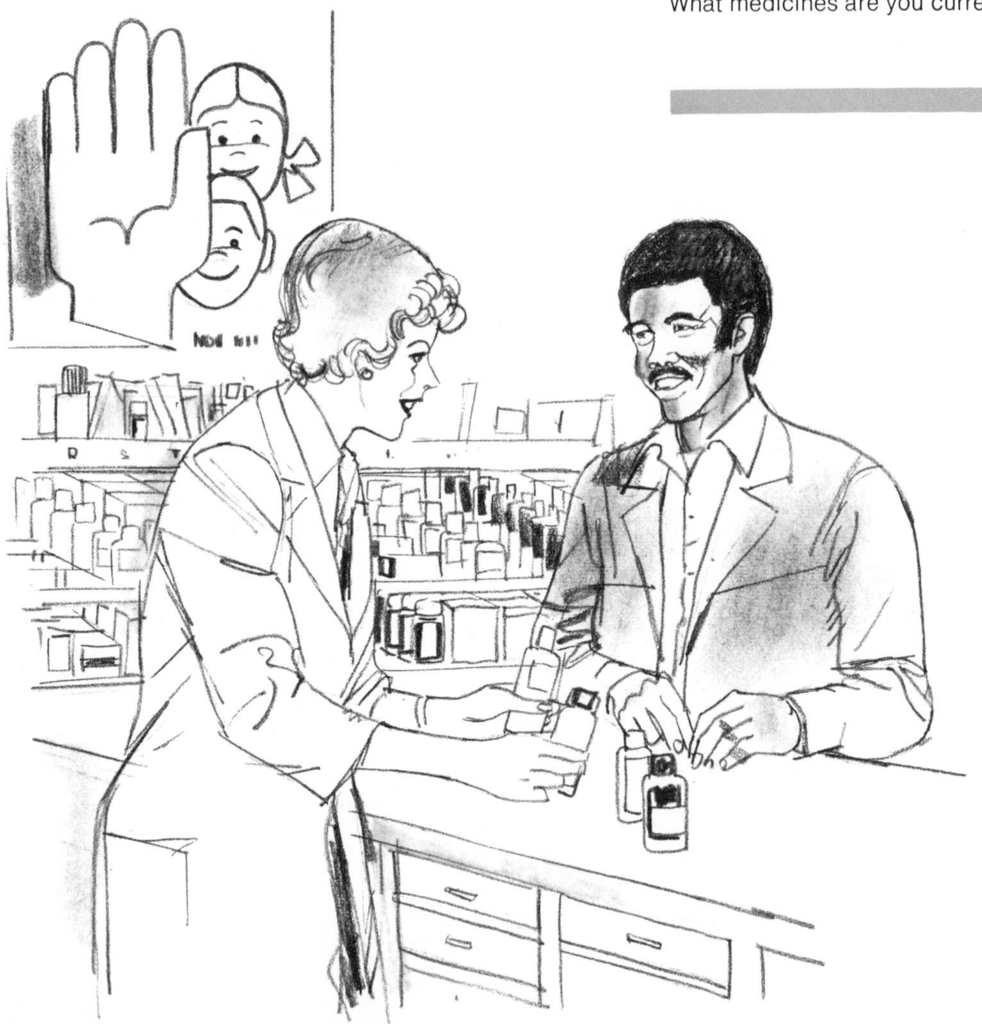

CHAPTER 5

Severe nausea and the realization that one is about to vomit are two of the more unpleasant symptoms an individual may have. However disagreeable the sensation, vomiting (emesis) may be an important body defense mechanism for ridding itself of a variety of toxins and poisons; it may also be an irritating accompaniment to travel or pregnancy. The over-the-counter antiemetics are used to prevent or control the symptoms of nausea and vomiting primarily due to motion sickness, pregnancy, and mild infectious diseases. Some OTC antiemetics are promoted for the relief of such vague symptoms as "upset stomach," "indigestion," and "distention" associated with excessive food indulgence, although their value in treating these complaints is not well documented. OTC emetic drugs are used to induce vomiting, or the oral expulsion of gastric contents, for the treatment of poisoning. Nausea and vomiting associated with radiation therapy, cancer chemotherapy, and the more serious metabolic and endocrine disorders are not appropriate diseases for self-medication and, thus, will not be addressed in this chapter.

The vomiting process

Vomiting is a complex process involving both the CNS and the GI system (Fig. 1). The central involvement includes two areas of the medulla oblongata—the vomiting center and the chemoreceptor trigger zone (CTZ). The CTZ cannot by itself produce vomiting but must act through stimulation of the vomiting center. Centrally acting emetics and antiemetics work primarily by stimulating or inhibiting the CTZ. In addition to stimuli from the CTZ, impulses from the GI tract and the labyrinth apparatus in the ear are received at the vomiting center. Stimuli are then sent to the abdominal musculature, the stomach, and the esophagus to initiate vomiting. (See Chapter 3 for the anatomy and physiology of the GI tract.)

Vomiting begins with a deep inspiration, closing of the glottis, and depression of the soft palate. A forceful contraction of the diaphragm and abdominal musculature occurs which produces an increase in intrathoracic and intra-abdominal pressure that compresses the stomach and raises esophageal pressure.[1-3] The body of the stomach and the esophageal musculature relax. The positive intrathoracic and intra-abdominal pressure move food into the esophagus and mouth. Several cycles of reflux into the esophagus occur before the actual vomiting.[3] Regurgitation is the casting up of stomach contents without oral expulsion. Food is expelled from the esophagus by a combination of increased intrathoracic pressure and reverse peristaltic waves.[1,2] Normally, the glottis closes off the trachea and prevents the vomitus from entering the airway. Aspiration of the vomitus may occur in some cases, e.g., in patients with significant CNS depression.

Vomiting is a symptom that may be produced by benign processes as well as significant, serious illnesses. It is important for the practitioner to be aware of the possibility that patients using OTC antiemetics may be self-treating the early stages of a serious illness. Nausea and vomiting may be symptomatic of digitalis toxicity, opiate use, or the ingestion of other drugs and chemicals. Knowledge of the patient's drug history is important in assessing the cause of nausea and vomiting. Nausea and vomiting may also be part of the symptomatology of diverse disorders such as acute appendicitis, cholecystitis, migraine headache, food allergy, radiation, and cancer chemotherapy.

Overstimulation of the labyrinth apparatus produces the nausea and vomiting of motion sickness. The three semicircular canals on each side of the head in the inner ear (labyrinth) are responsible for maintaining equilibrium. Postural adjustments are made when the brain receives nervous impulses initiated by the movement of fluid in the semicircular canals. Some individuals are more tolerant than others to the effect of a particular type of motion, but no one is immune. Moreover, it appears that individuals can vary in their susceptibility to various kinds of motion, such as flying, boat riding, etc.[4] Motion sickness may be produced by unusual motion patterns in which the head is rotated in two axes simultaneously. Mechanisms other than the stimulation of the semicircular canal are also important. Erroneous interpretation of stimuli by stationary subjects who watch a film taken from a roller coaster or an airplane doing aerobatics can produce motion sickness.

The genesis of vomiting, or "morning sickness," of pregnancy is not established. One-half of all pregnant women experience nausea, and about one-third of these suffer vomiting.[5] The increased levels of chorionic gonadotropin have been implicated as a cause of morning sickness; levels of this hormone are maximal during the early part of pregnancy, when nausea and vomiting are most common.[5,6] Nausea and vomiting of pregnancy are difficult symptoms to treat partly because no agent seems to be completely effective, but more importantly, because of the concern that drug use during pregnancy should be minimal.[6]

Acute transient attacks of vomiting, in association with diarrhea, are very common. Fever may be slight or absent. No precise figure is available for the incidence of this "viral gastroenteritis," although it can occur in sizeable outbreaks.[5] Research continues in order to uncover the precise etiologic agent in this usually harmless, self-limiting disorder.

Emetics

Incidence of poisoning

Emetics are most commonly used for the treatment of poisoning, both accidental and intentional. Poisoning is a relatively common occurrence and one that claims approximately 3,000 human lives each year.[7] Approximately half of these deaths are accidental, and about one-third occur in children under 5.[7] The number of poisoning fatalities is only a small percentage of total ingestions and in fact, Poison Centers throughout the U.S. reported 163,500 ingestions to the National Clearinghouse for Poison Control Centers during 1973 (the last year for which national statistics are available).[8] In addition, it has been estimated that only 1 ingestion in 10 is reported to a Poison Center.

Emergency treatment or an OTC emetic?

Emetics remove potentially toxic agents from the stomach. It is often difficult to decide whether a patient should be referred directly to an emergency treatment facility or should be given an OTC emetic and managed at home. Taking a good history, identifying the agent, and accurately assessing the condition of the patient are critical in making this decision. All ingestions where moderate to severe toxicity is expected must be referred to an emergency treatment facility. If minimal toxicity and no serious or life-threatening symptoms are anticipated, the administration of an OTC emetic at home by an alert adult may be all the treatment that is necessary. Many ingestions reported to Poison Centers fall into this category. For example, a child who ingests approximately 65 mg of aspirin/0.45 kg (1 lb) of body weight can usually be managed at home. To determine whether administration of an OTC emetic is appropriate or the patient should be referred, the following information must be obtained:

☐ *Name of product ingested.* The ingredients and the amount of each ingredient can be determined from the name of the ingested agent. Once this information is available, the potential toxicity of each ingredient must be investigated.

☐ *Amount ingested.* This information is not commonly available or easy to determine. For example, a child is found with an empty bottle of aspirin, and no one is quite sure how full the bottle was prior to ingestion. Often, a parent will underestimate the amount consumed. For example, a parent calls and says the child took two digoxin tablets. When asked "how do you know that it was two tablets?" the parent will often say that the child "was only alone for a few minutes and, therefore, couldn't have eaten very many," or "they don't taste very good, so I don't think the child would have eaten more than two." This type of information is very unreliable. Drugs can be both therapeutic agents and poisons, depending on the dose. Thus, a 2-year-old who takes two children's aspirin tablets would obviously require no treatment; the same child who takes 15 adult aspirin tablets may be severely poisoned.

☐ *Time since ingestion.* The amount of time since ingestion is important because an emetic will only be useful if a sufficient amount of the ingested agent remains in the stomach. Thus, for agents that are absorbed quickly, an emetic would not be recommended if several hours had elapsed after ingestion. For some agents that are slow to leave the stomach, e.g., anticholinergics and aspirin, the use of an emetic may be rational even many hours after ingestion.

☐ *Symptoms.* Certain symptoms (e.g., significant CNS depression) are contraindications to the use of emetics. In cases where significant symptoms—seizures, lethargy, ataxia, hallucinations, etc.—are present, an OTC emetic at home should not be considered; the patient should be immediately referred for treatment.

☐ *Patient's age and weight.* Much toxicity information is given on a dose/body weight basis. Thus, knowledge of the patient's weight is needed to determine which treatment is appropriate. The patient's age helps to determine the appropriateness of and the dose of an emetic.

This information should assist in answering the questions: Is an emetic indicated? Are there any contraindications to using an emetic? Can the emetic safely be administered outside of an emergency treatment facility? Poison Centers are available in most communities to help pharmacists answer these questions or handle referrals. Pharmacists should be aware of how to contact their local Poison Center. (A list of Poison Centers is available from the National Clearinghouse for Poison Control Centers, 5401 Westbard Ave., Bethesda, MD 20016.)

Treatment for poisoning

The mainstay of treatment in poisoning cases is symptomatic and supportive care. Support of vital functions, especially respiratory and cardiovascular, is critical. Treatment of specific symptoms such as seizures is also important. With symptomatic and supportive care alone, many patients will detoxify themselves and survive. Other specific treatment modalities, including emptying the stomach, administering adsorbents, cathartics, antidotes, etc., do not replace the need for symptomatic and supportive care.

Stomach contents may be removed by administering an emetic or by lavaging. Gastric lavage is a procedure in which a tube is placed in the stomach via the esophagus. Fluid is then instilled into the tube, allowed to mix with stomach contents and removed by the same tube. Boxer *et al.*[9] examined 20 patients between the ages of 12 and 20 months who had ingested salicylates. Each patient was lavaged and also given syrup of ipecac and the amount of salicylate returned was measured. Approximately one-half of the patients were lavaged first, and the others were given syrup of ipecac first. Ipecac was superior to lavage in removing salicylate, and in patients who had vomited with ipecac, little more stomach contents were removed by subsequent lavage. The patients were lavaged using a small nasogastric tube. Goldstein[10] reported on two adult patients who were first lavaged with 3 liters of normal saline through a small [20 Fr. (6.7 mm)] tube, 10 to 15 minutes after ingestion and then given syrup of ipecac. Twenty-five tablets from one patient and 10 to 15 from the other were included in the vomitus following ipecac. Arnold *et al.*[11] have shown that, under optimal conditions, dogs that had been given sodium salicylate returned 38 percent after lavage with a small [16 Fr. (5.3 mm)] tube and 45 percent after ipecac-induced emesis. In all of these studies, a lavage tube was used that was considerably smaller than the 26 to 50 Fr. (8.7 to 16.7 mm) orogastric tubes currently recommended by Rumack.[12] It has been suggested that the larger lavage tubes might return significantly more stomach contents than either the smaller tubes or ipecac alone. However, there are no data available to support this, and it is felt that emesis is preferred over lavage unless a contraindication to the induction of emesis exists.

Contraindications to emetics

Emetics are contraindicated in the following patients, most of whom should be treated in an emergency treatment facility:

☐ Patients who have significant CNS depression as evidenced by lethargy, loss of gag reflex, or unconsciousness. In these individuals, an emetic is not likely to produce vomiting. If vomiting is produced, the risk of aspiration of vomitus into the lungs is significant.

□ Patients who are experiencing seizures. They may aspirate vomitus if given an emetic. In addition, an emetic may produce seizures in susceptible patients or worsen an existing seizure.

□ Patients who have ingested a caustic. They should not vomit. Caustic agents are strong acids and bases that produce severe burns of the mucous membranes of the mouth and esophagus. If emesis is induced, these tissues will be reexposed to the caustic, and more damage may occur. In addition, if the esophagus is already damaged the force of vomiting may cause esophageal perforation.

□ Patients who have ingested antiemetics such as most phenothiazines. If an emetic is not given soon enough after ingestion, a significant emetic failure rate may result. If an emetic is given in the hospital setting and vomiting does not occur, gastric lavage may become necessary to remove the antiemetic substance. Emetics should be administered with caution to these patients.

□ Patients who have ingested petroleum distillates. Traditionally, they have not been given emetics. It was felt that inducing vomiting would increase the likelihood of aspiration of the petroleum distillate into the lungs. When small amounts of petroleum distillates (less than 30 ml or 1 ml/kg) have been ingested, emptying the stomach is unnecessary and emetics should not be considered. When large amounts have been taken, or in situations where a potentially dangerous chemical, e.g., some pesticides, are dissolved in a petroleum distillate base, emptying the stomach may be necessary.

In a retrospective study, Molinas [13] showed that, in patients who had ingested petroleum distillates, a lower percentage developed aspiration pneumonitis when vomiting was induced with ipecac than with either lavage or spontaneous vomiting. Ng *et al.*[14] have shown that evidence of aspiration pneumonitis is less likely in the initial radiographs of ipecac-treated patients than in those who were lavaged. Although initial radiographs are not generally considered good predictors of later pneumonitis, less than 10 percent of patients whose initial radiographs were negative were later found to be positive. The pneumonitis that developed in Ng's study was less severe in the ipecac-treated patients than in those who were lavaged.[14] Emetics may be used in petroleum distillate ingestions under medical supervision.

Ipecac syrup

Ipecac syrup is the emetic of choice for routine use. Syrup of ipecac is prepared from ipecac powder, a natural product derived from *Cephaelis ipecacuanha* or *acuminata,* and contains approximately 2.1 g of powdered ipecac/30 ml (1 oz). Vomiting is probably produced by both a local irritant effect on the GI mucosa and a central medullary effect (stimulation of the CTZ).[15] The central effect is probably caused by emetine and cephaeline, two alkaloids present in ipecac.

When a patient asks to purchase syrup of ipecac, the pharmacist should determine whether it is to be used immediately to treat a poisoning ingestion or if it is being purchased to keep in the home in case an ingestion occurs. If the purchase is for immediate use, the pharmacist should determine whether that use is appropriate. If the purchase is for later use, the pharmacist should discuss poison prevention with the patient, distribute poison prevention material, and provide the patient with the telephone number of a Poison Center. The patient must be warned that the syrup of ipecac must not be given without first consulting a pharmacist, physician, or Poison Center.

Ipecac toxicity. Toxicity following the administration of ipecac is rare. After therapeutic doses, diarrhea and slight CNS depression are common. Clinical experience has shown that the ingestion of 30 ml of ipecac syrup (the largest amount available OTC) is safe in children over 1. In significantly larger doses, ipecac may produce cardiovascular toxicity including bradycardia, atrial fibrillation, and hypotension.[16] Severe toxicity and death have occurred when fluidextract of ipecac was given by mistake. Fluidextract of ipecac is 14 times stronger than ipecac syrup and should no longer be found in any pharmacy.[17-20]

Dosages of ipecac. In children over 1, the recommended dose of ipecac is 15 ml (1 tbsp). Because children under 1 do not have a well-developed gag reflex, ipecac should not be administered without medical supervision. In addition, ipecac does not work well if the stomach is near empty. Therefore, it is recommended that at least 180 to 240 ml of fluid be given immediately after the ipecac. Vomiting should occur in 15 to 20 minutes. If vomiting has not occurred in 20 minutes, another 15 ml of ipecac syrup should be given.

The initial dose of ipecac for adults is 15 to 30 ml. One study suggests that the time to vomiting is longer when

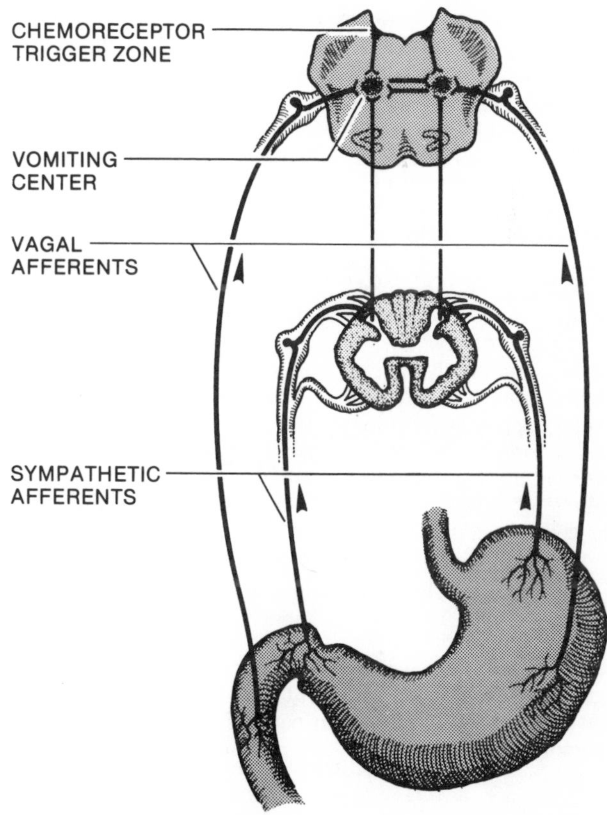

Figure 1. Mechanism of vomiting induction by emetics (apomorphine and ipecac). Adapted from A. C. Guyton, "Textbook of Medical Physiology," 5th Ed., Saunders, Philadelphia, Pa., 1976.

milk is given with the ipecac than when other fluids are used.[21] Other fluids, such as water, should be used instead of milk. The effect of other protein-containing substances that might be in the stomach when ipecac is given is not known. Syrup of ipecac is virtually 100 percent effective when 15 ml or more is given.[22,23] Patients who are ambulatory seem to vomit more quickly than those who are not. Stimulation of the posterior pharynx may help to initiate vomiting.

Drug interactions with ipecac. The only true drug interaction with syrup of ipecac involves activated charcoal. Activated charcoal is used as an adsorbent in many poisoning cases. When it is administered with ipecac, the ipecac is adsorbed by the charcoal and emesis is prevented. In addition, the adsorptive capacity of the charcoal is reduced. If both activated charcoal and ipecac are used, the charcoal must be given after successful vomiting has been produced by the ipecac.

Other methods of inducing vomiting

Vomiting may be produced in a number of ways. Syrup of ipecac is the only safe and effective OTC emetic. Home remedies other than ipecac used to induce vomiting are frequently ineffective and, in some cases, may be dangerous.

Mechanically induced vomiting is produced by giving fluids to and then gagging the patient with either a blunt object or a finger. Care must be taken not to injure the patient during this procedure. Dabbous *et al.*[24] have shown that the percentage of patients who vomit following this procedure is low and that the mean volume of vomitus is small compared to vomiting induced by syrup of ipecac.

Saltwater and powdered mustard in water are both unpalatable and unreliable emetics. Saltwater may be quite toxic and, in fact, fatalities have been produced in children and adults from the use of salt as an emetic.[25-29] If vomiting is not produced, severe hypernatremia may result. Saltwater should not be used under any circumstances, and mustard water should not be routinely recommended.

Copper and zinc sulfate have been used as emetics and act by producing direct gastric irritation. Hopefully, vomiting occurs before significant absorption of the metals takes place. In three children who vomited soon after the administration of copper sulfate as an emetic, only 54 to 67 percent of the dose was recovered in the vomitus.[30] In the same study, all six children who had been given copper sulfate as an emetic had significant increases in serum copper levels (15 to 105 μg/ml) as compared to one patient in the ipecac group. No evidence of copper intoxication, e.g., jaundice or oliguria, was noted. Copper sulfate administered to a patient with a 3/4 gastrectomy has caused death.[31]

Although apomorphine produces rapid emesis, it is available only by prescription and must be given parenterally. Apomorphine may produce or worsen already existing CNS and respiratory depression. Naloxone has been thought to reverse these effects. In several cases, significant respiratory and/or CNS depression unresponsive to naloxone developed in patients who had been given apomorphine.[32]

Antiemetics

Nausea and vomiting are symptoms common to many serious and minor disorders. The pharmacist should be very cautious about patient self-medication of these symptoms and should question the patient appropriately to be satisfied that referral is not indicated. Some of the more important considerations to determine whether an antiemetic is indicated are:

Age of the patient. Vomiting in newborns can result from a number of serious abnormalities, including obstruction of the GI tract and disorders of neuromuscular control, and may quickly lead to acid-base disturbances and dehydration. Pediatric referral is recommended for further workup of any vomiting in newborns. Simple causes of vomiting, such as overfeeding, feeding too quickly, or ineffective "burping" of the newborn, can obviously be resolved without drug therapy and should be excluded as causes in any evaluation.[33]

One of the more common causes of vomiting in children is acute gastroenteritis. Opinions vary on whether drug therapy should be directed at the symptom, vomiting; there are no acceptable data on the effects of OTC antiemetics on vomiting with gastroenteritis. Some sources question the safety of treating children with antiemetics in an acute, self-limited disorder.[34,35] It has been suggested that vomiting in gastroenteritis is a body defense that sheds the pathogen and should not be suppressed. This theory awaits confirmation.

Nondrug remedies such as coke syrup and carbonated beverages have been used to control vomiting, apparently on an empirical basis. Vomiting may be produced by acidosis and dehydration secondary to severe diarrhea and practitioners have noted that rehydration may control this vomiting.[36]

Sex of the patient. Nausea and vomiting may be one of the earliest symptoms of pregnancy. A woman who notes nausea and vomiting in the early part of the day and who has no other symptoms except a missed menstrual cycle and perhaps weight gain, should be referred for a pregnancy test and followup. Even if the woman is known to be pregnant, it is important to exclude "nonpregnant" causes of vomiting, such as urinary tract infections and appendicitis. Treatment of morning sickness has been characterized as "therapeutic nihilism" since the thalidomide tragedy, and most physicians are reluctant to prescribe any drug for a pregnant woman. OTC antiemetics have not been evaluated for, nor are they promoted for, use in nausea and vomiting of pregnancy. Some practitioners have suggested trying small frequent feedings to control morning sickness, although the benefits of this approach are not clear.[5,37]

Current drug use. Some drugs are known to cause nausea and vomiting as a side effect or as a toxic effect. For example, digitalis toxicity may be manifested as nausea and vomiting. One manifestation of congestive heart failure is visceral congestion which can also produce GI symptoms. Other drugs, such as tetracyclines, estrogens, and the opiate analgesics, can cause nausea and vomiting side effects.

Duration of vomiting and blood in the vomitus. A patient who vomits forcefully several times a day for 2 or 3 days or who has blood in the vomitus should be referred to a physician for diagnosis of the cause.

Other symptoms. Patients who complain of abdominal pain, vomiting, particularly projectile vomiting, and headache should be referred to a physician. Patients with vomiting and diarrhea of gastroenteritis in whom slight electrolyte imbalance may be critical, such as the newborn, should also be referred.

Ingredients in OTC products

"There is no ailment (motion sickness), with the possible exception of the common cold and hiccoughs, for which the general populace and medical profession alike have prescribed with greater assurance and originality. The remedies have been selected on the basis of hearsay, personal experience, accident or often apparently occult revelation. The treatments are generally uncontrolled, frequently amusing, and occasionally ingenious." [38]

The available OTC antiemetic preparations have been evaluated and are promoted only for nausea and vomiting of motion sickness (antihistamines and carbohydrates) and nausea associated with overeating or an "upset stomach" (bismuth compounds). Therefore, the pharmacologic properties of antiemetic agents pertinent only to relieving nausea and vomiting from these causes will be reviewed in depth.

The primary agents used to prevent or control motion sickness are the parasympatholytics, antihistamines, and phenothiazines. The compounds all have CNS activity, although the precise mechanism of action in preventing vomiting is unknown. Most compounds studied have varying success rates in controlling nausea and vomiting, according to the length of therapy, duration of pretreatment, duration and type of motion, as well as individual susceptibility to motion sickness. The ability of an agent to prevent motion sickness is not correlated with its potency as an antihistamine, anticholinergic, or phenothiazine tranquilizer.[4 38] Classic studies of the usefulness of antiemetics in motion sickness have identified scopolamine, particularly in conjunction with amphetamine, as probably the most effective agent in preventing vomiting.[39] However, these agents are available only by prescription and have produced significant side effects in therapeutic doses. Five agents have unquestionably been proved valuable in preventing motion sickness: scopolamine, promethazine, cyclizine, meclizine, and dimenhydrinate.[2 39] Only the last three are available OTC.

The OTC antihistaminic preparations have all been shown to be effective antiemetics under various conditions that induce motion sickness. There is little evidence of superiority of one agent over another in all cases.

Cyclizine and meclizine

Cyclizine and meclizine are members of the benzhydryl group of antihistamine compounds. They reportedly depress labyrinth excitability and have been shown to be safe and effective in the management of motion sickness.[39-42]

Dosages. Doses of meclizine for adults are 25 to 50 mg once daily, administered orally 1 hour before departure and repeated every 24 hours. The drug has a relatively long duration of action, and studies have suggested that it provides 24-hour protection against motion sickness.[43] Meclizine is not recommended for use in children under 12.

Adult doses of cyclizine are 50 mg up to 4 times a day.[39] For children 6 to 12 years old, the dose is 25 mg up to 3 times a day. The drug should be administered 30 minutes before departure.

Cautions. Drowsiness with therapeutic doses can occur, and patients should be cautioned not to drive a car or operate hazardous machinery while using meclizine or cyclizine. The effects are additive to those of other CNS depressants such as alcohol or tranquilizers. In large doses, these agents also produce anticholinergic effects, including blurred vision and dry mouth. Patients with narrow-angle glaucoma or prostatic enlargement should be cautioned about the potential exacerbation of their symptoms.

Since 1966, the FDA has required that products containing meclizine and cyclizine carry a warning against their use in pregnant women based on animal studies in several species that suggested the drug may have teratogenic or embryolethal potential. Subsequent epidemiologic studies of many pregnant women have not shown an increase in embryo deaths or malformations in children of women who used these drugs during early pregnancy.[44 45] The warning against the use of these drugs in pregnant women is no longer required, but pharmacists should note that these agents are not promoted for OTC use for morning sickness of pregnancy.

Dimenhydrinate

Dimenhydrinate is the 8-chlorotheophyllinate salt of the antihistamine, diphenhydramine. Both dimenhydrinate and diphenhydramine hydrochloride are effective antiemetics for motion sickness, although their precise mechanism is unknown.[41 43 46] Usual doses for adults are 50 to 100 mg, two to four times a day administered 30 minutes to 1 hour before departure.[39] The dose for children 2 to 5 years old is 12.5 to 25 mg up to 3 times a day.

Cautions. Drowsiness can occur at recommended doses, and patients should be cautioned about driving a car or operating hazardous machinery.[47] In doses of 50 mg, dimenhydrinate can cause anticholinergic side effects, e.g., dry mouth; [43] patients with narrow-angle glaucoma or prostatic hypertrophy should be cautioned about exacerbation of their symptoms. Cases of dimenhydrinate abuse have been reported where an individual took between 15 and 25 tablets of dimenhydrinate (50 mg) which caused delirium, visual and auditory hallucination, pupil dilation, and dry mouth.[48] In another case report, ten 50-mg tablets were ingested which caused cholinergic hypofunction and toxic psychosis.[49] Dimenhydrinate has been implicated in one case report as causing fixed drug eruptions.[50]

It is possible, although clinical examples are not available, that diphenhydramine salts mask the vestibular toxicity of aminoglycoside antibiotics (streptomycin, kanamycin, etc.).[51] A study of the control of vestibular toxic effects of streptomycin with dimenhydrinate suggests that the potential interaction warrants careful monitoring of the patient if both drugs are used.[52]

Phosphorated carbohydrate

Phosphorated carbohydrate solution is a mixture of levulose (fructose) and dextrose (glucose) with phosphoric acid added to adjust the pH to between 1.5 and 1.6. Studies evaluating its effectiveness in the vomiting of childhood, pregnancy, and motion sickness have been criticized as poorly designed.[53-56] The mechanism of action is suggested to be a delay in gastric emptying time because of the high osmotic pressure of the solution.[57] However, there is no evidence that an increase in gastric emptying time affects nausea and vomiting, particularly if it is due to a disturbance in the semicircular canals.

The usual adult dose of the phosphorated carbohydrate is 1 to 2 tbsp at 15-minute intervals until vomiting ceases. However, the FDA OTC Panel on Laxative, Antidiarrheal, Emetic, and Antiemetic Products has concluded that there is insufficient evidence available to establish the effectiveness of phosphorated carbohydrate and has recommended appropriate studies be done to document effectiveness within a 2-year period.[56]

Large doses of levulose may cause abdominal pain and diarrhea. Levels of uric acid in urine and serum have been reportedly increased in healthy volunteers when levulose (500 mg/kg) was given orally.[58]

Practitioners should be aware of the high glucose content of this product and associated problems with its use in diabetics.

Bismuth compounds

The OTC bismuth preparations are promoted for the relief of symptoms of nausea and upper GI distress, particularly related to the consumption of certain foods or excess quantities of food. The proposed mechanism of action is a "coating" effect of the bismuth preparation on the gastric mucosa, although this phenomenon has been questioned.[56] There is no evidence that bismuth compounds affect gastric emptying time, tone of the stomach wall, or intragastric pressure to relieve symptoms induced by overeating. Unpublished data suggest a consumer preference for this product in treating self-defined symptoms of "indigestion," "gas," "full stomach," etc.[59] However, no convincing objective data are available that bismuth compounds decrease nausea and vomiting from any cause. Nausea as a result of overeating is best treated prophylactically.

Bismuth salts appear to be poorly absorbed from the GI tract. Several studies report the absence of detectable bismuth in the urine of human subjects given high doses or doses over a long period. Detectable but unpredictable blood levels of salicylate have been reported after the ingestion of 30 to 45 ml of bismuth subsalicylate (equivalent to ingesting 357.5 to 536.3 mg of salicylic acid). Blood levels ranged from barely detectable to 6.2 mg/ 100 ml.[60]

The manufacturer's maximum recommended dose of bismuth subnitrate provides 5.6 g for adults and 0.475 g for children (3 to 6 years old) within 4 hours. There is a risk of methemoglobinemia in children under 2 due to absorption of nitrates from bismuth subnitrate.[60,61] Isolated cases of eruptions like those of pityriasis rosea due to bismuth injections have been reported, but no reaction to oral use of bismuth has been noted.[62]

Pharmacists should note that stools may darken with use of bismuth compounds.

Summary

Emetics are useful in cases of oral poisoning to remove gastric contents and to prevent further absorption of the ingested agent. Syrup of ipecac is the most effective and safest OTC emetic for this purpose. It should be kept in all homes with young children and used if an ingestion occurs.

OTC antiemetics are useful in limited, patient-diagnosed situations, such as prevention of motion sickness. The pharmacist should ascertain the reason for purchasing an OTC antiemetic and suggest referral if necessary, as discussed. Chronic unsupervised use of antiemetics, especially for an "upset stomach," should be discouraged and the patient encouraged to seek additional medical help for the continuous discomfort.

References

1. K. Isselbacher and J. Turner, in "Harrison's Principles of Internal Medicine," 7th ed., M. Winthrobe *et al.*, Eds., McGraw-Hill, New York, N.Y., 1974, p. 212.
2. J. Kirsner, in "Pathologic Physiology-Mechanisms of Diseases," 5th ed., W. Sodeman and W. Sodeman, Jr., Eds., Saunders, Philadelphia, Pa., 1974, p. 711.
3. T. R. Hendrix, in "Medical Physiology," vol. 2, 13th ed., V. Mountcastle, Ed., Mosby, St. Louis, Mo., 1974, p. 1225.
4. J. Brand and W. Perry, *Pharmacol. Rev.*, **18,** 895-924(1966).
5. I. Gordon *et al.*, in "Gastroenterologic Medicine," M. Paulson, Ed., Lea and Febiger, Philadelphia, Pa., 1969, pp. 468, 1233-1234.
6. "Williams Obstetrics," L. Hellman and J. Prichard, Eds., Meredith Corp., New York, N.Y., 1971, pp. 343-344.
7. J. Arena, *Mod. Treatm.*, **8,** 461(1971).
8. National Clearinghouse of Poison Control Centers Bulletin, U.S. Public Health Service, Washington, D. C., May-June, 1974, p. 7.
9. L. Boxer *et al.*, *J. Pediatr.*, **74,** 800(1969).
10. L. Goldstein, *J. Am. Med. Assoc.*, **208,** 2162(1969).
11. F. Arnold *et al.*, *Pediatrics*, **23,** 286(1959).
12. B. Rumack, "Poisindex," Micromedex, Denver, Co., 1975.
13. S. Molinas, National Clearinghouse for Poison Control Centers, U.S. Public Health Service, Washington, D. C., March-April, 1966.
14. R. Ng *et al.*, *Can. Med. Assoc. J.*, **111,** 537(1974).
15. I. M. Rollo, in "The Pharmacological Basis of Therapeutics," 5th ed., L. S. Goodman and A. Gilman, Eds., Macmillan, New York, N.Y., 1975, p. 1075.
16. J. McLeod, *N. Engl. J. Med.*, **268,** 146-147(1963).
17. J. Speer *et al.*, *Lancet*, **1,** 475(1963).
18. T. Bates and E. Grunwaldt, *Am. J. Dis. Child.*, **103,** 169-173(1962).
19. R. Allport, *Am. J. Dis. Child.*, **98,** 786(1959).
20. R. Smith and D. Smith, *N. Engl. J. Med.*, **265,** 23-25(1961).
21. R. Varipapa *et al.*, unpublished data (1976).
22. W. Robertson, *Am. J. Dis. Child.*, **103,** 58(1972).
23. W. MacLean, *J. Pediatr.*, **82,** 121-124(1973).
24. I. Dabbous *et al.*, *J. Pediatr.*, **66,** 952(1965).
25. J. Barer *et al.*, *Am. J. Dis. Child.*, **124,** 889(1973).
26. F. DeGenaro and W. Nyhan, *J. Pediatr.*, **78,** 1048(1971).
27. D. Ward, *Br. Med. J.*, **2,** 432(1963).
28. B. Lawrence and B. Hopkins, *Med. J. Aust.*, **1,** 1301-1303(1969).
29. W. Robertson, *J. Pediatr.*, **79,** 877(1971).
30. N. Holtzman and R. Haslam, *Pediatrics*, **42,** 189-193(1968).
31. R. Stein *et al.*, *J. Am. Med. Assoc.*, **235,** 801(1976).
32. J. Schofferman, *J. Am. Coll. Emerg. Phys.*, **5,** 22-25(1976).
33. A. Schaffer, *Surg. Clin. North Am.*, **50,** 853-861(1970).
34. O. Anderson, *Pediatrics*, **46,** 319-321 (1970).
35. M. Casteels *et al.*, *Arch. Dis. Child.* **45,** 130(1970).
36. H. Hirschhorn and W. B. Greenough, in "Davidson's Principles and Practices of Medicine," 19th ed., A. M. Harvey, Ed., Appleton-Century Crofts, New York, N.Y., 1976, p. 1264.
37. *Medical Letter*, **16,** 46-48(1974).
38. H. I. Chinn and P. K. Smith, *Pharmacol. Rev.*, **7,** 53-82(1955).
39. C. D. Wood and A. Graybiel, *Clin. Pharmacol. Ther.*, **11,** 621-627(1970).
40. L. B. Gutner *et al.*, *Arch. Otolaryngol.*, **59,** 503(1954).
41. H. I. Chinn *et al.*, *J. Am. Med. Assoc.*, **160,** 755-760(1956).
42. R. Trumball *et al.*, *Clin. Pharm. Ther.*, **1,** 280-283(1960).
43. H. I. Chinn *et al.*, *J. Pharmacol. Exp. Ther.*, **108,** 69-70(1953).
44. J. Yerushalmy and L. Milkovich, *Am. J. Obstet. Gynecol.*, **93,** 553-562(1965).
45. S. Shapiro, Unpublished data from Boston Collaborative Drug Surveillance Program, Testimony before OTC Panel, 1974.
46. S. W. Hanford *et al.*, *J. Pharmacol. Exp. Ther.*, **111,** 447-453(1954).
47. C. D. Wood *et al.*, *J. Am. Med. Assoc.*, **198,** 1155(1966).
48. J. Brown and H. Sigmundson, *Can. Med. Assoc. J.*, **101,** 49-50(1969).
49. S. A. Nigro, *J. Am. Med. Assoc.*, **203,** 301(1968).
50. C. Stritzler and A. W. Kopf, *J. Invest. Dermatol.*, **34,** 319-330(1960).
51. P. Hansten, "Drug Interactions," Lea and Febiger, Philadelphia, Pa., 1973, p. 128.
52. L. L. Titche and A. Nady, *Dis. Chest*, **20,** 324-326(1951).
53. J. E. Bradley *et al.*, *J. Pediatr.*, **38,** 41-44(1951).
54. A. B. Crunden, Jr. and W. A. Davis, *Am. J. Obstet. Gynecol.*, **65,** 311-313(1953).
55. H. A. Agerty, *Adult and Child*, **1,** 66(1969).

56. *Fed. Regist.*, **40,** 12935(March 21, 1975).
57. J. B. Houston and G. Levy, *J. Pharm. Sci.*, **64,** 1504-1507(1975).
58. J. Perkeentupa and K. Raivis, *Lancet,* **2,** 528(1967).
59. Norwich Pharmaceutical Company, unpublished data. Communication with OTC Panel on Laxative, Antidiarrheal, Emetics and Antiemetics, 1974.
60. R. E. Gosselin *et al.*, in "Clinical Toxicology of Commercial Products, Acute Poisoning," 4th ed., Williams and Wilkins, Baltimore, Md., 1976, pp. 251, 295.
61. "Accumulation of Nitrate," National Academy of Sciences, Washington, D. C., 1972, pp. 46-75.
62. W. L. Dobes and H. S. Alden, *South. Med. J.*, **42,** 572-579(1949).

Products **5** ANTIEMETIC

Product (manufacturer)	Dosage form	Active ingredients	Other
Bonine (Pfipharmecs)	chewable tablet	meclizine hydrochloride, 25 mg	—
Dramamine (Searle)	tablet liquid	dimenhydrinate, 50 mg/tablet 15 mg/5 ml	sucrose, 54% (liquid) ethanol, 5% (liquid) cherry pit flavor, 0.2% (liquid)
Eldodram (Elder)	tablet	dimenhydrinate, 50 mg	—
Emetrol (Rorer)	liquid	invert sugar, 3.74 g/5 ml phosphoric acid, 25 mg/5 ml	—
Ram (Scrip)	tablet	dimenhydrinate, 50 mg	—
Trav-arex (Columbia Medical)	tablet	dimenhydrinate, 50 mg	—
Vertrol (Saron)	tablet	meclizine hydrochloride, 12.5 mg	—

Hemorrhoidal Products

K. Richard Knoll

Questions to ask the patient

Has a physician diagnosed the problem as hemorrhoids?

Are you having minor discomfort (itching and mild irritation) or is there severe pain and bleeding?

Do you strain at the stool?

Are you pregnant?

Have you tried any products for the condition? Which ones? Were they helpful?

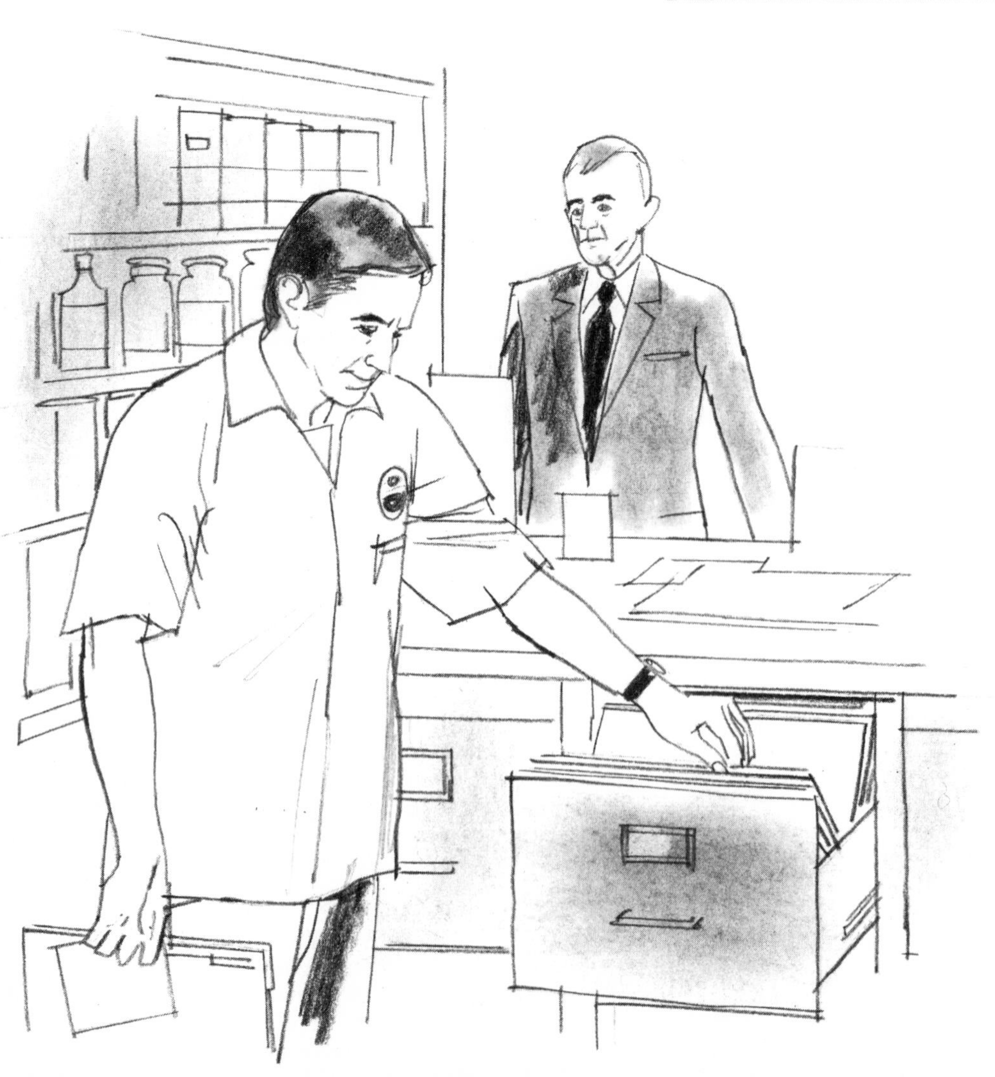

CHAPTER 6

Hemorrhoids (piles) are an anorectal condition. The terms "hemorrhoids" and "piles" are used interchangeably. Historically, hemorrhoids seem to have been one of the first conditions recognized as contributing to human discomfort. In ancient Egypt, the practice of proctology flourished. The Chester Beatty Papyrus essentially is a treatise on anal and rectal diseases, and the Ebers and Hearst Papyri are concerned with anal conditions. In ancient Greece, surgical treatment of hemorrhoids was practiced. Hippocrates believed that bile and phlegm caused hemorrhoids. Hemorrhoids also are mentioned in the Code of Hammurabi.[1-3]

Etiology

Many possible causes of hemorrhoids have been postulated, including hormones, genes, inflammation and/or infection, constipation, the erect stance, exercise, vascular stasis, diet, strain, laxation, loss of connective tissue elasticity with age, imbalance of the rectal sphincter mechanism, and anatomical peculiarities. Although hemorrhoids perhaps are not as serious as other rectal diseases, not many conditions are as annoying or produce as much discomfort as hemorrhoids.

The incidence of hemorrhoids is unknown because many hemorrhoids are asymptomatic and require no medical attention. The greatest incidence of symptoms from hemorrhoids occurs between the ages of 20 and 50. An epidemiological study of hemorrhoids notes that "Symptomatic hemorrhoids will only develop in susceptible individuals and are festered by socio-economic and cultural factors in both sexes and pregnancy in women . . . diet may be the means by which these forces manifest themselves. Pregnancy and constipation as causal factors are seriously questioned."[4] The significance of associated anorectal disease with hemorrhoids was studied and sex distribution was found to be equal.[5] In a group of 200 patients who had surgery primarily due to hemorrhoidal disease, associated anorectal diseases were found in 75.5 percent. The study concluded that hemorrhoids are not a single disease but part of group of anorectal diseases and cannot be ascribed to a particular cause. Possible predisposing factors include heredity and anatomical and physiological abnormalities. Contributory factors include constipation, diarrhea, straining at the stool, prolonged standing or straining at work or recreation, relaxation or deficiency of the anal fistula, cathartic abuse, certain foods, enemas, irritation of the rectal outlet, sedentary life, anal spasms, atony of the anal sphincter, rectal suppository abuse, vaginal pessaries, emmenagogues, obesity, and liver obstructions.

Medically, hemorrhoids are anorectal swellings, composed of varicosities involving one or more of the hemorrhoidal plexus of veins.[6] Pathologically, the process is a degeneration of the hemorrhoidal plexus, including dilation of the veins and thinning of their walls, resulting in complications such as inflammation, edema, ulceration, and thrombosis. Clinically, the process is characterized by bleeding and protrusion. The protrusions are globular or oblong and occur in the lowest portion of the rectum, in the anal canal, or at the anal margin. Hemorrhoids may appear red, purple, or black.

External hemorrhoids

External hemorrhoids (Fig. 1) involve the vein or veins of the inferior hemorrhoidal plexus and are located in the lower one-third of the canal or at the anal orifice. They usually are covered with skin, not mucosa, and may be painful.

Varicose. Varicose hemorrhoids are puffy folds in the anus. They indicate the presence of internal hemorrhoids.

Thrombotic. Thrombotic hemorrhoids, or anal hematomas, are similar to internal hemorrhoids, except that bleeding occurs under the skin, forming a bluish clot (thrombus). They range from pea to walnut size.

Cutaneous (skin tags). Skin tags (Fig. 1) are pieces of fibrous connective tissue covered by skin. They occur around the anal verge and may be single or multiple. They vary from a slight outgrowth of the skin to grossly projecting tags. Idiopathic skin tags are not caused by other conditions; secondary skin tags are associated with an anal fissure or pruritus ani.

Internal hemorrhoids

Internal hemorrhoids (Fig. 1) are swellings that involve varicosities of one or more veins of the superior hemorrhoidal plexus. They originate above the anorectal line and are covered by mucous membranes.

Prolapsed. A prolapsed hemorrhoid is one which, because of its size and distention, has descended below the anorectal line and outside the anal sphincter.

Thrombosed. A thrombosed hemorrhoid is one in which the blood has clotted.

Internal-external (mixed) hemorrhoids

A combination of external and internal hemorrhoids appears as a baggy swelling. These hemorrhoids are varicosities of both inferior and superior hemorrhoidal veins. Prolapsed mixed hemorrhoids are painful until the prolapse is reduced; bleeding may occur. Without prolapse, these hemorrhoids may bleed but are painless. Strangulated internal-external hemorrhoids are those that have prolapsed to such a degree and for so long that their blood supply is occluded by the constriction of the anal sphincter. These hemorrhoids are painful and usually become thrombosed.

Hemorrhoids also are classified according to their degree of development:

First degree. These hemorrhoids are not prolapsed. The number and size of the veins of the anal canal are increased and may bleed at the time of defecation.

Second degree. These are internal or mixed hemorrhoids that appear outside during defecation but return spontaneously to the anal canal where they remain until defecation.

Third degree. These internal and mixed hemorrhoids remain constantly outside the anal sphincter unless they are replaced by hand.

Fourth degree. These are hemorrhoids that have developed an edematous skin covering and have become so large that they cannot be returned into the anal canal. They remain as a permanent projection of the anal mucosa. Etiologically, hemorrhoids are divided into two categories:

Internal hemorrhoids. These are caused by a definite organic obstruction in the portal circulation. Obstructions include cirrhosis of the liver, thrombosis of the portal vein, and abdominal tumors.

Idiopathic hemorrhoids. This type is most common. These hemorrhoids show evidence of organic, venous obstruction. They cannot be ascribed to a particular cause, but many predisposing factors may play a part in their production.

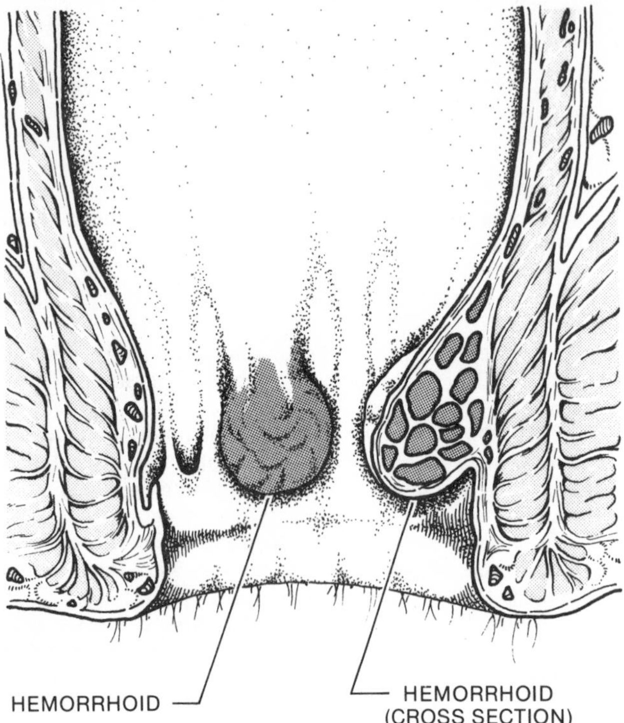

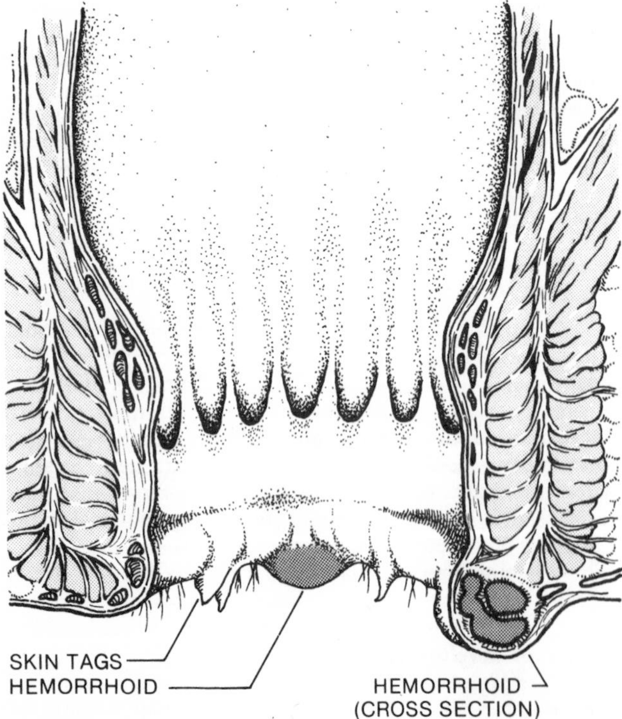

Figure 1. Hemorrhoids in the anal canal and anal orifice. Adapted from "The Ciba Collection of Medical Illustrations" by Frank H. Netter, M.D.

Signs and symptoms

External hemorrhoids. A thrombotic hemorrhoid is characterized by firm consistency, sudden and painful onset, and tenderness. If this type of hemorrhoid is left untreated and no complications develop, the pain diminishes after a few days; the lump recedes, often leaving a skin tag made of the external portion of the hemorrhoid. In some cases, however, a thrombosed hemorrhoid may not disappear so easily. Undue straining at the stool may result in a vein clot or rupture, producing an acute swelling. The degree of pain depends on the size and location of the clot and is intensified by walking and sitting. If the clot remains exposed, infection may develop and form an abscess or fistula.

Internal hemorrhoids. An internal hemorrhoid can remain asymptomatic for a long time. When symptoms do occur, bleeding and prolapse are the most common. Pain usually is not a symptom of uncomplicated internal hemorrhoids but may be severe if the hemorrhoids become prolapsed or thrombosed. The pain of thrombosis is dull, aching, and continuous. The discomfort of prolapsed hemorrhoids is caused by the temporary invasion of the hemorrhoid into the anal canal, which is supplied by sensory nerves. It disappears when the prolapsing hemorrhoid is reduced and returns to its usual location in the lower rectum. Other symptoms which may develop are a mucoid discharge, occurring most frequently with hemorrhoids that are in a permanently prolapsed condition, and perianal irritation caused by moisture from the discharge. Severe bleeding from internal hemorrhoids may result in secondary anemia characterized by breathlessness upon exertion, dizziness when standing up, lethargy, and pallor.

Mixed. A mixed hemorrhoid that has prolapsed is painful following defecation until the prolapse is reduced. Bleeding may occur, with or without prolapse, but there is no pain. If bleeding is continuous and excessive, severe anemia may develop. A strangulated mixed hemorrhoid that has prolapsed and become thrombosed produces severe, constant pain in the anal area, causing difficulty in sitting and walking.

Treatment of hemorrhoids

Treatment of hemorrhoids is confined to cases where symptoms hinder normal activity. Prophylactic measures for all types of hemorrhoids include avoidance of straining at the stool, heavy lifting, coughing, and excessive sneezing and proper control of constipation. The general therapy for treating hemorrhoids is medical, surgical, or injectional (Table 1). Medical treatment is nonspecific and treats symptoms only. Its main objectives are to reduce pain, itching, inflammation, and bleeding and to prevent further complications. Surgery is indicated where there is evidence of bleeding, thrombosis, infection, or ulceration. Injecting sclerosing agents directly into the hemorrhoid is effective but must be done by a physician. This procedure may result in scarring of the anal canal.[7]

The most recent method of treatment is a procedure called internal hemorrhoidectomy.[8] It consists of tying off hemorrhoids with rubber bands to cut off the blood supply and produce eventual sloughing of the lesions. It supposedly is more effective and less painful than surgery. This treatment is recommended instead of surgery for poor-risk, elderly patients and for those with recurrent hemorrhoidal disease after surgical treatment. Results are comparable to a hemorrhoidectomy and, because the operation can be performed in the physician's office, it saves time and money. The technique is contraindicated in the presence of fissures, fistulas, or strictures and is impractical for obese patients with a shortened anal canal. It should not be initiated casually because the bands must be carefully applied to avoid pain. Bleeding may be a complication, and necessary precautions must be taken.

Another alternative to hemorrhoidectomy for internal hemorrhoids is anal dilation. Lord[9] reported good results after anal dilation even for large prolapsed hemorrhoids. The first part of the treatment is carried out under general anesthesia and consists of forcible dilation of the lower rectum and anal canal. The second part is done by the patient and consists of using a special anal dilator and a combination of a mild laxative and fecal softener. The procedure is based on the theory that hemorrhoids are reversible and that they are caused by a narrowing of the lower rectum and/or canal. In a comparative study of anal dilation and rubber band ligation, there was no significant difference in the amount of discomfort caused by either method.[10] However, more patients were relieved of symptoms after rubber band ligation, and this method was recommended as a nonoperative treatment of internal hemorrhoids.

Another nonoperative procedure for treating hemorrhoids is cryodestruction. In this treatment, hemorrhoids are destroyed by freezing. This procedure does not require anesthesia and is painless.

Symptoms of hemorrhoids often are transient and respond to conservative treatment. Improvement of bowel function is important. Pharmacists should advise patients that an increase in fruit and cereal intake is helpful in regulating bowel function. A mild laxative, alone or in combination with a stool softener, may also be required. Sitz baths, as well as other forms of moist heat, provide symptomatic relief of hemorrhoids.

Treatment of other anorectal conditions

Some anorectal conditions may be confused with hemorrhoids. In some cases, hemorrhoids may be a contributing factor.

Pruritus ani. This syndrome, which involves the anal and perianal skin, is characterized by itching of varying intensity. It may be caused by local or systemic disease. The major causes of anogenital itching are parasitic infestation (most often pinworms), the use of broad-spectrum antibiotics (especially the tetracyclines), psoriasis and seborrheic dermatitis of the anogenital region, and possibly hemorrhoids or fissures; itching may be caused or aggravated by emotional factors.[11]

Various treatments can reduce the itching.[11] If the itching is persistent and has not been diagnosed, topical preparations may provide relief. Menthol and phenol are included in most OTC antipruritic preparations; if they are formulated in lotions, they may be useful. Some topical preparations contain antihistamines or local anesthetics. These ingredients are of little value and can cause allergic reactions if used repeatedly.

Prescription-only products may be more effective than OTC products in relieving itching. Antifungal medications (topical) containing nystatin are effective against *Candida* infections. Regardless of the cause, corticosteroids relieve itching.

Anal fissure. This slitlike ulcer occurs in the lining of the anal canal and is characterized by pain after defecation and bleeding which may be caused by the fissure itself or by associated hemorrhoids. The associated pain is relieved by topical anesthetic solutions such as procaine in oil or quinine and urea. Stools should be kept jellylike but should not leak, and the area should be kept clean and dry.

Cryptitis. Cryptitis is an inflammation and hypertrophy of the semilunar anal valve. It most likely originates in an anal gland, the duct of which opens into an anal crypt. Anal discomfort is the main symptom and is aggravated by defecation and walking. The use of stool softeners to lessen the pain of defecation, frequent hot baths, disposable wipes, and systemic antibiotics (e.g., penicillin) are the recommended methods of treatment.

Fistula. A fistula is a chronic lesion around the anus, characterized by a cavity. It usually is the result of an anorectal abscess or cryptitis. Symptoms include discharge, swelling, pain, and pruritus. Surgery is the only treatment that can cure a fistula.

Polyp. A benign tumor of the large bowel is called a polyp. Symptoms include bleeding, protrusion of a mass through the anus, and a feeling of fullness or pressure in the rectum. Surgical excision is the usual method of treatment.

Abscess. This perianal or intra-anal swelling is marked by a constant, throbbing pain. It usually is caused by the invasion by *Staphylococcus*, but other bacteria may also be involved. Antibiotic therapy may be used, but surgery is recommended.

Malignant neoplasm. Malignant neoplasms of the rectum, at times mistaken for hemorrhoids, are characterized by a progressively enlarging "lump" beside the anus and are accompanied by bleeding and pain. Surgical removal is usually indicated.

Ingredients in OTC products

More than 200 ointment and suppository products are used in the treatment of hemorrhoids. Total sales for 1975 were almost $30 million.[12] Hemorrhoids, one of the most common anorectal disorders, is one of the most frequently self-treated conditions affecting this region. Inhibition, fear, and embarrassment often prevent people with hemorrhoids from seeking medical attention. As a result, patients frequently self-medicate, undoubtedly influenced by the unsupported advertising claims made for hemorrhoidal preparations. Many preparations are available; some require a prescription, but many are OTC. Undue reliance on these preparations and failure to seek medical advice may have serious consequences.

Many hemorrhoidal preparations containing antiseptic or soothing ingredients relieve minor discomforts of hemorrhoids. Many of these products are combinations of traditional ingredients such as local anesthetics (benzocaine), vasoconstrictors (ephedrine), antiseptics (phenol, boric acid, oxyquinoline, or phenylmercuric nitrate), and mild astringents (bismuth subgallate, zinc oxide, or balsam Peru). Unfortunately, no documented evidence is available

Table 1. Methods of Treating Hemorrhoids

	Medical	Surgery	Injection
External hemorrhoids			
Skin tags	Bowel regulation, heat application (moist compress), soothing ointment.	Indicated if palliative measures are unsuccessful.	Not recommended.
Thrombotic	Bed rest, hot baths, astringent and/or local anesthetic ointment, mild laxative for constipation if necessary. Analgesic for pain (e.g., codeine).	Indicated where symptoms and conditions warrant.	Not recommended.
Internal hemorrhoids			
Nonprolapsing	Constipation control, bland diet.	Not recommended.	Applicable if uncomplicated (e.g., 5% phenol in olive oil; 5% aqueous solution quinine urea hydrochloride).
Prolapsing	Analgesic for pain (e.g., codeine).	Most satisfactory treatment.	Not recommended if prolapsed, if large thrombi are present, or if there is evidence of infection.
Internal-external hemorrhoids			
Nonstrangulated	Analgesic for pain (e.g., codeine).	Most satisfactory treatment.	Unsatisfactory; recommended only if debility or organic disease is present.
Strangulated	Ice bag, analgesic for pain (e.g., codeine).	Preferred treatment.	Not recommended.

regarding the effectiveness of these drugs, alone or in combination, in relieving the symptoms of anorectal disease.

Local anesthetics. If a local anesthetic is active on broken skin and mucous membranes and is present in sufficient concentration, it is useful in relieving anal pain and pruritus. There is a risk, however, of contact sensitization and hypersensitivity common to nearly all local anesthetics used; tetracaine, dibucaine, and benzocaine have most often caused sensitization.

Vasoconstrictors. The vasoconstrictors, including ephedrine and phenylephrine, are intended to reduce bleeding from hemorrhoids, but clinical evidence of their efficacy is not available. They produce capillary and arteriole constriction, but their effect on veins is negligible.

Antiseptics. The low concentrations of antiseptics in the available preparations have only a marginal effect on the high and constantly renewed bacterial population of the anus and rectum. Most antiseptics are harmless, but the risk of contact sensitization must be considered.[13]

Astringents. Astringents are locally applied protein precipitants that have low cell permeability. These agents reduce permeability of the cell membrane, causing a decrease in transcapillary movement of plasma protein, thereby reducing edema and inflammation. Most astringents also have some antiseptic properties. The astringents commonly used in OTC hemorrhoidal products include bismuth salts, zinc oxide, and hamamelis water (witch hazel).

Others. Other ingredients used in OTC hemorrhoidal preparations include those intended to promote skin healing. Vitamins A and D, balsam Peru, as well as "skin respiratory factors" from yeast and shark liver oil are included in this category. The value of these ingredients is questionable. One study, evaluating the effects of skin respiratory factor (SRF) on wound healing, showed that SRF contains substances capable of stimulating oxygen consumption, epithelialization, and collagen synthesis.[14] However, the effect of SRF on hemorrhoids has not been evaluated.

The Federal Trade Commission (FTC) has prohibited claims for a hemorrhoidal preparation as a cure, remedy, or effective treatment for hemorrhoids, or that a preparation will "end," "heal," "dry up," or give "lasting relief," or make operations unnecessary for hemorrhoids. Claims of palliative relief are permitted if they state that only temporary relief is provided for discomforts such as itching, burning, pain and soreness, and similar irritations caused by or associated with the symptoms of uncomplicated cases of hemorrhoids.

Product formulation

The preparations recommended for the relief of minor pain and itching associated with uncomplicated internal and external hemorrhoids are ointments and suppositories. These products provide only symptomatic relief; they do not remedy the underlying cause.

Suppositories, although they are widely advertised, are of little value for internal or external hemorrhoids.[15] A suppository goes past the site of painful external hemorrhoids into the rectum (pain-insensitive) before melting. Suppositories have no beneficial effect on bleeding internal hemorrhoids. The vasoconstrictor drugs in a suppository may reduce minor capillary bleeding but cannot stop the bleeding from a varicose vein. Ointments containing anesthetic drugs (e.g., benzocaine) may slightly relieve the pain of external hemorrhoids.

Many people who suffer from hemorrhoids also are constipated. Some preparations advertised for the treatment of hemorrhoids essentially are laxatives. Constipation is only one of the aggravating factors of hemorrhoids. Treatment of the constipation may be needed but does not assure against recurrence of the hemorrhoids because of the changes that may have taken place in the walls of the vessels and the structural tissue. Regular use of a laxative may aggravate the congestion and irritation of the hemorrhoidal area. The FTC requires advertisers of laxative preparations to stop promoting the products as beneficial in the treatment of hemorrhoids.

A comparison of the effectiveness of ointment and suppositories states, "Symptoms arising from the perianal skin and the anus itself, such as itching, soreness, and pain are more accessible to an ointment than to a suppository. Internal hemorrhoids and other rectal lesions are more accessible to drugs in a suppository unless the ointment is deposited inside the anus with an applicator. But the distribution of an ointment perianally is more controllable than that of a melted suppository in the rectum, where the vehicle is liable to spread over a large area and much of it will be diluted by feces. Very little drug from a suppository can reach the anal canal, especially if the anus is continent. However, the powerful psychological effect of a suppository may to some extent counterbalance the weak drug effect." [13]

Summary

OTC hemorrhoidal preparations provide only symptomatic relief of simple, inflammatory rectal conditions. Preparations requiring a prescription are used in the more acute phases of the disease, such as acute or chronic proctitis or pre- and postoperatively in hemorrhoidectomy. OTC products contain astringents, local anesthetics, antiseptics, emollients, and/or lubricating agents. They are intended to provide temporary relief of swelling, pain, and itching associated with simple hemorrhoids or other minor local irritations of the rectum. In recommending a product, the pharmacist should ascertain, whenever possible, whether the symptoms for which the patient is seeking relief indicate simple hemorrhoids or a more serious involvement not amenable to self-therapy. If self-medication is not indicated, the pharmacist should recommend that the patient see a physician.

References

1. C. C. Mettler, "History of Medicine," Blakiston, Philadelphia, Pa., 1947, p. 806.
2. H. Sigerist, "A History of Medicine," vol. 1, Oxford University Press, New York, N.Y., 1951, p. 335.
3. *South. Med. J.*, **39,** 536(1946).
4. L. Hyams and J. Philpot, *Am. J. Proctol.*, **21,** 177(1970).
5. J. J. Weinstein, *Med. Ann. D.C.*, **40,** 48(1971).
6. Information adapted from:
   H. E. Bacon *et al.*, "Proctology," Lippincott, Philadelphia, Pa., 1956.
   M. G. Spiesman and L. Malow, "Essentials of Clinical Proctology," 3d ed., Grune and Stratton, New York, N.Y., 1957.
   R. Turell, "Diseases of the Colon and Anorectum," vol. 2, Saunders, Philadelphia, Pa., 1959.
   C. W. Graham-Stewart, *Dis. Colon Rectum*, **6,** 333(1963).
   C. C. Jackson and E. Robertson, *Dis. Colon Rectum*, **8,** 185(1965).
   J. C. Goligher, "Surgery of the Anus, Rectum, and Colon," 2d ed., Charles C Thomas, Springfield, Ill., 1967.
7. K. L. Williams *et al.*, *Br. Med. J.*, **1,** 666(1973).
8. *Med. World News*, **7(29),** 36(1966).
9. Ph. H. Lord, *Br. J. Surg.*, **56,** 747(1969).
10. T. R. Hood and J. A. Williams, *Am. J. Surg.*, **122,** 545(1971).
11. *Med. Lett. Drugs Ther.*, **8,** 8(1966).
12. *Product Management*, 29(Aug., 1976).
13. *Drug Ther. Bull.*, **7,** 41(1969).
14. W. Goodson *et al.*, *J. Surg. Res.*, **21,** 125(1976).
15. Editors of *Consumer Reports*, "The Medicine Show," rev. ed., Pantheon Books, New York, N.Y., 1974, p. 106.

Products 6 HEMORRHOID

Product (manufacturer)	Dosage form	Anesthetic	Antiseptic	Astringent	Emollient/ Lubricant	Other
A-Caine (A.V.P.)	ointment	benzocaine, 2% diperodon hydrochloride, 0.25%	—	zinc oxide, 5% bismuth subcarbonate, 0.2%	cod liver oil base	phenylephrine, 0.255% pyrilamine maleate, 0.1%
Americaine (Arnar-Stone)	suppository ointment	benzocaine, 280 mg (suppository) 20% (ointment)	benzethonium chloride, 0.1%	—	polyethylene glycol base	—
Anusol (Warner-Chilcott)	suppository ointment	—	—	zinc oxide, 11% bismuth subgallate, 2.5% bismuth–resorcinol compound, 1.75% balsam Peru, 1.8%	vegetable oil base	benzyl benzoate, 1.2%
Aphco (Amer. Pharm.)	suppository ointment	benzocaine	boric acid	bismuth salts balsam Peru zinc oxide	—	—
BiCOZENE (Creighton)	cream	benzocaine, 6%	—	—	cream base	resorcinol, 1.67%

Product (manufacturer)	Dosage form	Anesthetic	Antiseptic	Astringent	Emollient/ Lubricant	Other
Blue-Gray (Columbia Medical)	suppository	benzocaine	boric acid	bismuth subgallate bismuth–resorcinol compound zinc oxide balsam Peru	—	—
Calmol 4 (Leeming)	suppository	—	—	bismuth subgallate zinc oxide balsam Peru	Norwegian cod liver oil cocoa butter base	—
Diothane (Merrell-National)	ointment	diperodon, 1%	benzoxyquine, 0.1%	—	propylene glycol	sorbitan sesquioleate
Eudicane (Rexall)	suppository	benzocaine, 130 mg	8-hydroxy-quinoline sulfate, 16.2 mg	zinc oxide, 260 mg bismuth subgallate, 64.8 mg balsam Peru, 64.8 mg	cocoa butter	ephedrine sulfate, 4.05 mg
Gentz Wipes (Philips Roxane)	medical pad	pramoxine hydro-chloride, 1%	cetylpyridinium chloride, 0.5%	hamamelis water, 50%	propylene glycol, 0.10%	aluminum chlorhy-droxyallantoinate, 0.2% fragrance
Hazel-Balm (Arnar-Stone)	aerosol	—	benzethonium chloride, 0.1%	hamamelis water, 79.9%	water-soluble lanolin derivative, 20%	—
Hemor-Rid (Columbia Medical)	ointment	diperodon hydro-chloride, 0.25%	—	zinc oxide, 5% bismuth sub-carbonate, 0.2%	cod liver oil petrolatum	phenylephrine hydrochloride, 0.25% pyrilamine maleate, 0.1%
Lanacane (Combe)	cream	benzocaine	phenylmercuric acetate, 0.02% chlorothymol	—	water wash-able base	resorcinol
Mamol (Abbott)	ointment	—	—	bismuth subnitrate, 40%	—	—
Manzan Ointment (DeWitt)	ointment	benzocaine, 1%	phenol, 0.5% menthol, 0.2%	tannic acid, 1.5%	—	allantoin, 0.5% ephedrine hydro-chloride, 0.2%
Manzan Stainless (DeWitt)	ointment	benzocaine, 1%	phenol, 0.5%	zinc oxide, 10%	—	allantoin, 0.5% ephedrine hydro-chloride, 0.2%
Manzan Supposi-tories (DeWitt)	suppository	benzocaine, 1%	phenol, 0.5% menthol, 0.2%	zinc oxide, 96%	—	allantoin, 0.2% phenylpropanolamine hydrochloride, 0.2%
Mediconet (Medicone)	medical pad	—	benzalkonium chloride, 0.02%	hamamelis water, 50%	ethoxylated lanolin, 0.5% glycerin, 10%	methylparaben, 0.15% perfume
Nupercainal Ointment (Ciba)	ointment	dibucaine, 1%	—	—	—	acetone sodium bisulfite, 0.5%
Nupercainal Sup-positories (Ciba)	suppository	dibucaine, 2.5 mg	—	zinc oxide bismuth subgallate	cocoa butter	acetone sodium bisulfite, 0.05%
Pazo (Bristol-Myers)	ointment suppository	benzocaine, 0.8%	camphor, 2.18% eucalyptus oil, 0.25%	zinc oxide, 4%	petrolatum, 87.57% (ointment) lanolin, 0.05% (ointment) hydrogenated vegetable oil (suppository)	ephedrine sulfate, 0.2%

Product (manufacturer)	Dosage form	Anesthetic	Antiseptic	Astringent	Emollient/ Lubricant	Other
PNS (Winthrop)	suppository	tetracaine hydrochloride, 10 mg	—	bismuth subcarbonate, 100 mg	—	tyloxapol, 25 mg phenylephrine hydrochloride, 5 mg
Pontocaine (Winthrop)	cream ointment	tetracaine hydrochloride (equivalent to 1% base) (cream) base, 0.5% (ointment)	menthol, 0.5% (ointment)	—	white petrolatum (ointment) white wax (ointment)	methylparaben (cream) sodium bisulfite (cream)
Preparation H (Whitehall)	ointment suppository	—	phenylmercuric nitrate, 0.01%	—	shark liver oil, 3%	live yeast cell derivative (supplying 2000 units of skin respiratory factor)
Proctodon (Rowell)	cream	diperodon hydrochloride, 1%	—	—	—	—
Proctofoam (Reed & Carnrick)	foam	pramoxine hydrochloride, 1%	—	—	petroleum mineral oil, 40%	—
Rantex (Holland-Rantos)	medical pad	—	benzalkonium chloride	hamamelis water, 50%	lanolin	methylparaben alcohol, 7%
Rectal Medicone Suppositories (Medicone)	suppository	benzocaine, 130 mg	8-hydroxyquinoline sulfate, 16.25 mg menthol, 9.3 mg	zinc oxide, 195 mg balsam Peru, 65 mg	cocoa butter vegetable and petroleum oils	—
Rectal Medicone Unguent (Medicone)	ointment	benzocaine, 20 mg	8-hydroxyquinoline sulfate, 5 mg menthol, 4 mg	zinc oxide, 100 mg balsam Peru, 12.5 mg	petrolatum, 625 mg lanolin, 210 mg	—
Tanicaine Ointment (Upjohn)	ointment	phenacaine hydrochloride, 325 mg/30 ml	camphor, 455 mg/30 ml phenol, 390 mg/30 ml menthol, 130 mg/30 ml	zinc oxide, 5.2 g/30 ml tannic acid, 1.6 g/30 ml	—	atropine, 16.25 mg/30 ml
Tanicaine Suppositories (Upjohn)	suppository	phenacaine, hydrochloride, 22 mg	phenol, 13 mg	zinc oxide, 390 mg tannic acid, 110 mg	—	atropine, 1 mg
Tucks Cream and Ointment (Fuller)	cream ointment	—	—	hamamelis water, 50%	lanolin petrolatum	—
Tucks Pads (Fuller)	medical pad	—	benzalkonium chloride, 0.003%	hamamelis water, 50%	glycerin, 10%	methylparaben, 0.1%
Vaseline Hemorr-Aid (Chesebrough-Pond)	ointment	—	—	—	white petrolatum, 100%	—
Wyanoid Ointment (Wyeth)	ointment	benzocaine, 2%	boric acid, 18%	zinc oxide, 5% balsam Peru, 1%	castor oil petrolatum	ephedrine sulfate, 0.1%
Wyanoid Suppositories (Wyeth)	suppository	—	boric acid, 543 mg	zinc oxide, 176 mg bismuth subcarbonate, 146 mg bismuth oxyiodide, 30 mg balsam Peru, 30 mg	cocoa butter	belladonna extract, 15 mg ephedrine sulfate, 3 mg

Ostomy Care Products

Michael L. Kleinberg

Questions to ask the patient

Are you experiencing any problems related to your ostomy such as diarrhea or gas?

What type of ostomy do you have? Where is it located?

How long have you had the ostomy?

What is the stoma size?

Do you irrigate or use a bag?

Do you have problems with the skin surrounding the stoma?

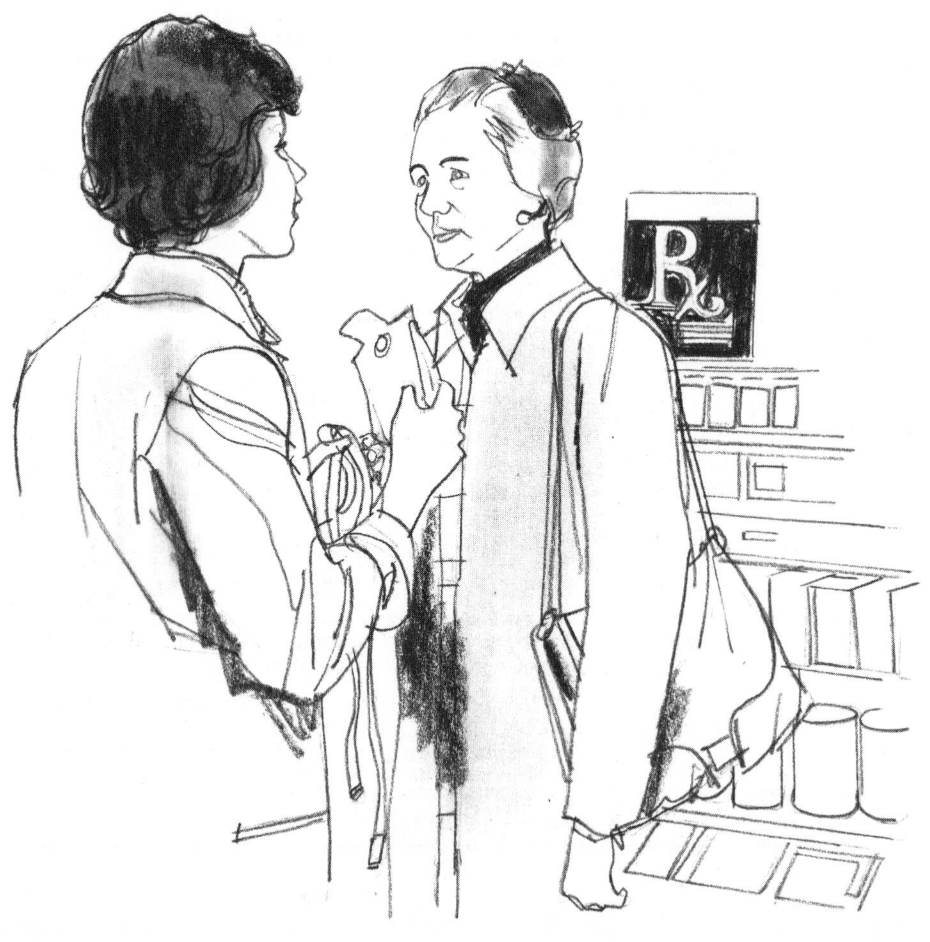

CHAPTER 7

An ostomy is the formation of an opening, or outlet, through the abdominal wall for the purpose of eliminating waste. It is usually made by passing the colon, small intestine, or ureters through the abdominal wall. The part of the intestine that is brought to the surface of the body is called the stoma.

Ostomy surgery necessitates the use of an appliance designed to collect the waste material normally eliminated via the bowel or bladder. Pharmacists involved in ostomy care must be familiar with the various types of ostomies and with the use and maintenance of the appliances for each type. In addition to information on ostomy products, the pharmacist should be prepared to provide patients with information on problems related to ostomy care such as skin care, diet, and drug therapy.

There are approximately 90,000 ostomies created annually in the U.S., and there are over 1 million patients who are living with established intestinal stomas.[1]

The idea of cutting into the abdominal cavity and creating an artificial opening is not new. This type of surgery was first suggested in 1710 by a French physician, Alexis Littre.[2] Since that time, the technique of ostomy surgery has been greatly refined. The surgical creation of an ostomy, however, is only the first step in the rehabilitation of an ostomate (a person with an ostomy). Complete recovery depends on how well ostomy patients understand their changed medical and physical circumstances and how completely they can subsequently adjust to and manage these changed conditions.

Because each ostomy patient is different, one patient may benefit from one type of appliance and another may develop problems with the same appliance. The ostomy patient should be familiar with the technique of applying and fitting an appliance that affords maximum benefit. Knowing the proper care of the skin or how to prevent skin irritation can prevent future problems. Proper patient counseling on diet, fluids, and medication is necessary to prevent complications.

The anatomy of the lower digestive tract is shown in Figure 1. The main function of the digestive system is the conversion of food into an assimilable form. Digestion begins in the mouth, then continues in the stomach and small intestine, and water absorption takes place in the large intestine. (See Chapter 3 for a complete discussion of digestion.)

Types of ostomies

Colostomy

A colostomy is the creation of an artificial opening using part of the large intestine or colon. Major indications for performing a colostomy include colon or rectum obstruction, cancer of the colon or rectum, genetic malformation, diverticular disease, trauma, and loss of anal muscular control.

When certain conditions are present in the lower bowel, it may be necessary to give that part a rest. A temporary colostomy is created for a period so that healing can take place. Depending on the healing process, it may take a few weeks, months, or years. Eventually the colon and rectum will be reconnected and bowel continuity will be restored. A permanent colostomy is formed when part of the colon is totally removed, and reconstruction of the bowel is impossible. A colostomy, permanent or temporary, can be made in any part of the colon but is most commonly made in the sigmoid colon.

Ascending colostomy. This ostomy appears on the right side of the abdomen (Fig. 2-A). Its discharge is semisolid and requires that the patient continually wear an appliance.

Transverse colostomy. This opening is usually created on the right side of the transverse colon (Fig. 2-B). The creation of this type of ostomy can be performed in two ways. The first method is to lift a loop of the transverse colon through the abdominal incision. A rod is then placed under the loop for a few days to give additional support (Fig. 2-C). The rod is removed after a few days. The second method is to divide the bowel completely and have two openings (double-barrel colostomy) (Fig. 2-D). In this case, the right ostomy discharges fecal material and the left one discharges small amounts of mucus. The consistency of the discharge from a transverse colostomy varies, depending on the distance from the small intestine to the opening. The rest of the colon assumes the concentrating function of effluent so that, in time, the stool takes on near-normal consistency. Management depends on the individual, but usually an appliance is worn continually.

Descending and sigmoid colostomies. These ostomies are on the left side of the abdomen (Fig. 2-E). They can be made as double-barrel (temporary) or single-barrel (permanent) openings. Because the fecal discharge is firm and can often be regulated by the patient, an appliance may not be needed. However, many patients prefer appliances to irrigation. There is no right or wrong method. Patient preference is the deciding factor.

Ileostomy

An ileostomy is a surgically created opening between the ileum and the abdominal wall. It usually is performed in cases of ulcerative colitis, Crohn's disease, trauma, multiple polyposis, or cancer. The entire colon is surgically removed and the ileum is brought to the surface of the abdomen (Fig. 2-F). The discharge is semisolid and contains pancreatic enzymes and, therefore, is irritating to the skin. An appliance is worn continually.

Urinary diversions

These diversions are performed as a result of loss of the bladder or bladder dysfunction usually due to cancer or genital malformation. An ileal conduit is created by implanting the ureters into the ileum and bringing the ileum to the surface of the abdomen (Fig. 2-G). An appliance is worn continually. A ureterostomy involves detaching the ureters from the bladder and bringing them to the outside of the abdominal wall. This procedure is performed less frequently than the ileal conduit because it is more difficult for the patient to take care of himself.

Types of ostomy appliances

The appliance is an extremely important aspect of the ostomate's well being. The ostomate has lost a normal functioning body process, and the appliance takes over that lost function and seemingly becomes a part of the body. The type of appliance depends on the type of surgery that was performed. An ileostomate may prefer to wear one type of appliance, and a colostomate another, or no appliance at all. An ideal appliance should be leakproof, comfortable, easily manipulated, odorproof, inconspicuous, inexpensive, and safe.[3] Unfortunately, there is no one appliance that meets all these criteria. Table 1 gives the major manufacturers of ostomy products.

Disposable (temporary)

A disposable appliance is usually a plastic bag that can be attached to the skin. It is usually transparent, which makes it easier for a surgeon to examine the stoma without removing the appliance. Disposable appliances save nursing time during appliance changes, are usually simple to apply and, therefore, are easier in self-instruction and care. They generally are used immediately after surgery until the stoma has healed and inflammation has subsided. Some ostomy patients continue to use this type of appliance because of its simplicity. Disadvantages are its fragility, relative lack of adhesiveness and cost.

Permanent

A permanent appliance has the advantage of strength, better adhesiveness, and a lower cost. Disadvantages include the extra care and additional supplies needed for using it. The appliance must be discarded after a few months due to its staining and retention of odor. It consists of two main parts: a pouch which can be emptied and a faceplate which is attached to the skin. These appliances are available in one piece (with the faceplate attached to the bag) or two pieces (with a removable faceplate).

Accessories

Foam pads. The foam pad is not an integral part of an appliance, but it can be very useful. It generally is made of closed-pore foam rubber and is nonabsorbable. The pad can be used to reduce the size of the appliance orifice and add comfort. It is cemented between the faceplate of the appliance and the skin. The foam pad may increase the number of days between appliance changes.

Belts. Special belts are made which can be attached to various appliances to give additional support to the appliance. Belts are made for specific appliances and are not interchangeable. They provide the pressure needed for a good bond and reassure the ostomy patient that the appliance will not fall off. Belts are optional, depending on the ostomate's preference. Patients must be careful not to wear a belt too tight. In moving, this could cause the faceplate to move, possibly damaging the stoma. Two fingers should fit under the belt when it is attached.

Cement. The cement that holds the appliance to the skin is usually made of latex, a hydrocarbon solvent, and a prophylactic additive such as zinc oxide. It is waterproof and protects the skin from irritation caused by fecal material. The cement itself may be irritating to the skin and should not be used until a patch test is performed. The test consists of placing a small piece of material (cement) to be tested on the abdomen (not near the stoma), covering it with tape, and leaving it for 48 hours. If redness, itching, or burning occurs during this period, the test is positive and the material should not be used. If there is no reaction, the material is safe to use. However, reactions may develop after 48 hours, and the patient should be instructed to watch for skin irritation.

Adhesive seals. Colly-Seal, Stomahesive, and Relia-

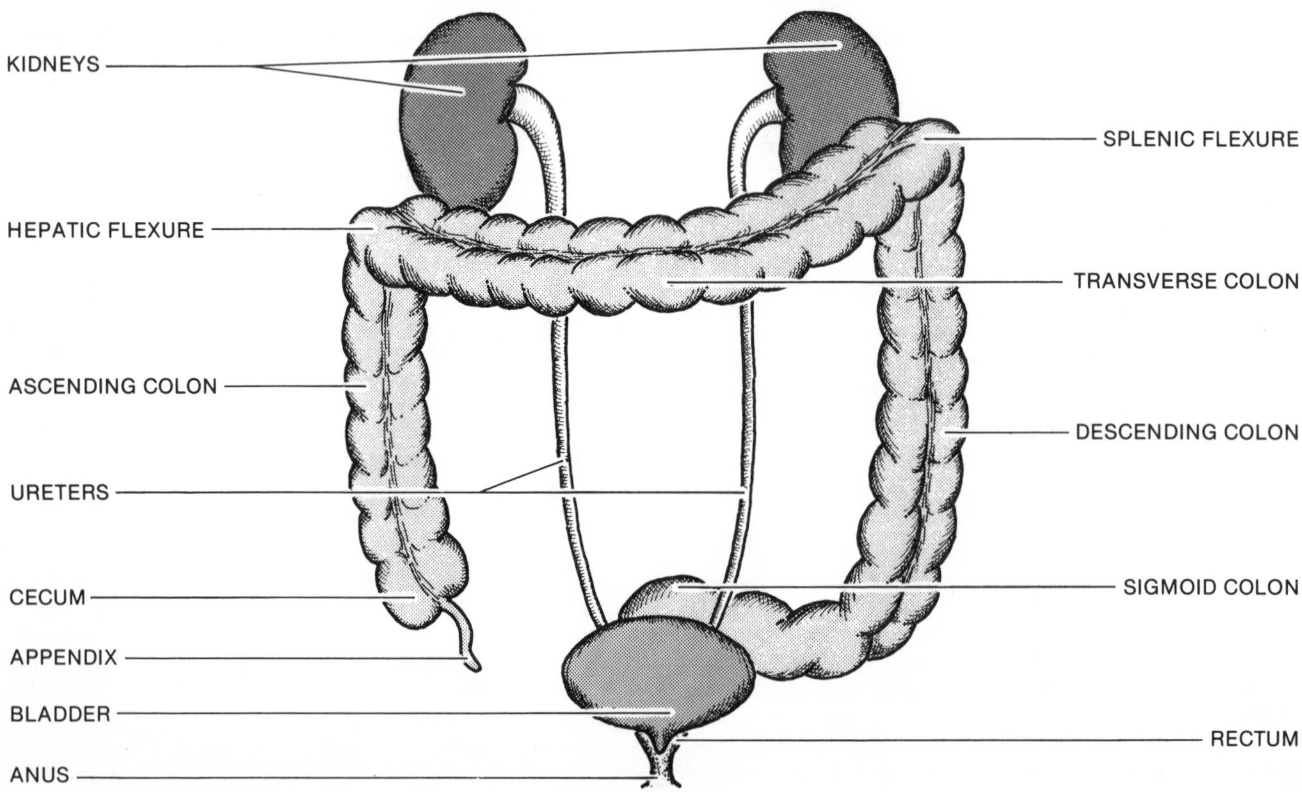

Figure 1. Anatomy of the lower digestive and urinary tracts.

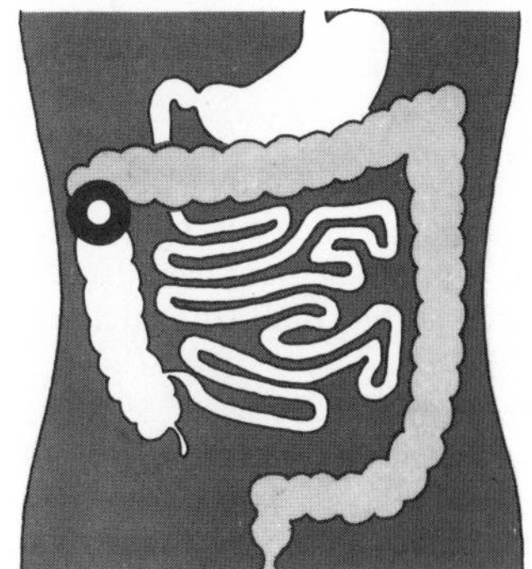

Figure 2-A.
Ascending colostomy.

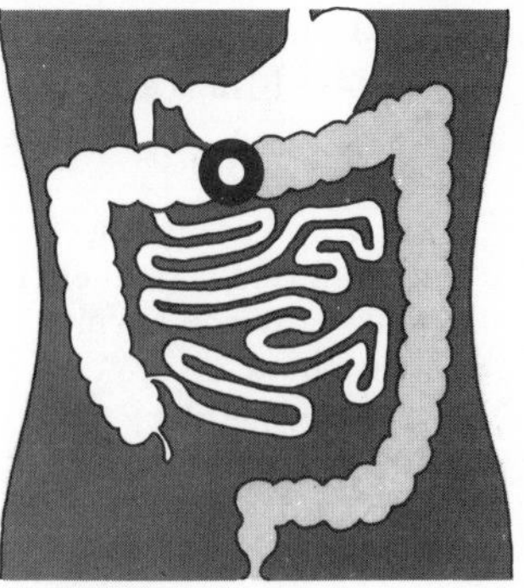

Figure 2-B.
Transverse colostomy.

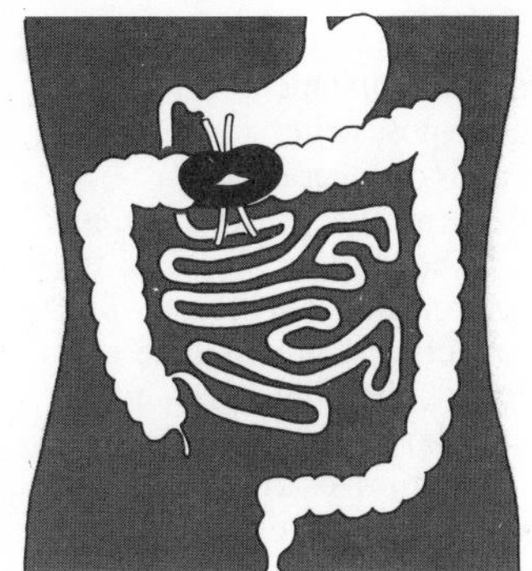

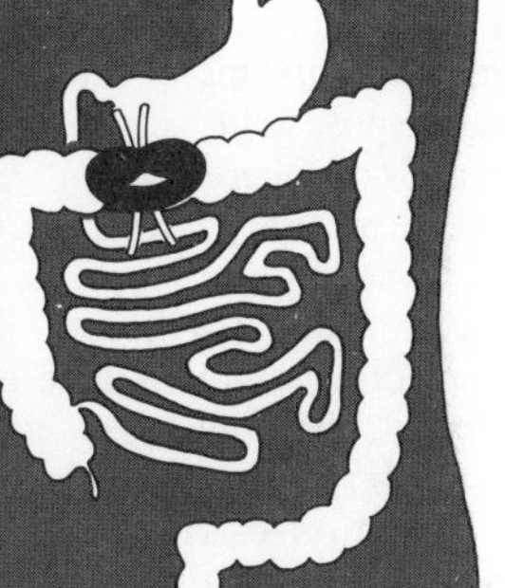

Figure 2-C.
Loop ostomy.

Adapted from J. R. Wuest, *J. Am. Pharm. Assoc.*, **NS15 (11)**, 626-628 (1975).

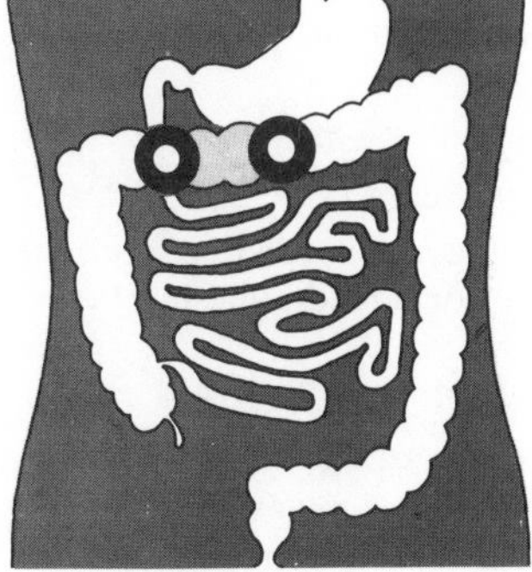

Figure 2-D.
Double-barrel colostomy.

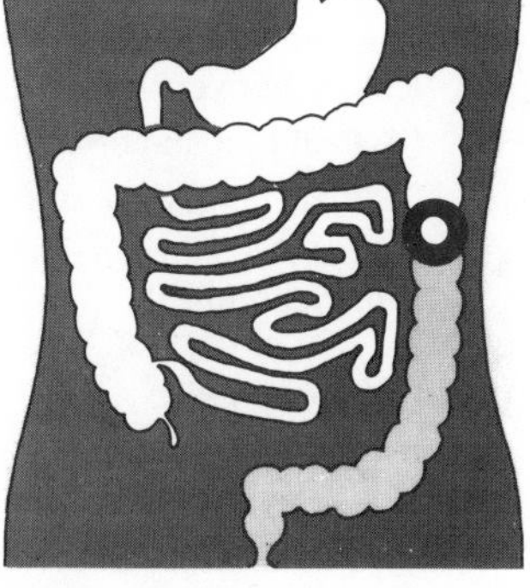

Figure 2-E.
Descending colostomy.

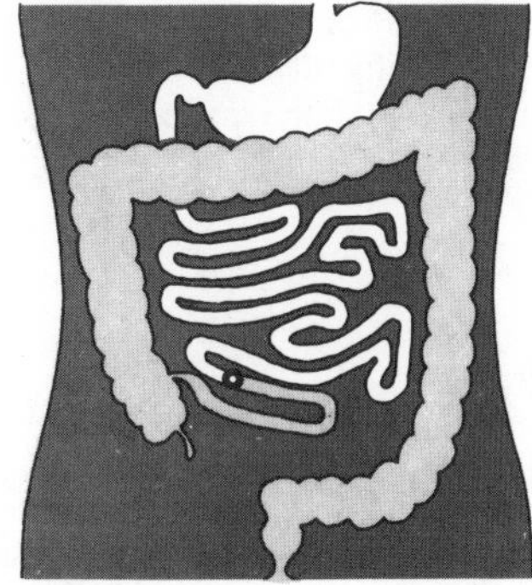

Figure 2-F.
Ileostomy.

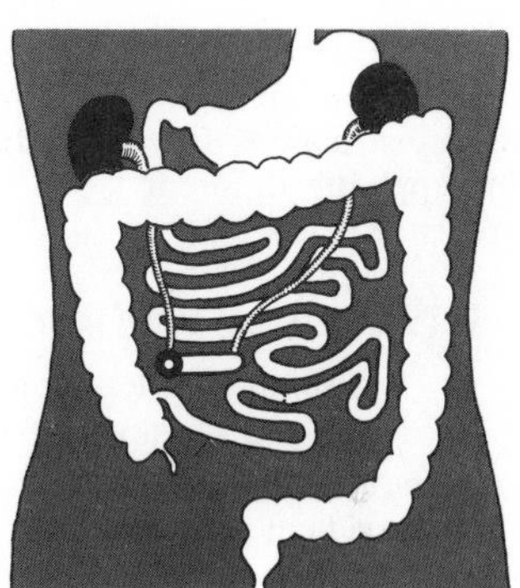

Figure 2-G.
Ileal conduit.

Seal are sometimes used instead of cement. The Colly-Seal contains karaya, and its adhesiveness may last longer than karaya powder. Stomahesive wafers are composed of gelatin, pectin, sodium carboxymethylcellulose, and polyisobutylene. They are nonallergenic and adhere to weepy skin. ReliaSeal is a combination foam pad and adhesive. For maximum effectiveness, it should be applied to dry skin.

Solvents. A solvent helps remove the cement from the appliance. It is applied between the appliance and the skin. This procedure allows easy removal of the appliance without pulling it, preventing possible skin irritation. The solvent is usually a hydrocarbon.

Karaya gum. Karaya gum powder is made from the resin of the *Sterculia urens* tree found in India. It is used by the ostomate for its adhesive and healing properties. Karaya becomes gelatinous when it is brought in contact with moisture. Instead of water, aluminum hydroxide gel can be mixed with the karaya to increase its healing properties. Some manufacturers produce karaya washers made of karaya mixed with glycerin and baked into a ring. The ring is moistened and stretched or cut to fit snugly around the stoma. Karaya may be placed over irritated or weeping areas for its healing properties.

Tape. Many kinds of tape provide additional appliance support and waterproof the cement-skin bond. A strip of tape is applied across the top and/or bottom of the faceplate, half on the faceplate and half on the skin.

Tincture of benzoin. Tincture of benzoin is used to make the skin more adhesive so that a better seal can be obtained. It also toughens the skin and helps prevent skin irritation. Tincture of benzoin is patted on the skin and allowed to dry. Cement is then placed over it. Some individuals may be allergic to tincture of benzoin. Tincture of benzoin compound should never be used as a substitute for tincture of benzoin because it will irritate the skin.

Irrigating sets. Colostomy management must be individualized. Some patients prefer to irrigate their colostomy to maintain bowel regularity. The irrigating set includes a reservoir for the irrigating fluid, a tube, irrigating tip, and a collection bag.

Frequency of irrigation depends on the colostomate's normal bowel habits. Basically, colostomy irrigation is the introduction of water into the colon through the stoma by means of a catheter or conical adapter. The water stimulates the intestinal wall, resulting in peristalsis, and softens the stool; this allows subsequent fecal evacuation. The patient should be very cautious in inserting the catheter because the mucosa of the colon is insensitive to pain, and perforation may occur without the patient knowing it. The catheter should be well lubricated and inserted without pressure. Patients may continue to wear the appliance after irrigation, or they may prefer to cover the stoma with a small piece of gauze between irrigations.

Deodorizers. Odor therapy is either local or systemic. Some agents (Banish, Odour-Guard, Uri-Kleen) are placed directly in the appliance to mask the odor of the fecal discharge. Chlorophyll and bismuth subgallate are taken internally. The mechanism of action of bismuth subgallate is unknown but may involve inhibition of bacterial fermentation. The dose of bismuth subgallate is 200 mg before each meal. A possible side effect of the agent is decreased peristaltic activity which is advantageous to an ostomate.

Appliance: fitting and application

Measuring the stoma to determine the proper fit of an appliance is an important part of ostomy care. Stress and irritation may be caused by an appliance which has an opening smaller than the stoma. An appliance which has an opening larger than necessary exposes the skin around the stoma and allows excoriation and/or ulceration.

Most appliance manufacturers provide stoma gauges to assure proper faceplate size. The gauges usually are pieces of cardboard with premeasured and cut holes. The ostomate determines the size by selecting a precut hole and placing it over the stoma. The size of the appliance should be one-sixteenth to one-eighth inch larger than the stoma. This allows for slight swelling or motion of the stoma or for an irregularly shaped stoma and prevents rubbing of the stoma against the faceplate edge.

Applying the appliance and accessories

The lack of uniformity in types of ostomies and ostomy equipment available makes it difficult to give standard instructions for application. Some of the procedures for applying different types of appliances and accessories are listed below.[4 5]

DISPOSABLE APPLIANCE

- ☐ Assemble the equipment.
- ☐ Remove the used appliance by gently peeling away the pouch from the skin. Solvent may be applied with a medicine dropper, one drop at a time, between the body and bag. Karaya can be removed with water.
- ☐ Measure the stoma (only when selecting an appliance, not routinely).
- ☐ Clean the skin around the stoma with soap and water. Be sure to remove all the soap. Pat dry.
- ☐ If a skin barrier is used, place it snugly around the stoma.
- ☐ Peel paper backing from adhesive. If appliance has a karaya backing, moisten with water.
- ☐ Grasp both sides of appliance and place center opening over stoma. Press gently around stoma.
- ☐ Close pouch by turning the bottom up twice. Secure with rubber band or clip supplied by manufacturer.
- ☐ Apply tape and belt, if desired.

REUSABLE APPLIANCE

- ☐ Assemble equipment.
- ☐ If using a two-piece appliance, attach the pouch to the faceplate by stretching the opening in the pouch over the faceplate. Secure the attaching device around the pouch.
- ☐ Old cement should be removed from the faceplate by rubbing with a cotton ball or gauze pad dipped in solvent.
- ☐ Apply two thin coats of cement to the clean faceplate, allowing each coat to dry thoroughly.
- ☐ Remove the used appliance in the same way as a disposable one.
- ☐ Clean the skin with soap and water. A little solvent may be used to remove excess cement. Allow to dry.
- ☐ Apply two thin coats of cement to the clean skin. Spread it slightly beyond area to be covered by faceplate. Allow each coat to dry thoroughly.
- ☐ If a skin barrier (e.g., karaya) is used, place it snugly around the stoma.
- ☐ Grasp both sides of appliance and place center opening over stoma. Press gently around stoma.
- ☐ Clamp the bottom of the pouch.
- ☐ Apply tape and belt, if desired.

KARAYA RING

- ☐ Cut karaya sheet into squares and cut hole one-eighth inch smaller than the stoma or use precut karaya washers which are one-eighth inch smaller than the stoma.
- ☐ Moisten the karaya with water.
- ☐ Stretch karaya around the stoma to fit snugly.
- ☐ Apply appliance as directed.

RELIASEAL

- ☐ Cut a hole in the ReliaSeal about the same size as the stoma. Use one pad per application.
- ☐ Peel white paper covering off of pad and apply ReliaSeal over the stoma.
- ☐ Peel blue paper covering off of pad.
- ☐ Place appliance over ReliaSeal.

(Note: An adhesive barrier may be needed between the ReliaSeal and the appliance for added adhesion.)

STOMAHESIVE

- ☐ Cut hole in wafer about the same size as the stoma. Use one wafer per application.
- ☐ Cut a hole in the double-faced adhesive disc the same size as the opening in the faceplate.
- ☐ Apply one side of adhesive disc to the shiny surface of the Stomahesive.
- ☐ Remove paper backing from the dull side of the Stomahesive and apply this side to the skin.
- ☐ Remove paper backing from the adhesive disc.
- ☐ Place the appliance over Stomahesive and adhesive disc.

The ostomate's diet

The diet for an ostomate should be individualized. Some ostomates are placed on a low-residue diet (a diet low in fruits and vegetables) the first few weeks following surgery. The purpose of this is to minimize the amount of waste discharged and to minimize intestinal obstruction. After this initial period, the ostomate may be allowed to eat all foods. It might be wise for the patient to try a different type of food each day. If the food causes cramps or diarrhea, he may want to avoid it in the future. Fish, onions, and eggs may produce odor, and the ostomate may want to voluntarily omit these from the diet. Cranberry juice, yogurt, and buttermilk may help in the reduction of odor. Peas, beans, asparagus, cabbage, radishes, cucumbers, and carbonated beverages may produce gas and, therefore, the ostomate may want to avoid them. Kidney stones may be a problem in patients with a urinary ostomy, ileostomy, or ascending colostomy. These patients must ensure an adequate amount of fluid in their diet to prevent or avoid the precipitation of crystals or stones in the urine.

Potential complications

The psychological complication from ostomy surgery may be postsurgical depression. This depression is variable and may depend on the patient's prior mental status and ability of the patient to take care of himself. There may also be the fear of not being able to engage in former work, participate in sports, perform sexually, or have children. The ostomate should be reassured that, in the majority of cases, the ability to carry out these activities or functions remains unchanged.

The physical complications are stenosis of the stoma, fistula formation, prolapse, retraction, and skin irritation.

Stenosis, or narrowing, of the stoma is caused by the formation of excess scar tissue. To overcome this problem, regular dilation of the stoma with a lubricated finger can be tried. Dilation should be done by a physician. If this does not work, surgery may be indicated.

The formation of an opening, or fistula, in the area projecting above the abdomen may also occur. This can be caused by an injury to the stoma, a poorly fitting appliance, or poor surgical technique. The fistula allows drainage directly on the skin which can lead to other problems. Treatment is surgical repair.

Prolapse is the abnormal extension of the bowel beyond the abdominal wall. A major cause of this complication is too large an opening in the abdominal wall. The danger of prolapse is the decrease in blood supply to the bowel outside the abdominal cavity. Treatment is by surgical intervention.

Retraction is the recession of the stoma to the length below normal and is caused by a stretched opening in the abdominal wall. It also can damage the skin surface. Treatment is by surgical intervention.

Skin irritation usually occurs when the correct methods of using an appliance are not followed. Irritation leads to leakage, and leakage causes more irritation. Karaya gum powder is useful in these cases. It can be applied to the inflamed skin, between the skin and the cement.

The ostomate's use of drugs

Because part or all of the colon is removed and because of the possible alteration in intestinal transit time, the ostomate may have difficulty in taking prescription or OTC medication.

Coated or sustained-release preparations may pass through the intestinal tract without being absorbed. It is feasible to assume that the ostomate may receive a subtherapeutic dose with these types of medication. Preparations that can be crushed or chewed before swallowing or liquid preparations are the best.

The ostomate must also be careful when taking antibiotics, diuretics, or laxatives. Antibiotics may alter the normal flora of the intestinal tract, resulting in a fungal infection of the skin surrounding the stoma. Nystatin powder may be prescribed by a physician to treat this condition. Because additional loss of fluid may cause dehydration, diuretics should be given with care, especially in patients with an ileostomy. Laxatives may be used in colostomy patients but only with close supervision. Ostomates tend to become obstructed, and the laxative's particular action may cause perforation in this situation. Ileostomates should never need a laxative.

United Ostomy Association

The United Ostomy Association was formed in 1962. It is made up of various ostomy organizations around the country whose main purpose is to help ostomy patients by giving moral and physical support and supplying information. The United Ostomy Association sponsors a yearly meeting and publishes a quarterly journal and other literature. The address is 1111 Wilshire Boulevard, Los Angeles, California 90017.

Table 1. Major Manufacturers for Ostomy Products

Manufacturer	Product
Atlantic Surgical	Appliances Karaya powder
Coloplast/Bard	Appliances
Davol	Appliances ReliaSeal
Duke	Double-backed adhesive
Eli Lilly	Oral deodorant (bismuth subcarbonate)
E. R. Squibb	Kenalog spray Mycostatin powder Stomahesive
Faultless Rubber Co.	One-piece permanent appliance
Hollister	Disposable pouches with built in karaya Karaya washers and paste Skin gel
Minnesota Mining and Manufacturing Co.	Hypoallergic adhesive products (Micropore paper tape and Blenderm tape) Double-faced adhesive disc (3M Stomaseal adhesive disc)
Nu-Hope	Appliances Supplies
Perma-Type Co.	Appliances Supplies
Requa	Charcoal deodorant

Summary

Pharmacy involvement in ostomy care is important. The American Pharmaceutical Association identifies ostomy care as a clinical role for the pharmacist in direct patient care.[6] Likewise, the American Society of Hospital Pharmacists specifies experience in ostomy care in the new accreditation standards for residency training.[7] Procurement and distribution of ostomy supplies and patient counseling are necessary services which can be provided by the pharmacist.

References

1. J. R. Benfielk *et al., Arch. Surg.,* **107**, 62(1973).
2. C. D. Cromar, *Dis. Colon Rectum,* **7(4)**, 256(1968).
3. M. Sparberg, "Ileostomy Care," Charles C Thomas, Springfield, Ill., 1971, p. 18.
4. L. Gross, "Ileostomy: A Guide," The United Ostomy Association, Inc., 1974, p. 28.
5. N. N. Gill *et al., Instructions for the Care of the Ileostomy Stoma,* Cleveland Clinic Foundation, Cleveland, Ohio.
6. *J. Am. Pharm. Assoc.,* **NS11**, 482(1971).
7. *Am. J. Hosp. Pharm.,* **32**, 192(1975).

Cold and Allergy Products

John F. Cormier
Bobby G. Bryant

Questions to ask the patient

How old are you?

What are the symptoms? Is there runny nose, sore throat, cough, fever, earache?

How long have the symptoms been present?

Do you have a history of allergies?

Do you have any respiratory disease such as asthma or bronchitis?

Do you have diabetes, glaucoma, heart disease, or high blood pressure?

What medications are you taking?

Which products have you used? Were they effective?

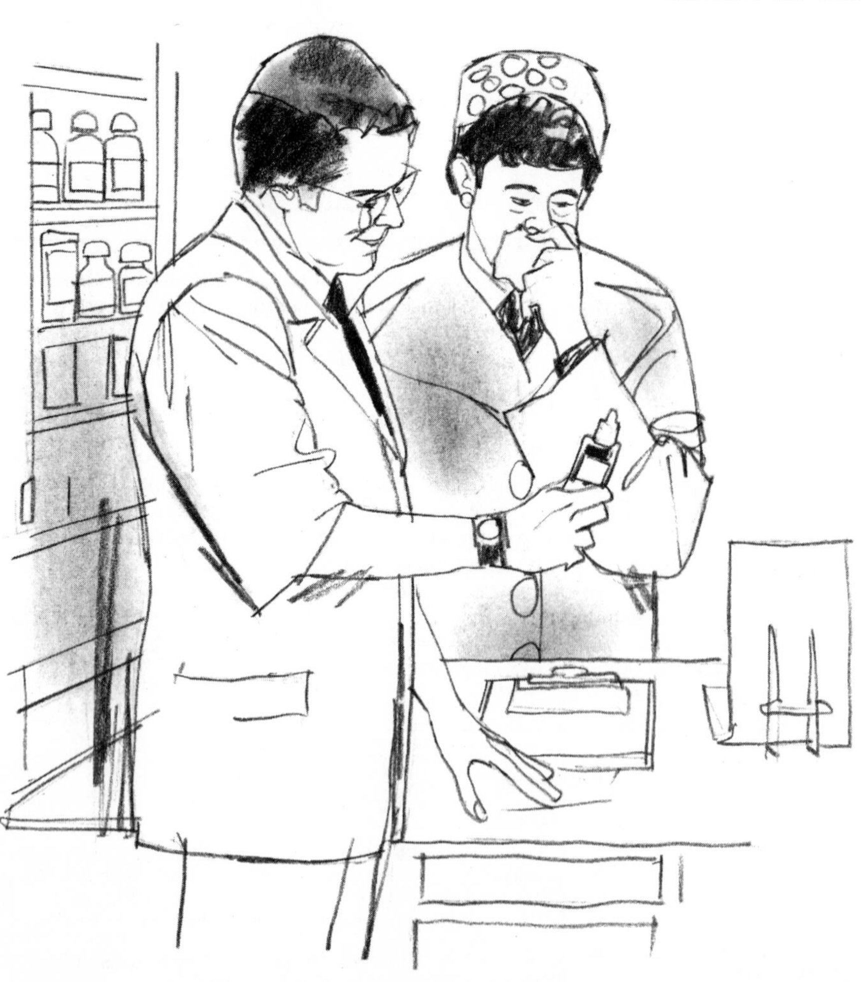

CHAPTER 8

Although the common cold and allergic rhinitis are etiologically different, they present similar symptoms and respond to similar approaches to management. Because of these similarities this chapter will attempt to provide the pharmacist and other health practitioners with the information necessary to identify and distinguish between these disorders, as well as other disorders which may mimic them.

The common cold is an acute, self-limiting viral infection of the upper respiratory tract (Fig. 1). It is also called a "cold," acute rhinitis, infectious rhinitis, coryza, or catarrh. The main anatomic sites of infection may vary, and therefore, a cold may present symptoms, individually or in combination, of the nose (rhinitis), throat (pharyngitis), larynx (laryngitis), or bronchi (bronchitis).

Allergic rhinitis is a specific allergic reaction of the nasal mucosa resulting from an antibody-mediated reaction to an inhaled antigen. It may be perennial due to the year-round presence of antigenic substances or it may be seasonal to correspond with the periodic appearance of offending antigens. Most commonly, allergic rhinitis is seasonal and is called hay fever or pollinosis.

Anatomy of the upper respiratory tract

The nose is an organ. As a passageway for airflow into and out of the lungs, it humidifies and warms inspired air and filters inhaled particles. Several anatomic features facilitate the performance of these functions. The nasal cavity is divided by a central septum and fingerlike projections (turbinates) which extend into the cavity, increasing the nasal surface area.

The surface of the nasal passageway is coated with a continuous thin layer of mucus, which is a moderately viscous, mucoproteinaceous liquid secreted continuously by the mucus glands. Under normal conditions, foreign bodies such as dust, bacteria, powder, and oil droplets are entrapped in the film and carried out of the nose into the nasopharynx. The turbinates may cause many eddies in the flowing air, forcing it to rebound in different directions before finally completing its passage through the nose. This rapid change in air flow enables air-suspended particles to precipitate against the nasal surfaces. High vascularity and resultant high blood flow within the nasal mucosa help warm and humidify the inspired air.

Nerve control of the nasopharyngeal vascular bed is derived from both divisions of the autonomic nervous system. Stimulation of the sympathetic fibers (or the action of sympathomimetic drugs) causes decreased activity of the mucus glands and vasoconstriction which reduces the size of the turbinates, widening the airway. Parasympathetic stimulation (or the action of cholinergic drugs) increases mucus production and narrows the airways by vasodilatation and vascular engorgement of the mucosal tissue.

The epithelium of the nasal passageways is ciliated. The constant beating of the cilia causes the mucus film to be continually moved toward the nasopharynx, carrying with it entrapped particles to be expectorated or swallowed.[1] Because this ciliary movement is one of the body's main defense mechanisms, care should be taken in the administration of agents which impair this movement. Oils, especially mineral oil, and the overuse of topically applied decongestants interfere with normal ciliary movement.

The mucus blanket is rich in lysozyme and contains glycoproteins and immunoglobulins.[2] Lysozyme of the mucus is an important defense against bacteria because it readily digests the lipid and carbohydrate cell wall of some bacteria. It is also responsible for the digestion of the cell wall of pollens and the subsequent release of antigenic substances. Glycoproteins of the mucus can temporarily inhibit some viruses by combining with the virus protein coat. The union of inhibitor and virus is reversible and, therefore, these inhibitors probably do no more than delay invasion of host cells by virus particles. Immunoglobulins of low molecular weight, mainly IgA and IgG, are also contained in the mucus secretion. Although present in low concentrations, they may also decrease the infectivity of certain viruses.

Viruses that attach to and invade host cells of the respiratory tract stimulate the infected cell to produce interferon. Interferon is active not only against the virus that caused its production, but also against other unrelated viruses. It protects neighboring, noninfected cells against subsequent viral infection.[3]

The cough reflex is an essential body defense mechanism by which the respiratory airways leading to the lungs are maintained free of foreign matter. It occurs in health, e.g., cigarette smoking, as well as disease and is frequently the symptom in a wide variety of pathologic states. All areas of the respiratory tract, i.e., the trachea, larynx, bronchi, and terminal bronchioles, are sensitive to foreign matter or other causes of irritation such as irritant corrosive gases and infection. A cough may be caused by the stimulation of receptors (mechanoreceptors and chemoreceptors) located in the mucosa of the airways and lungs. Afferent impulses pass along nerve pathways to the cough center in the medulla, which coordinates efferent impulses to the diaphragm and to the intercostal and abdominal muscles. The cough response is an automatic sequence of events leading to the rapid expulsion of air from the lungs designed to carry with it foreign bodies that have initiated the reflex. Localized bronchoconstriction may also play an important role in stimulation of the cough reflex. Although the evidence is inconclusive at this time, this "bronchomotor theory" is believed by some to be the mechanism whereby irritation causes bronchoconstriction which triggers the cough reflex.[4]

The sneeze reflex is very similar to the cough reflex, except that it is intended to clear the nasal passages instead of the lower regions of the respiratory tract. Irritation in the nasal passages is the initiating stimulus of the sneeze reflex. The afferent impulses from the nose travel to the medulla, where the reflex is triggered. A series of reactions similar to those for the cough reflex takes place. In addition to these reactions, the uvula is depressed so that large amounts of air pass rapidly through the nose, as well as through the mouth, helping to clear the nasal passages of foreign matter.[1]

The passageways of the trachea and lungs are lined with a ciliated, mucus-coated epithelium which aids in the removal of foreign matter. As in the nasal passageways, the cilia in the trachea and lungs also beat toward the pharynx, carrying mucus and entrapped particles out of the respiratory tract.

Differential diagnosis

Conditions that mimic the common cold

Other infectious diseases present initial manifestations identical to those of the common cold.[5] It is important that the pharmacist be aware of these disorders because some of them can have potentially serious implications for which a physician should be consulted. Using strictly palliative therapy in situations that may not be self-limiting would have little effect on the underlying problem. For example, a patient's complaint of a "sore throat," alone or in conjunction with other symptoms, may be caused by bacteria, by a virus, or by another irritative process. The only conclusive means by which bacterial pharyngitis may be excluded is by culture. This is not always practical, however, nor is it always needed. Table 1 can assist the pharmacist in evaluating a sore throat complaint in adults. It is the authors' opinion that a complaint of a sore throat in a child should be evaluated by a physician as soon as possible and that symptomatic therapy be employed only to provide relief until a physician can be seen. In this situation, if symptomatic therapy alone is recommended and the child is actually suffering from streptococcal pharyngitis, there is a possibility of rheumatic heart disease or glomerulonephritis developing due to inappropriate treatment, i.e., lack of antibiotic therapy.

Influenza. A viral infection of the respiratory tract that may mimic a cold is called influenza, or the "flu." The flu can usually be distinguished from the common cold by its epidemic occurrence and by fever, dry cough, and more significant general malaise. Although treatment for the flu is symptomatic, it usually is more vigorous than treatment for the cold, and complications, especially secondary bacterial infections, are more likely to develop. This is especially true in the elderly and debilitated patients, who should be referred to a physician when influenza is suspected.

Measles. The incidence of measles (rubeola) has been drastically reduced by immunization; when it does occur, it is associated with a prodrome (premonitory symptoms) which includes fever, rhinitis, dry cough, and conjunctivitis. Initially, it is difficult to rule out the common cold. However, in about 3 days, a red rash indicative of measles develops over the face, trunk, and extremities. The appearance of Koplik's spots is pathognomonic of

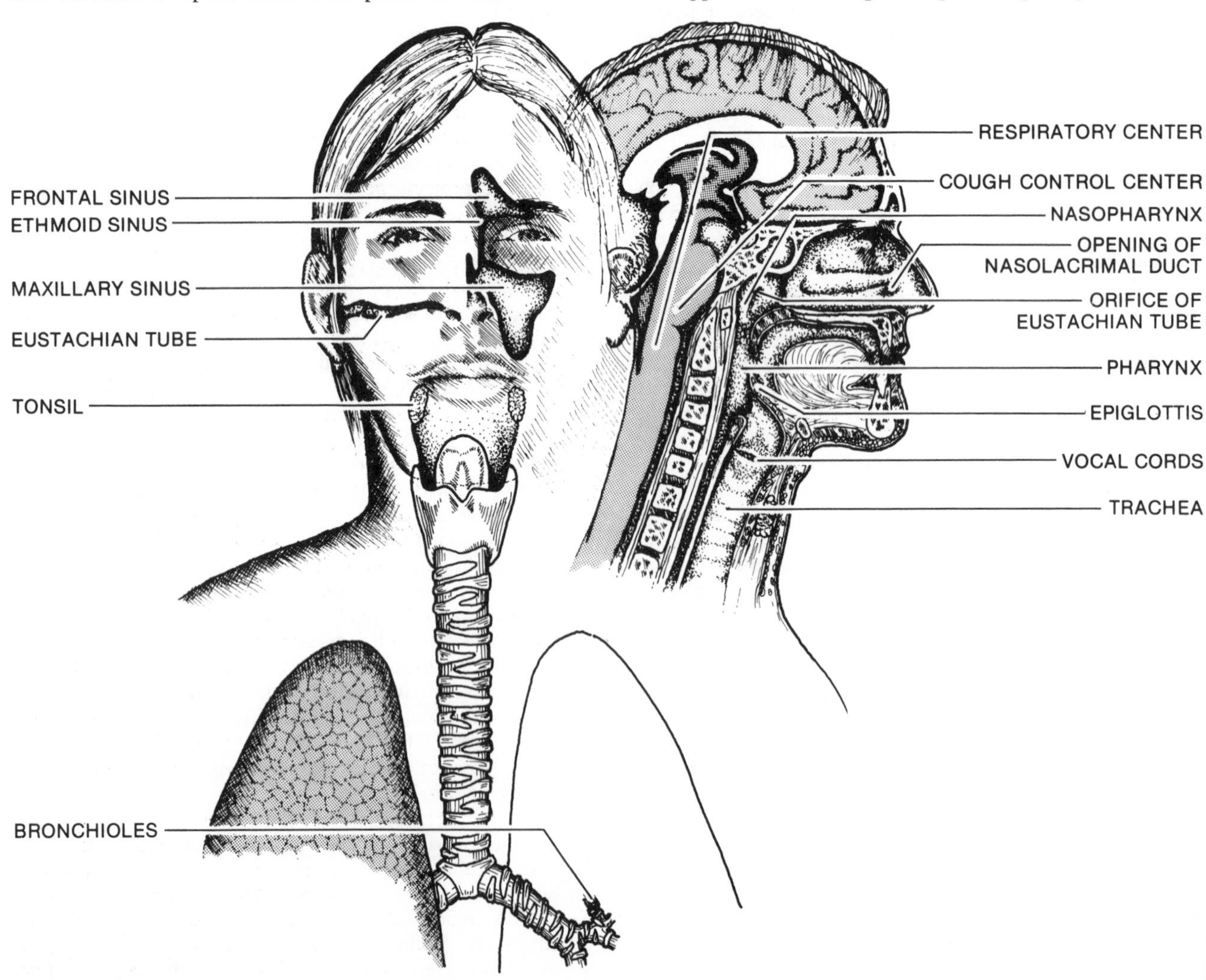

Figure 1. Anatomy of the respiratory passages.

measles. These spots usually appear a day or two prior to the rash as tiny "table salt crystals" on the mucous membranes of the cheek. Although the treatment of measles is symptomatic (along with patient isolation), a physician should be notified because secondary bacterial infections and a CNS complication (post-measles encephalitis) can develop. Also, local public health regulations may require reporting cases of the measles.

German measles. Another viral disease in which fever, malaise, and rhinitis coincide with the eruption of a fine red rash is German measles (rubella). It is recommended that this disorder also be brought to the attention of a physician because of possible complications. An important concern is the devastating effect that rubella can have on a fetus *in utero*. If a pregnant woman is exposed to a case of rubella (actual or suspected), she must be referred to a physician to determine her degree of immunity to the virus.

Allergy. A history of allergy and a review of symptoms help differentiate allergic rhinitis from the common cold. Hay fever may be suspected in young children who suffer from repeated coldlike symptoms. In evaluating a patient's complaints, the pharmacist must keep in mind that "all that sniffles is not a cold."

Conditions that mimic allergic rhinitis

It is also important for pharmacists to recognize common disease entities that may mimic signs or symptoms of allergic rhinitis. The main clinical entity in differential diagnosis of seasonal allergic rhinitis is infectious rhinitis. A mucopurulent discharge, the possibility of fever and other systemic symptoms, and the lack of pruritus often distinguish infectious from allergic rhinitis (Table 2). Chronic sinusitis, recurrent infectious rhinitis, abnormalities of nasal structures, and nonseasonal, nonallergic, noninfectious rhinitis of unknown etiology (vasomotor rhinitis) may be confused with perennial allergic rhinitis.[6] A physician should be consulted to differentiate between these conditions.

Other conditions that may mimic the symptoms of allergic rhinitis are rhinitis medicamentosa, reserpine rhinitis, foreign bodies in the nose, and cerebrospinal rhinorrhea. Rhinitis medicamentosa is a condition resulting from the overuse of topically applied vasoconstricting agents. The pharmacist may identify this condition by questioning the patient about the past use of nose drops or sprays for nasal congestion. Preparations containing reserpine or other sympatholytic antihypertensives have the potential of causing marked nasal congestion. Often, this side effect is transient and subsides with continued antihypertensive administration. However, if it persists and is bothersome, topical decongestant treatment may be necessary. Although a dosage reduction may be beneficial for nasal congestion, such a reduction may sacrifice blood pressure control. Another alternative is to try a different antihypertensive agent.

Rarely, the presence of a foreign body in the nose may be mistaken for chronic allergic rhinitis. Examination by a physician is necessary. Cerebrospinal rhinorrhea may follow a head injury; it is characterized by the unilateral discharge of a clear, watery fluid.

The common cold

The common cold has been rated as the most expensive single illness in the U.S. In fact, more time is lost from work and school because of the common cold than

Table 1. Characteristics of a Sore Throat—Bacterial vs. Nonbacterial[a]

Parameter	Bacterial sore throat	Nonbacterial sore throat
Onset	Rapid	Slower
Soreness	Marked	Seldom marked
Constitutional symptoms	Marked	Mild
Upper and lower respiratory symptoms	Present in 50% of cases	Usual
Lymph nodes	Large, tender	Slight enlargement, not tender

[a]Adapted from V. Bulteau, *Med. J. Aust.*, **2**, 1053-1055(1966).

from all other diseases combined. Among approximately 60 million industrial employees in the U.S., the common cold accounts for nearly 1 million person-years lost from work annually. This amounts to about one-half of all the absences and approximately one-fourth of the total work time lost each year in industry.[7]

The age of the patient is related to the incidence of the common cold and to its complications. Children 1 to 5 years old are most susceptible, and each child averages between 6 and 12 respiratory illnesses a year, most of which are common colds. Some practitioners feel that infants less than 6 months old are somewhat resistant to these viruses, but this finding may be attributed to the relative infrequency of exposure of infants to different environments. Individuals between 25 to 35 years old average about six respiratory illnesses a year; older adults average two or three. Young children are more prone to complications of the common cold, such as otitis media and pneumonia, than older cold sufferers. However, many adults also suffer from the sequelae of a cold (e.g., sinusitis).[2,7]

There is an apparent relationship between the season of the year and the common cold. It is not known what the exact relationship is, but it is usual to observe three peak seasons of common colds per year. One of these occurs in the autumn, a few weeks following the opening of schools; another occurs in mid-winter; and a third in the spring. These separate epidemics are associated with different viruses, each of which may have its own seasonal epidemiology. U.S. Public Health Service studies show that during the winter quarter of the year about 50 percent of the population experiences a common cold; during the summer quarter only about 20 percent.[7]

Chilling of the body or wet feet do not in themselves induce the common cold. However, if the virus is a recent invader, the effects of exposure probably are distinct contributory factors because such exposure is associated with a vasomotor effect that decreases the temperature of the nasal mucosa by several degrees. As a result of this temperature change many people experience symptoms of nasal irritation such as sneezing and serous discharge. These changes in the nasal mucosa and a subsequent change in the character of the mucus may then facilitate the invasion by the virus.[7] A poor state of nutrition, fatigue, and emotional disturbances are associated with a greater susceptibility to infection as well as increased severity of infection and a greater likelihood of complications.[7]

Table 2. Characteristics of Various Types of Rhinitis

Characteristic	Allergic		Infectious	Nonallergic (vasomotor)
	Seasonal	*Perennial*		
Etiology	IgE-mediated immunologic reaction	IgE-mediated immunologic reaction	Respiratory infection	Autonomic nervous system disorder
Seasonal pattern	Yes	Present year round	Often worse in winter	Worse in changing seasons
Recurrences	Mild symptoms between attacks	Mild symptoms between attacks	Clears completely	Frequently continuous
Family history of allergy	Common	Common	Occasional	Occasional
Systemic symptoms	Rare	Rare	Common	Rare
Other allergic symptoms (asthma, eczema)	Common	Common	Occasional	Occasional
Pruritus	Yes	Yes	No	Mild or absent
Fever	No	No	Occasional	No
Conjunctivitis	Yes	Yes	No	No
Discharge	Waterlike	Waterlike	Mucopurulent	Waterlike
Paroxysmal sneezing	Yes	Yes	No	Yes

The spread of respiratory disease such as the common cold is direct from person to person with no intermediate source of spread such as food, water, or animals. The only means by which spreading can be prevented is by isolating the infected individual. However, by the time a cold has been detected, the virus has undoubtedly already been transmitted via respiratory droplets to others.[3]

Allergic disorders involving the nasopharynx, e.g., hay fever, also seem to play a part in facilitating infection. The probable cause for this is the inflammatory changes occurring in the mucosa as a result of the antigen-antibody reaction which may facilitate subsequent virus invasion.

The American public buys approximately $400 to $500 million of OTC cough and cold preparations in pharmacies each year. These statistics illustrate the potential opportunities the pharmacist has to interact with and assist the self-medicating patient in proper product selection and administration.

Etiology

Viruses cause the common cold. More than 120 different viral strains which can produce symptoms of the common cold in humans have been isolated.[7] Known agents which may cause this syndrome include the rhinoviruses (approximately 60 different serologic types), adenoviruses, echoviruses, coxsackie viruses, influenza viruses, and parainfluenza viruses. Of these, the rhinoviruses comprise the largest etiologic group.[7] They probably account for more than one-half of all the common colds in adults. Five to ten percent of common colds are associated with more than one virus, and definite evidence of simultaneous infection with two viruses is not rare.[2,7]

Viruses differ from bacteria not only by their existence within the host cell but also by their chemical composition, their mode of replication, and their responsiveness to drug therapy.[3] The process of a viral infection is divided into three stages: entry into the host cell and release of nucleic acid; replication of the genome and synthesis of viral proteins; and assembly of new virus particles and their release from the cell to infect additional host cells.[8] There probably are several mechanisms by which the virus penetrates the host cell, but none is well defined. Once inside the host cell, the virus is attacked by host cell enzymes and possibly other substances, releasing the viral nucleic acid. In the second stage of infection, the virus uses metabolic pathways of the host cell itself to duplicate the viral genome and synthesize viral proteins. Finally, these components are assembled into new, mature virus particles and are released by the host cell. The release may be rapid and may be accompanied by lysis and death of the host cell, although cell death may not always result. The new virus particles can then infect adjacent cells by the same cycle.

When host cell injury or death occurs, the body's inflammatory defense mechanism is activated, causing pathological changes and subsequent symptoms. These clinical manifestations of infection are not evident, however, until extensive viral replication and inflammation have already occurred.

Pathophysiology and symptoms

The symptoms associated with the common cold are a manifestation of the pathologic changes (inflammation) that occur in the respiratory epithelium, secondary to viral invasion. The pathologic changes that make up the inflammatory response to one or more viruses are excess blood flow in the area (hyperemia), an abnormal accumulation of fluid in the intercellular spaces (edema), and profuse discharge from the mucous membrane of the nose (rhinorrhea).[7]

The severity of the cellular damage (hence, the degree of inflammation and symptoms) is related to the type and virulence of the infecting virus and the extent of the infection. Various strains of influenza virus, for example, do a great deal more damage to the respiratory epithelium than those that cause the cold. Therefore, the symptoms of the "flu" are usually more severe than those of the cold, and the predisposition to secondary bacterial complications is greater.

Although colds commonly involve the nasal structure, other sites along the respiratory tract may also be affected. This is due to the predilection of certain viruses for pharyngeal, laryngeal, or bronchial cells and to the extension of the infectious process from the original site of invasion.[3]

Because the incubation period for these viral infections is relatively short (1 to 4 days), patients often report a rapid onset and progression of symptoms. Virus shedding usually begins 1 or 2 days prior to the onset of symptoms and is associated with the sloughing and regeneration of the epithelium. A few days later, during the symptomatic phase, peak viral replication and host cell injury occur. Due to the intervention of body defenses, such as interferon, virus excretion ceases after several days and symptoms decrease.[2]

The clear, watery fluid that initially flows from the irritated nasal epithelium (nasal discharge or rhinorrhea) is the hallmark of the common cold. Although it is initially clear, it is followed shortly by a mucoid or purulent secretion which is much thicker and tenacious and is largely composed of dead epithelial cells and white blood cells. It is commonly assumed that these mucopurulent secretions are the result of secondary bacterial infection. This, however, is not always the case. Viruses can cause inflammatory reactions on their own, and the secretions occur even when there has been no change in the bacterial flora of the nose.[3]

Nasal congestion follows as the nasal turbinates become swollen (edematous), encroaching on the nasal lumen, which is also burdened with the increased secretions. Nasal discharge and congestion are the most commonly described discomforts associated with the common cold (Table 3).

The combination of nasal irritation, nasal discharge, and nasal congestion (which cause further irritation) give rise to sneezing. Sneezing is not as discomforting as the discharge and congestion and subsides with the clearing of the infection and secretions.

Pharyngitis may also occur during a cold. This throat symptom is usually described as a "dryness" or "soreness" rather than actual pain such as that associated with bacterial pharyngitis or acute tonsillitis. Pharyngitis is attributed to edema of the pharyngeal mucosa which activates sensory nerve fibers as the infection spreads to deeper tissue.

This irritation of the pharynx ("tickling") may also cause a nonproductive cough. The cough may also be caused by irritation of tracheal or bronchial mucous membranes due to the direct extension of the inflammation or by the dripping of infectious material from the nasopharynx (postnasal drip). At its onset, the cough is usually dry and nonproductive. Later stages of the common cold are characterized by heavy bronchial congestion resulting from the cellular debris of local phagocytic activity added to the respiratory tract fluids in the bronchial and nasal passage secretions and draining into the lower respiratory tract. Ciliary activity may not be sufficient to remove these congested fluids, and coughing is necessary to clear the lower tract of accumulated phlegm.

Another possible manifestation of the common cold is laryngitis, which is associated with hoarseness or loss of voice. It may also be caused by the spread of infection, or it may be an irritation secondary to drainage from the nasopharynx. A hot or warm sensation ("feverishness") is another fairly common complaint. There is usually little or no fever actually present. Headache, which usually occurs in the early stages of the cold, is caused by the infection and inflammation of the nasal passages and paranasal sinuses.

Complications

In an otherwise healthy individual, a virus-induced common cold is self-limiting in 5 to 7 days. It is not uncommon (but not inevitable) for complications to develop during or immediately following a common cold. The pharmacist should be familiar with possible complications, their causes, and how they are treated. Viral infection induces swelling and some exudation, but it causes no significant change in the bacterial flora of the nasopharynx. If the inflammatory changes are of sufficient magnitude, passages connecting the paranasal sinuses and middle ear become obstructed, and under these conditions, infection can occur from secondary bacterial growth.

The most common bacterial complications are sinusitis, otitis media, and pneumonia.[5] Obstruction of the various respiratory and auditory passages resulting in stasis of infected mucus is usually the predisposing factor to bacterial infection.

Young children are especially prone to otitis media and pneumonia. Children's eustachian tubes are short, relatively horizontal, and rather narrow. This facilitates fluid accumulation in the middle ear as well as rapid blockage in response to only a slight degree of inflammation. A child's bronchiole passages also are smaller in diameter than older children's and adults' and become blocked easily. The smaller passages and the child's lack of conscious effort to "cough up" accumulated fluids in the

Table 3. Frequency of Common Cold Symptoms

Symptoms	Frequency, %
Severe	
Nasal discharge	100
Nasal obstruction	99
Moderate	
Sore or dry throat	96
Malaise	81
Postnasal discharge	79
Headache	78
Cough	76
Mild	
Sneezing	97
Feverishness	49
Chilliness	43
Burning eyes and mucous membranes	28
Aching muscles	22

lower tract leads to stasis of the fluids, inflammation, and secondary bacterial infection. During the first few years of life, the "cold" problem can be a potentially serious one.

These complications usually manifest themselves by a worsening of local symptoms and signs (earache, headache, cough), the development of a fever, and failure of the cold to improve in the expected time. Such manifestations in a person with a history of a recent cold are probably caused by secondary bacterial invaders for which culture and sensitivity tests and appropriate prescribed antibiotic therapy are indicated.

Treatment of the common cold

Self-medication of the common cold is palliation of symptoms. There are no curative remedies, only drugs which bring temporary relief while the cold runs its course and the normal body defenses attempt to remove the viral invaders and repair the damage. In general, additional bed rest and the prevention of chilling add to the patient's comfort. Adequate fluid intake is necessary to prevent dehydration, and a well-balanced diet should be maintained.

Nasal congestion and nasal discharge. The symptomatic treatment of nasal stuffiness is of value in that it not only relieves the discomfort but also prevents excessive blowing of the nose which may further irritate mucous membranes and the nostrils. Excessive nose blowing may also force infected fluids into nasal sinuses and the eustachian tubes, extending the infection and discomfort.

Sympathomimetic amines (decongestants) applied topically to the nasal mucosa or administered systemically are effective vasoconstrictors which help decrease edema and swelling of the nasal mucosa. The decrease is not only comforting but also essential to an infant who must breathe through the nose while bottle or breast-feeding.

The watery nasal discharge found in the early stages of the common cold can possibly be minimized by the use of a decongestant.

Cough. The first step in attempting to control a cough is providing adequate fluids to the respiratory tract either by increasing oral fluid intake or by humidifying the inspired air. If the cough is dry, nonproductive, hyperactive, and annoying, a cough suppressant is indicated. An expectorant agent, by virtue of its action, is also useful in providing a demulcent effect. Practically, these two agents are given together anyway because there are very few cough suppressants available without an expectorant. If the cough is congested and productive and is not hyperactive, ensuring adequate fluid intake may be all that is needed. An expectorant agent may be recommended as adjunctive therapy to facilitate the removal of phlegm and to prevent the congested, productive cough from becoming hyperactive.

The "tickling" sensation perceived in the pharynx which causes a cough can be initially treated with a demulcent, e.g., hard candy or cough drop, but if the cough becomes more intense, a cough suppressant can be recommended.

Dry or sore throat. In the absence of definite pain and fever for a complaint of a sore throat, bacterial pharyngitis can probably be ruled out. However, a sore throat in a child is difficult to evaluate and should not be self-medicated; the child should be seen by a physician.

Lozenges and gargles containing antiseptics and/or topical anesthetics are promoted quite heavily for treating a sore throat. However, the use of an antibacterial lozenge or gargle is irrational because the antibacterial ingredients are not effective against viruses.

If the throat is dry or "raspy," hard, sour candy can be used to stimulate the flow of saliva, which acts as a demulcent. A frequently overlooked measure in soothing an inflamed throat is the regular use of a warm, normal saline gargle (2 tsp/qt of water). If these measures do not provide adequate relief, lozenges or sprays containing a local anesthetic (phenol, hexylresorcinol, benzocaine) may be used every 3 to 4 hours to provide symptomatic relief.

Laryngitis. Acute laryngitis presents a therapeutic problem—the only direct way to reach the inflamed laryngeal tissue is by the inspired air. Lozenges and gargles do little to relieve the hoarseness; their ingredients or the saliva that they stimulate do not reach this area in a sufficient amount to do any good. The inhalation of water vapor (steam or cool mist) several times a day has proven beneficial in acute laryngitis. Inhaling irritants (smoking) should be avoided, and the voice should be rested as much as possible.

Feverishness, headache, and malaise. Vague complaints of feverishness, headache, and malaise, although not necessarily occurring together, can be treated with the same remedies. Aspirin or acetaminophen, in the proper dosage, is usually effective. In conjunction with fluids and rest, aspirin or acetaminophen is very useful because of its analgesic/antipyretic properties as well as the "psychological" boost of these measures. Clinical fever is seldom associated with the common cold, and the benefit of the antipyretic property of aspirin and acetaminophen is doubtful. However, when fever is present and persists for over 24 hours, a physician should be consulted. In the interim, aspirin or acetaminophen (preferably acetaminophen in infants and small children, where there is a greater risk of aspirin toxicity) should be given. If fever persists in spite of these medical measures, the patient should be sponged or bathed in cool or tepid, not cold, water. The use of diluted isopropyl alcohol (e.g., 50:50 in water) has also been recommended as adjunctive antipyretic therapy. In spite of this sponging solution's proven effectiveness, its use has been associated with two drawbacks.[9] First, coma following acute alcohol poisoning has been reported in patients sponged with isopropyl alcohol, and second, it has been found that there is a significantly greater degree of discomfort associated with its use when compared to tepid water.[9, 10] It is the authors' opinion, therefore, that the most rational approach to fever reduction is aspirin (acetaminophen in children) followed by tepid water sponging.

The need for physician-directed treatment is usually unnecessary unless there is some concern that the patient has something other than a cold, the symptoms are severe, or secondary complications are present or suspected. Severely debilitated patients, however, should seek advice from their physicians as should patients with other chronic disorders (e.g., emphysema) in which a respiratory infection may pose serious problems or where the usual nonprescription remedies may be contraindicated.

Allergic rhinitis

Etiology and pathophysiology

Allergic rhinitis may begin at almost any age, although the incidence of first onset is greatest in children and young adults and decreases with increasing age. Heredity seems to play a role. Allergic rhinitis itself is not genetically transmitted; however, the heightened predisposition to become sensitized following exposure to adequate concentrations of an allergen is generally transferred.[6]

Pollens from plants that depend on the wind for cross-pollination and mold spores are the main agents responsible for seasonal allergic rhinitis. Ragweed pollen accounts for about 75 percent of seasonal rhinitis patients in the U.S.; grass pollens, 40 percent; and tree pollens, about 9 percent. Approximately 25 percent suffer from both grass and ragweed allergic rhinitis, and about 5 percent suffer from all three allergies.[11] The seasonal appearance of symptoms is a reflection of the pollen or spores in the air. Of the airborne mild spores, *Alternaria* and *Hormodendrum* are the most common and also may be causative agents of seasonal allergic rhinitis.[12] These spores are most prevalent from mid-March to late November. Tree pollination begins in late March and extends to early June. Grasses generally pollinate from mid-May to mid-July. Ragweed pollen has a long season, extending from early August to early October or to the first killing frost. For a particular plant in a given locale, the pollinating season is relatively constant from year to year. Weather conditions such as temperature and rainfall influence the amount of pollen produced but not the actual onset or termination of a specific season.[6] Thus, appearance of seasonal allergic rhinitis symptoms is influenced by the geographic location of the patient and the specific hypersensitivities.

Symptoms of perennial allergic rhinitis are usually caused by house dust, animal dander, and feathers. Occupational causes may include wheat flour, various grains, cotton and flax seeds, and enzymes used in detergents. The continued presence of the allergens results in patient symptoms which are persistent more or less year round.

The symptoms of allergic rhinitis may be due to many different etiological allergens. These allergens, which are primarily protein in nature, may, when deposited on the nasal mucosa, initiate an inflammatory response by the body and produce symptoms that are characteristic of allergic rhinitis. The pathologic inflammatory process of seasonal allergic rhinitis develops within minutes after an allergen is deposited on the mucous membrane of the nose of an allergy-prone individual. Pollen itself is not believed to be directly antigenic. However, the lysozyme component of nasal mucus has the ability to degrade the pollen cell wall to allow for the release of the proteinaceous contents. This released protein may be an antigen. The antigen stimulates lymphoid tissue in the respiratory tract to produce a specific type of immunoglobulin, IgE (reagin). These reaginic antibodies have a special affinity for circulating basophils and tissue mast cells. The cells pick up many IgE molecules on their surfaces and, thus, become sensitized. Subsequent exposure to the same antigen, by its deposition on nasal mucosa, causes an antigen-antibody reaction, resulting in the release of vasoactive chemical mediators. These mediators include histamine, slow-reacting substances of anaphylaxis, eosinophilic chemotactic factor, and possibly others.

The nasal mucosa is particularly vulnerable to this immediate type of allergic reaction because the allergen is deposited directly where it may act locally and because the mediators are very active vasodilators and are released in an area that is highly vascularized. The immediate effects are vasodilatation, increased vascular permeability, and increased secretion of mucus, all of which are responsible for the symptoms.

In the perennial form of the disease, the symptoms are more persistent. The histopathological changes that occur are initially identical to those found in seasonal allergic rhinitis. With the persistent disease, however, more chronic and irreversible changes such as thickening of the mucosal epithelium, connective tissue proliferation, loss of epithelial cilia, and development of polyps of the nose or sinuses may be noted.

Signs and symptoms

The major symptoms of allergic rhinitis are edema and those resulting from the engorgement of the nasal mucosa—sneezing, rhinorrhea, nasal pruritus, and nasal congestion are the most common. Sudden sneezing attacks may consist of 10 to 20 sneezes in rapid succession.

The rhinorrhea is typically a watery, thin discharge which might be quite profuse and continuous. Purulent discharge does not occur in uncomplicated allergic rhinitis; its presence indicates a secondary infection. The nasal congestion of allergic rhinitis is due to swollen turbinates. If the nasal obstruction is severe, it may result in headaches or earaches. With continuous, severe nasal congestion, a loss of smell and taste might occur. Itching of the nose might also be a prominent feature, particularly in children, and causes frequent rubbing of the nose.

Eye symptoms are commonly associated with allergic rhinitis. These conjunctival symptoms include itching and lacrimation. They are caused by the trapping of pollen grains in the conjunctival sac and subsequent antigen-antibody reaction as well as possible congestion of the lacrimal ducts caused indirectly by the nasal congestion. Patients with severe eye symptoms often complain of photophobia and sore, tired eyes. Dark circles or a greater than normal discoloration beneath the eyes is called "allergic shiners." This symptom is more common in perennial rhinitis than in the seasonal variant.

A characteristic of seasonal allergic rhinitis is the periodicity of its appearance. A careful history of the patient indicates when the symptoms first began and the intervals at which they were exacerbated. With seasonal rhinitis, the allergic reaction often begins with sneezing and progresses to rhinorrhea; the rhinorrhea may progress to severe nasal obstruction, at which time sneezing may be absent and rhinorrhea minimal. Perennial rhinitis is more likely to begin with nasal obstruction and postnasal discharge rather than sneezing and rhinorrhea.[13]

The symptoms of allergic rhinitis may exhibit periodicity even within the season. Most patients tend to exhibit more intense symptoms in the morning hours and on windy days due to the increased amount of pollen in the air. Symptoms may diminish when it is raining because of the clearing of pollen from the air.

It is more difficult to associate perennial rhinitis than seasonal rhinitis with the environment; the patient history is not as helpful in these cases. The most common perennial allergens are house dust and dander of household pets which may be in contact with the patients during all seasons.

Generally, allergic rhinitis tends to show an increase in its severity of symptoms for 2 to 3 years until a somewhat stabilized condition is reached. With seasonal allergic rhinitis, symptoms then tend to be exacerbated annually. There is no effective means of predicting if symptoms will increase or decrease in severity. In fact, for reasons that are not well understood, hypersensitivity may disappear after several years. The pharmacist can differentiate seasonal allergic rhinitis from the perennial allergic rhinitis by questioning the patient concerning the appearance and disappearance of symptoms. The treatment is similar with both of these conditions. Most commonly, however, patients experiencing the perennial allergic rhinitis are under the care of a physician due to the duration of symptoms.

Complications

Patients with allergic rhinitis may develop complications due to chronic nasal inflammation including recurrent otitis media with hearing loss, sinusitis, and nasal or sinus polyps. Complications of allergic rhinitis seem to be more prominent in children. Nasal allergy in children also leads to bony structural changes in the palate and a depression of the prominence of the cheek bones. The resulting crowding of incisor teeth is called the "Gothic Arch." Children with chronic, recurrent rhinitis may develop a hearing impairment because of the involvement of the eustachian tubes and middle ear. Often a child develops a characteristic manner of rubbing the nose to relieve the itching and to spread the nasal wall to produce better nasal ventilation. This persistent rubbing is called the "allergic salute."

Another possible complication of seasonal rhinitis, especially in children, is its progression to asthma or other atopic disorders. Although asthma is difficult to predict, allergic rhinitis and asthmatic attacks can often be precipitated by the same agents. If the symptoms of allergic rhinitis are prolonged, a slight cough and a feeling of constriction in the chest or asthmatic wheezing may follow. These are dangerous signals—a warning of the possible onset of asthma. Because one-third or more of all patients with allergic rhinitis may develop asthma, these signs should be the basis for directing the patient to a physician for diagnosis and treatment.[14] Perennial allergic rhinitis is associated with chronic symptoms which may lead to anatomical changes within the nasal and sinus cavities. The resulting complications include loss of epithelial cilia and development of nasal polyps. Because of the chronic nature of the symptoms and the development of these complications, all perennial allergic rhinitis sufferers should be under a physician's care.

Treatment

The treatment of allergic rhinitis involves the avoidance of allergens to prevent the immunologic response; immunological treatment to alter the immunologic response to the allergens; and pharmacological treatment to minimize or counteract the consequences of the immunologic response once it has occurred. In most cases of allergic rhinitis, total avoidance of the allergen is difficult because airborne allergens are so widely distributed and, in most cases, patients are sensitive to more than one allergen. However, avoidance of certain situations (burning leaves, sleeping with bedroom windows open, driving in the countryside at those times of the year when pollen counts are especially high) decreases exposure to environments or situations which increase the possibility of encountering potential allergens. If they are changed regularly (e.g., monthly), the mechanical filters in most air conditioners help reduce the number of allergens if doors and windows are kept closed and the air is recirculated. An electrostatic precipitator in conjunction with a central heating and air conditioning unit is even more effective in reducing house dust and other potential allergens.

When a brief exposure to an allergen cannot be avoided, a proper face mask will effectively filter the inhaled air. Such masks are sold by industrial or scientific supply firms for protection against noxious dust. Gauze masks which are commonly used are useless. The pharmacist can reinforce or educate the patient concerning specific measures mentioned above that decrease the likelihood of exposure to the offending allergen.

Immunotherapy attempts to raise a person's threshold for symptoms following exposure to the allergen. Although the mechanisms of immunotherapy are not completely understood, it is believed that blocking antibodies are produced by allergen injections which result in an increased allergen tolerance. The indications for immunotherapy, a relatively long-term treatment modality, are relative rather than absolute. For example, if a patient's symptoms are mild and last only for a few weeks, the patient may be well managed by symptomatic therapy alone. For those whose reaction to the allergens is much more severe or who cannot tolerate symptomatic treatment, immunotherapy may be considered.

Immunotherapy begins with the proper identification of the offending allergen. This is most commonly done by skin tests that measure the patient's response to the intracutaneous introduction of test allergens. Following the identification of the offending allergen, an extract is administered by injection to the patient in small amounts at frequent intervals. Most studies indicate that in pollen allergy 70 to 80 percent of the patients treated with immunotherapy experience beneficial results.[6, 15, 16] Immunotherapy does not cure the disease but reduces the number of symptoms, making it easier to control the allergy by symptomatic medication. Patients who experience allergic rhinitis symptoms throughout the year, whose allergic reactions tend to be severe, and who do not demonstrate a beneficial response from self-medication may be candidates for immunotherapy and should be advised by the pharmacist to seek the aid of a physician.

During the hay fever season, patients who have not received specific immunotherapy or have not obtained adequate relief require drug treatment designed to lessen the discomfort. The pharmacological classes of agents that are most commonly used are antihistamines, decongestants, and corticosteroids. The antihistamines are valuable because they counteract the effects of histamine released as a result of the allergen-antibody reaction. Decongestants provide relief from the nasal congestion that accompanies the rhinitis.

Ingredients in OTC products

Antihistamines

Histamine is a common biogenic amine found in every tissue in the body; most, however, is found in the mast cells. In these cells, histamine is localized and stored in granules and generally becomes active only when the cells are lysed. It can be released and exert its effects as a result of an antigen-antibody reaction (e.g., allergy) or physical damage (e.g., trauma, infection). The most significant effects of histamine are on the cardiovascular system, exocrine glands, and smooth muscles. Its major effects in the common cold and allergic rhinitis are the ability to cause profound vasodilatation, increased capillary permeability, and edema. These effects of histamine are more pronounced in highly vascularized areas such as the nose.

Histamine is released in both the common cold and allergy, but the actual cause of its release and the amount released is different and, therefore, the magnitude of its contribution to the symptoms is different between the two disorders. In the case of hay fever, the antigen-antibody reaction leads to cellular damage of specific sensitized cells (e.g., mast cells) and consequent release of histamine that initiates the local, inflammatory response. In the case of a cold, the local inflammatory response results from widespread cell injury caused by virus particle invasion. Therefore, the vasodilatation and resultant edema associated with a cold cannot be attributed solely to histamine release but also (and perhaps predominantly) to the body's inflammatory defense and the release of inflammatory mediators other than histamine.

Antihistamines are chemical agents that exert their effect in the body primarily by preventing or blocking the actions of histamine at receptor sites.[17 18] They are, therefore, classified as "pharmacological antagonists" of histamine with a mechanism of action analogous to other pharmacological antagonists such as the antiadrenergics and anticholinergics. They do not prevent histamine release and, because they act by competitive inhibition, if the histamine concentration at the receptor site exceeds the concentration of the drug, the effects of histamine occur. Although the antihistaminic activity is the dominant effect of these agents, the antihistamines possess a structural similarity to other pharmacologic classes of drugs (e.g., anticholinergic, local anesthetic, ganglionic-blocking, and adrenergic-blocking agents) and exert various combinations and degrees of side effects. In some cases the side effects have been used to achieve a therapeutic goal, e.g., CNS depression for insomnia and local anesthetic effects for pruritus. However, these side effects, especially drowsiness, can be bothersome and potentially dangerous.

The most commonly used nonprescription antihistamines and their usual dosage are shown in Table 4. Brompheniramine maleate (which has been recommended for OTC status), chlorpheniramine maleate, methapyrilene hydrochloride, phenindamine tartrate, pheniramine maleate, doxylamine succinate, and pyrilamine maleate are recognized by the FDA OTC Panel on Cold, Cough, Allergy, Bronchodilator, and Anti-Asthmatic Drugs as safe for OTC use and effective in suppressing the symptoms of allergic rhinitis when taken in the dosage specified. Conclusive evidence is still lacking as to the safety and effectiveness of phenyltoloxamine. *(This chapter contains references to the Panel's report. The reader should be aware that the FDA Commissioner has disagreed with some of the Panel's recommendations. Proposed regulations based on the Panel's report have not been published by FDA as of this writing.)*

The antihistamines are most effective in controlling seasonal allergic rhinitis.[19] They are less effective in perennial allergic rhinitis and are rarely effective in vasomotor rhinitis.

Some people who regularly take antihistamines may find that they do not obtain the same degree of relief after a period of weeks or months. The reason for this apparent decreased effectiveness is that some antihistamines are capable of hepatic enzyme induction, resulting in an increase of metabolism in the liver. The enzyme induction has also implicated antihistamines as a possible cause of diminished effectiveness of several other types of drugs. However, the clinical significance of such interactions is open to question. The various classes of antihistamines differ in their capacity to induce hepatic enzymes. Therefore, because only a few antihistamines have been studied in this regard, when tolerance develops, switching to a different antihistamine is a practical recommendation.

In spite of the fact that antihistamines have no ability to prevent or abort the common cold, they are found in almost all cold remedies. Their widespread inclusion in these products probably stems from their anticholinergic action, which decreases the amount of mucus secretion, relieving the rhinorrhea. Although some people experience this "drying" effect, the anticholinergic activity of the antihistamines is actually very weak, and this action may be insignificant at the dosage levels of the various nonprescription preparations.

In general, the antihistamines possess a high therapeutic index (toxic dose/therapeutic dose), and serious toxicities are seldom noted in adults. At recommended labeled doses the antihistamines are also safe for use in children. As with most drugs, however, accidental overdose in children can lead to profound symptoms. Symptoms of antihistamine overdose in children are excitement, ataxia, incoordination, muscular twitching, generalized convulsion with pupillary dilation, and flushing of the skin. The treatment of acute overdose of antihistamine is symptomatic and usually requires supportive therapy with artificial respiration.

The major contraindication to the use of an antihistamine—the sedative properties of the agent—is a relative one. There are varying degrees of drowsiness associated with all antihistamines depending on the chemical class of the agent. The ethanolamines (e.g., diphenhydramine hydrochloride) have a pronounced tendency to induce sedation. The alkylamines (e.g., chlorpheniramine maleate), on the other hand, possess minimal sedative properties, and the ethylenediamines (e.g., pyrilamine maleate, methapyrilene hydrochloride) are approximately intermediate in their sedative properties.[19] Although most individuals acquire a tolerance to this effect, it would appear that the alkylamine group would, in most cases, be the more suitable agents for daytime use.[19] Should drowsiness persist, a dosage reduction or switching to another antihistamine may alleviate the problem. If a person's job or other activities require a high degree of mental alertness, these drugs must be used cautiously until their effect can be determined by the individual. The effects of alcohol and other CNS depressants including hypnotics, sedatives, analgesics, and antianxiety agents can be potentiated by the antihistamines. If concurrent administration is necessary, caution must be exercised due to the increased possibility of drowsiness.[19 20]

The anticholinergic properties of an antihistamine may predominate in some individuals. A paradoxical effect is frequently seen in children in which CNS stimulation rather than depression predominates, causing insomnia, nervousness, and irritability. For this reason antihistamines must be used cautiously in children who have convulsive disorders.[16] Antihistamines can cause dry mouth, blurred vision, urinary retention (in older males suffering from an enlarged prostate), and constipation as a result of their anticholinergic effects; these effects, however, are usually associated with high doses. Because of the drying effect on respiratory secretions and potential airway obstruction, some practitioners believe that antihistamines should not be given to asthmatics.[21] The agents may be useful, however, in special situations.[2] The cholinergic-blocking properties of the antihistamines may pose a problem for patients whose glaucoma is being controlled with an anticholinesterase. Such an effect is unpredictable, but because of the potential consequences, a patient being treated for narrow-angle glaucoma should probably receive antihistamines only when prescribed by a physician.

The cholinergic-blocking effect of the antihistamines has an additive effect with anticholinergic drugs. Although the effects of excessive cholinergic blockade are usually of minor clinical significance, effects such as urinary retention, constipation, and dry mouth may be bothersome.

Hypersensitivity reactions may develop with the antihistamines, but this is more common with topical application than with oral use.[19]

Topical decongestants

Various sympathomimetic amines have been used to provide relief from the nasal stuffiness of colds and allergic rhinitis. These drugs, which differ primarily in their duration of action, are contained in many of the nonprescription products promoted for hay fever and colds. Nasal decongestants stimulate the α-adrenergic receptors of the vascular smooth muscle, constricting the dilated network of arterioles within the nasal mucosa and reducing the flow of blood in the engorged edematous nasal area. This constriction results in a shrinkage of the engorged mucous membranes which promotes drainage, improves nasal ventilation, relieves the feeling of stuffiness, and helps to diminish pain resulting from nasal engorgement.

The ideal topical decongestant agent should have a prompt and prolonged effect. It should not produce systemic side effects, irritation to the mucosa with resultant harmful effects on the cilia of the respiratory tract, or rebound congestion. An ideal, topical sympathomimetic amine has not yet been found.[22]

The intranasal application of commercially available decongestants provides a prompt and dramatic decrease of the nasal congestion. The shrinking of the mucous

Table 4. Antihistamine Dosage[a]

Drug (by chemical class) and category	Dosage		
	Adults	*Children* 6–12 years	2–6 years
Ethanolamines			
Diphenhydramine hydrochloride (I)	25–50 mg every 4–6 hr (not to exceed 300 mg/24 hr)	12.5–25 mg every 4–6 hr (not to exceed 150 mg/24 hr)	6.25 mg every 4–6 hr (not to exceed 37.5 mg/24 hr)
Doxylamine succinate (I)	7.5-12.5 mg every 4-6 hr (not to exceed 75 mg/24 hr)	3.75–6.25 mg every 4–6 hr (not to exceed) 37.5 mg/24 hr)	Professional labeling only: 1.9 - 3.125 mg every 4-6 hr (not to exceed 18.75 mg / 24 hr)
Phenyltoloxamine citrate (III)	50 mg every 4–6 hr (not to exceed 300 mg/24 hr)	Information inadequate to establish dosage	
Ethylenediamines			
Methapyrilene (I)	50 mg every 4–6 hr (not to exceed 300 mg/24 hr)	25 mg every 4–6 hr (not to exceed 150 mg/24 hr)	12.5 mg every 4–6 hr (not to exceed 75 mg/24 hr)
Pyrilamine maleate (I)	25–50 mg every 6–8 hr (not to exceed 200 mg/24 hr)	12.5–25 mg every 6–8 hr (not to exceed 100 mg/24 hr)	6.25–12.5 mg every 6–8 hr (not to exceed 50 mg/24 hr)
Thonzylamine hydrochloride (I)	50–100 mg every 4–6 hr (not to exceed 600 mg/24 hr)	25–50 mg every 4–6 hr (not to exceed 300 mg/24 hr)	12.5–25 mg every 4–6 hr (not to exceed 150 mg/24 hr)
Alkylamines			
Pheniramine maleate (I)	12.5–25 mg every 4–6 hr (not to exceed 150 mg/24 hr)	6.25–12 mg every 4–6 hr (not to exceed 75 mg/24 hr)	3.125–6.25 mg every 4–6 hr (not to exceed 37.5 mg/24 hr)
Brompheniramine maleate (I)	4 mg every 4–6 hr (not to exceed 24 mg/24 hr)	2 mg every 4–6 hr (not to exceed 12 mg/24 hr)	1 mg every 4–6 hr (not to exceed 6 mg/24 hr)
Chlorpheniramine maleate (I)	4 mg every 4–6 hr (not to exceed 24 mg/24 hr)	2 mg every 4–6 hr (not to exceed 12 mg/24 hr)	1 mg every 4–6 hr (not to exceed 6 mg/24 hr)
Miscellaneous			
Phenindamine tartrate (I)	25 mg every 4–6 hr (not to exceed 150 mg/24 hr)	12.5 mg every 4–6 hr (not to exceed 75 mg/24 hr)	6.25 mg every 4–6 hr (not to exceed 37.5 mg/24 hr)

[a] As proposed by the FDA OTC Panel on Cold, Cough, Allergy, Bronchodilator, and Anti-Asthmatic Drugs.

membrane not only makes breathing easier but also permits the sinus cavities to drain. Unfortunately, the OTC topical sympathomimetic vasoconstrictors provide only temporary relief.

It is very important that the patient follow the label directions as to frequency and duration of use. The topical application of these drugs is often followed by a rebound phenomenon (rhinitis medicamentosa)—the nasal mucous membranes become even more congested and edematous as the vasoconstrictor effect of the drug subsides. This secondary congestion is believed to result from ischemia caused by the drug's intensive local vasoconstriction and local irritation of the topically applied agent itself. If the use of a topical nasal decongestant is restricted to 3 or 4 days or less, the rebound congestion is minimal; with chronic use and/or overuse of these agents, rebound nasal stuffiness can become quite pronounced. This rebound phenomenon represents a vicious cycle because it leads to more frequent use of the agent that causes it. To determine the possible existence of this condition, the pharmacist should question a patient concerning the prior use of nasal sprays, drops, or inhalants. If, in the pharmacist's judgment, the patient experiences this rebound phenomenon, topical decongestant therapy should be discontinued and systemic decongestants and/or an isotonic saline drop should be used.

The patient should be instructed on the proper administration of topical decongestants to obtain maximum relief without encountering side effects from the systemic absorption of the drug. Nasal decongestant sprays are packaged in flexible plastic containers that produce a fine mist when squeezed. The patient should administer nasal sprays in the upright position, squeezing once into each nostril. The nose should be blown to remove the mucus 3 to 5 minutes after the initial administration of the spray. If there is still some congestion, another dose should be administered at this time which should reach further into the nasal cavities and to the surfaces of the turbinates.

Some people may prefer to administer the decongestant solution with a nasal atomizer. Most commercial spray containers are designed to deliver the approximate dose with one squeeze; the atomizer, however, is not so calibrated. Also, using an atomizer may increase the possibility of contamination of the solution. If the patient prefers to use a nasal atomizer, instructions should be provided as to the proper use of the particular atomizer including the liquid level and proper placement within the nostril. The patient should be instructed to remove the solution and rinse the atomizer after use to guard against solution contamination. Naphazoline solutions should not be used in atomizers containing aluminum parts because a degradation of the drug may result.

Nasal drops usually do not cover the entire nasal mucosa and may pass to the pharynx where they may be swallowed. Although systemic absorption from the nasal mucosa is minimal due to the local vasoconstriction induced by the drug, if an excess amount drains through the nasal passage and is swallowed, absorption and systemic effects are then possible. Swallowing the medication may be minimized by proper administration. To administer nasal drops, the patient should recline on a bed with the head tilted back over the edge or recline on the side, holding the head lower than the shoulders. The drops should be placed in the lower nostril without touching the nasal surface with the dropper. After the drops have been instilled into each nostril, the patient should breathe through the mouth and remain in the reclining position for about 5 minutes. To ensure spread of the medication, the head may be turned from side to side while reclining. The pharmacist should realize that a topical decongestant in a spray form is probably more convenient for adults and older children. Sprays may also afford better decongestion by reaching greater areas of the mucous membranes. Drops are the most effective means of administering a topical decongestant to infants and children under 6 because of their smaller nostril openings.

There are several agents commonly used as topical nasal decongestants. The primary difference lies in their intensity and duration of action.

Phenylephrine hydrochloride. Phenylephrine hydrochloride is one of the most effective OTC topical nasal decongestants.[23] It is commonly applied as three or four drops or one or two sprays of a 0.25- to 0.5-percent solution every 4 hours. This agent may produce a marked irritation of the nasal mucosa in some individuals. The irritation is additional to the irritation already present from the pathological condition of the allergic disorder or cold.

Phenylephrine hydrochloride is also commercially available as an aqueous jelly. A small amount of the jelly is placed in each nostril and snuffed well back into the nasal passage. This procedure is not convenient and is not widely used. Nasal decongestants in jelly form are used most commonly by otolaryngologists for office examination or treatment. A more prolonged decongestant effect may be achieved with nasal jellies, which may have an emollient and protective action on the nasal mucosa.[24]

Naphazoline hydrochloride. Naphazoline hydrochloride is a more potent vasoconstrictor than phenylephrine hydrochloride. It produces CNS depression rather than stimulation when it is absorbed systemically. This agent is not recommended for use with children, who commonly swallow nasally administered medications (especially drops). Naphazoline hydrochloride is available as a 0.05- to 0.1-percent solution. It is commonly administered as one to three drops every 4 to 6 hours. It is irritating to the mucosa and may sting when administered.

Oxymetazoline and xylometazoline hydrochlorides. Longer acting topical nasal decongestants, such as oxymetazoline hydrochloride and xylometazoline hydrochloride, have a decongestant effect which may last for as long as 6 hours, with a gradual decline thereafter.[25] [26] Due to their longer duration, these agents are less likely to be overused. Because they are used only twice a day, the incidence of rebound congestion and the development of rhinitis medicamentosa are decreased. These two long-acting agents have been recommended for OTC status by the Panel.[27]

Levodesoxyephedrine and propylhexedrine. These sympathomimetic amines are commonly used in inhalants. They cause constriction of the vessels in the nasal mucosa. There is a lack of controlled studies that compare the efficacy and safety of these aromatic amines to other nasal decongestants. The use of these volatile substances through an inhaler seems to be an efficient and convenient way of reaching the desired areas of the nasal mucosa, provided there is some airflow through the nose.

One problem is the loss of the agent when the cap is not properly replaced. Also, there may not be sufficient nasal airflow to distribute the agent throughout the nasal cavity. These agents have been implicated as being irritating to the nasal mucosa and as interfering with ciliary action. When overused, they share the side effects of local irritation and rebound congestion with the other topical amines.

Oral decongestants

The oral administration of the sympathomimetic amines distributes the drug via the systemic circulation to the vascular bed of the nasal mucosa. The oral decongestant agents have the advantage of a longer duration of action. However, they cause less intense vasoconstriction than the topically applied sprays or drops. The oral agents have not been associated with rebound congestion or rhinitis medicamentosa because of their lesser degree of vasoconstriction and the lack of local drug irritation.[19]

These agents, of course, do not exert their action exclusively on the vasculature of the nasal mucosa; in doses large enough to bring about nasal decongestion, they also affect other vascular beds.[19] Although the vasoconstriction produced by oral decongestants usually does not increase blood pressure, individuals who are predisposed to hypertension may experience a change in blood pressure. These decongestants may cause cardiac stimulation and the development of arrhythmias in individuals predisposed to these conditions. In a prediabetic or a brittle or juvenile diabetic, the administration of sympathomimetics may be a problem because they increase the blood sugar level. Labeling instructions on products containing sympathomimetics should indicate that patients with hypertension, hyperthyroidism, diabetes mellitus, or ischemic heart disease should use these products only on the advice of a physician (see section on patient considerations). Sympathomimetic amines should not be administered to patients on monoamine oxidase inhibitor (MAOI) therapy because a hypertensive crisis may result. They should be used cautiously in hypertensive patients who are stabilized on guanethidine, bethanidine, or debrisoquin sulfate.[28] These warnings pertain only to the oral agent, not to topically applied drugs.

Ephedrine, phenylpropanolamine hydrochloride, phenylephrine hydrochloride, and pseudoephedrine are sympathomimetic amines commonly incorporated into cold and allergy products.

Ephedrine. Ephedrine is more effective as a bronchodilator for asthma than as a nasal decongestant. It has oral nasal decongestant activity, but it is much more effective used topically. Orally, in doses of 25 to 50 mg every 3 to 4 hours, ephedrine relieves nasal congestion associated with hay fever and relaxes muscle spasm in bronchial asthma. These effects usually appear within 30 minutes to 1 hour following oral administration. Ephedrine has CNS stimulatory effects. Several commercial preparations incorporate a mild CNS depressant in the formulation to overcome this side effect.

Phenylpropanolamine hydrochloride. Phenylpropanolamine hydrochloride resembles ephedrine in its action but is somewhat more active as a vasoconstrictor and less active as a CNS stimulant and bronchodilator. Oral doses of 25 to 50 mg three times daily are recommended for the symptomatic treatment of nasal congestion. The peak effect occurs approximately 3 hours after administration.

Phenylephrine hydrochloride. Phenylephrine hydrochloride in doses of 10 mg every 4 hours is recommended. This drug is rapidly hydrolyzed in the GI tract, and the amount delivered to the bloodstream via the oral route is hard to predict. For this reason, it is more commonly used topically than orally.[23]

Pseudoephedrine. Pseudoephedrine is another effective vasoconstrictor. It has less vasopressor action than ephedrine and causes little CNS stimulation. The dose for adults and older children is 60 mg three or four times daily; for children 6 to 12 years old, it is 30 mg three or four times daily; and for those 2 to 5 years old, 15 mg three or four times daily. The peak effect of a 60-mg dose occurs approximately 4 hours after administration.

Antitussives: expectorants, suppressants

The cough associated with the common cold may be either productive or nonproductive (dry cough).

The productive cough is useful and essential if it facilitates the removal of accumulated secretions and debris (phlegm) from the lower tract. It is worth noting that, although it is expected, a patient with "chest congestion" does not necessarily expectorate phlegm ("productive" cough) during coughing. It would be inappropriate, however, to describe the cough as "nonproductive" because this description usually is related to dry, noncongested coughing. For the sake of distinction in this section as well as rationale for product selection later, a cough will be either:

- ☐ Congested/productive: cough associated with the expectoration of phlegm.
- ☐ Congested/nonproductive: cough associated with chest congestion and scant expectoration of phlegm.
- ☐ Dry/nonproductive: cough not associated with chest congestion.

By referring to these categories the pharmacist will be able to determine when and which type of an antitussive agent should be used.

Excessive coughing, particularly if it is dry and nonproductive, is not only discomforting but also tends to be self-perpetuating because the rapid air expulsion further irritates the tracheal and pharyngeal mucosa. The general types of antitussive agents available for self-medication are expectorants and cough suppressants. Table 5 indicates the sites at which the cough reflex can be blocked as well as the mechanism of the agents.

Expectorants. These agents are administered orally to stimulate the flow of respiratory tract secretions.[19 29] They are indicated when there is difficulty in removing endobronchial secretions or accumulated phlegm. By stimulating the flow of mucus, the thickened accumulated secretions in the lower tract are diluted, decreasing their viscosity and facilitating their removal via ciliary action and coughing. Such an effect also provides a soothing, demulcent coating to irritated mucosal areas. The removal of the accumulations and the demulcent effect on irritated mucous membranes indirectly promote cough suppression.

Fluid intake and maintaining adequate humidity of the inspired air are important to respiratory tract fluid production, and, therefore, constitute an essential component of the therapy of a cold. These measures can be accomplished by increasing fluid intake and by using a cool mist or hot steam vaporizer, especially for a congested cough.

Expectorant drugs are thought to act by direct stimulation (terpin hydrate) of secretory glands of the lower respiratory tract and by reflex stimulation (ammonium chloride, ipecac, and guaifenesin) of respiratory secretions by a direct irritating effect on the gastric mucosa. Potassium iodide, although not used for self-medication, is thought to act both reflexly and directly.[19]

The use of expectorants in clinical practice is a highly controversial issue revolving around doubts as to their therapeutic efficacy. This controversy stems from the lack of objective experimental data that show that an expectorant decreases sputum viscosity or eases expectoration more than a placebo. In fact, in spite of the widespread use of guaifenesin, one study states that "from a scientific point of view . . . , (this drug) probably has no rational use in clinical medicine as an expectorant."[29] Other literature also questions the efficacy of expectorants, stating that "the use of expectorants is based primarily on tradition and the widespread subjective clinical impression that they are effective."[19] The apparent difficulty in accumulating objective evidence stems from: a) insufficient evidence as to which physicochemical property of respiratory secretions correlates best with ease of expectoration and b) lack of appropriate techniques and instrumentation.[30]

Subjective findings constitute the basis for the continued use of expectorants. In fact, the FDA OTC Panel on Cold, Cough, Allergy, Bronchodilator and Anti-Asthmatic Drugs has stated that "until such objective methods become available, the Panel will consider well-controlled, double-blind subjective studies in the assessment of efficacy."[31] Using these subjective data, Table 6 lists the usual dose and dosage range of the most commonly used expectorants.

There are no apparent absolute contraindications to the use of orally administered expectorants. The toxicity associated with expectorant drugs varies between agents. In general, the most common adverse effect to anticipate is gastric upset. Guaifenesin (glyceryl guaiacolate) is seldom associated with gastric upset and nausea. When it is used in doses larger than those recommended by the manufacturer, it has been shown to reduce the ability of platelets to agglutinate (*in vitro*), resulting in longer clotting time, but this does not seem to be clinically significant.[27,29]

Ammonium chloride can cause serious illness in a healthy person if 50 g or more is ingested. In the presence of renal, hepatic, or chronic heart disease, doses of 5 g have caused severe poisoning.[32] A relative contraindication exists when using ammonium chloride in patients with hepatic, renal, or pulmonary insufficiency; larger than recommended doses may be predisposing to metabolic acidosis. Due to ammonium chloride's ability to acidify the urine, it has the potential for affecting the excretion of other drugs from the body.[28] This probably is not significant because the usual daily dosage range as a systemic acidifier is 4 to 12 g.[33]

Cough suppressants. Suppressants are indicated when a cough becomes hyperactive, especially when it is the dry/nonproductive type.[19,34] The mechanism by which the narcotic and nonnarcotic agents affect the intensity and frequency of a cough is a relatively selective depressant effect on the cough control center in the medulla.

Codeine. Codeine is considered the most useful narcotic antitussive agent and is the drug of choice.[15] The dependence liability of codeine is much less than that of morphine, but tolerance and addiction can occur when taken in excessive amounts. The average adult antitussive dose is 15 mg (with a range of 10 to 20 mg). At this dosage codeine provides effective cough relief. (See Table 7 for children's dosage.) Stringent controls have been placed on codeine-containing nonprescription products as a result of their abuse potential. When used in recommended amounts for short periods, the danger of psychological and physical dependence is minimal. The respiratory depressant effect of codeine is about one-fourth that of morphine. Even when the dose is increased, commensurate increase in respiratory depression does not necessarily occur. In doses commonly used for cough in an otherwise healthy person, the effects on respiration are not apparent. Codeine exerts a drying effect on the respiratory mucosa which may be an advantage during the common cold; in asthma or emphysema, this drying effect may be detrimental due to increased viscosity of respiratory fluids.[34]

In clinical practice the adverse effects most commonly encountered with codeine include nausea, drowsiness, and constipation. Allergic reactions and pruritus may also occur but are not as common. In general, antitussive doses of codeine are well tolerated by adults and children.

Codeine may enhance the effects of oral anticoagulants, but this is probably not significant with short-term antitussive doses. The CNS depressant effect of codeine is additive to that of other CNS depressants, and such agents should be used cautiously when given concurrently.

The contraindications to the use of codeine include its use in individuals with chronic pulmonary disease, where mucosal drying and slight respiratory depression (unlikely at recommended doses) can be detrimental. Codeine should be avoided by patients who have experienced codeine-induced allergic manifestations (e.g., pruritus, rash). In summary, codeine is safe and effective when used as directed for cough.

Dextromethorphan hydrobromide. Dextromethorphan is a derivative of levorphanol, but, unlike its analgesic counterpart, it has no significant analgesic properties and does not depress respiration or predispose to addiction.[34] Some investigators believe that dextromethorphan and codeine are equipotent; others give a slight edge to codeine.[34] Unlike codeine, increasing the dose of dextromethorphan to 30 mg does not increase its antitussive effects but does prolong the effects over a period of 8 to 12 hours.[34] Such an effect is especially beneficial when a hyperactive cough interrupts sleep.

Adverse effects produced by dextromethorphan hydrobromide are mild and infrequent. Drowsiness and GI upset are the most common complaints. Accidental poisonings in children have resulted in stuporousness and disturbances in gait, with rapid recovery after emesis.[34]

Dextromethorphan hydrobromide is a safe and effective antitussive for which there are no apparent contraindications unless, of course, the patient is hypersensitive to it.[27]

Diphenhydramine hydrochloride. Diphenhydramine hydrochloride, a potent antihistamine, is a safe and effective antitussive.[27] The OTC Panel has recommended that it be available as an OTC cough suppressant.

Objective results of clinical studies have indicated that diphenhydramine, in 25- and 50-mg doses, significantly reduced coughing in chronic cough patients.[35] The recommended adult dose is 25 mg every 4 hours, not to exceed 150 mg in 24 hours (see Table 7).

The adverse effects associated with diphenhydramine hydrochloride are typical of other antihistamines. The most commonly encountered adverse effects are sedation and anticholinergic effects [diphenhydramine hydrochloride (Benadryl) also has FDA approval as a sedative and antiparkinsonian agent]. Because of these properties, diphenhydramine hydrochloride should not be taken by individuals in whom anticholinergics are contraindicated (those with narrow-angle glaucoma or prostatic hypertrophy) or in situations where mental alertness is required (e.g., driving a car).

Diphenhydramine should be used cautiously in individuals taking "tranquilizers," sedatives, or hypnotics, due to its additive CNS depressant effect. Likewise, ingesting alcohol will have additive depressant effects, and caution must be exercised while taking diphenhydramine hydrochloride. Diphenhydramine hydrochloride should not be given to patients receiving monoamine oxidase inhibitors and should be used cautiously in patients taking other anticholinergic drugs because of additive effects.[36] It should be used cautiously, if at all, in patients with a history of asthma, due its anticholinergic properties. Diphenhydramine hydrochloride, like codeine and dextromethorphan hydrobromide, is a safe and effective antitussive but has a propensity for side effects, which must be kept in mind when recommending it.

Noscapine. Noscapine is an alkaloid of opium and is related to papaverine. It is contained in only a few nonprescription preparations. Noscapine's limited availability is not an indication of its effectiveness—it has been shown to reduce the frequency and severity of allergic cough.[33 34] Nevertheless, the FDA Panel has suggested additional testing of noscapine to clearly establish its effectiveness.[27] Its antitussive effectiveness is dose related, and, although some investigators believe it is equipotent on a weight basis to codeine, dosages range from 5 to 90 mg two to four times a day.[34]

In therapeutic doses noscapine shows little or no effect on the CNS or respiratory system and has neither analgesic properties nor addictive liabilities. Constipation and other GI reactions have not been encountered to a significant degree. Noscapine is an apparently safe and effective antitussive and has no contraindications to its use.

Bronchodilators

The involvement of bronchoconstriction has been implicated as a cause of the cough reflex. Drugs known to inhibit bronchoconstriction may have antitussive action. It is on the basis of the "bronchomotor theory" that some investigators contend that a sympathomimetic bronchodilator is indicated and would be a rational addition to an antitussive preparation. This consideration requires further investigation.

Oral antibacterials and anesthetics

Pharyngitis, or sore throat, is a symptom of the common cold and, less commonly, of allergic rhinitis. In allergic rhinitis, it may result from the drying effect of constant mouth breathing caused by the nasal congestion or as a result of swelling in the pharynx from a pollen sensitivity reaction. Treatment of the nasal congestion and the administration of antihistamines help diminish the pharyngitis in this condition. With the common cold, pharyngitis is usually the result of the infectious process. Most commonly, the symptom is soreness or dryness rather than actual pain as in the more severe cell injury and inflammation of bacterial infections. Pharyngitis is also believed to be the result of continuous postnasal discharge of mucus impinging on the pharynx.

The pharmacist should be aware of the environmental factors which may lead to complaints of pharyngitis. The overuse of tobacco products, ingestion of large amounts of concentrated alcohol-containing beverages, or other irritating substances have been associated with pharyngeal irritation and the development of a sore throat. More rarely, inhalation of irritant gases has also been an etiological factor.

Diseases in which pharyngitis may be a symptom include not only the common cold but also strep throat, scarlet fever, tonsillitis, influenza, measles, and smallpox. It is important that the etiology of the pharyngitis be uncovered so that appropriate measures can be taken. An acute sore throat which accompanies a nonbacterial infection has a much slower onset than bacterial pharyngitis. The soreness and the constitutional symptoms are milder, temperature is usually normal or only slightly elevated, and there is a dry, raspy, possibly tickling sensation in the throat when swallowing.

A sore throat may be indicative of a more serious disease process that demands medical attention (e.g., streptococcal pharyngitis), and the pharmacist should exercise caution in recommending self-treatment which may mask the symptoms. When the pharmacist suspects that the sore throat symptom is not related to environmental factors, to allergic rhinitis, or to a cold, physician referral is indicated. Failure to consult a physician may result in a worsening of the condition and development of complications. If, in the pharmacist's opinion, the sore throat symptoms can be self-medicated, there are many products to choose from which are promoted for relief. Most of these products are lozenges or mouthwashes (gargles, throatwashes).

The primary purpose of a mouthwash is to cleanse and soothe. Most mouthwashes are promoted for bad breath with the suggestion that these products kill germs. The Council on Dental Therapeutics does not recognize substantial contributions to oral health by using medicated mouthwashes.[37] Much of the controversy that surrounds the use of these products stems from the problems associated with substantiating germicidal or germistatic claims. There is no method available that effectively compares the germicidal activity in the test tube with that in the oral cavity. There is also no adequate evidence that individuals benefit from a nonspecific change in the flora of the oral cavity; it is possible that alteration of the normal oral cavity flora may actually allow invasion by pathogenic organisms. In addition, most infectious sore throats are viral in origin, and using a lozenge or gargle promoted as an "antibacterial" does not influence the viral pharyngitis.

The antimicrobial substances contained in most commercial mouthwashes are phenols, alcohol, quaternary ammonium compounds, volatile oils, oxygenating agents, and iodine-containing preparations. These agents are believed to be of little value in the treatment of sore throat symptoms.

A possible benefit of oral mouthwashes and gargles is derived from the anesthetic compounds they contain. These agents temporarily desensitize the sensory nerves located in the mucosa of the pharynx, affording transient relief. The danger remains, however, in masking a symptom of a condition which potentially is harmful. Many commercially available lozenges also are promoted for the treatment of sore throat symptoms. They usually contain an antibacterial agent in combination with a local anesthetic. The beneficial effect of this combination is probably caused by the anesthetic agent.

There is much controversy surrounding the effectiveness of the different anesthetic ingredients included in lozenges and mouthwashes promoted for sore throats. The value and effectiveness of a local anesthetic agent are usually established by animal and human skin testing, not pharyngeal tests. Consequently, patient satisfaction is probably the best indicator of effectiveness of these products.

Benzocaine. Benzocaine is beneficial in diminishing sore throat symptoms in concentrations of 5 to 20 percent. Concentrations of less than 5 percent are not considered beneficial. At present, the authors are not aware of commercial preparations which contain an effective concentration of benzocaine.

Phenol and phenol-containing salts. These agents are included in several OTC lozenges. They are effective in concentrations of 0.5 to 1.5 percent.

Benzyl alcohol. Benzyl alcohol is an effective oral

anesthetic agent when used in concentrations of as much as 10 percent.

The pharmacist should recommend a product that contains an effective dose of a local anesthetic and a minimum of extraneous compounds of doubtful effectiveness or value. The pharmacist should also try to follow up on patient response to recommended agents for future suggestions as to proper OTC therapy for pharyngeal soreness.

Anticholinergics

Some nonprescription cold remedies contain atropine or a mixture of belladonna alkaloids. The rationale for their inclusion is that their drying effect provides symptomatic relief from the "runny nose" associated with the cold and allergic rhinitis.

Although anticholinergics have the potential to dry the excess secretions in the nose, the doses commonly found in nonprescription remedies (e.g., 0.06 to 0.2 mg total alkaloids) do little to accomplish this objective. To make up for this therapeutic shortcoming, these agents are usually found in products which also contain an antihistamine. The additive anticholinergic effect obtained from such a combination may have an occasional palliative effect on the common cold by helping to reduce secretions. Such a combination exposes the patient to the unwanted sedative effects of the antihistamine. It hardly seems rational to combine the therapeutic effect of one drug (in subtherapeutic amounts) with the unpredictable side effect of another, in an attempt to achieve the effects obtainable with a larger (therapeutic) dose of the former.

Drug interactions involving anticholinergics are unlikely at the doses in a cold or allergy remedy. However, hypersensitivity to these relatively small amounts does occur. If a hypersensitive individual also suffers from asthma, narrow-angle glaucoma, or enlarged prostate, a physician should be contacted before taking a preparation containing an anticholinergic.

Pending further definitive data on dosage, the anticholinergics available in OTC products should not be considered significant contributors to the relief of cold or allergy symptoms. Therefore, their presence in a product should not be a criterion for product selection.

Table 5. Blockade of Cough Reflex[a]

Site of blockade	Mechanism of blockade	Blocking agents
Sensory nerves	Reduction of primary irritation; inhibition of bronchoconstriction; inhibition of afferent impulses	Demulcents/ expectorants; bronchodilators; local anesthetics
Cough center (medulla)	Depression	Opiate and nonopiate suppressants
Motor nerves	Inhibition of efferent impulses	Local anesthetics

[a]Adapted from H. Salem and D. M. Aviado, *Drug Inform. J.*, **8**, 111 (Oct.-Dec., 1974).

Antipyretic analgesics

In the case of the common cold, there is seldom an actual clinical fever present. More often it is a feeling of warmth but with little or no temperature elevation. The usefulness of aspirin or acetaminophen in the uncomplicated common cold is in relieving the discomforts of generalized aches and pains or malaise associated with the viral infection.

In adults, 325 to 650 mg of aspirin or acetaminophen every 4 to 6 hours should help relieve discomfort and slight fever. In children, aspirin may be given as follows: 65 mg per year of age up to a maximum of 650 mg for a 10-year-old or older, every 4 to 6 hours. Some practitioners may prefer to avoid possible aspirin toxicity in small children and recommend acetaminophen. The doses of acetaminophen for children are: under 1 year, 60 mg; 1 to 2 years, 60 to 120 mg; 3 to 6 years, 120 mg; 6 to 12 years, 240 mg. They should be repeated every 4 to 6 hours.[38]

Table 6. Expectorant Dosage[a]

Drug and category	Dosage		
	Adults	*Children* 6–12 years	2–6 years
Ammonium chloride (III)	300 mg every 2-4 hr	150 mg every 2-4 hr	75 mg every 2-4 hr
Guaifenesin (III)	200-400 mg every 4 hr (not to exceed 2,400 mg/24 hr)	100-200 mg every 4 hr (not to exceed 1,200 mg/24 hr)	50-100 mg every 4 hr (not to exceed 600 mg/24 hr)
Ipecac syrup (III)	0.5-1.0 ml (of syrup containing not less than 123 mg and not more than 157 mg of total ether-soluble alkaloids of ipecac/100 ml) 3 or 4 times a day	0.25-0.5 ml (of syrup containing not less than 123 mg and not more than 157 mg of total ether-soluble alkaloids of ipecac/100 ml) 3 or 4 times a day	Not recommended
Terpin hydrate (III)	200 mg every 4 hr (not to exceed 1,200 mg/24 hr)	100 mg (of terpin hydrate alone or in a nonalcoholic mixture, not the elixir for children under 12) every 4 hr (not to exceed 600 mg/24 hr)	50 mg every 4 hr (not to exceed 300 mg/24 hr)

[a]As proposed by the FDA OTC Panel on Cold, Cough, Allergy, Bronchodilator, and Anti-Asthmatic Drugs.

Both aspirin and acetaminophen have been reported to increase the response to oral anticoagulants, although any effect from acetaminophen is likely to be small and not clinically significant.[28 39] Although acetaminophen might be preferred when an analgesic-antipyretic is indicated for a patient also taking an oral anticoagulant, it should not be added to the regimen without first ensuring adequate follow-up of clinical and laboratory parameters by first checking with the patient's physician.

Patients taking either probenecid or sulfinpyrazone to control their serum uric acid levels should avoid aspirin because of its inhibitory effect on the uricosuric action of these drugs.[28] Aspirin has also been shown to diminish the effectiveness of indomethacin and should likewise be avoided when conditions such as rheumatoid arthritis are treated with the latter.[39]

In cases of patients with a history of peptic ulcer disease, aspirin should be avoided and acetaminophen recommended. Patients with a history of asthma or hay fever and nasal polyps should avoid aspirin because it has been established that some of these individuals are allergic (hypersensitive) to aspirin.[19]

Adverse reactions to acetaminophen are rare; GI disturbances are common with aspirin.

It is important when considering patients with the aforementioned problems that many combination products incorporate both aspirin and acetaminophen in the same product.

Vitamin C (ascorbic acid)

The claim that vitamin C is effective in preventing and treating the common cold is controversial. Linus Pauling,[40] who popularized the use of vitamin C for the cold, recommends 1 to 5 g daily as a prophylactic measure and as much as 15 g daily to treat a cold. Many studies have been conducted, and, although some have shown trends in favor of vitamin C's effectiveness, they have not shown the vitamin to be unequivocally effective in any dosage in either preventing or reducing the severity or duration of colds.[41]

The potential for adverse effects associated with these large doses of vitamin C is also a debated issue. The most frequently noted adverse effect of large doses is diarrhea. Precipitation of urate, oxalate, or cystine stones in the urinary tract has been seen, although the potential incidence of this problem at these higher doses remains to be clearly documented. The effects on the urinary excretion of other drugs must also be investigated because of vitamin C's ability to acidify the urine.[42]

Acidification of the urine increases the possibility of aminosalicylic acid crystalluria in patients receiving aminosalicylic acid in the free-acid form. It also increases the excretion of drugs that are weak bases (e.g., amphetamines), reducing their effect, and increases renal tubular reabsorption of salicylate, increasing plasma salicylate concentrations. Vitamin C, in doses large enough to acidify the urine (4 to 12 g daily) should not be given with aminosalicylic acid and should be used cautiously when salicylates are taken in large doses (e.g., 3 to 5 g daily). There is no apparent problem in taking vitamin C with amphetamines as long as the decreased effect of the amphetamines is anticipated.[28]

Vitamin C has been implicated in an interaction with warfarin in which the hypoprothrombinemic effect of the anticoagulant was diminished.[28 39] The reports were of isolated incidents, however, and it is felt that the interaction was either dose dependent or occurred only in certain patients. Until further clarification is provided, practitioners should be aware of this possible interaction and inquire about vitamin C intake in patients who respond erratically to an anticoagulant. The possibility of an exaggerated hypoprothrombinemic response must also be kept in mind when these patients stop taking the vitamin C.

Diabetics taking vitamin C and testing the urine by the glucose oxidase "dip" test may encounter false negative results; the copper reduction method may produce false positive results.[28]

Humidification

The inhalation of water vapor is an adjunctive therapeutic measure that provides a demulcent action on the respiratory mucosa and adds to and dilutes respiratory tract fluid, decreasing its viscosity.[34 43] Humidifying the inspired

Table 7. Cough Suppressant Dosage[a]

Drug and category	Dosage		
	Adults	*Children* 6–12 years	2–6 years
Codeine (I)	10–20 mg every 4–6 hr (not to exceed 120 mg/24 hr)	5–10 mg every 4–6 hr (not to exceed 60 mg/24 hr)	2.5–5 mg every 4–6 hr (not to exceed 30 mg/24 hr)
Dextromethorphan (I)	10–20 mg every 4 hr or 30 mg every 6–8 hr (not to exceed 120 mg/24 hr)	5–10 mg every 4 hr or 15 mg every 6–8 hr (not to exceed 60 mg/24 hr)	2.5–5 mg every 4 hr or 7.5 mg every 6–8 hr (not to exceed 30 mg/24 hr)
Diphenhydramine hydrochloride (I)	25 mg every 4 hr (not to exceed 150 mg/24 hr)	12.5 mg every 4 hr (not to exceed 75 mg/24 hr)	6.25 mg every 4 hr (not to exceed 37.5 mg/24 hr)
Noscapine hydrochloride (III)	15–30 mg every 4–6 hr (not to exceed 180 mg/24 hr)	7.5–15 mg every 4–6 hr (not to exceed 90 mg/24 hr)	3.75–7.5 mg every 4–6 hr (not to exceed 45 mg/24 hr)

[a]As proposed by the FDA OTC Panel on Cold, Cough, Allergy, Bronchodilator, and Anti-Asthmatic Drugs.

air usually aids in relieving cough and hoarseness that is associated with laryngitis. Humidification may be a prophylactic measure against upper respiratory infections when people are exposed to low relative humidities. This is usually the case during the winter months, when doors and windows are closed and the heat is on. With inspiration of dry air, the viscosity of the mucus increases, and irritation of the respiratory mucosa may develop, creating a predisposition to viral or bacterial invasion.

The oldest method of humidifying the air involves the generation of steam from a pot of boiling water or more commonly from an electric steam vaporizer. A newer method of humidification involves a cool-mist vaporizer from which fine droplets of water are formed by pumping water through a fine screen. Therapeutically, the steam vaporizer does not seem to offer an advantage over the cool-mist type. The cool-mist type vaporizers are safe in that they do not generate heat or hot water; however, they are noisier, and they humidify somewhat more slowly than the steam vaporizers. It is important to follow the manufacturer's directions for cleaning the unit to avoid bacterial overgrowth (a problem not encountered with steam vaporizers).

If it is desired to supplement the humidification with a volatile substance (menthol, compound benzoin tincture), the steam vaporizer must be used. It has not been established whether these volatile substances are of therapeutic value and, therefore, may have no advantage over the inhalation of plain water vapor.

As an adjunctive measure humidification of the inspired air is important. Either a steam-generated unit or a cool-mist vaporizer can be used as prophylaxis and should be used at the onset of the cold. It is also important to increase oral fluid intake to prevent dehydration during a cold.

Product selection

Patient considerations

The effectiveness of many products available for self-medication of colds may be questionable, but they are generally safe when used as directed. The treatment of allergic rhinitis provides comfort until the acute symptoms subside. Past experience may influence a person's selection of a product which has proven effective in the past. Nevertheless, the pharmacist must be prepared to recognize the common cold and allergic rhinitis based on the symptoms; recognize complications that may arise or have arisen; and recommend the proper approaches for control of the symptoms (i.e., self-medicate or consult a physician), including drugs, adjunctive measures, and duration of treatment.

When presented with the symptoms usually associated with the common cold, recognition of the underlying disorder is not difficult. However, recognition of the allergic rhinitis condition is often more involved. In both conditions the pharmacist should conduct a brief but careful history of the present illness. This history should provide information that is useful in distinguishing one disorder from another, identifying those disorders which should or should not be self-medicated. Specific points which should be investigated are:

☐ Abruptness of onset. Have you felt this coming on, or did it develop spontaneously?

☐ Intensity. How severe are the symptoms? Have they gotten worse?

☐ Duration. How long have you had the problem?

☐ Recurrence. Do the symptoms come and go? Do they recur when you stop taking the medication?

The onset of the common cold is generally associated with a prodrome (e.g., "running nose," dry throat); in fact, it is very common for people to predict that they are "coming down with a cold." Allergic rhinitis is much more abrupt in onset—the condition develops immediately after exposure to the allergen. It is usually initially manifested by a paroxysmal attack of repetitive sneezing.

Early in the development of a cold, the intensity of symptoms is minor. As the infection runs its course, the symptoms may get worse, but this is subject to patient variability and varies with the infecting organism. The intensity of symptoms in allergic rhinitis is based on the amount of allergen encountered and the degree of individual hypersensitivity. Generally, the symptoms are most intense following allergen exposure and subside over time unless additional exposures are encountered.

Duration of cold symptoms is a very important detail in deciding which course of action should be taken. Typically, the common cold lasts 4 to 7 days. If the problem persists beyond this time with no apparent improvement or if the cold symptoms tend to be recurrent, a physician should be consulted for an evaluation. Duration of allergic rhinitis symptoms is extremely variable due, in part, to the individual sensitivity to the allergen. If the patient has received no relief in 10 days of self-treatment, physician followup evaluation and proper management are indicated.

The recurrent nature of seasonal allergic rhinitis is a hallmark in the differentiation of this condition from other nonallergic respiratory conditions. The recurrence of symptoms often follows the patterns of high pollen counts or patient activities which result in increased allergen exposure. If the symptomatology is present throughout the year or if it persists after the first killing frost, the condition may be perennial allergic rhinitis. Referral to a physician is desirable with perennial allergic rhinitis because of the prolonged duration of symptoms and the potential for developing complications.

Information on medications which have already been tried will aid the pharmacist not only in assessing the patient's current status but also in selecting a product. If, in the judgment of the pharmacist, the measures were appropriate and were not effective, the patient should be encouraged to see a physician. If no medication has been tried or if measures were taken that were inadequate or inappropriate, the pharmacist should recommend a more appropriate course of therapy. When a patient seeks the pharmacist's assistance in selecting a cold or allergy remedy, the pharmacist should question the individual as to the presence of other acute or chronic illnesses. This can identify those patients for whom many preparations should be used cautiously, if at all.

Orally administered preparations containing sympathomimetics should be given only on the advice of a physician to patients with hyperthyroidism (the patient is already predisposed to tachycardia and arrhythmias); with hypertension (especially moderate to severe, where additional peripheral vasoconstriction may cause significant blood pressure elevation); with diabetes mellitus (especially in diabetics who are insulin dependent and where glycogenolysis may cause the diabetes to go out of control); and with ischemic heart disease or angina (where an increase in heart rate can precipitate an acute angina attack and, possibly, a subsequent myocardial infarction). These concerns center primarily around the oral administration of sympathomimetic decongestants, where systemic effects are predictable. Judiciously administered drops, spray, or inhalation of a decongestant can provide a local intranasal action without significant concern of systemic absorption.

Theoretically, all of these effects can occur when the sympathomimetics reach the systemic circulation. In actual practice, however, the effect on a diabetic has not been a particular problem, except in an extremely unstable (brittle) diabetic. Should a diabetic patient take a liquid cough/cold preparation containing sugar? The syrup vehicle may contain as much as 85 percent (w/v) sucrose, and each gram of sucrose has about 4 cal (17 cal/tsp). If 4 tsp (about 70 cal) were taken in 1 day, the additional (nondietary) calories may be clinically significant in a brittle diabetic. Consequently, a sugar-free preparation would be preferred. In a stable diabetic, however, these additional calories would probably be of little concern.

Another factor that pharmacists should take into consideration when dealing with a diabetic patient is the alcohol contained in the product. Alcohol, like sucrose, also will provide calories—more calories, in fact, than an equal weight of sucrose. Because most liquid cough remedies contain alcohol (from 1 to 25 percent, with each gram providing about 7 cal), it is clear that a brittle diabetic taking a "usual" dose might experience some difficulty with diabetes control.

The anticholinergic properties of antihistamines are usually not prominent in OTC preparations. However, the anticholinergic effects of atropine and other belladonna alkaloids in some allergy and cold remedies pose a potential problem. In cases of glaucoma or urinary retention secondary to prostatic hypertrophy, preparations containing anticholinergic agents should be used only on advice of a physician.

The pharmacist should have a medication history to avoid possible drug interactions and to identify and avoid drug allergies or idiosyncrasies. In addition, a history of chronic use of a topical nasal decongestant may help identify rhinitis medicamentosa.

Product considerations

In view of the number of available preparations (single-entity and combinations), it is important that the pharmacist become familiar with a few preparations, especially those found from experience as useful, and recommend these preferentially. In trying to single out a preparation, it is necessary to know what effect is sought, which drug entity will produce this effect, how much of the drug is necessary to produce this effect, and which nonprescription product satisfactorily meets these needs.

If only one effect is sought (e.g., nasal decongestion), a preparation with a single agent in a full therapeutic dose should be used. When more than one effect is desired, selection becomes more complex. Several single-entity products can be used, but this is not usually acceptable to the patient—a combination product is preferred. The pharmacist should be selective in recommending a combination because many of these preparations carry the idea of "shotgun therapy" to its extreme. One study states that "the numerous compounded remedies, including those with vitamins, bioflavonoids, quinine, alkalinizers, multiple analgesics, antihistamines, decongestants, and tranquilizers, are developed for sales profit in a large market of uninformed and uncritical people and are not for the benefit of the patient. . . ."[2]

The selection of a combination product should be based on the presence of the desired agents in full therapeutic doses, with as few additional ingredients as possible. This goal, however, can seldom be achieved. The pharmacist must decide which effect is most important and select the combination on the basis of the agent that will produce this effect. For example, the efficacy of the antihistamines in treating the common cold is doubtful, and this is magnified by the subtherapeutic doses contained in most nonprescription remedies. An antihistamine-decongestant, therefore, should be selected on the basis of the decongestant with only secondary consideration given to the antihistamine. The opposite is probably indicated when selecting a combination product for allergic rhinitis. There is no proven evidence that the incorporation of other ancillary agents or other preparations of the same pharmacological class in a subtherapeutic dose provides more relief or even as much relief as one agent in its full therapeutic dose.

It is the authors' opinion that combination products containing analgesic-antipyretic agents should not be recommended. Their routine use carries the risk of masking a fever which may be an indication of a bacterial infection. Also, in the case of aspirin, significant blood loss may occur if taken regularly over a 5- to 7-day period. Such agents should be administered separately and only when needed. Similarly, preparations that do not disclose the amounts of ingredients on the package should not be recommended. It would be difficult to justify a pharmacist recommending a product for the amelioration of a symptom when there is no indication as to the amount of the active ingredient in the product.

The use of timed-release preparations provides for better patient compliance, increased patient convenience, and lower incidence and/or severity of side effects. However, some practitioners feel that these advantages may be outweighed by the fact that bioavailability of the drug or drugs in this type of a dosage form may be neither uniform nor reliable.[19] The recommendation of a timed-release preparation by the pharmacist should be based on the presence of indicated agents in therapeutic doses and, in the pharmacist's experience, the product's success record.

There is much controversy concerning the advantages of oral nasal decongestants over the topical agents. Proponents of oral decongestants state that these agents have the ability to affect all respiratory membranes, that they are unaffected by the character of mucus, that they do not induce pathological changes in the nasal mucosa, and that they relieve nasal obstruction without the additional irritation of locally applied medication. It is also true that these oral agents provide a greater duration of therapeutic effect.

There is also evidence to support the value of topically applied vasoconstrictors. Although the administration of these agents through sprays and drops does not represent the ideal dosage form, the relief is rapid. Because the relief is so dramatic, the patient tends to overuse topical agents, resulting in drug-induced irritation to the nasal mucosa, alteration of the ciliary movement of the mucosa, and possibly rhinitis medicamentosa.

The combination of topical therapy with oral decongestant therapy is also controversial. In the opinion of the authors, there is definite advantage to the judicious use of an oral decongestant which is proven safe and effective along with the application of a rapid-acting topical agent. With this combination, the patient experiences rapid relief from the topically applied decongestant and a longer duration of action via the systemic circulation from the oral agent if given in an adequate dose.

Patient consultation

In almost all cases of self-medication, the pharmacist is the first and only knowledgeable professional who is contacted. If the pharmacist takes the time to identify the patient's problem and ensure proper product selection, advice regarding proper use must also be considered essential to fulfilling professional responsibility.

Patients cannot always be depended on to read and/or follow the package instructions. There is a tendency to believe in the philosophy that "if one is good, two are better." This is not always the case, especially with medication. Pharmacists should caution against increasing the dose and/or frequency of administration of any medication. This is especially true of antihistamines and topical decongestants.

Even when antihistamines are taken in recommended amounts, they may cause transient drowsiness. Patients should be advised of this, especially if they are taking a prescription medication which also depresses the CNS. They should be advised as to the possible effects and should determine what effect the medication has on them before engaging in activities requiring mental alertness.

Nasal solutions can become contaminated. The pharmacist should recommend that the tip of the dropper or the spray applicator be rinsed in hot water after use, that only one person use the spray or drop applicator, and that the bottle or spray be discarded when the medication is no longer needed. Contamination of the nasal dropper can also be minimized by not touching the nose or the nasal surface with the dropper itself.

Nondrug measures (humidification, increased fluid intake, and local heat) can be recommended, and, although these suggestions may not seem acceptable to the patient who desires a medication, they can also be quite beneficial in combination with a medication. The recommendation by the pharmacist that the patient use humidification and/or increase fluid intake is in the patient's best interest. Normal saline gargles several times a day help relieve an inflamed throat, and a cool water sponge bath in conjunction with aspirin or acetaminophen usually causes a dramatic fall of an elevated temperature.

It is important that the patient realize that a cold will go away in spite of the medication recommended, that the medication is only intended to relieve discomfort, and that relief should occur in a week or less. The concern for duration of self-medication does not stem solely from the potential adverse effects of some of the medications but also from the minority of the cold sufferers who may develop complications, such as secondary bacterial infections. By not stipulating a time limit for therapy, patients will unknowingly continue self-medicating with little effect, prolonging their discomfort and delaying the time for a physician's diagnosis and appropriate treatment.

A cold usually lasts for 7 days. The duration of therapy depends on which day in the course of the cold the medication is begun. If symptoms persist beyond the arbitrary, yet fairly reliable, 7-day limit in spite of adequate therapy, consideration should be given to seeking a physician's appraisal of the condition. Most people want to continue self-medication for another "day or two" before calling a physician. Realizing that it will be almost impossible to convince them otherwise, the pharmacist should insist that another "day or two" be the absolute limit. If after 2 or 3 days of therapy the symptoms become more intense or if a fever, a very painful sore throat, or a cough productive of a mucopurulent sputum develops, the patient should seek the physician's diagnosis.

Duration of treatment for allergic rhinitis is less distinct. Usually, seasonal sufferers self-medicate throughout those periods when the allergen count is high. They should be cautioned about the overuse of topical nasal decongestants. Perennial sufferers should be referred to a physician for management of symptoms.

Product selection must be based not only on the presence of an effective agent in a therapeutic amount but also on underlying disorders which may be adversely influenced by the recommended therapy. Having chosen the product, the pharmacist must then ensure that the patient knows how to take the medication and what to expect from it with regard to symptomatic relief as well as adverse effects. The patient must be told for how long the medication should be taken. Realizing that questions may arise later, the patient should be encouraged to return to or call the pharmacist.

Summary

By evaluating the presenting symptoms, the pharmacist can usually distinguish the common cold from disorders such as the "flu" or allergic rhinitis and offer proper suggestions for treatment. The pharmacist also can offer the allergic rhinitis sufferer medications to provide symptomatic relief. By conducting a careful history and recognizing the pertinent symptoms, a partial diminution of the symptoms can be achieved through advice and medication.

Recommendations for the treatment of common cold and allergic rhinitis should be directed at the relief of the symptoms. The endorsement by the pharmacist of a "shotgun" remedy is irrational, unless the patient suffers from all of the symptoms for which the product was promoted. Recommendation of a particular product is also irresponsible if it contains agents in less than therapeutic amounts.

In the case of the common cold, the objectives of treatment are drying nasal secretions, opening congested nasal passages, stifling a cough, soothing a sore throat, overcoming the hoarseness of laryngitis, and relieving feverishness, headache, and malaise. For allergic rhinitis, the treatment is directed at blocking or competing with the effect of released histamine, relieving nasal congestion, and palliation of secondary symptoms such as pharyngitis and headache. For nasal congestion, topically applied (preferably as the spray) phenylephrine hydrochloride (0.25 to 0.5 percent) is one of the most effective decongestants when it is used every 4 hours, if needed. To augment the duration of the topical decongestant, an oral nasal decongestant may also be recommended. Pseudoephedrine, 60 mg three times a day, or phenylpropanolamine hydrochloride, as much as 50 mg three times a day, is usually effective for this purpose.

Very few oral nasal decongestants are available as a single-entity product. When nasal decongestion is the effect sought, a combination product with a minimum of added ingredients and with the decongestant in full therapeutic amount should be recommended. Topically applied products should contain only the decongestant. For example, antihistamines add no beneficial effect to a topical decongestant preparation. Oral antihistamines in combination with nasal decongestants may be indicated in allergic rhinitis.

A hyperactive, dry cough in colds can usually be controlled by humidification of the inspired air (vaporizers), a demulcent/expectorant to the mucosa (hard candy or cough drop), and/or a cough suppressant (codeine, dextromethorphan hydrobromide). Humidification should be started early in the course of a cold and continued throughout. Most products contain a cough suppressant in combination with an expectorant. In the case of a dry cough, the dose of the cough suppressant is the criterion by which a product is selected. Administration of 15 mg of codeine or dextromethorphan hydrobromide usually decreases the frequency and intensity of a cough.

A patient with a congested cough may benefit from expectorants in conjunction with humidification to facilitate removal of thickened secretions. Guaifenesin, 200 to 400 mg every 4 hours, can be used. If the congested cough becomes hyperactive, it also can be treated with a cough suppressant.

The dry, sore throat present in colds and to a lesser extent in allergic rhinitis may be relieved by dissolving a piece of hard candy in the mouth to stimulate saliva flow. Frequent, warm, normal saline gargles can relieve symptoms. Topical antibacterials for a viral infection or allergic rhinitis are unwarranted. Significant relief can be obtained with the use of a lozenge or throat spray containing an anesthetic such as hexylresorcinol or phenol in a sufficient concentration.

Laryngitis can be managed by the inhalation of water vapor, by voice rest, and by the avoidance of inhaled irritants (e.g., smoking). Dissolving lozenges in the mouth or gargling do little to reach the inflamed tissues of the larynx.

Relief from feverishness, malaise, and headache in both conditions may be provided by the use of the analgesic/antipyretics, aspirin or acetaminophen. Products containing these agents in combination with several other ingredients are not recommended. The regular administration of aspirin or acetaminophen during the common cold or acute allergic rhinitis will mask the possible development of a fever, which would be an indication of a secondary bacterial infection. An antipyretic agent should be used to bring relief only as needed.

Antihistamines are effective in allergic rhinitis; their role in treatment of common colds is at best only adjunctive by virtue of mild, anticholinergic drying effects. Chlorpheniramine maleate, administered orally in doses of as much as 4 mg, is effective and only slightly sedative. There is marked individual variability to the different antihistamines. The pharmacist should be aware of this variability and be prepared to suggest an alternative if relief is not obtained with the original agent. As with the nasal decongestants, most antihistamines are found in combination with other ingredients in commercial preparations. The only rational combination for the treatment of allergic rhinitis is an oral antihistamine with an oral nasal decongestant. Other ingredients found in OTC products are of dubious efficacy.

The duration of therapy depends on when during a cold the patient decides to start treatment. In any case, treatment should be able to be stopped on the sixth or seventh day of the cold. Slight symptoms, e.g., cough, may persist for another day or so and, if necessary, should be treated.

The duration of treatment of allergic rhinitis should be limited to 3 to 5 days when topical nasal decongestants are used, in order to minimize the chances of rhinitis medicamentosa. Generally, oral decongestant therapy should be limited to 10 days. The need of the patient for the oral agents for longer than 10 days may indicate the development of complications, and the patient should be referred to a physician. An antihistamine product may be used prophylactically in acute allergic rhinitis. The duration of antihistamine therapy should coincide with the appearance and disappearance of the particular allergen.

Patients who have a common cold or allergic rhinitis offer the pharmacist many opportunities to be involved. Although pharmacists often cannot counsel every cold and/or hay fever sufferer, they should be available upon request and voluntarily as other professional responsibilities permit.

References

1. A. C. Guyton, "Textbook of Medical Physiology," Saunders, Philadelphia, Pa., 1976, pp. 525-527.
2. G. G. Jackson, in "Cecil-Loeb Textbook of Medicine," P. B. Beeson and W. McDermott, Eds., Saunders, Philadelphia, Pa., 1975, pp. 184-187, 829.
3. A. G. Christie, "Infectious Disease—Epidemiology and Clinical Practice," Churchill Livingstone, New York, N.Y., 1974, pp. 316-318, 359-360, 363.
4. H. Salem and D. M. Aviado, *Drug Inform. J.*, October/December, 111(1974).
5. "Current Medical Diagnosis and Treatment," M. A. Krupp and M. J. Chatton, Eds., Lange Medical Publications, Los Altos, Calif., 1976, p. 96.
6. J. I. Tennenbaum, in "Allergic Diseases—Diagnosis and Management," R. Patterson, Ed., Lippincott, Philadelphia, Pa., 1972, pp. 161-195.
7. *Medical Notes on the Common Cold,* Burroughs Wellcome, Research Triangle Park, N.C., 1972.
8. W. B. Pratt, "Fundamentals of Chemotherapy," Oxford University Press, New York, N.Y., 1972, p. 232.
9. R. W. Steele *et al.*, *J. Pediatr.*, **77,** 824(1970).
10. S. W. McFadden and J. E. Haddow, *Pediatrics,* **43,** 622(1969).
11. W. B. Sherman, "Hypersensitivity Mechanisms and Management," Saunders, Philadelphia, Pa., 1968.
12. J. M. O'Loughlin, *Drug Ther.*, 47-55(1974).
13. P. M. Seebohm, *Postgrad. Med.*, 52-56(1973).
14. L. Tuft, "Allergy Management in Clinical Practice," Mosby, St. Louis, Mo., 1973, pp. 185-238.
15. A. W. Frankland, *Int. Arch. Allergy Appl. Immunol.*, **6,** 45-52(1955).
16. L. H. Criep, *J. Am. Med. Assoc.*, **166,** 572-577(1965).
17. F. E. Roth and I. I. A. Tabachnick, in "Drill's Pharmacology in Medicine," J. R. DiPalma, Ed., McGraw-Hill, New York, N.Y., 1971, pp. 1003-1015.
18. "International Encyclopedia of Pharmacology and Therapeutics," vol. 1, section 74, Schachter, Ed., Pergamon Press, New York, N.Y., 1973, p. 127.
19. "AMA Drug Evaluations," 2d ed., Publishing Sciences Group, Acton, Mass., 1973, pp. 199, 467, 469, 475, 481, 491, 492.
20. "Evaluations of Drug Interactions," 2d ed., American Pharmaceutical Association, Washington, D. C., 1976.
21. E. C. Boedeker and J. H. Dauber, "Manual of Medical Therapeutics," 21st ed., Little, Brown, Boston, Mass., 1974, p. 177.
22. B. Levy and R. Ahlquist, in "Drill's Pharmacology in Medicine," J. R. DiPalma, Ed., McGraw-Hill, New York, N. Y., 1971, p. 655.
23. D. M. Aviado, "Sympathomimetic Drugs," Charles C Thomas, Springfield, Ill., 1970, pp. 282, 288, 382.
24. E. W. Martin, "Techniques of Medication," Lippincott, Philadelphia, Pa., 1969, p. 91.
25. J. T. Connell, *Ann. Allergy,* **27,** 541-546(1969).
26. G. Aschan and B. Drettner, *Eye Ear Nose Throat Mon.*, **43,** 66-74(1964).
27. *Fed. Regist.* **41(176),** 38312-38424(1976).
28. P. D. Hansten, "Drug Interactions," Lea and Febiger, Philadelphia, Pa., 1973.
29. S. R. Hirsch, *Drug Ther.*, **5(4),** 179(1975).
30. Summary Minutes of Meeting 4, FDA OTC Panel on Cold, Cough, Allergy, Bronchodilator, and Anti-Asthmatic Drugs, Division of OTC Drug Evaluation, Bureau of Drugs, Department of Health, Education and Welfare, Rockville, Md., Feb. 28 and March 1, 1973.
31. Summary Minutes of Meeting 5, FDA OTC Panel on Cold, Cough, Allergy, Bronchodilator, and Anti-Asthmatic Drugs, Division of OTC Drug Evaluation, Bureau of Drugs, Department of Health, Education and Welfare, Rockville, Md., April 5 and 6, 1973.
32. C. J. Polson and R. N. Tattersall, "Clinical Toxicology," Lippincott, Philadelphia, Pa., 1969, p. 92.
33. "The United States Dispensatory," 27th ed., A. Osol and R. Pratt, Eds., Lippincott, Philadelphia, Pa., 1973, p. 794.
34. H. A. Bickerman, in "Drugs of Choice, 1974-1975," W. Modell, Ed., Mosby, St. Louis, Mo., 1974, p. 399.
35. Parke, Davis and Company, product information, 1976.
36. Parke, Davis and Company, package literature.
37. "Accepted Dental Therapeutics," 36th ed., American Dental Association, Chicago, Ill., 1975.
38. H. C. Shirkey, "Pediatric Dosage Handbook," American Pharmaceutical Association, Washington, D. C., 1973.
39. "Evaluations of Drug Interactions," 2d ed., American Pharmaceutical Association, Washington, D. C., 1976.
40. L. Pauling, "Vitamin C and the Common Cold," Freeman, San Francisco, Calif., 1970.
41. *Med. Lett. Drugs Ther.*, **16(21),** 85-86(1974).
42. *Med. Lett. Drugs Ther.*, **12(26),** 105(1970).
43. E. M. Boyd, in "Drill's Pharmacology in Medicine," J. R. DiPalma, Ed., McGraw-Hill, New York, N.Y., 1971, pp. 1021-1028.

The authors wish to acknowledge the invaluable assistance of Robert K. Chalmers in organizing the material for this chapter and that of Charlene Douglass, Phyllis Mansfield, and Stacy MacLeod in the preparation of this manuscript.

Product [a] (manufacturer)	Cough suppressant	Expectorant	Sympathomimetic	Antihistamine	Other
Actol Expectorant (Beecham Labs)	noscapine, 30 mg/5 ml	guaifenesin, 200 mg/5 ml	—	—	alcohol, 12.5% fruit flavoring
Alamine (North American)	—	—	phenylephrine hydrochloride, 5 mg/5 ml	chlorpheniramine maleate, 1 mg/5 ml	menthol, 1 mg/5 ml alcohol, 5% green mint flavor
Alamine-C (North American)	codeine phosphate,[b] 5 mg/5 ml	—	phenylephrine hydrochloride, 10 mg/5 ml	chlorpheniramine maleate, 2 mg/5 ml	menthol, 1 mg/5 ml alcohol, 5% grape flavor
Alamine Expectorant (North American)	codeine phosphate,[b] 5 mg/5 ml	guaifenesin, 100 mg/5 ml	phenylephrine hydrochloride, 10 mg/5 ml	chlorpheniramine maleate, 2 mg/5 ml	menthol, 1 mg/5 ml alcohol, 5% grape flavor
Alo-Tuss Tablets (North American)	dextromethorphan hydrobromide, 10 mg	—	phenylephrine hydrochloride, 5 mg	chlorpheniramine maleate, 2 mg	—
Amonidrin Tablets (O'Neal, Jones & Feldman)	—	ammonium chloride, 200 mg guaifenesin, 100 mg	—	—	—
Atussin D.M. Expectorant (Amfre-Grant)	dextromethorphan hydrobromide, 15 mg/5 ml	guaifenesin, 100 mg/5 ml	phenylephrine hydrochloride, 5 mg/5 ml phenylpropanolamine hydrochloride, 5 mg/5 ml	chlorpheniramine maleate, 2 mg/5 ml	—
Atussin Expectorant [c] (Amfre-Grant)	—	guaifenesin, 100 mg/5 ml	phenylpropanolamine hydrochloride, 5 mg/5 ml phenylephrine hydrochloride, 5 mg/5 ml	chlorpheniramine maleate, 2 mg/5 ml	—
Baby Cough Syrup (DeWitt)	—	ammonium chloride, 13 mg/5 ml	—	—	glycerin, 343 mg/5 ml licorice extract, 12 mg/5 ml
Breacol (Glenbrook)	dextromethorphan hydrobromide, 10 mg/5 ml	—	phenylpropanolamine hydrochloride, 37.5 mg/5 ml	chlorpheniramine maleate, 4 mg/5 ml	alcohol, 10%
Broncho-Tussin [c] (First Texas)	codeine phosphate,[b] 65 mg/30 ml	terpin hydrate, 260 mg/30 ml	—	—	alcohol, 40%
C3 Capsules (Menley & James)	dextromethorphan hydrobromide, 30 mg	—	phenylpropanolamine hydrochloride, 50 mg	chlorpheniramine maleate, 4 mg	—
Cerose DM [c] (Ives)	dextromethorphan hydrobromide, 10 mg/5 ml	potassium guaiacolsulfonate, 86 mg/5 ml ipecac fluidextract, 0.17 min./5 ml	phenylephrine hydrochloride, 5 mg/5 ml	phenindamine tartrate, 5 mg/5 ml	sodium citrate, 195 mg/5 ml citric acid, 65 mg/5 ml glycerin, 40 min./5 ml alcohol, 2.5%
Cheracol (Upjohn)	codeine phosphate,[b] 11 mg/5 ml	guaifenesin, 115 mg/5 ml	—	—	alcohol, 3% wild cherry bark white pine bark

Product [a] (manufacturer)	Cough suppressant	Expectorant	Sympathomimetic	Antihistamine	Other
Cheracol D (Upjohn)	dextromethorphan hydrobromide, 9.86 mg/5 ml	guaifenesin, 15 mg/5 ml	—	—	alcohol, 3% wild cherry bark white pine bark
Chlor-Trimeton Expectorant (Schering)	—	ammonium chloride, 100 mg/5 ml guaifenesin, 50 mg/5 ml	phenylephrine hydrochloride, 10 mg/5 ml	chlorpheniramine maleate, 2 mg/5 ml	sodium citrate, 50 mg/5 ml alcohol, 1%
Chlor-Trimeton Expectorant with Codeine (Schering)	codeine,[b] 10 mg/5 ml	ammonium chloride, 100 mg/5 ml guaifenesin, 50 mg/5 ml	phenylephrine hydrochloride, 10 mg/5 ml	chlorpheniramine maleate, 2 mg/5 ml	sodium citrate, 50 mg/5 ml alcohol, 1%
Cidicol [c] (Upjohn)	ethylmorphine hydrochloride,[b] 16.25 mg/30 ml	potassium guaiacolsulfonate, 520 mg/30 ml	—	—	alcohol, 5% potassium citrate citric acid
Codimal DM [c] (Central)	dextromethorphan hydrobromide, 10 mg/5 ml	potassium guaiacolsulfonate, 83.3 mg/5 ml	phenylephrine hydrochloride, 5 mg/5 ml	pyrilamine maleate, 8.33 mg/5 ml	sodium citrate, 216 mg/5 ml citric acid, 50 mg/5 ml alcohol, 4%
Codimal Expectorant (Central Pharmacal)	—	potassium guaiacolsulfonate, 100 mg/5 ml	phenylpropanolamine hydrochloride, 25 mg/5 ml	—	sodium citrate, 216 mg/5 ml citric acid, 50 mg/5 ml
Codimal PH (Central)	codeine phosphate,[b] 10 mg/5 ml	potassium guaiacolsulfonate, 83.3 mg/5 ml	phenylephrine hydrochloride, 5 mg/5 ml	pyrilamine maleate, 8.33 mg/5 ml	sodium citrate, 216 mg/5 ml citric acid, 50 mg/5 ml
Colrex [c] (Rowell)	dextromethorphan hydrobromide, 10 mg/5 ml	potassium guaiacolsulfonate, 80 mg/5 ml ammonium chloride, 80 mg/5 ml	phenylephrine hydrochloride, 5 mg/5 ml	chlorpheniramine maleate, 1 mg/5 ml	cherry flavor
Colrex Expectorant [c] (Rowell)	—	guaifenesin, 100 mg/5 ml ammonium chloride, 50 mg/5 ml	—	—	alcohol, 4.7%
Conar [c] (Beecham Labs)	noscapine, 15 mg/5 ml	—	phenylephrine hydrochloride, 10 mg/5 ml	—	mint flavor
Conar Expectorant (Beecham Labs)	noscapine, 15 mg/5 ml	guaifenesin, 100 mg/5 ml	phenylephrine hydrochloride, 10 mg/5 ml	—	citrus flavor
Conex (O'Neal, Jones & Feldman)	—	guaifenesin, 50 mg/10 ml	phenylpropanolamine hydrochloride, 25 mg/10 ml	chlorpheniramine maleate, 2 mg/10 ml	methylparaben, 0.13% propylparaben, 0.03%
Conex c Codeine (O'Neal, Jones & Feldman)	codeine phosphate,[b] 10 mg/10 ml	guaifenesin, 50 mg/10 ml	phenylpropanolamine hydrochloride, 25 mg/10 ml	chlorpheniramine maleate, 2 mg/10 ml	methylparaben, 0.13% propylparaben, 0.03%
Consotuss (Merrell-National)	dextromethorphan hydrobromide, 15 mg/5 ml	—	—	doxylamine succinate, 3.75 mg/5 ml	alcohol, 10%
Coricidin (Schering)	—	ammonium chloride, 100 mg/5 ml guaifenesin, 50 mg/5 ml	phenylpropanolamine hydrochloride, 12.5 mg/5 ml	chlorpheniramine maleate, 2 mg/5 ml	—

Product [a] (manufacturer)	Cough suppressant	Expectorant	Sympathomimetic	Antihistamine	Other
Coryban-D [c] (Pfipharmecs)	dextromethorphan hydrobromide, 7.5 mg/5 ml	guaifenesin, 50 mg/5 ml	phenylephrine hydrochloride, 5 mg/5 ml	—	alcohol, 7.5% acetaminophen, 120 mg/5 ml
Cosanyl DM Improved Formula (Parke-Davis)	dextromethorphan hydrobromide, 15 mg/5 ml	—	pseudoephedrine hydrochloride, 30 mg/5 ml	—	alcohol, 6% peach flavor
Creomulsion (Creomulsion Co.)	—	creosote ipecac	—	—	beechwood, white pine, menthol, cascara, wild cherry, alcohol
Creo-Terpin (Roberts)	—	creosote, 133 mg/30 ml terpin hydrate, 131 mg/30 ml	—	—	sodium glycerophosphate, 263 mg/30 ml alcohol, 25%
DayCare (Vick)	dextromethorphan hydrobromide, 20 mg/30 ml	—	phenylpropanolamine hydrochloride, 25 mg/30 ml	—	acetaminophen, 600 mg/30 ml alcohol, 7.5%
Dimocol Liquid and Capsules (Robins)	dextromethorphan hydrobromide, 15 mg/5 ml or capsule	guaifenesin, 100 mg/5 ml or capsule	pseudoephedrine hydrochloride, 30 mg/5 ml or capsule	—	alcohol, 4.75% (liquid)
DM-4 Children's Cough Control (DeWitt)	dextromethorphan hydrobromide, 4 mg/5 ml	ammonium chloride, 40 mg/5 ml potassium guaiacolsulfonate, 38 mg/5 ml	—	—	glycerin, 75 mg/5 ml alcohol, 1.5%
DM-8 (DeWitt)	dextromethorphan hydrobromide, 8 mg/5 ml	ammonium chloride, 80 mg/5 ml potassium guaiacolsulfonate, 75 mg/5 ml	—	—	alcohol, 3%
Dondril Anticough Tablets (Whitehall)	dextromethorphan hydrobromide, 10 mg	guaifenesin, 50 mg	phenylephrine hydrochloride, 5 mg	chlorpheniramine maleate, 1 mg	—
Dorcol Pediatric (Dorsey)	dextromethorphan hydrobromide, 7.5 mg/5 ml	guaifenesin, 37.5 mg/5 ml	phenylpropanolamine hydrochloride, 8.75 mg/5 ml	—	alcohol, 5%
Dr. Drake's (Roberts)	—	ipecac fluidextract	—	—	castor oil
Dristan (Whitehall)	dextromethorphan hydrobromide, 7.5 mg/5 ml	—	phenylephrine hydrochloride, 5 mg/5 ml	chlorpheniramine maleate, 1 mg/5 ml	sodium citrate alcohol, 12%
Duad Capsules (Hoechst-Roussel)	dextromethorphan hydrobromide, 10 mg	—	—	—	sodium citrate, 50 mg benzocaine, 3 mg
Efricon (Lannett)	codeine phosphate,[b] 10.96 mg/5 ml	ammonium chloride, 90 mg/5 ml potassium guaiacolsulfonate, 90 mg/5 ml	phenylephrine hydrochloride, 5 mg/5 ml	chlorpheniramine maleate, 2 mg/5 ml	sodium citrate, 60 mg/5 ml lemon flavor
Endotussin-NN (Endo)	dextromethorphan hydrobromide, 10 mg/5 ml	ammonium chloride, 40 mg/5 ml	—	pyrilamine maleate, 7.5 mg/5 ml	alcohol, 4%

Product [a] (manufacturer)	Cough suppressant	Expectorant	Sympathomimetic	Antihistamine	Other
Endotussin-NN Pediatric (Endo)	dextromethorphan hydrobromide, 5 mg/ml	ammonium chloride, 60 mg/ml	—	—	alcohol, 4%
Fedahist Expectorant (Dooner)	—	guaifenesin, 100 mg/5 ml	pseudoephedrine hydrochloride, 30 mg/5 ml	chlorpheniramine maleate, 2 mg/5 ml	—
Formula 44-D (Vick)	dextromethorphan hydrobromide, 20 mg/10 ml	guaifenesin, 100 mg/10 ml	phenylpropanolamine hydrochloride, 25 mg/10 ml	—	alcohol, 10%
2/G (Dow)	—	guaifenesin, 100 mg/5 ml	—	—	alcohol, 3.5% corn derivatives
2/G-DM (Dow)	dextromethorphan hydrobromide, 15 mg/5 ml	guaifenesin, 100 mg/5 ml	—	—	alcohol, 5% corn derivatives
GG-Cen Capsules and Syrup (Central Pharmacal)	—	guaifenesin, 200 mg/capsule 100 mg/5 ml	—	—	alcohol, 10% (syrup)
G G Tussin (Vitarine)	—	guaifenesin, 100 mg/5 ml	—	—	alcohol, 3.5%
Halls (Warner-Lambert)	dextromethorphan hydrobromide, 15 mg/10 ml	—	phenylpropanolamine hydrochloride, 37.5 mg/10 ml	—	menthol; eucalyptus oil; alcohol, 22%; glycerin
Histadyl EC (Lilly)	codeine phosphate,[b] 64.8 mg/30 ml	ammonium chloride, 660 mg/30 ml	ephedrine hydrochloride, 30 mg/30 ml	methapyrilene fumarate, 81 mg/30 ml	menthol alcohol, 5%
Histivite-D (Vitarine)	dextromethorphan hydrobromide, 30 mg/30 ml	ammonium chloride, 518 mg/30 ml	ephedrine sulfate, 24.3 mg/30 ml	methapyrilene fumarate, 75 mg/30 ml	menthol alcohol, 4.8%
Hytuss Tablets [c] (Hyrex)	—	guaifenesin, 100 mg	—	—	—
Hytuss 2X Capsules (Hyrex)	—	guaifenesin, 200 mg	—	—	—
Kiddies Pediatric (Vitarine)	—	potassum guaiacolsulfonate ammonium chloride	—	—	cocillana bark extract menthol alcohol, 2% wild cherry flavor
Kleer Chewable Tablets (Scrip)	dextromethorphan hydrobromide, 2.5 mg	—	phenylephrine hydrochloride, 5 mg	chlorpheniramine maleate, 2 mg	—
Lanatuss [c] (Lannett)	—	guaifenesin, 100 mg/5 ml	phenylpropanolamine hydrochloride, 5 mg/5 ml	chlorpheniramine maleate, 2 mg/5 ml	sodium citrate, 197 mg/5 ml citric acid, 60 mg/5 ml
Naldetuss (Bristol)	dextromethorphan hydrobromide, 15 mg/5 ml	—	phenylpropanolamine hydrochloride, 17.5 mg/5 ml	phenyltoloxamine citrate, 7.5 mg/5 ml	acetaminophen, 162 mg/5 ml
Neophiban Tablets (O'Neal, Jones & Feldman)	—	guaifenesin, 50 mg	phenylpropanolamine hydrochloride, 12.5 mg	phenyltoloxamine citrate, 25 mg	acetaminophen, 195 mg

Product [a] (manufacturer)	Cough suppressant	Expectorant	Sympathomimetic	Antihistamine	Other
Noratuss (North American)	codeine phosphate,[b] 20 mg/30 ml	ammonium chloride, 194.4 mg/30 ml potassium guaiacolsulfonate, 32.4 mg/30 ml terpin hydrate, 32.4 mg/30 ml	—	—	cocillana extract, 26.6 mg/30 ml sodium benzoate, 0.1% cherry flavor
Nortussin (North American	—	guaifenesin, 100 mg/30 ml	—	—	alcohol, 3.5% cherry flavor
Novahistine DH (Dow)	codeine phosphate,[b] 10 mg/5 ml	—	phenylpropanolamine hydrochloride, 18.75 mg/5 ml	chlorpheniramine maleate, 2 mg/5 ml	alcohol, 5%
Novahistine DMX (Dow)	dextromethorphan hydrobromide, 10 mg/5 ml	guaifenesin, 100 mg/5 ml	pseudoephedrine hydrochloride, 30 mg/5 ml	—	alcohol, 10%
Novahistine Expectorant (Dow)	codeine phosphate,[b] 10 mg/5 ml	guaifenesin, 100 mg/5 ml	phenylpropanolamine hydrochloride, 18.75 mg/5 ml	chlorpheniramine maleate, 2 mg/5 ml	alcohol, 7.5%
Nyquil (Vick)	dextromethorphan hydrobromide, 15 mg/30 ml	—	ephedrine sulfate, 8 mg/30 ml	doxylamine succinate, 7.5 mg/30 ml	acetaminophen, 300 mg/30 ml alcohol, 25%
Ornacol Capsules and Liquid (Smith Kline & French)	dextromethorphan hydrobromide, 30 mg/capsule 15 mg/5 ml	—	phenylpropanolamine hydrochloride, 25 mg/capsule 12.5 mg/5 ml	—	alcohol, 8% (liquid)
Orthoxicol (Upjohn)	dextromethorphan hydrobromide, 10 mg/5 ml	—	methoxyphenamine hydrochloride, 17 mg/5 ml	—	—
Pediaquil (Philips Roxane)	—	potassium guaiacolsulfonate, 389 mg/30 ml	phenylephrine hydrochloride, 15 mg/30 ml	—	squill, 105 mg/30 ml sorbitol corn syrup currant and caramel flavors
Pertussin 8-Hour (Chesebrough-Pond)	dextromethorphan hydrobromide, 30 mg/20 ml	—	—	—	alcohol, 9.5%
Pertussin Wild Berry (Chesebrough-Pond)	dextromethorphan hydrobromide, 14 mg/20 ml	guaifenesin, 100 mg/20 ml	—	—	alcohol, 8.5%
Pinex Regular & Concentrate (Roberts)	—	potassium guaiacolsulfonate	—	—	pine tar oil, eucalyptus oil, grindelia extract, glycerin
Prunicodeine [c] (Lilly)	codeine sulfate,[b] 65 mg/30 ml	terpin hydrate, 175 mg/30 ml	—	—	wild cherry, white pine, sanguinaria, alcohol
Quelidrine (Abbott)	dextromethorphan hydrobromide, 10 mg/5 ml	ammonium chloride, 40 mg/5 ml ipecac fluidextract, 0.005 ml/5 ml	ephedrine hydrochloride, 5 mg/5 ml phenylephrine hydrochloride, 5 mg/5 ml	chlorpheniramine maleate, 2 mg/5 ml	alcohol, 2%
Queltuss Tablets (O'Neal, Jones & Feldman)	dextromethorphan hydrobromide, 15 mg	guaifenesin, 100 mg	—	—	—

Product [a] (manufacturer)	Cough suppressant	Expectorant	Sympathomimetic	Antihistamine	Other
Quiet-Nite (Rexall)	dextromethorphan hydrobromide, 15 mg/30 ml	—	ephedrine sulfate, 10 mg/30 ml	chlorpheniramine maleate, 2 mg/30 ml	acetaminophen, 600 mg/30 ml alcohol, 25%
Rem (Block)	—	ammonium chloride, 0.7% ipecac, 0.07%	—	—	alcohol, 1.2%; white pine, 0.47%; squill, 0.14%; lobelia, 0.08%; horehound, 0.08%; sanguinaria, 0.07%; tar, 0.07%; menthol, 0.05%; tolu, 0.004%
Robitussin (Robins)	—	guaifenesin, 100 mg/5 ml	—	—	alcohol, 3.5%
Robitussin A-CV (Robins)	codeine phosphate,[b] 10 mg/5 ml	guaifenesin, 100 mg/5 ml	—	—	alcohol, 3.5%
Robitussin-CF (Robins)	dextromethorphan hydrobromide, 10 mg/5 ml	guaifenesin, 50 mg/5 ml	phenylpropanolamine hydrochloride, 12.5 mg/5 ml	—	alcohol, 1.4%
Robitussin-DM (Robins)	dextromethorphan hydrobromide, 15 mg/5 ml	guaifenesin, 100 mg/5 ml	—	—	alcohol, 1.4%
Robitussin-PE [c] (Robins)	—	guaifenesin, 100 mg/5 ml	pseudoephedrine hydrochloride, 30 mg/5 ml	—	alcohol, 1.4%
Romex (Amer. Pharm.)	dextromethorphan hydrobromide, 10 mg/5 ml	guaifenesin, 33 mg/5 ml	phenylephrine hydrochloride, 5 mg/5 ml	chlorpheniramine maleate, 1 mg/5 ml	—
Romilar III (Block)	dextromethorphan hydrobromide, 5 mg/5 ml	guaifenesin, 50 mg/5 ml	phenylpropanolamine hydrochloride, 12.5 mg/5 ml	—	alcohol, 10% flavor
Romilar Capsules (Block)	dextromethorphan hydrobromide, 15 mg	—	phenylephrine hydrochloride, 5 mg	chlorpheniramine maleate, 1 mg	acetaminophen, 120 mg
Romilar CF (Block)	dextromethorphan hydrobromide, 15 mg/5 ml	—	—	chlorpheniramine maleate, 1 mg/5 ml	acetaminophen, 120 mg/5 ml alcohol, 10%, 0.5 ml/5 ml flavor
Romilar Chewable Tablets for Children (Block)	dextromethorphan hydrobromide, 7.5 mg	—	—	—	benzocaine, 2 mg cherry flavor
Romilar Children's (Block)	dextromethorphan hydrobromide, 7.5 mg/5 ml	guaifenesin, 25 mg/5 ml	—	—	sodium citrate citric acid grape flavor
Ryna-Tussadine Expectorant Liquid and Tablets (Mallinckrodt)	—	guaifenesin, 100 mg/5 ml and tablet	phenylpropanolamine hydrochloride, 6.25 mg/5 ml and tablet phenylephrine hydrochloride, 3.75 mg/5 ml and tablet	pyrilamine maleate, 6.25 mg/5 ml and tablet chlorpheniramine maleate, 1 mg/5 ml and tablet	alcohol, 3%
Silence Is Golden (Bristol-Myers)	dextromethorphan hydrobromide, 10 mg/5 ml	—	—	—	honey flavor

Product [a] (manufacturer)	Cough suppressant	Expectorant	Sympathomimetic	Antihistamine	Other
Silexin Cough Syrup and Tablets (Otis Clapp)	dextromethorphan hydrobromide	guaifenesin (syrup)	—	—	benzocaine (tablet)
Soltice (Chattem)	—	ammonium chloride, 170 mg/10 ml	phenylpropanolamine hydrochloride, 25 mg/10 ml	—	sodium citrate, 170 mg/10 ml cetylpyridinium chloride, 0.10 mg/10 ml
Sorbutuss [c] (Dalin)	dextromethorphan hydrobromide, 10 mg/5 ml	guaifenesin, 100 mg/5 ml ipecac fluidextract, 0.003 ml/5 ml	—	—	potassium citrate, 85 mg/5 ml citric acid, 35 mg/5 ml mint flavor glycerin–sorbitol vehicle
St. Joseph Cough Syrup for Children (Plough)	dextromethorphan hydrobromide, 7.5 mg/5 ml	—	—	—	sodium citrate menthol alcohol, 0.38%
Supercitin [c] (Vitarine)	dextromethorphan hydrobromide, 20 mg/10 ml	—	—	chlorpheniramine maleate, 2 mg/10 ml	acetaminophen, 120 mg/10 ml sodium citrate, 100 mg/10 ml
Toclonol Expectorant [c] (Cenci)	carbetapentane citrate, 7.25 mg/5 ml	terpin hydrate, 16.65 mg/5 ml	—	—	sodium citrate, 66.15 mg/5 ml citric acid, 6.65 mg/5 ml glycerin, 2.8 ml/5 ml menthol, 0.83 mg/5 ml alcohol, 7.2%
Toclonol with Codeine [c] (Cenci)	codeine,[b] 10 mg/5 ml carbetapentane citrate, 7.25 mg/5 ml	terpin hydrate, 16.65 mg/5 ml	—	—	sodium citrate, 66.15 mg/5 ml citric acid, 6.65 mg/5 ml glycerin, 2.8 ml/5 ml menthol, 0.83 mg/5 ml alcohol, 7.2%
Tolu-Sed [c] (First Texas)	codeine phosphate,[b] 60 mg/30 ml	guaifenesin, 600 mg/30 ml	—	—	alcohol, 10%
Tolu-Sed DM [c] (First Texas)	dextromethorphan hydrobromide, 10 mg/5 ml	guaifenesin, 100 mg/5 ml	—	—	alcohol, 10%
Tonecol (A.V.P.)	dextromethorphan hydrobromide, 10 mg/5 ml	guaifenesin, 25 mg/5 ml	phenylephrine hydrochloride, 5 mg/5 ml	chlorpheniramine maleate, 1 mg/5 ml	sodium citrate, 15 mg/5 ml alcohol, 7% cherry flavor
Triaminic Expectorant (Dorsey)	—	guaifenesin, 100 mg/5 ml	phenylpropanolamine hydrochloride, 12.5 mg/5 ml	pheniramine maleate, 6.25 mg/5 ml pyrilamine maleate, 6.25 mg/5 ml	alcohol, 5%
Triaminic Expectorant with Codeine (Dorsey)	codeine phosphate,[b] 10 mg/5 ml	guaifenesin, 100 mg/5 ml	phenylpropanolamine hydrochloride, 12.5 mg/5 ml	pheniramine maleate, 6.25 mg/5 ml pyrilamine maleate, 6.25 mg/5 ml	alcohol, 5%
Triaminicol (Dorsey)	dextromethorphan hydrobromide, 15 mg/5 ml	ammonium chloride, 90 mg/5 ml	phenylpropanolamine hydrochloride, 12.5 mg/5 ml	pheniramine maleate, 6.25 mg/5 ml pyrilamine maleate, 6.25 mg/5 ml	—

Products 8 ANTITUSSIVE

Product (manufacturer)	Cough suppressant	Expectorant	Sympathomimetic	Antihistamine	Other
Trind (Mead Johnson)	—	guaifenesin, 50 mg/5 ml	phenylephrine hydrochloride, 2.5 mg/5 ml	—	acetaminophen, 120 mg/5 ml alcohol, 15%
Trind-DM (Mead Johnson)	dextromethorphan hydrobromide, 7.5 mg/5 ml	guaifenesin, 50 mg/5 ml	phenylephrine hydrochloride, 5 mg/5 ml	—	acetaminophen, 120 mg/5 ml alcohol, 15%
Troutman's (Troutman)	dextromethorphan hydrobromide, 10 mg/5 ml	—	—	—	alcohol, ammonium chloride, corn syrup, sucrose, caramel, horehound, menthol, peppermint
Tussagesic Suspension (Dorsey)	dextromethorphan hydrobromide, 15 mg/5 ml	terpin hydrate, 90 mg/5 ml	phenylpropanolamine hydrochloride, 12.5 mg/5 ml	pheniramine maleate, 6.25 mg/5 ml pyrilamine maleate, 6.25 mg/5 ml	acetaminophen, 120 mg/5 ml
Tussagesic Tablets (Dorsey)	dextromethorphan hydrobromide, 30 mg	terpin hydrate, 180 mg	phenylpropanolamine hydrochloride, 25 mg	pheniramine maleate, 12.5 mg pyrilamine maleate, 12.5 mg	acetaminophen, 325 mg
Tussar-2 (Armour)	codeine phosphate,[b] 10 mg/5 ml carbetapentane citrate, 7.5 mg/5 ml	guaifenesin, 50 mg/5 ml	—	chlorpheniramine maleate, 2.0 mg/5 ml	sodium citrate, 130 mg/5 ml citric acid, 20 mg/5 ml methylparaben, 0.1% alcohol, 5%
Tussar-SF [c] (Armour)	codeine phosphate,[b] 10 mg/5 ml carbetapentane citrate, 7.5 mg/5 ml	guaifenesin, 50 mg/5 ml	—	chlorpheniramine maleate, 2.0 mg/5 ml	sodium citrate, 130 mg/5 ml citric acid, 20 mg/5 ml methylparaben, 0.1% alcohol, 12%
Tusscapine (Fisons)	noscapine, 15 mg/5 ml	—	—	—	lime flavor
Tussciden Expectorant (Cenci)	—	guaifenesin, 100 mg/5 ml	—	—	—
Vicks (Vick)	dextromethorphan hydrobromide, 3.5 mg/5 ml	guaifenesin, 25 mg/5 ml	—	—	sodium citrate, 200 mg/5 ml alcohol, 5%

[a] Liquid unless specified otherwise.
[b] Schedule V drug: OTC sale forbidden in some states.
[c] Sugar free.

Products 8 LOZENGE

Product (manufacturer)	Anesthetic	Antibacterial	Other
Axon (McKesson)	benzocaine, 5 mg	cetylpyridinium chloride, 2.5 mg	—
Cepacol (Merrell-National)	—	cetylpyridinium chloride, 1:1500	benzyl alcohol, 0.3%
Cepacol Troches (Merrell-National)	benzocaine, 10 mg	cetylpyridinium chloride, 1:1500	—
Cherry Chloraseptic (Eaton)	—	phenol, sodium phenolate (total phenol, 1.4%) (these ingredients are also anesthetic)	—
Chloraseptic (Eaton)	—	phenol, sodium phenolate (total phenol, 1.4%) (these ingredients are also anesthetic)	—

Product (manufacturer)	Anesthetic	Antibacterial	Other
Colrex Troches (Rowell)	benzocaine, 10 mg	cetylpyridinium chloride, 2.5 mg	—
Conex (O'Neal, Jones & Feldman)	benzocaine, 5 mg	cetylpyridinium chloride, 0.5 mg	methylparaben, 2 mg propylparaben, 0.5 mg
Creozets (Creomulsion Co.)	—	—	beechwood creosote; ipecac; menthol; licorice; white pine; wild cherry; cascara; ascorbic acid
Hold (Calgon)	benzocaine	—	dextromethorphan hydrobromide
Listerine (Warner-Lambert)	—	hexylresorcinol, 2.4 mg	eucalyptol, menthol
Listerine Cough Control (Warner-Lambert)	benzocaine, 2.5 mg	—	dextromethorphan hydrobromide, 7.5 mg
Meloids Pastilles (Cunningham)	—	—	licorice, 98 mg; sugar, 48 mg; capsicum, 2 mg; menthol, 1.8 mg
Oracin (Vick)	benzocaine, 6.25 mg	—	menthol, 0.10%; sorbitol base
Oradex-C (Commerce)	benzocaine, 10 mg	cetylpyridinium chloride, 2.5 mg	—
Robitussin-DM Cough Calmers (Robins)	—	—	dextromethorphan hydrobromide, 7.5 mg guaifenesin, 50 mg
Romilar Cough Discs (Block)	—	—	dextromethorphan hydrobromide, 5 mg benzyl alcohol, 0.5%
Semets (Beecham Labs)	benzocaine, 3 mg	cetylpyridinium chloride, 1:1500	—
Sepo (Otis Clapp)	benzocaine	—	—
Silence Is Golden (Bristol-Myers)	—	—	dextromethorphan hydrobromide, 5 mg honey flavor
Spec-T Sore Throat Anesthetic (Squibb)	benzocaine, 10 mg	—	—
Spec-T Sore Throat/Cough Suppressant (Squibb)	benzocaine, 10 mg	—	dextromethorphan hydrobromide, 10 mg
Spec-T Sore Throat/Decongestant (Squibb)	benzocaine, 10 mg	—	phenylephrine hydrochloride, 5 mg phenylpropanolamine hydrochloride, 10.5 mg
Spongiacaine (Otis Clapp)	benzocaine	—	—
Sucrets (Calgon)	—	hexylresorcinol, 2.4 mg	—
Synthaloids (Buffington)	benzocaine	calcium–iodine complex	—
Teeds (Warren-Teed)	benzocaine, 10 mg	—	chlorophyll
Thantis (Hynson, Westcott & Dunning)	—	meralein sodium, 8.1 mg	salicyl alcohol, 64.8 mg
Throat Discs (Parke-Davis)	—	—	capsicum, peppermint, anise, cubeb, glycyrrhiza extract, linseed
Trocaine (North American)	benzocaine, 5 mg	—	—
Trokettes (Vitarine)	benzocaine, 10 mg	cetylpyridinium chloride, 1:3000 cetalkonium chloride, 1:3000	orange flavor
Vicks Cough Silencers (Vick)	benzocaine, 1 mg	—	dextromethorphan hydrobromide, 2.5 mg/drop; menthol; anethole; peppermint oil
Vicks Formula 44 Cough Discs (Vick)	benzocaine, 1.25 mg	—	dextromethorphan hydrobromide, 5 mg; menthol; anethole; peppermint oil
Vicks Medi-trating (Vick)	benzocaine, 5 mg	cetylpyridinium chloride, 1.66 mg	menthol, camphor, eucalyptus oil

Products 8 COLD AND ALLERGY

Product (manufacturer)	Dosage form	Sympathomimetic	Antihistamine	Analgesic	Other
Alka-Seltzer Plus (Miles)	effervescent tablet	phenylpropanolamine bitartrate, 24.08 mg	chlorpheniramine maleate, 2.0 mg	aspirin, 324 mg	—
Allerest (Pharmacraft)	time capsule	phenylpropanolamine hydrochloride, 50 mg	pyrilamine maleate, 15 mg methapyrilene fumarate, 10 mg	—	—
Allerest Regular and Children's (Pharmacraft)	tablet	phenylpropanolamine hydrochloride, 18.7 mg 9.4 mg (children's)	chlorpheniramine maleate, 2 mg 1 mg (children's)	—	—
Allergesic (Bryant-Vitarine)	tablet	phenylpropanolamine hydrochloride, 25 mg	methapyrilene fumarate, 10 mg chlorpheniramine maleate, 1 mg	—	—
Anodynos Forte (Buffington)	tablet	phenylephrine hydrochloride, 10 mg	chlorpheniramine maleate, 2 mg	salicylamide acetaminophen	caffeine
Apcohist Allergy Tablets (Amer. Pharm.)	tablet	phenylpropanolamine hydrochloride, 25 mg	methapyrilene fumarate, 5 mg chlorpheniramine maleate, 1 mg	—	—
Bayer Children's Cold Tablets (Glenbrook)	tablet	phenylpropanolamine hydrochloride, 3.125 mg	—	aspirin, 81 mg	—
Bayer Decongestant (Glenbrook)	tablet	phenylpropanolamine hydrochloride, 18.75 mg	chlorpheniramine maleate, 2 mg	aspirin, 325 mg	—
BC All Clear (Block)	tablet	phenylephrine maleate, 10 mg	chlorpheniramine maleate, 2 mg	aspirin, 648 mg salicylamide, 194 mg	caffeine, 32 mg cellulose povidone
Cenagesic (Central)	tablet	phenylephrine hydrochloride, 5 mg	pyrilamine maleate, 12 mg	salicylamide, 250 mg phenacetin, 120 mg	ascorbic acid, 30 mg caffeine, 15 mg
Chlor-Trimeton Decongestant (Schering)	tablet	pseudoephedrine, 60 mg	chlorpheniramine maleate, 4 mg	—	—
Codimal (Central Pharmacal)	tablet capsule	pseudoephedrine hydrochloride, 30 mg	chlorpheniramine maleate, 2 mg	salicylamide, 150 mg acetaminophen, 150 mg	—
Colrex (Rowell)	capsule	phenylephrine hydrochloride, 5 mg	chlorpheniramine maleate, 2 mg	acetaminophen, 300 mg	ascorbic acid, 200 mg
Conex DA (O'Neal, Jones & Feldman)	tablet	phenylpropanolamine hydrochloride, 50 mg	phenyltoloxamine citrate, 50 mg	—	—
Conex Plus (O'Neal, Jones & Feldman)	tablet	phenylpropanolamine hydrochloride, 25 mg	phenyltoloxamine citrate, 25 mg	acetaminophen, 250 mg	—
Congespirin (Bristol-Myers)	chewable tablet	phenylephrine hydrochloride, 1.25 mg	—	aspirin, 81 mg	—
Contac (Menley & James)	time capsule	phenylpropanolamine hydrochloride, 50 mg	chlorpheniramine maleate, 4 mg	—	belladonna alkaloids, 0.2 mg
Coricidin (Schering)	tablet	—	chlorpheniramine maleate, 2 mg	aspirin, 325 mg	—
Coricidin "D" (Schering)	tablet	phenylpropanolamine hydrochloride, 12.5 mg	chlorpheniramine maleate, 2 mg	aspirin, 325 mg	—

Product (manufacturer)	Dosage form	Sympathomimetic	Antihistamine	Analgesic	Other
Coricidin Demilets (Schering)	children's chewable tablet	phenylephrine hydrochloride, 2.5 mg	chlorpheniramine maleate, 0.5 mg	aspirin, 80 mg	—
Coricidin Medilets (Schering)	children's chewable tablet	—	chlorpheniramine maleate, 0.5 mg	aspirin, 80 mg	—
Coryban-D (Pfipharmecs)	capsule	phenylpropanolamine hydrochloride, 25 mg	chlorpheniramine maleate, 2 mg	—	caffeine, 30 mg
Cotylenol (McNeil)	tablet	pseudoephedrine hydrochloride, 30 mg	chlorpheniramine maleate, 2 mg	acetaminophen, 325 mg	—
Co Tylenol Cold Formula for Children (McNeil)	liquid	pseudoephedrine hydrochloride, 7.5 mg/5 ml	chlorpheniramine maleate, 0.5 mg/5 ml	acetaminophen, 120 mg/5 ml	alcohol, 7%
Covanamine (Mallinckrodt)	liquid	phenylpropanolamine hydrochloride, 6.25 mg/5 ml phenylephrine hydrochloride, 3.75 mg/5 ml	pyrilamine maleate, 6.25 mg/5 ml chlorpheniramine maleate, 1 mg/5 ml	—	—
Covangesic (Mallinckrodt)	liquid tablet	phenylpropanolamine hydrochloride, 6.25 mg/5 ml 12.5 mg/tablet phenylephrine hydrochloride, 3.75 mg/5 ml 7.5 mg/tablet	pyrilamine maleate, 6.25 mg/5 ml 12.5 mg/tablet chlorpheniramine maleate, 1.0 mg/5 ml 2.0 mg/tablet	acetaminophen, 120 mg/5 ml 275 mg/tablet	alcohol, 7.5% (liquid)
Decapryn (Merrell-National)	syrup	—	doxylamine succinate, 6.25 mg/5 ml	—	—
Demazin (Schering)	syrup repetabs	phenylephrine hydrochloride, 2.5 mg/5 ml 20 mg/repetab	chlorpheniramine maleate, 1.0 mg/5 ml 4 mg/repetab	—	alcohol, 7.5% (syrup)
D-Feda (Dooner)	syrup	pseudoephedrine hydrochloride, 30 mg/5 ml	—	—	—
Dristan (Whitehall)	tablet	phenylephrine hydrochloride, 5 mg	phenindamine tartrate, 10 mg	aspirin	caffeine aluminum hydroxide magnesium carbonate
Dristan (Whitehall)	time capsule	phenylephrine hydrochloride, 20 mg	chlorpheniramine maleate, 4 mg	—	—
Duadacin (Hoechst-Roussel)	capsule	phenylephrine hydrochloride, 5 mg	pyrilamine maleate, 12.5 mg chlorpheniramine maleate, 1 mg	salicylamide, 200 mg acetaminophen, 120 mg	ascorbic acid, 50 mg caffeine, 30 mg
Duradyne-Forte (O'Neal, Jones & Feldman)	tablet	phenylephrine hydrochloride, 5 mg	chlorpheniramine maleate, 2 mg	salicylamide, 225 mg acetaminophen, 160 mg	caffeine, 30 mg
Emagrin Forte (Otis Clapp)	tablet	phenylephrine hydrochloride, 5 mg	—	aspirin salicylamide	atropine sulfate, 0.06 mg caffeine
Endecon (Endo)	tablet	phenylpropanolamine hydrochloride, 25 mg	—	acetaminophen, 325 mg	—
Euphenex (O'Neal, Jones & Feldman)	tablet	—	phenyltoloxamine citrate, 25 mg	acetaminophen, 300 mg	caffeine, 15 mg

Product (manufacturer)	Dosage form	Sympathomimetic	Antihistamine	Analgesic	Other
Extendac (Vitarine)	extended-action capsule	phenylpropanolamine hydrochloride, 50 mg	pheniramine maleate, 12.5 mg chlorpheniramine maleate, 1 mg	—	belladonna alkaloids, 0.2 mg
Fedahist (Dooner)	tablet syrup	pseudoephedrine hydrochloride, 60 mg/tablet 30 mg/5 ml	chlorpheniramine maleate, 4 mg/tablet 2 mg/5 ml	—	—
Fedrazil (Burroughs Wellcome)	tablet	pseudoephedrine hydrochloride, 30 mg	chlorcyclizine hydrochloride, 25 mg	—	—
Fendol (Buffington)	tablet	phenylephrine hydrochloride, 10 mg	—	salicylamide acetaminophen	caffeine
Ginsopan (O'Neal, Jones & Feldman)	tablet	phenylpropanolamine hydrochloride, 25 mg phenylephrine hydrochloride, 2.5 mg	pyrilamine maleate, 12.5 mg chlorpheniramine maleate, 1 mg	—	—
Hista-Compound No. 5 (North American)	tablet	phenylephrine hydrochloride, 4 mg	chlorpheniramine maleate, 2 mg	salicylamide, 227.5 mg phenacetin, 162.5 mg	caffeine, 32.5 mg
Hot Lemon (Rexall)	tablet	phenylephrine hydrochloride, 10 mg	chlorpheniramine maleate, 2 mg	acetaminophen, 600 mg	ascorbic acid, 60 mg
Inhiston (Plough)	tablet	—	pheniramine maleate, 10 mg	—	—
Kiddisan (O'Neal Jones & Feldman)	chewable tablet	phenylephrine hydrochloride, 1.25 mg	chlorpheniramine maleate, 0.5 mg	salicylamide, 80 mg	ascorbic acid, 30 mg
Midran Decongestant (Columbia Medical)	tablet	phenylephrine hydrochloride, 5 mg	chlorpheniramine maleate, 2 mg	salicylamide, 97.5 mg acetaminophen, 32.5 mg	caffeine, 32.5 mg
Naldegesic (Bristol)	tablet	pseudoephedrine, 15 mg	—	acetaminophen, 325 mg	—
Nazac Timed-Disintegration Decongestant (Columbia Medical)	time capsule	phenylpropanolamine hydrochloride, 50 mg	pheniramine maleate, 12.5 mg chlorpheniramine maleate, 1 mg	—	belladonna alkaloids, 0.16 mg
Neo-Synephrine Compound (Winthrop)	tablet	phenylephrine hydrochloride, 5 mg	thenyldiamine hydrochloride, 7.5 mg	acetaminophen, 150 mg	caffeine, 15 mg
Novafed (Dow)	syrup	pseudoephedrine hydrochloride, 30 mg/5 ml	—	—	alcohol, 7.5%
Novafed A (Dow)	syrup	pseudoephedrine hydrochloride, 30 mg/5 ml	chlorpheniramine maleate, 2 mg/5 ml	—	alcohol, 5%
Novahistine Elixir (Dow)	syrup	phenylpropanolamine hydrochloride, 18.75 mg/5 ml	chlorpheniramine maleate, 2 mg/5 ml	—	alcohol, 5%
Ornex (Smith Kline & French)	capsule	phenylpropanolamine hydrochloride, 18 mg	—	acetaminophen, 325 mg	—
Pyrroxate (Upjohn)	capsule tablet	methoxyphenamine hydrochloride, 25 mg	chlorpheniramine maleate, 2 mg	aspirin, 227.5 mg phenacetin, 162.5 mg	caffeine, anhydrous, 32.5 mg

Product (manufacturer)	Dosage form	Sympathomimetic	Antihistamine	Analgesic	Other
Rhinidrin (Central Pharmacal)	tablet	phenylpropanolamine hydrochloride, 25 mg	phenyltoloxamine citrate, 25 mg	acetaminophen, 150 mg phenacetin, 150 mg	—
Sinacet (Meyer)	tablet	pseudoephedrine hydrochloride, 15 mg	—	acetaminophen, 325 mg	—
Sinarest (Pharmacraft)	tablet	phenylephrine hydrochloride, 5 mg	chlorpheniramine maleate, 1 mg	acetaminophen, 300 mg	caffeine, 30 mg
Sine-Off (Menley & James)	tablet	phenylpropanolamine hydrochloride, 18.75 mg	chlorpheniramine maleate, 2 mg	aspirin, 325 mg	—
Sinulin (Carnrick)	tablet	phenylpropanolamine hydrochloride, 37.5 mg	chlorpheniramine maleate, 2 mg	acetaminophen, 325 mg salicylamide, 250 mg	homatropine methylbromide, 0.75 mg
Sinurex (Rexall)	tablet	phenylpropanolamine hydrochloride, 25 mg	chlorpheniramine maleate, 0.5 mg methapyrilene fumarate, 6.25 mg	salicylamide, 300 mg	—
Sinustat (Vitarine)	tablet	phenylpropanolamine hydrochloride, 25 mg	phenyltoloxamine dihydrogen citrate, 22 mg	acetaminophen, 325 mg	—
Sinutab (Warner-Chilcott)	tablet	phenylpropanolamine hydrochloride, 25 mg	phenyltoloxamine dihydrogen citrate, 22 mg	acetaminophen, 325 mg	—
Sinutab II (Warner-Chilcott)	tablet	phenylpropanolamine hydrochloride, 25 mg	—	acetaminophen, 325 mg	—
Soltice Decongestant–Analgesic (Chattem)	tablet	phenylpropanolamine hydrochloride, 12.5 mg	—	acetaminophen, 325 mg	—
Spantac (North American)	capsule	phenylpropanolamine hydrochloride, 50 mg	chlorpheniramine maleate, 4 mg	—	belladonna alkaloids, 0.2 mg
St. Joseph Cold Tablets for Children (Plough)	chewable tablet	phenylpropanolamine hydrochloride, 3.125 mg	—	aspirin, 81 mg	—
Sudafed (Burroughs Wellcome)	tablet syrup	pseudoephedrine hydrochloride, 30 mg/tablet or 5 ml	—	—	—
Super Anahist (Warner-Lambert)	tablet	phenylpropanolamine hydrochloride, 25 mg	phenyltoloxamine citrate, 6.25 mg thonzylamine hydrochloride, 6.25 mg	acetaminophen, 325 mg aspirin, 227 mg phenacetin, 97.2 mg	caffeine
Timed Cold Capsules (Amer. Pharm.)	time capsule	phenylpropanolamine hydrochloride, 50 mg	chlorpheniramine maleate, 1 mg pheniramine maleate, 12.5 mg	—	belladonna alkaloids, 0.16 mg
Triaminic (Dorsey)	syrup	phenylpropanolamine hydrochloride, 12.5 mg/5 ml	pheniramine maleate, 6.25 mg/5 ml pyrilamine maleate, 6.25 mg/5 ml	—	—
Triaminicin (Dorsey)	tablet	phenylpropanolamine hydrochloride, 25 mg	chlorpheniramine maleate, 2 mg	aspirin, 450 mg	caffeine, 30 mg
Triaminicin Chewables (Dorsey)	chewable tablet	phenylpropanolamine hydrochloride, 6.25 mg	chlorpheniramine maleate, 0.5 mg	—	—
Ursinus (Dorsey)	in-lay tablet	phenylpropanolamine hydrochloride, 25 mg	pheniramine maleate, 12.5 mg pyrilamine maleate, 12.5 mg	calcium carbaspirin (equiv. to 300 mg of aspirin)	—

Products 8 COLD AND ALLERGY

Product (manufacturer)	Dosage form	Sympathomimetic	Antihistamine	Analgesic	Other
Valihist (Otis Clapp)	capsule	phenylephrine hydrochloride, 10 mg	pyrilamine maleate, 12.5 mg chlorpheniramine maleate, 1 mg	acetaminophen	caffeine
Vasominic TD (A.V.P.)	tablet	phenylpropanolamine hydrochloride, 50 mg	pheniramine maleate, 25 mg pyrilamine maleate, 25 mg	—	—
Ventilade (Warren-Teed)	syrup	phenylpropanolamine hydrochloride, 75 mg	methapyrilene fumarate, 25 mg pyrilamine maleate, 25 mg pheniramine maleate, 25 mg	—	alcohol, 5%
4-Way Cold Tablets (Bristol-Myers)	tablet	phenylephrine hydrochloride, 5 mg	—	aspirin, 324 mg	magnesium hydroxide, 125 mg white phenolphthalein, 15 mg

Products 8 TOPICAL DECONGESTANT

Product (manufacturer)	Application form	Sympathomimetic	Preservative/ Antiseptic	Other
Afrin (Schering)	nasal spray nose drops	oxymetazoline hydrochloride, 0.05%	benzalkonium chloride, 0.2 mg/ml phenylmercuric acetate, 0.02 mg/ml	sorbitol, 40 mg/ml glycine, 3.8 mg/ml sodium hydroxide
Alconefrin (Alcon)	nose drops	phenylephrine hydrochloride	—	—
Allerest (Pharmacraft)	nasal spray	phenylephrine hydrochloride, 0.5%	benzalkonium chloride	edetate disodium sodium bisulfite saline phosphate buffer
Benzedrex (Smith Kline & French)	inhaler	propylhexedrine, 250 mg	—	aromatics
Biomydrin (Warner-Chilcott)	nasal spray	phenylephrine hydrochloride, 0.25%	—	thonzonium bromide, 0.05%
Contac Nasal Mist (Menley & James)	nasal spray	phenylephrine hydrochloride, 0.5%	cetylpyridinium chloride, 0.02% thimerosal, 0.011%	methapyrilene hydrochloride, 0.2%
Coricidin (Schering)	nasal spray	phenylephrine hydrochloride, 0.5%	—	—
Coryban-D (Pfipharmecs)	nasal spray	phenylephrine hydrochloride, 0.5%	benzalkonium chloride, 0.02%	—
Dristan (Whitehall)	inhaler nasal spray	propylhexedrine (inhaler) phenylephrine hydrochloride (spray)	benzalkonium chloride (spray)	pheniramine maleate (spray) menthol eucalyptol methyl salicylate
Duration (Plough)	nasal spray	oxymetazoline hydrochloride, 0.05%	phenylmercuric acetate, 0.002%	—
Forthane (Lilly)	inhaler	methylhexaneamine, 250 mg	—	menthol, 32 mg aromatics
Hydra (North American)	nasal spray	phenylephrine hydrochloride, 0.25%	cetyltrimethylammonium bromide, 0.25% chlorobutanol, 0.25%	methapyrilene hydrochloride, 0.20%

Product (manufacturer)	Application form	Sympathomimetic	Preservative/ Antiseptic	Other
I-Sedrin Plain (Lilly)	nose drops	ephedrine, 1%	chlorobutanol, 0.5%	gluconic acid
Isophrin Hydrochloride (Riker)	nasal spray nose drops	phenylephrine hydrochloride, 0.125, 0.25, 0.5, and 1%	—	—
Naso Mist (Vitarine)	nasal spray	phenylephrine hydrochloride, 0.5%	benzalkonium chloride, 0.02%	methapyrilene hydrochloride, 0.15%
Neo-Synephrine Hydrochloride (Winthrop)	nasal spray nose drops nasal jelly	phenylephrine hydrochloride, 0.25 and 0.5% (spray) 0.125, 0.25, 0.5, and 1% (drops) 0.5% (jelly)	benzalkonium chloride, 0.02% (spray and 0.125% drops) methylparaben, propylparaben, sodium bisulfite (other drops) phenylmercuric acetate (jelly)	—
NTZ (Winthrop)	nose drops nasal spray	phenylephrine hydrochloride, 0.5%	benzalkonium chloride, 1:5,000	thenyldiamine hydrochloride, 0.1%
Privine (Ciba)	nose drops nasal spray	naphazoline hydrochloride, 0.05%	benzalkonium chloride, 1:5,000	—
Sine-Off Once-A-Day (Menley & James)	nasal spray	xylometazoline hydrochloride, 0.1%	—	menthol eucalyptol camphor methyl salicylate
Sinex-L.A. (Vick)	nasal spray	xylometazoline hydrochloride, 0.1%	thimerosal, 0.001%	—
Sinutab (Warner-Chilcott)	nasal spray	phenylephrine hydrochloride, 0.5%	—	thonzonium bromide, 0.05%
Soltice (Chattem)	nasal spray	phenylephrine hydrochloride, 2.6 mg/100 ml	—	methapyrilene hydrochloride, 600 mg/100 ml
Super Anahist (Warner-Lambert)	nasal spray	phenylephrine hydrochloride, 0.25%	thimerosal, 0.002%	alcohol, 0.038%
Triaminicin (Dorsey)	nasal spray	phenylpropanolamine hydrochloride, 0.75% phenylephrine hydrochloride, 0.25%	benzalkonium chloride, 1:10,000	pheniramine maleate, 0.125% pyrilamine maleate, 0.125%
Tuamine (Lilly)	inhaler	tuaminoheptane (equiv.), 325 mg	—	menthol, 32 mg aromatics
Tyrohist (Columbia Medical)	nasal spray	phenylephrine hydrochloride, 0.25%	cetalkonium chloride, 0.04%	pyrilamine maleate, 0.15%
Va-Tro-Nol (Vick)	nose drops	ephedrine sulfate, 0.35%	thimerosal, 0.001%	methapyrilene hydrochloride, 0.15% menthol eucalyptol camphor methyl salicylate
Vicks (Vick)	inhaler	levodesoxyephedrine, 50 mg	—	menthol camphor methyl salicylate bornyl acetate
Vicks Sinex (Vick)	nasal spray	phenylephrine hydrochloride, 0.50%	cetylpyridinium chloride, 0.04% thimerosal, 0.001%	methapyrilene hydrochloride, 0.12% menthol eucalyptol camphor methyl salicylate
4-Way (Bristol-Myers)	nasal spray	phenylephrine hydrochloride, 0.05% naphazoline hydrochloride, 0.05% phenylpropanolamine hydrochloride, 0.2%	—	pyrilamine maleate, 0.2%

Asthma Products

Lawrence J. Hak

Questions to ask the patient

Has a physician diagnosed the condition as asthma?

How old is the patient (if not adult)?

Are you under the care of a physician?

Do you have heart disease, high blood pressure, or diabetes?

What medications are you taking?

Which asthma products have you used before? Were they effective?

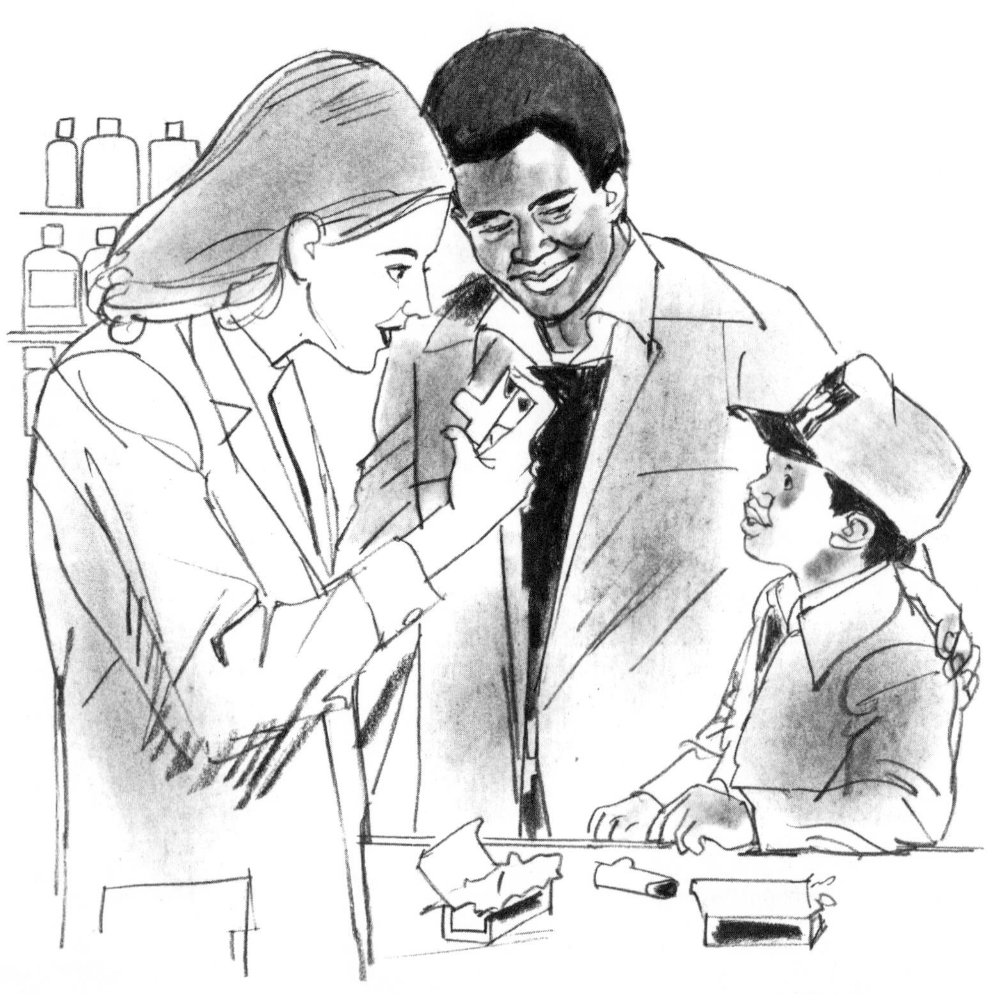

CHAPTER 9

The American Thoracic Society defines bronchial asthma as "a disease characterized by an increased responsiveness of the trachea and bronchi to various stimuli and manifested by a widespread narrowing of the airways that changes in severity either spontaneously or as a result of therapy." [1]

The overall incidence of asthma in the U.S., reported in the 1958 United States National Health Survey, is 2.3 percent.[2] About 50 percent of asthmatic patients developed the disease before age 10, and another 30 percent before age 30. However, asthma may develop even in old age. Before age 10, the incidence is twice as common in males as in females; by age 30 the incidence is equal. Although asthma is a common childhood disease, many children "grow out" of it by adulthood. Rackemann and Edwards,[3] in a long-term, followup study of childhood asthma, reported that 20 years later, 70 percent of the patients were symptom free.

Asthma attacks generally are precipitated by an allergic response to inhaled allergens such as pollen, dust, mold, pollutants, etc.; a respiratory tract infection; or a psychophysiologic response to stress.[4] One or more of these factors can interact in varying degrees to precipitate an attack. An allergic response is the major precipitating factor in about 30 percent of people who have asthma, and respiratory infections are a major factor in about 40 percent.

Although patients are generally characterized as having either extrinsic or intrinsic asthma, many patients present characteristics of both. A history of allergy to environmental allergens, a family history of allergic disorders, seasonal variation in the symptoms, positive skin tests, and elevated circulating levels of immunoglobulin E (IgE) are characteristics of extrinsic asthma. Patients with intrinsic asthma usually have a negative family history of allergy, negative skin tests, normal levels of IgE, and frequently develop nasal polyps and aspirin sensitivity.[5-7] About 2 to 10 percent of asthmatic patients will develop an acute attack of asthma after taking as little as 300 mg of aspirin.[8] Snyder and Siegel [9] have used the phrase "asthma triad" in referring to people with intrinsic asthma, nasal polyps, and aspirin intolerance.

Physiology of the respiratory system

The respiratory system is a series of airways ending in air sacs. The mouth and nasal passages lead to the pharynx which branches into the esophagus and the trachea. The trachea divides into two large bronchi, each supplying air to one lung. Each bronchus progressively divides into smaller branches (bronchioles) which give rise to alveolar ducts, alveolar sacs, and alveoli (Fig. 1).[10]

When an airway branches, its walls become thinner; at the level of the alveoli, all that remains is a thin layer of cells surrounded by pulmonary capillaries. The process of respiration, which is an exchange of gases, occurs in the alveoli. Oxygen passes across the alveolar walls into the capillaries, and carbon dioxide diffuses in the opposite direction.

The lungs are essentially elastic air sacs which are suspended in the airtight thoracic cavity. The movable walls of this cavity are formed by the sternum, ribs, and diaphragm. As the thoracic cavity becomes enlarged the pressure within the cavity becomes less than the atmospheric pressure and air will enter, expanding the lungs. The process of enlarging the thoracic cavity is accomplished via two simultaneous mechanisms. The diaphragm, when relaxed, is a dome-shaped muscle which extends upward into the thoracic cavity. As the diaphragm contracts, it becomes flattened and moves downward into the abdomen causing an increase in the longitudinal size of the thoracic cavity. The ribs are attached to the vertebrae and protrude forward and downward to the sternum. Contraction of the external intercostal muscles raises the ribs upward, causing an elevation and forward movement of the sternum and an increase in the anterior-posterior diameter of the chest cavity. During inspiration, the movement of the diaphragm and ribs occurs simultaneously, thus increasing the size of the thoracic cavity, and the lungs fill with air.

During quiet breathing, relaxation of the above processes and recoil of the lungs and abdominal wall provide sufficient pressure to cause expiration. For labored breathing, as occurs with exercise, contraction of the internal intercostal muscles and several abdominal muscles provides sufficient pressure on the thoracic cavity to cause the forceful expiration of air.

In order for respiration to function efficiently, inhaled air must be cleaned and humidified before it is delivered to the alveoli. The nasal cavities are lined with highly vascular mucous membranes and ciliated epithelial cells. As air passes over these areas, it is warmed, humidified, and filtered. Dust particles, bacteria, and other foreign matter are trapped in the mucus and propelled toward the pharynx by the movement of the nasal cilia. Humidification and filtration continue as air passes through the trachea, bronchi, and bronchioles which are also lined by a ciliated mucous membrane. Trapped particles are moved upward by the wavelike movement of the cilia and are deposited in the oral cavity where they are either expelled or swallowed.

Bronchial smooth muscle tone is under neural and humoral control.[11] β-Adrenergic receptors, specifically β_2 receptors, are found in the bronchioles; their stimulation causes bronchodilation. Bronchial smooth muscle is also under the control of the parasympathetic system via the vagus nerves. Stimulation of this system causes bronchoconstriction.

Pathophysiology of asthma

The mechanism by which asthma attacks occur is not completely understood. There are indications that both allergy and an imbalance of autonomic nervous functions are involved.[12] Patients with an allergic component (extrinsic asthma) have markedly elevated levels of IgE.[13,14] Plasma cells that produce IgE have been identified in the tonsils, adenoids, bronchial and peritoneal lymph nodes, and mucosa of the respiratory and GI tracts.[15] With antigenic stimulation, IgE is produced and becomes fixed to mast cells in the pulmonary tissue. These sensitized cells, upon subsequent exposure to an antigen, release chemical mediators such as histamine, bradykinin, and slow-reacting substance of anaphylaxis (SRS-A) into surrounding tissue, causing bronchoconstriction.

Patients with intrinsic asthma do not have increased levels of IgE but seem to exhibit an imbalance in autonomic function.[8] Although this disorder has not been fully elucidated, Kaliner [16] showed that the release of the chemical mediators is modulated by intracellular concentrations of the cyclic nucleotides, 3′,5′-guanosine monophosphate (cyclic GMP) and 3′,5′-adenosine monophosphate (cyclic AMP). Cyclic GMP enhances release of the mediators, and cyclic AMP inhibits it. The intracellular concentration of these nucleotides seems to be under autonomic control—cholinergic stimulation increases cyclic GMP, and β-adrenergic stimulation increases cyclic AMP. Gold *et al.*[17] have shown that bronchoconstriction is mediated through reflex cholinergic pathways via the vagus nerve. Szentivanyi [18 19] has proposed a relative decrease in β-adrenergic activity as the mechanism for bronchoconstriction. Thus, the hypersensitivity of bronchiolar smooth muscle in asthmatics may result from either overactive vagal reflexes or a deficiency in the β-adrenergic control.[12]

The hallmark of the asthmatic attack is obstruction of airways. However, there is some question as to whether or not this results entirely from bronchospasm.[20] Dunnill [21] reported that bronchospasm plays little or no role in the pathogenesis of asthma. In the statement of the American Thoracic Society, excessive contraction of bronchial smooth muscle and hypersecretion of mucus are the major pathologies seen in asthma.[1] Whatever the initiating factor, autopsy findings in patients who have died of asthma include mucus plugs which block terminal bronchioles, increased number and size of goblet cells, thickening of the basement membrane, hypertrophied smooth muscle of the preterminal bronchioles, and inflammatory infiltration of the submucosa of the bronchioles.[1]

Signs and symptoms

Asthma characteristically occurs in episodes which last from a few minutes to several hours. Between attacks, pulmonary function is essentially normal, and there are no symptoms. Attacks, which often occur in the middle of the night, usually begin with tightness in the chest; coughing and wheezing occur and become more severe over time. Dyspnea is severe, and expiration is more difficult than inspiration. In prolonged or severe attacks, overinflation of the lungs occurs, and there is audible wheezing and physical exhaustion. The sputum is viscid and difficult to expectorate.

Ingredients in OTC products

There is general agreement that the quantity of chemical mediators which is released is modulated by the intracellular concentration of cyclic AMP, and that increased levels of cyclic AMP result in bronchial smooth muscle relaxation. Therefore, agents that augment the intracellular concentration of cyclic AMP are useful in the therapy of asthma. Two main classes of pharmacologic agents have this effect—the sympathomimetic agents (β-adrenergic stimulators) and the methylxanthines. These β-adrenergic agents, by stimulating β receptors, increase cyclic 3′,5′-AMP. Phosphodiesterase, a normally occurring intracellular enzyme, rapidly destroys cyclic 3′,5′-AMP by converting it to 5′-AMP (Fig. 2).

The methylxanthines exert their activity by inhibiting

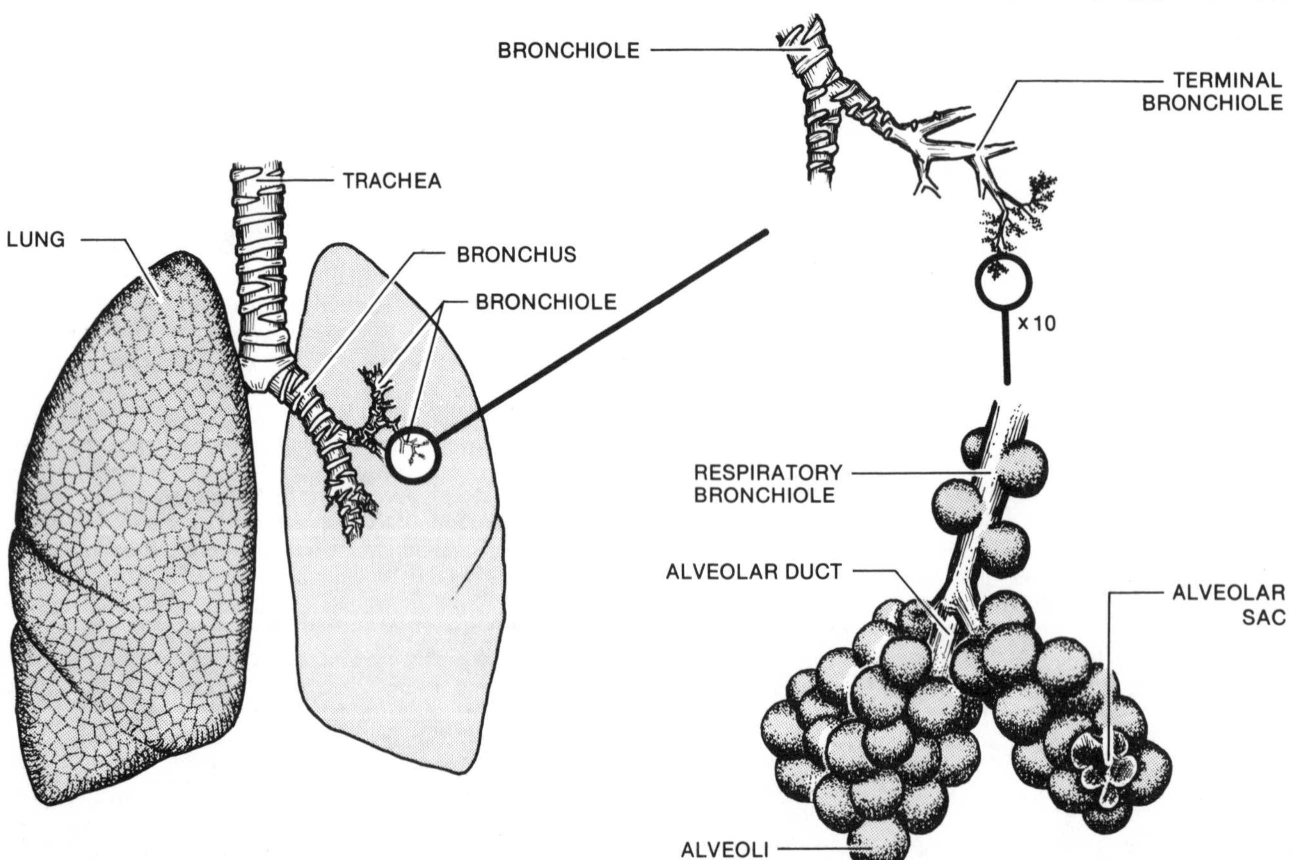

Figure 1. Anatomy of the upper and lower respiratory passages and the bronchial tree.

phosphodiesterase, thereby allowing intracellular concentrations of cyclic AMP to accumulate. Until the introduction of adrenergic agents, e.g., metaproterenol, which have mainly β_2 activity, it was necessary to treat asthma with drugs that had mixed activity. Although this therapy was effective, it also was the source of many side effects. For example, epinephrine stimulates β_1, β_2, and α receptors. Thus, parenteral administration produces bronchodilation, tachycardia, and increased blood pressure; tachycardia and increased blood pressure may be detrimental to asthmatic patients with cardiovascular disease. It should be noted that repeated use of sympathomimetic amines at shorter than recommended intervals reduces the ability of the receptor to respond to subsequent stimulation; tolerance to the drug action may develop. The methylxanthines, by virtue of their ability to increase intracellular concentrations of cyclic AMP, also can cause undesired effects including cardiac, CNS, and skeletal muscle stimulation.

The ideal agent for the therapy of asthma should be orally effective; should produce minimal CNS stimulation, tachycardia, and hypertension; and should have prolonged action.[22] Such an agent has not yet been found; therefore, in choosing a drug for an asthmatic patient, the side effects of each agent as well as the current physical status of the patient must be considered.

Ephedrine

Since the early work of Miller [23] and Chen *et al.*, [24-27] ephedrine has been widely used in the therapy of asthma. It is effective orally and is partially metabolized by the liver, but about 75 percent of the dose is excreted unchanged in the urine.[28] Its onset of action occurs in 30 to 60 minutes with a duration of 2 to 3 hours.[25 29-31] Ephedrine has direct α and β receptor stimulating activity.[28 32] It also acts indirectly by causing the release of norepinephrine from peripheral sympathetic fibers. Ephedrine is used for asthma because of its β-stimulating activity, which results in bronchodilation. As with most sympathomimetic amines, tolerance develops with rapidly repeated doses.

Because ephedrine crosses the blood brain barrier, it often causes tenseness, nervousness, tremors, and sleeplessness.[22 32] Peripheral effects include tachycardia, palpitations, and elevation of systolic and diastolic blood pressure. Urinary retention may also occur, especially in older male patients with prostatic hypertrophy.[22 28 32] Overdosage results in exaggeration of these side effects. Normal doses may produce a significant and potentially dangerous rise in blood pressure if MAO inhibitors are taken concurrently because these agents inhibit the metabolism of norepinephrine.

Because of its slow onset, prolonged action, and decreased potency as compared to epinephrine, ephedrine is used to prevent attacks in patients with milder forms of asthma rather than as acute therapy for moderate to severe asthma.[5 33] For adults, doses of 12.5 to 25 mg, not more often than every 4 hours, not to exceed 150 mg in 24 hours are effective in relieving bronchoconstriction.[34] For children 12 or under, the FDA OTC Panel on Cold, Cough, Allergy, Bronchodilator, and Antiasthmatic Drugs has recommended that no dosage be included in OTC labeling. (Professional labeling recommends that for children 6 to 12 years, the dosage is 6.25 to 12.5 mg, not more often than every 4 hours, not to exceed 75 mg in 24 hours; for children 2 to 6, it is 0.3-0.5 mg/kg, not more often than every 4 hours, not to exceed 2 mg/kg in 24 hours.) [34] If symptoms occur which are not relieved within 1 hour after taking a dose, additional ephedrine should not be taken; a physician should be consulted immediately.

The systemic administration of sympathomimetic amines may affect glucose metabolism, resulting in increased serum glucose levels. Diabetics should be informed of this possibility and instructed to closely monitor urine sugars while taking ephedrine-containing products. People with heart disease, high blood pressure, or thyroid disease should use ephedrine only as directed by a physician.

Methoxyphenamine hydrochloride

Methoxyphenamine hydrochloride is a sympathomimetic amine which is structurally related to ephedrine. It is most effective when used chronically for the prevention of asthmatic attacks and for the relief of mild symptoms. Acute attacks are better treated with more potent agents. Methoxyphenamine hydrochloride produces antiasthmatic effects similar to ephedrine but may exhibit fewer side effects.[35-37] Improvement of symptoms begins about 1 hour after oral administration and continues for 2 to 3 hours.[22 31 35]

The most common side effects of methoxyphenamine hydrochloride are dry mouth and, occasionally, mild anorexia, nausea, light-headedness, dizziness, and drowsiness. Methoxyphenamine hydrochloride causes little or no CNS stimulation and no increase in blood pressure or heart rate.[35 36] In an oral dose of 200 mg, it is therapeutically equivalent to 30 mg of ephedrine. No data are currently available on the use of methoxyphenamine hydrochloride in children under 12; in this age group it should only be used on the advice of a physician. The usual adult dose is 100 mg every 4 to 6 hours, not to exceed 600 mg in 24 hours.[38]

Epinephrine

Epinephrine is effective only when given parenterally or via inhalation because of its instability in gastric fluids and metabolism by enzymes in the gut wall.[28] Because it has a profound effect on the cardiovascular system, it is given parenterally in severe attacks after other means of therapy have failed. All OTC aerosol products used for asthma contain epinephrine or one of its salt forms. When they are used correctly, these products deliver a small quantity of epinephrine directly to the bronchioles, where the drug exerts its effect. There are few side effects because significant systemic absorption does not occur. However, overuse of the aerosols may cause enough systemic absorption to produce side effects.

Epinephrine exerts α- and β-stimulating effects which cause both bronchodilation and vasoconstriction of the vessels that supply the bronchial mucosa. Vasoconstriction probably causes a decrease in bronchial mucosal edema and a decrease in systemic absorption of the drug.[5 32] Relief usually occurs in 5 to 10 minutes after administration of epinephrine, but because of its short duration of action (about 30 to 40 minutes), relapse frequently occurs within a few hours.[5 31-33]

As with all sympathomimetics, frequent use leads to tolerance. This especially is a problem with epinephrine inhalation; patients with moderate to severe attacks increase their use of epinephrine, delaying the time before seeking professional help and often causing the precipitation of a serious attack, i.e., status asthmaticus. Rees *et al.*[39] reported that, although the administration of epinephrine rapidly relieved airway obstruction, hypoxemia persisted for as long as 1 hour, even though the patient was breathing comfortably. This probably results from increased ventilation of areas of the lung that are poorly perfused by blood. For this reason, it is advisable for patients to refrain from exercise for at least 1 hour after an asthmatic attack.

The main side effects of epinephrine are tremors, nervousness, restlessness, insomnia, and palpitations.[32] Dry mouth and throat and gastric irritation also are common, probably resulting from vasoconstriction of vessels caused by a local effect of the drug reaching these areas. These effects may be alleviated by gargling after each use of an aerosol epinephrine preparation.[32,33] Tilting the head back to form a straight passageway for the inhaled drug has also been suggested to prevent the dryness.

One to three inhalations of a 1-percent aqueous solution via nebulizer or an equivalent amount of aerosolized epinephrine may be used not more than once every 3 hours except on the advice of a physician. The same dosage may be used in children over 4, if they are able to use aerosol dosage forms. Epinephrine by inhalation should not be used by people with congestive heart failure, cardiac arrhythmias, or high blood pressure except on the advice of a physician. It also should not be used for the treatment of asthma, unless a diagnosis of asthma has been made by a physician.

Epinephrine by inhalation has been used for many years without question concerning its safety. In the early 1960's, aerosol products containing isoproterenol and metaproterenol (orciprenaline) became widely used also with little concern for their safety. There were reports of a rapidly rising mortality rate from asthma, especially in children between 10 and 14 years.[40,41] Deaths were sudden and unexpected, and patients were often found clasping an empty aerosol container.[40] Greenberg and Pines[41] were the first to suggest that sympathomimetic aerosols may have been the causative agent when they wrote: "We suspect that patients with asthma may be killing themselves by the excessive use of sympathomimetic agents in the form of metered or pressurized aerosols containing isoprenaline, orciprenaline, or adrenaline." These reports prompted investigators to examine drug use patterns and mortality rates in England and Wales.[42-46]

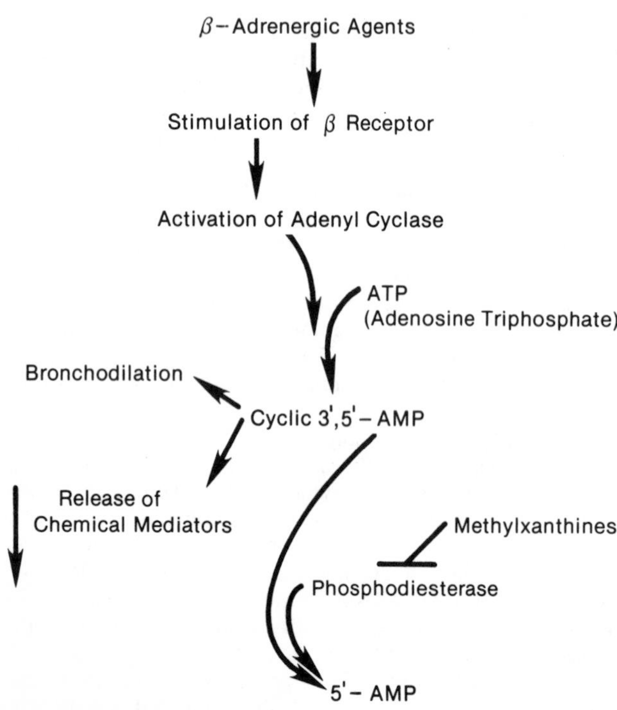

Figure 2. β-Adrenergic agents.

These investigations brought forward several interesting observations. During this period, aerosols containing sympathomimetic agents were available as OTC products in the United Kingdom. Between 1961 and 1967, the estimated percent of total sales of aerosolized sympathomimetics in England was: isoetharine, 1 percent; epinephrine, 4 percent; metaproterenol, 8 percent; isoproterenol in doses of 0.2 mg or less, 59 percent; and isoproterenol in doses of more than 0.2 mg, 28 percent. Thus, 87 percent of total sales contained isoproterenol. After the publication in both professional and lay literature in 1966 and 1967 of the possible hazards of these products, a significant downward trend in mortality began. Between 1967 and 1968, sales of epinephrine, metaproterenol, and isoetharine changed little. However, sales of isoproterenol declined by about 30 percent in 1968 alone. In December, 1968, new poison regulations in England became effective, eliminating the OTC sale of these products.

Although these data are subject to interpretation (many factors can affect mortality in asthma), the evidence strongly implicates the use of isoproterenol as a causative factor. There are no such reports implicating epinephrine. Although there were increasing rates of mortality reported in England, no such increases occurred in the U.S. The difference may possibly have been due to the English preparations containing as much as five times the concentration of isoproterenol as did the U.S. products.

Epinephrine stimulates α and β receptors, causing constriction of the mucosal blood vessels of the bronchioles. This property may possibly allow for a decreased rate of absorption of epinephrine into the systemic circulation, causing less toxicity. Isoproterenol (predominantly a β stimulator) would be expected to produce vasodilation which may increase its own rate of absorption. The significance of this hypothesis, although not firmly established, may be inferred by the rapid onset of tachycardia upon inhalation of isoproterenol. The evidence seems to indicate that epinephrine by inhalation, when used according to instructions, is a safe OTC preparation.

Theophylline

With the exception of dyphylline, which exerts its own action, theophylline is the pharmacologically active derivative of xanthines used in the therapy of asthma.[32] It is also the most potent xanthine with respect to its effects on the bronchi and cardiovascular system. The main effects of theophylline are stimulation of skeletal muscle, relaxation of smooth muscle and bronchiolar tone, coronary artery dilation, and decreased peripheral vascular resistance.[47] A transient increase in cardiac output also occurs, resulting in an increase in glomerular filtration rate and a diuresis of short duration.

The half-life of theophylline is highly variable among patients (2.5 to 9.5 hours).[48-50] Doses of 400 to 3,200 mg/day may be necessary to maintain therapeutic plasma concentrations—between 10 and 20 μg/ml.[48] Toxicity usually occurs at levels of more than 20 μg/ml, and there is no toxicity at less than 13 μg/ml. Absorption is slowed by food, but in chronic use, accumulation occurs and therapeutic levels are maintained even when the drug is taken with food.[48-51] The xanthines are partly metabolized and excreted as methyluric acids or methylxanthines. None is completely metabolized to uric acid; therefore, their use in patients with gout is not contraindicated.[5]

The main side effects of theophylline are anorexia, nausea, and vomiting. Severe toxicity involving CNS stimulation leading to convulsions, coma, and cardiovascular collapse has been reported in children.[52] Most of these cases occurred in pediatric patients receiving suppositories in combination with oral or parenteral theophylline preparations. Usual adult doses of aminophylline are 100 to 200 mg orally every 6 hours not to exceed 800 mg in 24 hours; aminophylline should not be used in children under 12 except on the advice of a physician. When using other derivatives, the dosage should be calculated according to the amount of theophylline base present: aminophylline (85 percent), theophylline olamine (75 percent), choline oxtriphylline (65 percent), and dyphylline (70 percent).

Theophylline became popular as an oral bronchodilator in the 1930's, and pharmaceutical manufacturers began production of a multitude of dosage forms and fixed combination products. Weinberger and Riegelman [53] stated: "This plethora of preparations may have been either a cause or a result of the irrational use of theophylline."

Early use of theophylline resulted in nausea and GI irritation; thus, enteric-coated tablets and rectal suppositories were introduced. However, Jenne *et al.*[48] have shown that the GI side effects occurred with greater frequency when "trough" plasma levels were above 20 μg/ml. They suggest that some mechanism mediated through blood levels rather than direct irritation of the gastric mucosa is responsible for these symptoms. Waxler and Schack [54] reported significantly lower blood levels with enteric-coated as compared to uncoated tablets. Rectal suppositories containing aminophylline have also been shown to be slowly and erratically absorbed as compared to oral tablets and liquid.[51,54] The use of theophylline olamine as a retention enema has been shown to produce reliable therapeutic levels, although they are somewhat lower than those expected with oral uncoated tablets.[55]

Several investigators have demonstrated that theophylline in hydroalcoholic solution provides equivalent or slightly higher blood levels when compared to oral tablets.[56,57] Herxheimer [58] suggests that the rapid absorption from hydroalcoholic solutions may allow the use of oral therapy for moderately severe attacks, making hospital admission unnecessary. Although this reasoning has some merit in acute situations, such rapid absorption offers no advantage and may actually be undesirable when chronic sustained levels are the goal.[59] Usual doses of hydroalcoholic elixirs range from 30 to 60 ml, making it cumbersome for patients to carry a day's supply of medication.

Many pharmaceutical manufacturers have introduced combination products usually containing theophylline (100 to 130 mg), ephedrine (24 mg), and phenobarbital (8 mg). The dose of theophylline in these combinations is subtherapeutic, but ephedrine, the weaker bronchodilator, is present in therapeutic concentrations. Phenobarbital is added to decrease the CNS stimulation caused by ephedrine; however, with chronic use, CNS effects are minimal, and 8 mg of phenobarbital is probably of no benefit. Barbiturates can depress respiratory centers and may potentially aggravate ventilation. Weinberger and Bronsky [60,61] studied theophylline alone, in combination with ephedrine, and in conventional fixed dose combinations. Their data indicate that theophylline in individualized doses provides control of asthmatic symptoms. The addition of ephedrine provided no additional benefit; however, the combination caused an increase in the incidence of insomnia, nervousness, and GI complaints. Fixed dose combinations were relatively ineffective in these studies.

Other agents

Antihistamines. Many combination asthma products contain antihistamines to antagonize the effects of histamine. However, they have no effect on bradykinin and SRS-A and thus are ineffective as therapeutic agents for asthma. Antihistamines also have anticholinergic activity, resulting in a reduction of watery secretions in the bronchi. This leads to the formation of thicker mucus which is more difficult to expectorate. Because mucus plugs are a main cause of airway obstruction, antihistamines may actually worsen an asthmatic attack.

Expectorants. Many asthma products contain expectorants, especially guaifenesin (glyceryl guaiacolate) and potassium iodide. These agents probably are not more effective as expectorants than an adequate intake of water. Therefore, their use in asthma is questionable.

Antitussives. Antitussives such as codeine and dextromethorphan hydrobromide are occasionally used in asthma products. Coughing is the major mechanism for removing bronchial secretions and mucus plugs. Therefore, antitussives generally should not be used for asthma.

Water. Water remains a major therapeutic agent in the treatment of asthma, a fact which should be stressed with all patients. Adequate hydration increases the watery secretions in the bronchioles which thins mucus secretions. This thinning allows for easier removal of mucus and decreased formation of mucus plugs. Effective delivery of water to the lungs depends on adequate oral intake. Additional benefit may be gained from vaporizers and cool-mist humidifiers. Care should be taken to keep the cool-mist humidifier clean to prevent the growth of mold on the atomizing mechanism.

Specialized dosage forms

Administration of bronchodilators via inhalation provides rapid and effective treatment of acute symptoms of asthma. The drug is delivered directly to its site of action (the bronchioles), eliminating delays in absorption and distribution found with other routes of administration. Proper formulation and use of aerosols is the key to effective therapy and prevention of complications. In order for the inhaled mist to be be deposited in the bronchioles, the particle size must range from 0.5 to 5 micrometers (μm).[62,63] Particles larger than 5 μm are deposited in the upper airways; those smaller than 0.5 μm are exhaled. Most commercially available aerosol preparations are in this range. Conventional nebulizers, although somewhat less reliable than aerosols in their ability to deliver an accurate dose of appropriate particle size, are adequate when they are used properly.

Patient consultation

It is important that the pharmacist determine whether symptoms of dyspnea, cough, and wheezing are asthma or another disease. Chronic bronchitis and emphysema have similar symptoms; however, they are continuous rather than episodic, as with asthma. Patients with congestive heart failure may awake in the middle of the night with dyspnea and cough resulting from pulmonary edema. Airway obstruction may also occur in people with pulmonary emboli, infection, and cancer.

Although it is not the responsibility of the pharmacist to make a differential diagnosis, certain information can help determine whether to recommend an OTC product or physician referral. If the symptoms are new and the patient has not been diagnosed by a physician as having asthma, physician referral for evaluation is essential. OTC medication for the relief of asthma should never be used unless a diagnosis of asthma has been established by a physician. This information is important in order to rule out other causes of pulmonary symptoms, establish a baseline for the severity of the disease, explore the etiology of the patient's asthma in hopes that the causative factor may be removed, and avoid OTC medications which can worsen other conditions. If a diagnosis of asthma has been established, it is important to determine which self-treatment approaches have been tried. If aminophylline and an aerosol bronchodilator are currently used but dyspnea is becoming worse, a severe attack is imminent, and the patient should see a physician immediately. In this situation OTC products would be useless. If, on the other hand, the dyspnea is mild, intermittent, and does not worsen, recommendation of an OTC asthma product is appropriate.

Education in the use of medications for asthma is as important as the choice of the drug. Improper use of aerosol agents can decrease effectiveness and increase side effects. The patient should be instructed to hold the aerosol upside down, close the lips and teeth around the mouthpiece, forcefully expel as much air as possible, then deeply inhale through the mouthpiece. Shortly after inhalation begins, the bottle should be pressed down to activate the spray and inhalation should continue. The patient should then pause for a few seconds and slowly exhale. An alternative method is for the patient not to close the teeth and lips around the mouthpiece but to hold the mouthpiece at the level of the lips, with the mouth open. It is important to position the tongue away from the mainstream of the mist, otherwise the medication will be deposited in the oral cavity and upper airways. If symptoms are not relieved in 20 minutes, a physician should be consulted. If headache, nervousness, or palpitations occur, the medication should be discontinued. The mouthpiece should be washed daily with warm water to prevent clogging, and it should always be kept free of particles. Gargling after each use prevents dry mouth and throat irritation.

Doses of oral sympathomimetics or xanthines should be spaced evenly throughout the day; the last dose should be taken at bedtime because many attacks occur during the night. The pharmacist should stress that these oral medications should be taken regularly to prevent the occurrence of asthma symptoms and will probably be of little value in treating an acute attack. Patients should be informed that nervousness or insomnia may occur during the initiation of therapy with these agents but will usually disappear in a few days. If symptoms persist beyond a few days, the patient should consult a physician. Patients with aspirin sensitivity should be cautioned that some asthma preparations contain aspirin. However, the FDA Panel has recommended that no aspirin be included in products used for asthma.[64] If nausea, vomiting, or restlessness occurs after taking xanthine preparations, the dosage should be reduced. OTC xanthine medications should not be taken with prescription medication containing theophylline salts or with theophylline rectal suppositories. Adequate hydration, humidification of room air, rest, and the avoidance of allergens and stressful situations are also important considerations which should be discussed. When stressful situations, e.g., cold air or exercise, are unavoidable, prophylactic use of an aerosol prior to exposure may prevent an asthmatic attack.

Considerations in product selection

Before recommending an OTC product for asthma, it is important for the pharmacist to have a good understanding of the patient's condition. A complete patient profile alerts the pharmacist to conditions such as heart disease, diabetes, hypertension, aspirin sensitivity, and to prescription medications being taken which can duplicate or interact with OTC products. It may also provide an indication concerning the patient's compliance with drug regimens. The patient can help determine whether OTC medications are providing sufficient relief without bothersome side effects or whether prescription medications might be more appropriate.

Summary

Asthma is currently an intensively studied disease. However, its pathogenesis is not completely understood. Evidence indicates that several factors interrelate in variable degrees in the precipitation of an attack. These include allergy, infection, autonomic nervous system balance, and psychophysiological response to stress.

The choice of agents in the therapy of asthma is also complex. The severity of the disease, existence of other diseases, previous response to therapy, and current medications for both asthma and other diseases are important considerations which should be known before recommendations for OTC asthma products are made. Continuous oral therapy should be used for the prevention and control of asthmatic symptoms. In mild cases, ephedrine (12.5 to 25 mg) or methoxyphenamine (100 mg) every 4 to 6 hours may provide adequate protection. Theophylline or one of its derivatives is the oral therapy of choice in individuals with more severe asthma. However, unless appropriate blood levels are obtained, this agent usually provides unsatisfactory results. Because individuals vary in their ability to metabolize theophylline, individualized dosage regimens are required. Appropriate theophylline plasma levels are highly effective with relatively little toxicity. Levels below 10 μg/ml are usually ineffective, and those above 20 μg/ml are usually toxic. Theophylline should be used correctly or not at all.

If exacerbation of the disease occurs, oral therapy should be supplemented with inhalation of aerosol bronchodilators. In patients who have mild asthma without concurrent cardiovascular disease, OTC products that contain epinephrine may provide adequate therapy. In severe asthma, the more potent prescription-only bronchodilators, such as isoproterenol or metaproterenol, should be used. Patients should be cautioned that overuse of aerosol bronchodilators may lead to tolerance, cardiovascular toxicity, or progression of the attack to life-threatening severity by delaying the time before a physician is consulted.

Water provides a major therapeutic modality in the treatment of all asthmatic patients. It is important that patients be instructed in maintaining an adequate oral intake of fluids and in the proper use of humidifiers and vaporizers.

References

1. American Thoracic Society, *Am. Rev. Respir. Dis.*, **85**, 762-768 (1962).
2. U.S. National Health Survey, U.S. Public Health Service Publication No. 584-B12, Washington, D.C., U.S. Government Printing Office, 1958.
3. F. M. Rackemann and M. C. Edwards, *N. Engl. J. Med.*, **246**, 815-823, 858-863(1952).
4. "Harrison's Principles of Internal Medicine," M. M. Wintrobe *et al.*, Eds., McGraw-Hill, New York, N.Y., 1974, pp. 371-374.
5. A. L. Sheffer and M. D. Valentine, *Med. Clin. North Am.*, **53(2)**, 239-248(1969).
6. R. P. McCombs, *N. Engl. J. Med.*, **286**, 1186-1194(1972).
7. D. A. Mathison *et al.*, *J. Am. Med. Assoc.*, **224**, 1134-1139(1973).
8. R. F. Lockey *et al.*, *Ann. Intern. Med.*, **78**, 57-63(1973).
9. R. D. Snyder and G. L. Siegel, *Ann. Allergy*, **25**, 377-380(1967).
10. P. M. Penna, *J. Am. Pharm. Assoc.*, **NS13**, 690-697(1973).
11. G. N. Beall *et al.*, *Ann. Intern. Med.*, **78**, 405-419(1973).
12. W. A. Mahon, *Can. Med. Assoc. J.*, **110**, 376(1974).
13. T. Berg and S. G. Johansson, *Int. Arch. Allergy Appl. Immunol.*, **36**, 219(1969).
14. K. Ishizaka and T. Ishizaka, *J. Immunol.*, **99**, 1187-1198(1967).
15. "Pathologic Basis of Disease," S. L. Robbins, Ed., Saunders, Philadelphia, Pa., 1974, p. 803.
16. M. Kaliner, *Can. Med. Assoc. J.*, **110**, 431-435(1974).

17. W. M. Gold *et al.*, *J. Appl. Physiol.*, **3,** 719(1972).
18. A. Szentivanyi, *J. Allergy,* **42,** 203-232(1968).
19. A. Szentivanyi, *Ann. Allergy,* **24,** 253(1966).
20. A. S. Rebuck, *Drugs,* **7,** 344-369(1974).
21. M. S. Dunnill, *J. Clin. Pathol.,* **13,** 27-33(1960).
22. M. C. S. Kennedy and S. L. O. Jackson, *Br. Med. J.,* **2,** 1506(1963).
23. T. G. Miller, *Am. J. Med. Sci.,* **170,** 157(1925).
24. W. S. Middleton and K. K. Chen, *Arch. Intern. Med.,* **39,** 385(1927).
25. K. K. Chen and C. F. Schmidt, *Medicine,* **9(1),** 339-357(1930).
26. K. K. Chen and C. F. Schmidt, *J. Pharmacol. Exp. Ther.,* **24,** 339-351(1924).
27. K. K. Chen, *Arch. Intern. Med.,* **39,** 404-411(1927).
28. "The Pharmacological Basis of Therapeutics," L. S. Goodman and A. Gilman, Eds., Macmillan, New York, N.Y., 1970, pp. 507-513.
29. A. H. Beckett *et al., J. Pharm. Pharmacol.,* **Suppl. 24,** 65P-70P(1972).
30. G. R. Wilkinson and A. H. Beckett, *J. Pharm. Sci.,* **57,** 1933-1938 (1968).
31. E. Bresnick *et al., J. Clin. Invest.,* **28,** 1182-1189(1949).
32. C. G. Blumstein, *Semin. Drug Treat.,* **2(4),** 385-401(1973).
33. F. Sadik *et al., J. Am. Pharm. Assoc.,* **NS15,** 247-250(1975).
34. *Fed. Regist.,* **41(176),** 38371(1976).
35. J. J. Curry *et al., J. Allergy,* **20,** 104-110(1949).
36. R. S. B. Pearson, *Br. Med. J.,* **2,** 905-907(1958).
37. E. C. Roy *et al., J. Allergy,* **20,** 364-368(1949).
38. *Fed Regist.,* **41(176),** 38372(1976).
39. H. A. Rees *et al., Lancet,* **2,** 1164-1167(1967).
40. J. M. Smith, *Lancet,* **1,** 1042(1966).
41. M. J. Greenberg and A. Pines, *Br. Med. J.,* **1,** 563(1967).
42. P. J. D. Heaf, *Br. Med. Bull.,* **26,** 245-247(1970).
43. W. H. W. Inman and A. M. Adelstein, *Lancet,* **2,** 279-285(1969).
44. F. E. Speizer *et al., Br. Med. J.,* **1,** 335-339(1968).
45. F. E. Speizer and R. Doll, *Br. Med. J.,* **3,** 245(1968).
46. F. E. Speizer *et al., Br. Med. J.,* **1,** 339-343(1968).
47. T. G. Tong, *Drug Intell. Clin. Pharm.,* **7,** 156-167(1973).
48. J. J. Jenne *et al., Clin. Pharm. Ther.,* **13,** 349-360(1972).
49. P. A. Mitenko and R. I. Ogilvie, *Clin. Pharmacol. Ther.,* **14,** 509-513(1973).
50. P. A. Mitenko and R. I. Ogilvie, *Clin. Pharmacol. Ther.,* **13,** 329-335(1972).
51. L. P. Lillehei, *J. Am. Med. Assoc.,* **205,** 530-533(1968).
52. H. L. Bacal *et al., Can. Med. Assoc. J.,* **80,** 6(1959).
53. M. Weinberger and S. Riegelman, *N. Engl. J. Med.,* **291,** 151-153(1974).
54. S. H. Waxler and J. A. Schack, *J. Am. Med. Assoc.,* **143,** 736-739(1950).
55. J. W. Yunginger *et al., Ann. Allergy,* **24,** 469-483(1966).
56. J. T. McGinn, *Curr. Ther. Res.,* **7,** 110-115(1965).
57. J. Schluger *et al., Am. J. Med. Sci.,* **233,** 296-302(1957).
58. H. Herxheimer, *N. Engl. J. Med.,* **291,** 1192(1974).
59. M. Weinberger and S. Riegelman, *N. Engl. J. Med.,* **291,** 1193(1974).
60. M. Weinberger and E. Bronsky, *Clin. Pharm. Ther.,* **17,** 585-592 (1975).
61. M. M. Weinberger and E. A. Bronsky, *J. Pediatr.,* **84,** 421-427 (1974).
62. "The Theory and Practice of Industrial Pharmacy," L. Lachman *et al.,* Eds., Lea and Febiger, Philadelphia, Pa., 1970, p. 614.
63. M. Lippmann and R. E. Albert, *Am. Ind. Hyg. Assoc. J.,* **30,** 257(1969).
64. *Fed. Regist.,* **41(176),** 38326(1976).

Products 9 ASTHMA

Product (manufacturer)	Dosage form	Ephedrine	Epinephrine	Theophylline	Other
Amodrine (Searle)	tablet	25 mg (as racemic hydrochloride)	—	—	aminophylline, 100 mg phenobarbital, 8 mg
Asma-Lief (Columbia Medical)	tablet	24 mg (as hydrochloride)	—	130 mg	phenobarbital, 8 mg
Asthma Haler (Norcliff-Thayer)	oral inhalant	—	7 mg/ml (as bitartrate)	—	—
Asthma Nefrin (Norcliff-Thayer)	inhalant solution	—	2.25% (as racemic hydrochloride)	—	chlorobutanol, 0.5%
Breatheasy (Pascal)	inhalant	—	2.2% (as hydrochloride)	—	benzyl alcohol, 1% isotonic salts, 0.5%
Bronitin (Whitehall)	tablet	24 mg	—	130 mg	guaifenesin, 100 mg methapyrilene, 16 mg
Bronkaid (Breon)	tablet	24 mg (as sulfate)	—	100 mg (anhydrous)	guaifenesin, 100 mg magnesium trisilicate, 74.52 mg
Bronkaid Mist (Breon)	inhalant	—	0.5%	—	ascorbic acid, 0.07% alcohol, 34% hydrochloric and nitric acid buffers
Bronkotabs (Breon)	tablet	24 mg (as sulfate)	—	100 mg	guaifenesin, 100 mg phenobarbital, 8 mg
Phedral (North American)	tablet	24.3 mg	—	129.6 mg	phenobarbital, 8.1 mg
Primatene M (Whitehall)	tablet	24 mg (as hydrochloride)	—	130 mg	methapyrilene, 16 mg
Primatene P (Whitehall)	tablet	24 mg	—	130 mg	phenobarbital, 8 mg
Tedral (Warner-Chilcott)	tablet elixir suspension	24 mg/tablet 6 mg/5 ml elixir 12 mg/5 ml suspension (all as hydrochloride)	—	130 mg/tablet (anhydrous) 32.5 mg/5 ml elixir 65 mg/5 ml suspension	phenobarbital, 8 mg/tablet 2 mg/5 ml elixir 4 mg/5 ml suspension
Thalfed (Beecham Labs)	tablet	25 mg (as hydrochloride)	—	120 mg (hydrous)	phenobarbital, 8 mg
Vaponefrin Solution (Fisons)	inhalant	—	2.25% (as racemic hydrochloride)	—	chlorobutanol, 0.5%
Verequad (Knoll)	tablet suspension	24 mg/tablet 12 mg/5 ml (as hydrochloride)	—	130 mg/tablet 65 mg/5 ml (as calcium salicylate)	guaifenesin, 100 mg/tablet 50 mg/5 ml phenobarbital, 8 mg/tablet 4 mg/5 ml

Internal Analgesic Products

W. Kent Van Tyle

Questions to ask the patient

Do you now have or have you ever had asthma, other allergic diseases, or ulcers?

Are you now taking medication for gout, arthritis, or diabetes? If so, what?

Are you now taking any medication which affects the clotting of your blood?

Have you ever had any problem with your blood being slow to clot?

Have you ever had an allergic reaction to aspirin?

What type of pain do you have, and how long have you had it?

Do you have any other symptoms which you feel might be associated with the pain you have?

(If appropriate) How high is your fever, and how long have you had fever?

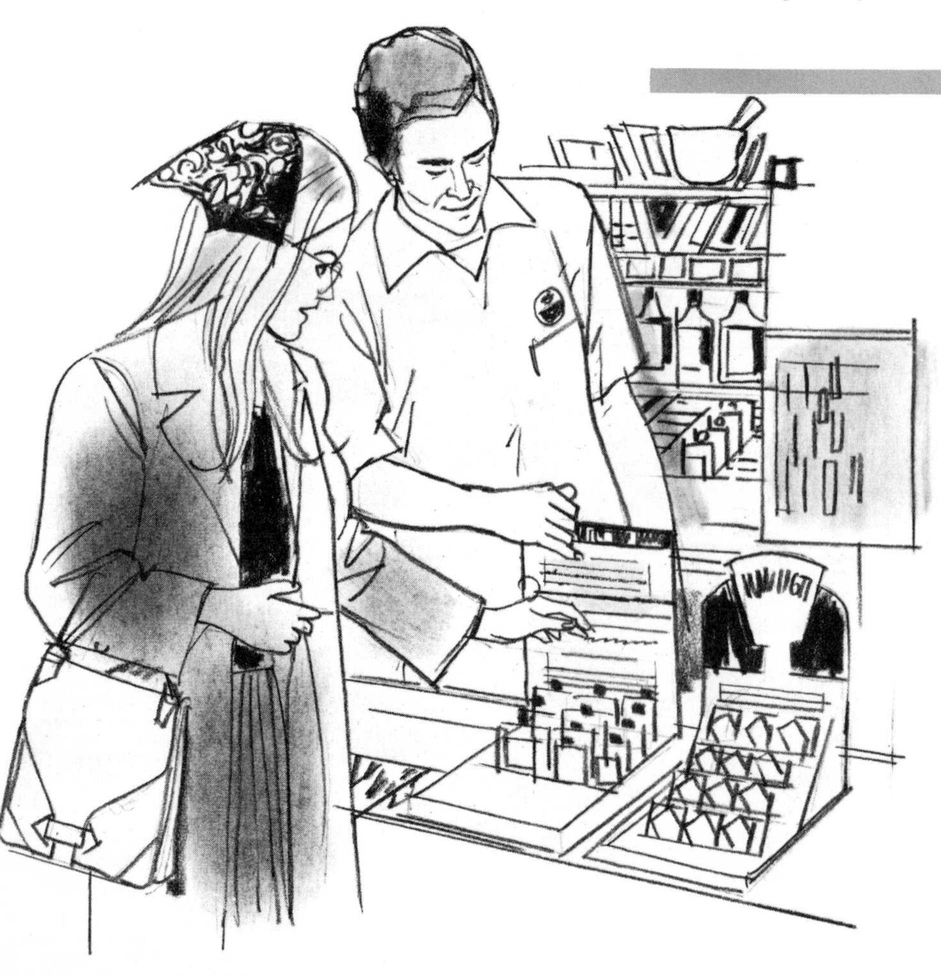

CHAPTER 10

Internal analgesics are drugs that are ingested to relieve pain. Although classification as analgesics would seem to exclude their use for other purposes, certain compounds in this group also possess pharmacologic activities which make them valuable for reducing elevated body temperature and for ameliorating various inflammatory conditions.

Even though pain is a common experience, it is not a simple condition to define. Pain is a sensation, but it is also an interpretation of that sensation which can be influenced by many factors. Fatigue, anxiety, fear, and the anticipation of more pain all affect the perception of and reaction to pain. Haslam [1] has shown that various personality types experience pain differently; the introverted personality has a lower pain threshold than the extrovert. In addition, the perception of pain can be significantly modified by suggestion. Studies indicate that approximately 35 percent of patients suffering pain from a variety of causes report their pain as being "satisfactorily relieved" by placebo.[2]

Pain is usually a protective mechanism, occurring when tissue is damaged or when cells are altered by pain stimuli which threaten to produce tissue damage. Pain that is the result of a functional disturbance or pathology is called "organic" pain. In contrast, "psychogenic" pain is a symptom of an underlying behavioral disturbance and is not a consequence of organic pathology. Organic pain is the type of pain usually presented to the pharmacist when advice is sought on nonprescription analgesics. This type of pain is amenable to treatment with internal analgesics.

Origin and perception of pain

Pain is categorized, according to its origin, as either somatic or visceral. Somatic pain arises from the musculoskeletal system or skin; visceral pain originates from the organs or viscera of the thorax and abdomen.

Free nerve endings serve as pain receptors to initiate nerve impulses which travel via specialized pain fibers through the spinal cord and/or brain stem to specific receiving areas of the brain. These receptors are found throughout the superficial layers of the skin and in certain deeper tissues such as the membranous covering of bones, the arterial walls, muscles, tendons, joint surfaces, and membranes lining the skull.[3] Pain-evoking stimuli have in common the ability to injure cells and to cause the release of a proteolytic enzyme which produces polypeptides from the globulins found in intercellular fluid. Polypeptides produced in this way stimulate nerve endings at the site of injury or trauma and thus initiate the pain impulse.[4]

Pain fibers enter the dorsal roots of the spinal cord and interconnect with other nerve cells which cross to the opposite side of the cord and ascend to the brain. A pain impulse terminates in the thalamus, where conscious perception of pain appears to be localized, or in well-defined areas of the cerebral cortex, where recognition and interpretation of the nature and location of the pain impulse occur.

Pain initiation, transmission, and perception are essentially the same for both visceral and somatic pain. One important distinction, however, is that highly localized visceral damage rarely causes severe pain. Diffuse stimulation of nerve endings throughout an organ is required to produce significant visceral pain. Conditions producing visceral pain include ischemia of organ tissue, chemical destruction of visceral tissue, spasm of visceral smooth muscle, and physical distention of an organ or the stretching of its associated mesentery.[3]

In evaluating the etiology and therapy of pain, it is important to recognize the potential for referred pain, or pain seeming to be in a part of the body that is not the actual body part initiating the pain signal. Unlike somatic pain, visceral pain cannot be localized by the brain as coming from a specific organ. Instead, most visceral pain is interpreted by the brain as coming from various skin segments, or it is "referred" to various body surface areas (Table 1). When advising as to the need of or potential benefit to be derived from nonprescription analgesic products, an appreciation for the sites of referred visceral pain is invaluable. Failure to recognize the possibility of referred visceral pain could mean that a serious visceral pathology might go undiagnosed and untreated while ineffective self-medication with nonprescription analgesics is attempted.

Response of pain to nonprescription analgesics

The analgesic products available for self-medication are more effective in treating musculoskeletal, or somatic, pain than pain of visceral origin.[5] Nonprescription analgesic therapy is most frequently used for headache or for pain associated with either peripheral nerves (neuralgia), joints (arthralgia), or muscles (myalgia).

Headache. The most common form of pain is headache. Estimates are that each week, 15 percent of the population experiences headache pain.[6] Wolff [7] has classified headache as either intracranial or extracranial, depending on the area of initiation of the pain. Intracranial headache results from inflammation or traction of sensitive intracranial structures, primarily vascular. Its etiology includes tumor, abscess, hematoma, or infection. Intracranial headache is an uncommon situation, but because of the potential seriousness of its underlying causes, it requires immediate medical attention.

Because headache may be a symptom of a serious underlying pathology, the pharmacist should evaluate the potential for headache of intracranial origin and should be prepared to recommend medical attention when appropriate. Intracranial headache produced by tumor or meningeal traction is "deep, aching, steady, dull, and seldom rhythmic or throbbing." [8] The pain may be continuous, is generally more intense in the morning, and may be associated with nausea and vomiting. Pain location cannot be used to differentiate headache of intracranial origin. Concomitant disturbances in sensory function such as blurred vision, dizziness, or hearing loss, or changes in personality, behavior, speech patterns, or memory are signals to seek immediate medical attention.

The more common forms of headache are all of extracranial origin and are of diverse etiology. Vascular headaches of the migraine type vary greatly in intensity, frequency, and duration. Although the exact cause of migraine is not completely understood, it is thought that emotion and tension contribute to the production of vasospasm in the arteries supplying the brain, causing localized ischemia. The ischemia produces a loss of vascular tone in these arteries, and they begin to pulsate with the rising and falling intravascular pressure.[3] The stretching of the arterial walls or associated meninges then produces the intense pain characteristic of migraine. The pain of migraine is usually throbbing, often unilateral, and often preceded by a variety of sensations including nausea, loss of vision in part of the visual field, and visual aura.

The "tension" headache is the result of spasms of the somatic musculature of the neck and scalp. Symptoms include a feeling of tightness or pressure at the base of the head or in the muscles of the back of the neck. Localization of pain with a tension headache is often in the forehead or at the base of the skull.

The "sinus" headache can be characteristically distinguished from headache of other etiology because its location is restricted to the frontal areas of the forehead and scalp and behind or around the eyes. Accompanying symptoms include rhinorrhea, nasal congestion, and a feeling of pressure in the sinuses. Irritation and edema of the mucous membranes of the nose and sinuses as a consequence of infection or allergy are the underlying causes.

In addition to being a symptom of sinus headache, pain around or behind the eyes may be caused by uncorrected visual problems associated with difficulty in focusing on near or far objects. Tonic contraction of the ciliary muscles in an attempt to gain clear vision can result in muscle spasm and referred retro-orbital pain. If retro-orbital headache recurs persistently, referral for ophthalmic examination is indicated. Similarly, recurrent facial or mandibular pain may indicate the need for professional dental examination and treatment.

Table 1. Body Surface Areas Associated with Referred Visceral Pain[a]

Origin of visceral pain	Localization of pain on body surface
Appendix	Around umbilicus localizing in right lower quadrant of abdomen
Bladder	Lower abdomen directly over bladder
Esophagus	Pharynx, lower neck, arms, midline chest region
Gallbladder	Upper central portion of abdomen; lower right shoulder
Heart	Base of neck, shoulders and upper chest; down arms (left side involvement more frequent than right)
Kidney and ureters	Regions of lower back over site of affected organ; anterior abdominal wall below and to the side of umbilicus
Stomach	Anterior surface of chest or upper abdomen
Uterus	Lower abdomen

[a] Summarized from A. C. Guyton, "Textbook of Medical Physiology," 4th ed., Saunders, Philadelphia, Pa., 1971, pp. 577-591 and L. Zetzel, in "Textbook of Medicine," vol. 1, 13th ed., P. B. Beeson and W. McDermott, Eds., Saunders, Philadelphia, Pa., 1971, p. 1327.

Neuralgia. Pain in the distribution of a sensory nerve is called neuralgia. The trigeminal nerve is frequently affected, and trigeminal neuralgia is characterized by sharp, stabbing pain in the face or jaw region occurring in brief, agonizing episodes. The cause of trigeminal neuralgia is unknown, but it apparently is not the result of organic damage to the nerve.[9,10] Because of the intense pain of trigeminal neuralgia, therapy with drugs that are more potent than those available in nonprescription medications usually is required.

Dull, aching facial pain localized in the area of the trigeminal nerve may occur in association with or during recovery from an upper respiratory tract infection. Although the pain often is described as "neuralgia," the exact etiology usually is unknown. Nevertheless, nonprescription analgesics are frequently helpful in alleviating this type of facial pain.

Myalgia. Pain from skeletal muscle, or myalgia, is common. The most frequent cause is strenuous exertion by the untrained person. However, prolonged tonic contraction produced by tension or the maintenance of a certain body position for extended periods can also produce muscle pain.[7] Myalgia responds well to nonprescription analgesics and adjunctive treatment with rubefacients, counterirritants, and heat. (See Chapter 26 for a complete discussion of external analgesics.)

Arthralgia. The most frequent cause of joint pain is inflammation of the synovial membrane (arthritis) or the associated bursa (bursitis). Joints that require free movement between two bones are constructed to maintain the articulating ends of the bones bathed in a lubricating synovial fluid. The two opposing bone ends are held in position by tough, fibrous tissue which forms an enclosure around the bone ends. The inner lining of this fibrous enclosure is the synovial membrane which produces the lubricating synovial fluid.[11] Bursae are saclike structures which contain fluid formed at sites of joint friction, e.g., where a tendon passes over a bone.

Rheumatoid arthritis is a chronic inflammation of synovial membranes, often occurring at multiple sites throughout the body and having a predilection for smaller joints such as those of the hands, fingers, wrists, feet, and toes. Characteristic symptoms include joint stiffness, especially pronounced after arising in the morning, pain with joint motion, and swelling and tenderness of affected joints. Studies indicate that approximately 2.5 to 3 percent of the adult population is afflicted with this condition, the highest incidence occurring in people over 40.[12] Although the cause of rheumatoid arthritis is obscure, hereditary influence has been demonstrated and an immunologic mechanism has been proposed.

Because of the slow, subtle nature of the onset of rheumatoid arthritis, many people attempt self-medication in the initial stages based on the belief that advancing age inevitably brings aches and pains. As the disease progresses, it is a common practice to voluntarily increase the dosage of nonprescription analgesics to maintain relief from arthritic pain. The pharmacist should caution about the potential for chronic toxicity or drug interaction and should be on guard for symptoms that indicate overmedication. Also, because rheumatoid arthritis is a progressive, degenerative disease, medical attention must be encouraged to institute physical therapy and exercise to maintain the maximum possible mobility of affected joints.

Bursitis. This condition may be caused by trauma, gout, infection, or rheumatoid arthritis. Although the most common site of bursa inflammation is the shoulder, the knee (Housemaid's Knee) and the elbow (Tennis Elbow) can also be affected. Common symptoms include pain and limitation of motion of the affected joint, and, depending upon the severity, the pain will usually respond to analgesic therapy. Limitation of motion of the affected joint often hastens recovery.[13 14]

Mechanisms of normal thermoregulation and fever

In a normothermic individual, the internal temperature of the body is maintained within 1° F of its normal mean temperature by a complex thermoregulatory system. Although the normal mean body temperature is 98.6° F (37° C) when measured orally, normal body temperature can range from approximately 97° F (36.1° C) to more than 99° F (37.2 C°). When measured rectally, these normal values are 1° F higher.[12]

In order to maintain a constant body temperature, the thermoregulatory system must balance heat production with heat loss. Thermoregulation is accomplished by continually keeping the temperature control center in the hypothalamus apprised of body temperature. Temperature-sensitive neurons located in the hypothalamus and skin relay body temperature information to the hypothalamus. Responding to this information, the hypothalamus can either initiate responses to conserve heat and to increase heat production or to increase heat loss.

The skin is the primary site of heat loss from the body. Heat is carried by the blood from internal structures to the body surface where it is lost to the surroundings by processes of radiation, conduction, and evaporation. The rate of heat loss from the skin is directly related to the rate of cutaneous blood flow which in turn is a reflection of the degree of tone in the cutaneous vasculature. Consequently, the hypothalamic thermoregulatory center can change the rate of heat loss by altering the degree of vasoconstriction in the cutaneous vasculature. It also facilitates cooling by stimulating sweating which increases the rate of evaporative heat loss from the skin. Heat production can be enhanced by hormonally mediated increases in cellular metabolism and by increased muscle tone and shivering.

Fever, or the elevation of body temperature above normal, may be an indication that the body's defenses have been overwhelmed by bacterial invasion. Although there are other causes of elevated body temperature such as drugs, dehydration, brain tumor, and heat stroke, the production of fever by these causes is of secondary importance when considering the antipyretic activity of analgesic products. Pyrogens, or fever-producing substances, are produced by pathogenic bacteria or by the degeneration of leukocytes. It has been shown that during the course of bacterial invasion, bacterial toxins interact with leukocytes to produce endogenous or leukocyte pyrogen. When pyrogenic bacterial toxins are not present, the destruction of polymorphonuclear leukocytes during the disease process also releases leukocyte pyrogen. Whichever the source, the leukocyte pyrogen is the common causal factor in fever.[15 16] Once it is produced, the leukocyte pyrogen travels in the blood to the hypothalamic areas controlling body temperature. There, the pyrogen elevates the setpoint of the hypothalamus above normal and produces fever.

Using mechanisms of heat conservation and production, the hypothalamus directs the reestablishment of body temperature to correspond to the new elevated setpoint. Within hours, the body temperature reaches this new setpoint and a febrile condition results. During the period of upward temperature readjustment, symptoms of chills, shivering, and feeling cold are experienced, even though the body temperature is elevated above normal. These are all manifestations of peripheral heat conservation and production mechanisms, e.g., vasoconstriction and increased skeletal muscle tone with shivering.

Fever produces a clouding of intellectual function, disorientation, and possibly delirium. Headache is common in a febrile individual and is thought to be the result of dilation and stretching of the larger arteries at the base of the brain. Tachycardia often occurs concomitantly with fever and is usually of little concern unless there is a history of impaired cardiovascular function.[16]

Fever itself does not require therapy unless there is a possibility of CNS damage, cardiovascular insufficiency, or significant discomfort to the patient. Temperatures of as high as 105° F (40.6° C) are usually tolerated by adults. However, children are more prone to convulsions with temperatures in this range. When body temperature rises above 106° F (41.1° C), tissue damage begins. The brain is acutely sensitive to temperatures in this range because brain tissue does not regenerate. Body temperatures above 110° F (43.3° C) are fatal within hours.[15 17]

Ingredients in OTC products

The salicylates

By virtue of their historical significance, extent of use, and spectrum of pharmacological activity, the salicylates represent the standard prototype of nonnarcotic analgesics. They produce their pharmacological effects through the production of salicylate ion in the body. Salicylic acid, sodium salicylate, methyl salicylate, and acetylsalicylic acid (aspirin) are all salicylates. However, only aspirin and sodium salicylate are used internally. Although it is chemically related, salicylamide is not a salicylate.[18]

The salicylates have analgesic, antipyretic, and anti-inflammatory activity and are most effective in treating mild to moderate pain of the dull, aching type that originates in somatic structures. In doses of 325 to 650 mg, "controlled experiments have repeatedly shown aspirin to be superior to placebo in pathologic pain of a wide variety of etiologies."[18] Salicylates produce analgesia both centrally, by acting on hypothalamic structures, and peripherally, by inhibiting pain impulse production in pain receptors.[5 19] Recent studies suggest that the inhibition of prostaglandin synthesis by aspirin is involved in this peripheral mechanism. Prostaglandin E_1 sensitizes peripheral pain receptors, making them more sensitive to chemical or mechanical initiation of pain impulses.[20] Aspirin inhibits prostaglandin synthesis and desensitizes pain receptors to the initiation of pain impulses by decreasing prostaglandin production at sites of inflammation and trauma.[21]

Therapeutic doses of aspirin will effectively reduce an elevated body temperature. Aspirin therapy for fever reduction is most frequently initiated in children because of their propensity for fever-induced convulsions. The recommended pediatric dose is 65 mg (1 gr) per year of age up to a maximum of 650 mg for a 10-year-old or older, repeated not more than once every 4 hours.[22] With this dose, peak antipyretic action is reached between 2 and 3 hours and is sustained for at least 4 hours.[23] Salicylates reduce elevated body temperature by acting on the hypothalamic thermoregulatory center to reestablish a normal setpoint. Heat production is not inhibited, but rather heat loss is augmented by increasing cutaneous blood flow and sweating.[5] Recent studies suggest that prostaglandins are involved in the production of fever and that aspirin exerts its antipyretic effect by inhibiting prostaglandin synthesis in the hypothalamus.[5,24]

Although the efficacy of aspirin in treating inflammatory conditions such as rheumatic fever and rheumatoid arthritis is well established, the mechanism by which these beneficial effects are produced is not. Studies show that the anti-inflammatory effect of salicylates is the result of their inhibition of prostaglandin synthesis.[21,25] Prostaglandins are formed at sites of inflammation, and the injection of either prostaglandin E_1 or E_2 (dinoprostone) produces many of the manifestations of inflammation and intensifies the effects of histamine and bradykinin, known chemical mediators of inflammation.[5,21,25]

Doses of aspirin in the range of 4 to 6 g daily are effective in the management of rheumatoid arthritis. Proposed nonprescription labeling regulations for aspirin direct the patient not to exceed 12 tablets (4 g) in a 24-hour period and to use aspirin for arthritis only under a doctor's supervision.[26] Consequently, self-medication with aspirin for arthritis is inadequate therapy because the dose of aspirin required for efficacy is greater than that deemed safe for self-medication.

Contraindications. Salicylates can compromise hemostasis by inhibiting platelet aggregation and by reducing plasma prothrombin levels. In a normal individual, a single dose of 650 mg (10 gr) of aspirin approximately doubles the mean bleeding time for a period of 4 to 7 days.[5,27] This increase in the bleeding time is not due to hypoprothrombinemia but rather to the inhibition of platelet aggregation. The exact mechanism of inhibition of platelet aggregation is unclear. However, the consequence is a reduction in the rate of formation of a platelet-fibrin plug to occlude blood vessels at points of injury. Salicylate doses of more than 6 g/day are required to reduce plasma prothrombin levels, and the minimal prolongation of prothrombin time that occurs with these doses is rarely clinically significant.[5] Salicylates reduce plasma prothrombin levels by interfering with the use of vitamin K for prothrombin synthesis.[28]

The use of aspirin should be avoided by individuals with hypoprothrombinemia, vitamin K deficiency, or hemophilia and by those with a history of peptic ulcer or GI bleeding. Also, aspirin therapy should be discontinued at least 1 week prior to surgery. Neither sodium salicylate nor acetaminophen significantly affects platelet aggregation and bleeding time.[27,29] Therefore, they are useful in cases where concern about hemostasis contraindicates the use of aspirin.

Salicylates affect the secretion and reabsorption of uric acid by the renal tubules. In low doses of 1 to 2 g/day, salicylates inhibit tubular secretion of uric acid without affecting reabsorption. Consequently, low doses of salicylate reduce urate excretion by the kidney, elevate plasma urate levels, and may precipitate an acute attack of gout. For this reason, self-medication with salicylates by individuals with a history of gout should be discouraged.

Dyspepsia with heartburn, epigastric distress, and nausea or vomiting occurs in approximately 5 percent of patients taking aspirin.[30] More common than dyspepsia is mild GI bleeding which occurs following aspirin ingestion in 40 to 70 percent of patients. GI blood loss usually is in the range of 2 to 6 ml/day, but as much as 10 ml/day has been reported.[31,32] Gastroscopic examination in salicylate-treated patients often reveals ulcerative and hemorrhagic lesions of the gastric mucosa, although lesions are not always visible in those experiencing blood loss.[5,6,33]

Massive GI bleeding characterized by the vomiting of blood (hematemesis) or the presence of large amounts of digested blood in the stools (melena) has been linked to the ingestion of aspirin. Approximately 30 to 40 percent of hospital admissions for hematemesis and/or melena can be attributed to the prior use of salicylates.[34-36] Individuals who take aspirin at least 4 days a week during a 12-week period have a significantly greater likelihood of suffering major GI bleeding than the less frequent user or nonuser of aspirin. The incidence rate of hospital admissions for major upper GI bleeding attributable to the regular use of aspirin is estimated to be about 15/100,000/year.[37] Aspirin is contraindicated in individuals having a history of peptic ulcer disease due to its potential for activating latent ulcers or aggravating existing ones. In addition, the concomitant ingestion of alcohol with aspirin increases GI bleeding, and patients taking aspirin daily should be advised of the potential hazards of alcohol ingestion.[38]

In predisposed individuals, aspirin can produce a hypersensitivity reaction characterized by skin rash and/or anaphylactic symptoms of bronchoconstriction with respiratory difficulty, edema, and shock. Aspirin hypersensitivity occurs most frequently in individuals having a history of allergic disease, especially asthma. Although the overall incidence of aspirin hypersensitivity is 0.2 to 0.9 percent, the incidence of aspirin hypersensitivity is higher among asthmatics.[5] Estimates indicate that 3 to 5 percent of all asthmatics exhibit aspirin hypersensitivity.[39,40] Aspirin hypersensitivity probably involves acetylation of protein in the body to produce an antigenic material, making cross-sensitivity to sodium salicylate or acetaminophen uncommon.[5,41] Many aspirin-hypersensitive individuals are also hypersensitive to indomethacin.[5,41] A history of asthma or other allergic disease is a relative contraindication for aspirin. However, demonstrated hypersensitivity to aspirin or indomethacin absolutely contraindicates self-medication with aspirin. In these situations, sodium salicylate or acetaminophen is the indicated alternative. Also, individuals with known aspirin hypersensitivity should be cautioned about the use of other nonprescription medications which may contain aspirin.

Drug interactions. Uricosuric agents such as sulfinpyrazone and probenecid are effective in the treatment of gout because they block the tubular reabsorption of uric acid. Salicylates inhibit the uricosuric effects of both drugs by blocking this inhibitory effect on uric acid reabsorption.[42,43] Consequently, the concurrent administration of salicylates with either probenecid or sulfinpyrazone should be avoided because of the possibility of precipitating acute gouty attacks, hyperuricemia, or urate stone formation.

Because of their effects on hemostasis and GI mucosa, salicylates have the potential for producing hemorrhaging if administered with oral anticoagulants. The effect of oral anticoagulants on bleeding time may be enhanced by the salicylates, and the severity of salicylate-induced GI bleeding may be augmented as a result of the impairment of hemostasis by anticoagulant drugs. Although it is not an absolute contraindication, it is advised that the concurrent administration of aspirin and oral anticoagulants be avoided. For analgesic-antipyretic activity, acetaminophen is recommended for self-medication in patients on oral anticoagulant therapy.

Several reports suggest that the lowering of blood-glucose levels by the sulfonylurea oral hypoglycemics can be enhanced by the concurrent administration of aspirin.

Salicylates displace tolbutamide and chlorpropamide from plasma protein binding sites and have intrinsic hypoglycemic activity when administered to diabetics.[5 44] Controlled clinical studies documenting the significance of this interaction are lacking. However, in view of existing evidence, it is advisable to monitor closely diabetics who are receiving both salicylates and a sulfonylurea hypoglycemic agent. When recommending a nonprescription analgesic for concurrent administration, acetaminophen seems to have less potential for interaction than the salicylates.

Salicylate toxicity. Mild salicylate toxicity may occur in adults after repeated administration of large doses or in young children as a result of therapeutic overdosage. Symptoms consist of dizziness, ringing in the ears, difficulty in hearing, nausea, vomiting, diarrhea, mental confusion, and lassitude.[5] Skin eruptions may appear if salicylates are continued for a week or longer, and more pronounced CNS symptoms may develop, e.g., incoherent speech, delirium, or hallucinations.

Salicylates are consistently involved in more accidental poisonings in children under 5 than any other single drug or household product.[45 46] The limitation of 36 children's aspirins to a bottle and the use of childproof safety closures are positive steps taken to prevent accidental salicylate ingestion. However, in spite of such measures, fatalities from salicylate poisoning continue.[46]

The mean lethal dose of aspirin in adults is between 20 and 30 g, and the toxic dose for children is 0.15 g/kg.[47 48] Symptoms of salicylate poisoning include those cited for mild toxicity and hyperventilation, dimness of vision, mental confusion, delirium, hallucinations, convulsions, and coma. Acid-base disturbances are prominent and vary from respiratory alkalosis to metabolic acidosis. Initially, salicylate effects on the respiratory center in the medulla produce hyperventilation and respiratory alkalosis. In severely intoxicated adults and in most children under 5, respiratory alkalosis rapidly changes to metabolic acidosis.[5 48]

Salicylate poisoning affects other physiological functions. Metabolic rate is increased, resulting in increased heat production and fever. Children are more prone to develop high fever in salicylate poisoning than are adults.[47] Hypoglycemia results from increased tissue use of glucose and may be especially serious in children.[5] Bleeding may occur from the GI tract due to erosion of the mucosal lining or hemorrhaging from other sites may occur as a consequence of salicylate inhibition of platelet aggregation.[47 48]

Emergency management of aspirin poisoning is designed to delay absorption of the drug and to remove it from the stomach. If the person is conscious and able to swallow, give one or two glasses of milk or water to dilute the drug, delay gastric emptying, and slow absorption. However, the volume of liquid given to children should not exceed 50 ml/10 kg. Because of the rapid absorption of salicylates from the GI tract, emptying of the stomach at home or en route to an emergency medical facility is advised. Vomiting should be induced even if the child or adult has vomited spontaneously. Syrup of ipecac is recommended in doses of 15 ml for children or 30 ml for adults. The administration of liquids to a person convulsing or to one who is not completely conscious is absolutely contraindicated.[47-49]

Biopharmaceutics of aspirin-containing products. The rate-limiting step for achieving therapeutic blood levels with solid dosage forms of aspirin is dissolution into rather than absorption from GI fluids.[50] Factors affecting the rate of dissolution include the degree of GI motility, the pH of gastric fluid, and the pH of the diffusion layer (the region of high salicylate concentration surrounding the dissolving aspirin particles). The dissolution rate of aspirin is increased by raising the pH of the surrounding medium.[51] The inclusion of alkaline buffering agents in the tablet formulation produces an elevated pH in the diffusion layer, increasing the rate of aspirin dissolution. If formulated properly, buffered aspirin has a significantly greater rate of dissolution and absorption than nonbuffered aspirin.[52-54] However, there is no evidence from controlled clinical studies that buffered aspirin provides a more rapid onset or greater degree of pain relief than nonbuffered aspirin.[52 54]

The degree of salicylate-induced gastric irritation and erosion is a function of the salicylate concentration and the duration of exposure at the gastric mucosal surface. Although solutions of aspirin can also produce GI erosion, undissolved aspirin particles are thought to be primarily responsible for gastric mucosal damage because they produce high concentrations of salicylate at mucosal surfaces in the region of their diffusion layer.[55] Buffered aspirin tablets have been shown to produce less GI bleeding than nonbuffered tablets presumably because they dissolve more rapidly, reducing the exposure time of the gastric mucosa to the offending aspirin particles.[52 56]

When administered in solution, aspirin is absorbed more rapidly than from either buffered or nonbuffered tablets because the dissolution factor is eliminated.[53] Highly buffered aspirin solutions having a neutralizing capacity of at least 20 mEq of hydrochloric acid significantly decrease the amount of gastric bleeding.[54 57 58] However, the effervescent-type buffered aspirin solutions achieve their buffering action at the expense of a high sodium content. For this reason, their use by patients on restricted sodium intake should be avoided. In addition, there is no valid evidence that highly buffered aspirin solutions produce more rapid or effective analgesia than either plain or buffered aspirin tablets.[52]

Enteric-coated aspirin is specially formulated to prevent tablet dissolution until it reaches the more alkaline pH of the small intestine, preventing the gastric distress associated with dissolution in the stomach. However, absorption of aspirin from enteric-coated tablets may be highly erratic. Tablets sometimes dissolve prematurely in the stomach or possibly not at all.[59] The variable absorption of aspirin from enteric-coated tablets is also caused by differences in the gastric retention time of the tablets.[60 61]

Timed-release aspirin is a formulation using encapsulation techniques attempting to prolong the product's duration of action. Such products are not useful for rapid pain relief because their absorption is delayed. However, the prolonged absorption may make timed-release aspirin useful as a bedtime medication. Hollister[62] reported that at 6 and 8 hours after ingestion of a single 1,300-mg aspirin dose, the total salicylate concentration in serum is significantly higher with the timed-release product tested than with regular tableted aspirin. Timed-release aspirin has been implicated in the production of hemorrhagic gastritis,[63] but definitive clinical studies are not available.[64]

The *p*-aminophenols

Analgesic compounds in this class include phenacetin and acetaminophen. These compounds are analgesic-antipyretic and are effective in treating mild to moderate pain such as headache, neuralgia, and pain of musculoskeletal origin.[18 65] The major part of a dose of phenacetin is biotransformed in the body to acetaminophen which is thought to be primarily responsible for the compound's analgesic-antipyretic activity.[66] However, phenacetin also has been shown to have intrinsic analgesic-antipyretic activity in laboratory animals.[66 67] The mechanism and site of analgesic action of these compounds have not been definitely established.[5]

Studies document the analgesic efficacy of phenacetin and acetaminophen in doses of 300 to 600 mg.[68-71] The recommended dose of acetaminophen is 325 to 650 mg every 4 hours for adults and older children, not to exceed a total daily dose of 2.6 g. The single dose for young children is 60 to 120 mg, depending on age and weight, and should not exceed a total daily dose of 1.2 g.[5] Although comparative effectiveness of analgesic products is difficult to establish due to the nature of existing clinical testing procedures, acetaminophen and phenacetin are about as potent as aspirin as analgesics and antipyretics.[18] However, Huskisson [72] has reported that a single 1,000-mg dose of acetaminophen is less effective than 600 mg of aspirin in relieving pain associated with rheumatoid arthritis when it is given as an analgesic supplement to regular anti-inflammatory drug therapy.

Both phenacetin and acetaminophen are effective antipyretic agents, and both reduce fever by acting on the hypothalamic thermoregulatory center to increase dissipation of body heat. Acetaminophen reduces fever by inhibiting the action of endogenous pyrogen on the hypothalamus, probably by inhibiting prostaglandin synthesis.[24 73 74] In febrile individuals, both compounds begin to reduce body temperature about 30 minutes after administration and produce their peak effect in 2 to 4 hours.[68] Clinical studies indicate that acetaminophen and aspirin are equally effective as antipyretics.[75-77]

Although there are reports of minimal anti-inflammatory activity with acetaminophen, the *p*-aminophenols have no therapeutic use as anti-inflammatory drugs in the treatment of rheumatoid arthritis.[5 18 65 78]

p-Aminophenol toxicity. Although methemoglobin production contributes to the toxicity of phenacetin in acute overdose, therapeutic doses of phenacetin in the range of 1 to 2 g/day cause only minimal methemoglobinemia which is of no clinical significance.[5] Phenacetin-induced hemolytic anemia has been most frequently associated with chronic ingestion of the drug; however, clinically significant hemolysis can occur with the administration of a single dose of phenacetin. Phenacetin produces hemolytic anemia in an individual deficient in glucose 6-phosphate dehydrogenase or in an immunologically sensitive individual.[79] Glucose 6-phosphate dehydrogenase deficiency is a genetically transferable enzyme deficiency which predisposes a person to acute, drug-induced hemolytic episodes. This deficiency occurs rarely in Americans of West European genetic origin but has an incidence of about 13 percent in American Negroes.[80] By contrast, acetaminophen does not produce hemolytic anemia and produces almost no methemoglobin formation.[81 82]

Because it lacks many undesirable effects produced by aspirin, acetaminophen is gaining favor in this country as the "common household analgesic." [5] However, there is also growing concern that increasing household availability and the public's lack of recognition of acetaminophen's acute toxicity will produce a new health hazard.[83-86] Acetaminophen poisoning can produce fatal hepatic necrosis. In adults, symptoms of acute toxicity occur following the ingestion of more than 7 g.[87] A single dose of 10 to 15 g (200 to 250 mg/kg) may produce hepatotoxicity, and a dose of more than 25 g is potentially fatal.[5] The progression of symptoms with acetaminophen poisoning include: vomiting within a few hours; anorexia, nausea, and stomach pain within 24 hours; evidence of liver injury in 2 to 4 days with jaundice; death at any time from 2 to 7 days.[5 87] In addition, kidney damage, disturbances in clotting mechanisms, metabolic acidosis, hypoglycemia, and myocardial necrosis may occur.[5 84 85] In nonfatal cases, the hepatic damage is reversible.[5] Emergency first aid treatment of acetaminophen overdoses includes delaying absorption by giving water or milk and inducing vomiting.[5 88] The same cautions apply regarding maximum fluid volume in children and the induction of vomiting as described for the management of salicylate poisoning.

Salicylamide

Although it is structurally similar to salicylates, salicylamide is not converted to salicylate in the body, and its pharmacological activity resides in the salicylamide molecule itself.[89] It is rapidly absorbed from the GI tract, and peak plasma levels of the drug are reached 30 to 60 minutes after ingestion, approximately 2 hours sooner than aspirin.[90] Because of its rapid metabolism to the sulfate and glucuronide conjugates, free salicylamide disappears rapidly from plasma, and the peak plasma levels are lower than for the same dose of salicylate.[90-92] The unusual pharmacokinetic character of salicylamide metabolism complicates interpretation of the compound's efficacy and formulation factors. It is possible to overwhelm the metabolizing system for salicylamide and to dramatically increase peak plasma levels. The critical dose for achieving this effect is between 1 and 2 g because it has been shown that the peak plasma concentration is 20 times greater for 2 g than for 1 g.[93]

Many animal studies indicate that salicylamide is at least as potent an analgesic as either aspirin or acetaminophen.[94 95] However, well-controlled clinical studies demonstrate that in humans, salicylamide is a less effective analgesic than either aspirin or acetaminophen.[18 96-98] Salicylamide has consistently proven to be inferior to aspirin as an antipyretic in both animal and human studies.[18 99 100] Individuals who are allergic to aspirin are usually not sensitive to salicylamide, and salicylamide does not increase prothrombin time.[97 98 101]

Although an effective analgesic dose of salicylamide has not been conclusively established, the manufacturers' suggested dosage is 460 to 600 mg three or four times daily for adults.[98] The efficacy of the small amounts of salicylamide in some nonprescription analgesics is questionable.

Analgesic renal toxicity

Reports first appeared in the 1950's linking the chronic use of analgesic products to the production of renal papillary necrosis and interstitial nephritis.[102-105] The syndrome is characterized by asymptomatic sloughing of renal papillary tissue, sometimes with the elimination of "brown lumps" of necrotic tissue in the urine. Tissue necrosis may be accompanied by oliguria, nausea and vomiting, massive diuresis, or hematuria. Anemia may be present as the syndrome progresses, and final stages include renal insufficiency, hypertension, and death.[106]

Although early clinical reports of analgesic nephrotoxicity implicated phenacetin, current opinion is that phenacetin is not the sole causative agent.[107-109] Abel [110] concludes in a critical analysis of analgesic nephrotoxicity that "it is mixtures of analgesics—particularly aspirin, phenacetin, and caffeine—which are nephrotoxic rather than any single component."

In healthy adult volunteers, aspirin, phenacetin, and caffeine citrate given separately in divided total doses of 3.6 g, 3.6 g, and 2.4 g, respectively, all produce an increase in the number of renal tubule cells in urine; this is probably indicative of renal tubule necrosis.[111] In laboratory animals, renal lesions can be produced with aspirin, phenacetin, and caffeine combinations, but attempts to produce nephrotoxic effects with phenacetin alone have largely been unsuccessful.[105 107 112 113] A salicylate-induced alteration in phenacetin metabolism may contribute to the renal toxicity of aspirin-phenacetin combinations.[114]

Analgesic nephrotoxicity is well-documented, although the identity of the causative agent(s) remains uncertain. The pharmacist should advise that the chronic consumption of a nonprescription analgesic should be avoided and that if pain is frequent or recurring, medical attention must be sought.

Comparison of products

In evaluating the relative merits of nonprescription internal analgesic products, the choices are aspirin or acetaminophen and the formulation of the product. Aspirin is the most frequently used nonprescription analgesic except when specifically contraindicated due to its effects on hemostasis, GI erosion, or in cases of allergic hypersensitivity. Buffered aspirin has the advantage of producing less GI distress but retains the other contraindications of aspirin. Highly buffered aspirin solutions produce less GI erosion, but they contain large amounts of sodium and should not be used by individuals on low-sodium diets. Enteric-coated aspirin products reduce the likelihood of GI erosion but have a longer onset of action due to their delayed and possibly incomplete absorption. The delayed onset of such products precludes their use in acute pain such as headache, when prompt relief is desired.

Attempts to increase salicylate solubility and its rate of absorption have produced a number of salicylate delivery forms including choline salicylate and calcium carbaspirin. Choline salicylate is the choline ester of salicylic acid and calcium carbaspirin is the urea complex of calcium acetylsalicylate. Both compounds are more soluble in water than is aspirin. In spite of a substantially greater dissolution rate, calcium carbaspirin is equipotent with regular aspirin.[18] Choline salicylate is a highly soluble salicylate and is supplied as a solution. However, compared to aspirin in solution, there is no significant difference in absorption rates.[115] Current opinion is that neither form of salicylate offers a significant advantage over aspirin.[18 116]

In many cases, acetaminophen is the drug of choice. It is much less likely to trigger asthmalike symptoms in asthmatics, but hypersensitivity reactions have been reported to the drug.[117] Because acetaminophen does not cause gastric mucosal erosion and does not affect platelet function, it can be recommended for individuals with a history of peptic ulcer disease.[118] Although acetaminophen in a dose of 650 mg four times daily for a 2-week period significantly increases prothrombin time, two 650-mg doses 4 hours apart do not.[119 120] Consequently, the intermittent use of acetaminophen by individuals on oral anticoagulant therapy should present no serious interaction. Because of its lack of anti-inflammatory activity, acetaminophen is not an acceptable substitute for aspirin in the treatment of rheumatoid arthritis and similar inflammatory conditions. Acetaminophen is the nonprescription analgesic of choice for patients taking uricosuric drugs because it does not antagonize the uricosuric effect.[117] In addition, the stability of acetaminophen in liquid dosage forms provides a convenient and palatable pediatric analgesic-antipyretic.

The rationale for the inclusion of caffeine in many analgesic combinations remains obscure. The FDA panel evaluating nonprescription internal analgesics has concluded that "there is weak evidence that the combination of caffeine and aspirin is more effective than aspirin alone" and that well-controlled clinical studies are needed to prove the efficacy, if any, of this combination.[54] An evaluation of analgesic combinations in the treatment of cancer pain showed that 65 mg of caffeine did not significantly increase the analgesic efficacy of 650 mg of aspirin.[121]

Recent claims promoting "extra strength pain relievers" require clarification. Such products are usually combinations of several analgesic ingredients and may include acetaminophen, salicylamide, and aspirin. Because the total analgesic ingredients may be more than 325 mg, or 5 gr, the implication in these products' promotional materials is that they are "stronger" and hence, more effective. These claims only confuse the consumer because combinations have not been proved to be more effective than the sum of their individual ingredients. In most controlled clinical trials, pain relief provided by analgesic combinations has not been superior to that of aspirin alone.[5]

Determination of product efficacy

There are three general methods for determining the effectiveness of an analgesic drug: testing the effect of the drug in animals subjected to painful stimuli; measuring the analgesia produced in humans subjected to experimentally induced pain; and determining the degree of analgesia reported by human subjects experiencing pain from disease or trauma. The first two do not predict with any consistency the clinical performance of the analgesics used in nonprescription formulations.[18] Consequently, the FDA Panel on OTC Internal Analgesics states that "the appraisal of real analgesic power must be based on the capacity of the agent to relieve pain present as a consequence of disease or trauma."[122]

The FDA Panel also recommends that the clinical evaluation of antipyretic efficacy be done in several different types of patients, including those suffering fever secondary to cancer, fever in children with acute infections, and fever in adults with acute infections. The antipyretic effect should be evaluated by determining the patient's temperature at least every hour for a 4- to 6-hour period following drug administration and comparing this to predrug temperatures.

Antirheumatic efficacy should be evaluated in human subjects suffering inflammatory rheumatic conditions. Induced inflammatory conditions in laboratory animals do not respond to analgesics in a way that consistently predicts the efficacy of the drug in humans. FDA recommendations for demonstrating clinical antirheumatic efficacy include: grouping patients according to disease; conducting a double-blind crossover design using aspirin as the standard reference drug; and using objective indices of joint inflammation such as grip strength, joint circumference, number of swollen or tender joints, or the determination of walking time for a specified distance.[122]

Table 2. Factors Influencing the Choice of Analgesic Agents

Patient	Drug
Condition being treated	**Efficacy of drug**
type of pain accompanying symptoms frequency of dose and duration of treatment	analgesic potency antipyretic and anti-inflammatory potency onset and duration of effect formulation factors
Patient profile	**Untoward effects of drug**
age of patient drug allergy or idiosyncrasies pathological conditions or susceptibility to untoward effects concomitant use of other drugs, therapeutic diets or diagnostic procedures	general acute and chronic toxicity allergenic potential and cross-sensitivity with other drugs relative tendency to produce untoward effects potential to modify pharmacologic activities of other drugs or endogenous compounds

Summary

The appropriate choice of an analgesic agent involves a consideration of both patient and drug factors (Table 2). In determining the drug of choice for recommendation, the pharmacist must consider the condition being treated; the nature and origin of the pain or fever; accompanying symptoms; a past history of asthma or other allergic disease, hypersensitivity reactions, peptic ulcer, or clotting disorders; and the concomitant use of other medication. In addition, product selection must include evaluation of the proven efficacy of the product for the condition being treated, formulation factors which may give the patient more prompt relief or fewer side effects, and the potential for adverse effects from the product ingredients.

References

1. D. R. Haslam, *Br. J. Psychol.*, **58**, 139(1967).
2. H. K. Beecher, in "Nonspecific Factors in Drug Therapy," K. Rickels, Ed., Charles C Thomas, Springfield, Ill., 1968, p. 27.
3. A. C. Guyton, "Textbook of Medical Physiology," 4th ed., Saunders, Philadelphia, Pa., 1971, pp. 577-591.
4. V. B. Mountcastle, "Medical Physiology," vol. 1, 13th ed., Mosby, St. Louis, Mo., 1974, pp. 348-381.
5. D. M. Woodbury and E. Fingl, in "The Pharmacological Basis of Therapeutics," 5th ed., L. S. Goodman and A. Gilman, Eds., Macmillan, New York, N.Y., 1975, pp. 325-358.
6. M. L. Tainter and A. J. Ferris, "Aspirin in Modern Therapy," Sterling Drug Inc., New York, N.Y., 1969, p. 43.
7. H. G. Wolff, "Headache and Other Head Pain," 2d ed., Oxford University Press, New York, N.Y., 1963.
8. F. Plum, in "Textbook of Medicine," 13th ed., P. B. Beeson and W. McDermott, Eds., Saunders, Philadelphia, Pa., 1971, p. 156.
9. A. G. Swanson, in "Textbook of Medicine," 13th ed., P. B. Beeson and W. McDermott, Eds., Saunders, Philadelphia, Pa., 1971, pp. 149-154.
10. "The Merck Manual," 12th ed., D. N. Holvey, Ed., Merck, Sharp, and Dohme Research Laboratories, Rahway, N.J., 1972, p. 1304.
11. W. S. Gilmer, Jr., in "Concepts of Disease," J. B. Brunson and E. A. Gall, Eds., Macmillan, New York, N.Y., 1971, p. 746.
12. W. D. Robinson, in "Textbook of Medicine," 13th ed., P. B. Beeson and W. McDermott, Eds., Saunders, Philadelphia, Pa., 1971, p. 1884.
13. "The Merck Manual," 12th ed., D. N. Holvey, Ed., Merck, Sharp, and Dohme Research Laboratories, Rahway, N.J., 1972, p. 1222.
14. W. D. Robinson, in "Textbook of Medicine," 13th ed., P. B. Beeson and W. McDermott, Eds., Saunders, Philadelphia, Pa., 1971, p. 1910.
15. A. C. Guyton, "Textbook of Medical Physiology," 4th ed., Saunders, Philadelphia, Pa., 1971, pp. 831-843.
16. F. Allison, Jr., in "Concepts of Disease," J. G. Brunson and E. A. Gall, Eds., Macmillan, New York, N.Y., 1971, p. 443.
17. "Manual of Medical Therapeutics," 20th ed., M. G. Rosenfeld, Ed., Little, Brown, Boston, Mass., 1971, p. 236.
18. W. T. Beaver, *Am. J. Med. Sci.*, **250**, 577(1965) and **251**, 576(1966).
19. R. K. S. Lim *et al.*, *Arch. Int. Pharmacodyn. Ther.*, **152**, 25(1964).
20. S. H. Ferreira, *Nature New Biol.*, **240**, 200(1972).
21. J. R. Vane, *Nature New Biol.*, **231**, 232(1971).
22. W. M. Wallace, *Q. Rev. Pediatr.*, **9**, 135(1954).
23. A. A. Mintz, *Clin. Med.*, **71**, 865(1964).
24. R. J. Flower, *Am. Heart J.*, **86**, 844(1973).
25. S. H. Ferreira and J. R. Vane, *Annu. Rev. Pharmacol.*, **14**, 57(1974).
26. Food and Drug Administration, Summary Minutes of OTC Panel on Internal Analgesics, Including Antirheumatic Drugs, Fifteenth Meeting, July 8-10, 1974.
27. J. H. Weiss, in "Aspirin, Platelets and Stroke," W. S. Fields and W. K. Hass, Eds., Warren H. Green, St. Louis, Mo., 1971, p. 51.
28. K. P. Link *et al.*, *J. Biol. Chem.*, **147**, 463(1943).
29. A. H. Sutor *et al.*, *Mayo Clin. Proc.*, **46**, 178(1971).
30. A. Muir, in "Salicylates—An International Symposium," A. St. J. Dixon *et al.*, Eds., J. & A. Churchill Ltd., London, England, 1963, p. 230.
31. L. Th. F. L. Stubbe, *Br. Med. J.*, **2**, 1062(1958).
32. M. I. Grossman *et al.*, *Gastroenterology*, **40**, 383(1961).
33. H. E. Paulus and M. W. Whitehouse, *Annu. Rev. Pharmacol.*, **13**, 107(1973).
34. A. Muir and I. A. Cossar, *Br. Med. J.*, **2**, 7(1955).
35. H. F. Lange, *Gastroenterology*, **33**, 778(1957).
36. A. S. Alvarez and W. H. J. Summerskill, *Lancet*, **2**, 920(1958).
37. M. Levy, *N. Engl. J. Med.*, **290**, 1158(1974).
38. K. Goulston and A. R. Cooke, *Br. Med. J.*, **4**, 664(1968).
39. F. H. Chafee and G. A. Settipane, *J. Allergy Clin. Immunol.*, **53**, 193(1974).
40. G. A. Settipane and F. H. Chafee, *J. Allergy Clin. Immunol.*, **53**, 200(1974).
41. H. Kreithen, *Semin. Drug Treat.*, **2**, 431(1973).
42. T. F. Yu *et al.*, *J. Clin. Invest.*, **42**, 1330(1963).
43. "Physicians' Desk Reference," 28th ed., Medical Economics, Oradell, N.J., 1974, p. 1005.
44. H. Wishinsky *et al.*, *Diabetes (Suppl.)*, **11**, 18(1962).
45. H. J. Verhulst and J. J. Crotty, *J. Clin. Pharmacol.*, **7**, 10(1967).
46. "Deaths from Accidental Poisonings," Bulletin of the National Clearinghouse for Poison Control Centers, U.S. Department of Health, Education, and Welfare, September-October, 1975.
47. M. N. Gleason *et al.*, "Clinical Toxicology of Commercial Products," 3d ed., Williams and Wilkins, Baltimore, Md., 1969, pp. 209-214.
48. H. B. Andrews, *Am. Fam. Physician*, **8**, 102(1973).
49. H. R. Dreisbach, "Handbook of Poisoning: Diagnosis and Treatment," 8th ed., Lange Medical Publications, Los Altos, Calif., 1974, pp. 13-19, 258-263.
50. G. Levy and J. R. Leonards, in "The Salicylates—A Critical Bibliographic Review," M. J. H. Smith and P. K. Smith, Eds., Interscience, New York, N.Y., 1966, pp. 5-47.
51. G. Levy, in "Salicylates—An International Symposium," A. St. J. Dixon *et al.*, Eds., J. & A. Churchill Ltd., London, England, 1963, pp. 9-16.
52. *Med. Lett. Drugs Ther.*, **16**, 57(1974).
53. J. R. Leonards, *Clin. Pharmacol. Ther.*, **4**, 476(1963).
54. Food and Drug Administration, Summary Minutes of OTC Panel on Internal Analgesics, Including Antirheumatic Drugs, Eighteenth Meeting, December 9-10, 1974.
55. K. W. Anderson, in "Salicylates—An International Symposium," A. St. J. Dixon *et al.*, Eds., J. & A. Churchill Ltd., London, England, 1963, pp. 217-223.
56. J. R. Leonards and G. Levy, *Arch. Intern. Med.*, **129**, 457(1972).
57. J. R. Leonards and G. Levy, *Clin. Pharmacol. Ther.*, **10**, 571(1969).
58. P. H. N. Wood *et al.*, *Br. Med. J.*, **1**, 669(1962).
59. L. Th. F. L. Stubbe *et al.*, *Br. Med. J.*, **1**, 675(1962).
60. E. Nelson, *Clin. Pharmacol. Ther.*, **4**, 283(1963).
61. J. R. Leonards and G. Levy, *J. Am. Med. Assoc.*, **193**, 99(1965).
62. L. E. Hollister, *Clin. Pharmacol. Ther.*, **13**, 1(1972).
63. J. R. Hoon, *J. Am. Med. Assoc.*, **229**, 841(1974).
64. R. John, *J. Am. Med. Assoc.*, **230**, 823(1974).
65. L. O. Randall, in "Physiological Pharmacology," vol. 1, W. S. Root and F. G. Hofmann, Eds., Academic Press, New York, N.Y., 1963, pp. 356-369.

66. B. B. Brodie and J. Axelrod, *J. Pharmacol. Exp. Ther.*, **97**, 58(1949).
67. A. H. Conney *et al.*, *J. Pharmacol. Exp. Ther.*, **151**, 133(1966).
68. P. K. Smith, "Acetophenetidin—A Critical Bibliographic Review," Interscience, New York, N.Y., 1958.
69. F. B. Flinn and B. B. Brodie, *J. Pharmacol. Exp. Ther.*, **94**, 76(1948).
70. S. L. Wallenstein and R. W. Houde, *Fed. Proc.*, **13**, 414(1954).
71. D. R. L. Newton and J. M. Tanner, *Br. Med. J.*, **2**, 1096(1956).
72. E. C. Huskisson, *Br. Med. J.*, **4**, 196(1974).
73. W. G. Clark and S. G. Moyer, *J. Pharmacol. Exp. Ther.*, **181**, 183(1972).
74. R. J. Flower and J. R. Vane, *Nature*, **240**, 410(1972).
75. A. N. Eden, *Am. J. Dis. Child.*, **114**, 284(1967).
76. M. T. Colgan and A. A. Mintz, *J. Pediatr.*, **50**, 552(1957).
77. L. Tarlin *et al.*, *Am. J. Dis. Child.*, **124**, 880(1972).
78. J. Hajnal *et al.*, *Ann. Rheum. Dis.*, **18**, 189(1959).
79. M. Swanson, *Drug Intell. Clin. Pharm.*, **7**, 6(1973).
80. P. A. Parks and J. Banks, *Ann. N.Y. Acad. Sci.*, **123**, 198(1965).
81. "AMA Drug Evaluations," 2d ed., Publishing Science Group, Acton, Mass., 1973, pp. 266-267.
82. L-O. Boreus and F. Sandberg, *Acta Physiol. Scand.*, **28**, 261(1953).
83. J. R. Dipalma, *Am. Fam. Physician*, **13**, 142(1976).
84. E. Sutton and L. F. Soyka, *Clin. Pediatr.*, **12**, 692(1973).
85. H. Matthew, *Clin. Toxicol.*, **6**, 9(1973).
86. R. Goulding, *Pediatrics*, **52**, 883(1973).
87. A. T. Proud and W. N. Wright, *Br. Med. J.*, **3**, 557(1970).
88. R. H. Dreisbach, "Handbook of Poisoning: Diagnosis and Treatment," 8th ed., Lange Medical Publications, Los Altos., Calif., 1974, pp. 264-266.
89. D. C. Brodie and I. J. Szekely, *J. Am. Pharm. Assoc. (Sci. Ed.)*, **40**, 414(1951).
90. J. H. Wiekel, Jr., *J. Am. Pharm. Assoc. (Sci. Ed.)*, **47**, 477(1958).
91. H. G. Mandel *et al.*, *J. Pharmacol. Exp. Ther.*, **106**, 433(1952).
92. V. P. Seeberg *et al.*, *J. Pharmacol. Exp. Ther.*, **101**, 275(1951).
93. W. H. Barr, *Drug Inf. Bull.*, **3**, 27(1969).
94. E. R. Hart, *J. Pharmacol. Exp. Ther.*, **89**, 205(1947).
95. E. M. Bavin *et al.*, *J. Pharm. Pharmacol.*, **4**, 872(1952).
96. R. Houde *et al.*, in "Analgetics, Chemistry and Pharmacology," G. de Stevens, Ed., Academic Press, New York, N.Y., 1965, p. 75.
97. D. M. Woodbury, in "The Pharmacological Basis of Therapeutics," 3d ed., L. S. Goodman and A. Gilman, Eds., Macmillan, New York, N.Y., 1965, p. 330.
98. "AMA Drug Evaluations," 2d ed., Publishing Science Group, Acton, Mass., 1973, p. 265.
99. A. J. Vignec and M. Gasparik, *J. Am. Med. Assoc.*, **167**, 1821(1958).
100. M. P. Borovsky, *Am. J. Dis. Child.*, **100**, 23(1960).
101. A. J. Quick, *J. Pharmacol. Exp. Ther.*, **128**, 95(1960).
102. O. Spuhler and H. N. Zollinger, *Z. Klin. Med.*, **151**, 1(1953).
103. L. F. Prescott, *J. Pharm. Pharmacol.*, **18**, 331(1966).
104. J. H. Shelley, *Clin. Pharmacol. Ther.*, **8**, 427(1967).
105. M. H. Gault *et al.*, *Ann. Intern. Med.*, **68**, 906(1968).
106. B. Koch *et al.*, *Can. Med. Assoc. J.*, **98**, 9(1968).
107. J. J. Haley, *J. New Drugs*, **6**, 193(1966).
108. L. F. Prescott, *Anesth. Analg.*, **45**, 303(1966).
109. A. Gilman, *Am. J. Med.*, **36**, 167(1964).
110. J. A. Abel, *Clin. Pharmacol. Ther.*, **12**, 583(1971).
111. L. F. Prescott, *Lancet*, **2**, 91(1965).
112. E. Clausen, *Lancet*, **2**, 123(1964).
113. R. S. Nanra and P. Kincaid-Smith, *Br. Med. J.*, **3**, 559(1970).
114. R. L. Smith and J. A. Timbrell, *Xenobiotica*, **4**, 503(1974).
115. "American Hospital Formulary Service," American Society of Hospital Pharmacists, Washington, D.C., 1974, Section 28:08.
116. "Drugs of Choice, 1974-75," W. Modell, Ed., Mosby, St. Louis, Mo., 1974, pp. 183-184.
117. *Med. Lett. Drugs Ther.*, **13**, 74(1971).
118. C. H. Mielke, Jr., and A. F. Britten, *N. Engl. J. Med.*, **282**, 1270(1970).
119. A. M. Antlitz *et al.*, *Curr. Ther. Res.*, **10**, 501(1968).
120. A. M. Antlitz and L. F. Awalt, *Curr. Ther. Res.*, **11**, 360(1969).
121. C. G. Moertel *et al.*, *J. Am. Med. Assoc.*, **229**, 55(1974).
122. Food and Drug Administration, Summary of Minutes of OTC Panel on Internal Analgesics, Including Antirheumatic Drugs, Thirteenth Meeting, April 10-11, 1974.

Products 10 INTERNAL ANALGESIC

Product[a] (manufacturer)	Aspirin	Phenacetin	Salicylamide	Acetaminophen	Caffeine	Other
Actamin (Buffington)	—	—	—	NS[b]	—	—
Act-On (Keystone)	—	—	129.6 mg	—	—	sodium salicylate, 194.3 mg potassium iodide sodium bicarbonate
Alka-Seltzer Effervescent Pain Reliever and Antacid (Miles)	324 mg	—	—	—	—	sodium bicarbonate, 1.904 g citric acid, 1.0 g
Amphenol (O'Neal, Jones & Feldman)	—	—	—	325 mg	—	—
Anacin (Whitehall)	400 mg	—	—	—	32.5 mg	—
Anodynos (Buffington)	NS[b]	—	NS[b]	NS[b]	NS[b]	—
Apamide (Dome)	—	—	—	300 mg	—	—
Arthralgen (Robins)	—	—	250 mg	250 mg	—	—
Arthritis Pain Formula (Whitehall)	486 mg (micronized)	—	—	—	—	aluminum hydroxide magnesium hydroxide
Arthritis Strength Bufferin (Bristol-Myers)	486 mg	—	—	—	—	magnesium carbonate, 145.8 mg aluminum glycinate, 72.9 mg
Arthropan Liquid (Purdue Frederick)	—	—	—	—	—	choline salicylate, 870 mg/5 ml (equivalent to 648 mg of aspirin)

Product[a] (manufacturer)	Aspirin	Phenacetin	Salicylamide	Acetaminophen	Caffeine	Other
A.S.A. Compound Capsules (Lilly)	227 mg	160 mg	—	—	32.5 mg	—
A.S.A. Enseals (Lilly)	325 and 650 mg	—	—	—	—	enteric coating
Ascriptin (Rorer)	325 mg	—	—	—	—	magnesium hydroxide, 75 mg aluminum hydroxide gel, dried, 75 mg
Ascriptin A/D (Rorer)	325 mg	—	—	—	—	magnesium hydroxide, 150 mg aluminum hydroxide gel, dried, 150 mg
Aspergum (Plough) (gum tablet)	228 mg	—	—	—	—	—
B-A (O'Neal, Jones & Feldman)	325 mg	—	—	—	—	aluminum hydroxide, 100 mg magnesium hydroxide, 30 mg
Bancap Capsule (O'Neal, Jones & Feldman)	—	—	200 mg	300 mg	—	—
Bayer Aspirin (Glenbrook)	324 mg	—	—	—	—	—
Bayer Children's Aspirin (Glenbrook)	81 mg	—	—	—	—	—
Bayer Non-Aspirin Pain Reliever (Glenbrook)	—	—	—	325 mg	—	—
Bayer Timed-Release Aspirin (Glenbrook)	650 mg	—	—	—	—	—
BC Tablet and Powder (Block)	320 mg/tablet 648 mg (powder)	—	96 mg/tablet 194 mg (powder)	—	16 mg/tablet 33 mg (powder)	potassium chloride, 96 mg (powder)
Bromo-Seltzer (Warner-Lambert) (granules)	—	130 mg/capful	—	325 mg/capful	32.5 mg/capful	sodium bicarbonate and citric acid to yield 2.8 g of sodium citrate/capful
Buffaprin (Buffington)	NS[b]	—	—	—	—	magnesium carbonate
Bufferin (Bristol-Myers)	324 mg	—	—	—	—	magnesium carbonate, 97.2 mg aluminum glycinate, 48.6 mg
Calurin (Dorsey)	—	—	—	—	—	calcium carbaspirin equivalent to 300 mg of aspirin
Cama (Dorsey) (in-lay tablet)	600 mg	—	—	—	—	magnesium hydroxide, 150 mg aluminum hydroxide gel, dried, 150 mg
Capron Capsules (Vitarine)	227 mg	162 mg	—	65 mg	32 mg	—
Comeback (Norcliff-Thayer)	—	—	150 mg	150 mg	100 mg	—
Congespirin Chewable (Bristol-Myers)	81 mg	—	—	—	—	phenylephrine hydrochloride, 1.25 mg

Product[a] (manufacturer)	Aspirin	Phenacetin	Salicylamide	Acetaminophen	Caffeine	Other
Cope (Glenbrook)	421.2 mg	—	—	—	32 mg	magnesium hydroxide, 50 mg aluminum hydroxide, 25 mg methapyrilene fumarate, 12.5 mg
Cystex (Smith, Miller & Patch)	—	—	NS[b]	—	—	methenamine sodium salicylate benzoic acid
Dolcin (Dolcin Corp.)	240.5 mg	—	—	—	—	calcium succinate, 182 mg
Dolor (Geriatric Pharmaceutical)	230 mg	—	—	230 mg	30 mg	calcium carbonate, 100 mg dry skim milk powder, 50 mg
Dularin Syrup (Dooner)	—	—	—	120 mg/5 ml	—	—
Duradyne (O'Neal, Jones & Feldman)	230 mg	150 mg	—	30 mg	15 mg	—
Duragesic (Meyer)	325 mg	—	—	—	—	salicylsalicylic acid, 162.5 mg
Ecotrin (Smith Kline & French)	300 mg	—	—	—	—	enteric coating
Emagrin (Otis Clapp)	NS[b]	—	NS[b]	—	NS[b]	—
Empirin Compound (Burroughs Wellcome)	227 mg	162 mg	—	—	32 mg	—
Excedrin (Bristol-Myers)	194.4 mg	—	129.6 mg	97 mg	64.8 mg	—
Excedrin P.M. (Bristol-Myers)	194.4 mg	—	129.6 mg	162 mg	—	methapyrilene fumarate, 25 mg
Febrinol (Vitarine)	—	—	—	325 mg	—	—
Felsol Tablets and Powder (American Felsol)	—	—	—	—	—	antipyrine, 325 mg/tablet 975 mg (powder)
Fendon Tablets and Elixir (Amer. Pharm.)	—	—	—	324 mg/tablet 120 mg/5 ml	—	alcohol, 10% (elixir)
Fizrin Powder (Glenbrook)	325 mg/packet	—	—	—	—	sodium bicarbonate, 1.825 g/packet citric acid, 1.449 g/packet sodium carbonate, 400 mg/packet
Goody's Headache Powder (Goody's)	455 mg	325 mg	—	—	32.5 mg	—
Liquiprin Suspension (Norcliff-Thayer)	—	—	—	60 mg/1.25 ml	—	—
Magan (Warren-Teed)	—	—	—	—	—	magnesium salicylate, 325 mg
Maranox (Dent)	—	100 mg	150 mg	60 mg	15 mg	—
Measurin (Breon) (time-release)	660 mg	—	—	—	—	—
Medache (Organon)	—	—	150 mg	150 mg	32 mg	phenyltoloxamine dihydrogen citrate, 44 mg

Product[a] (manufacturer)	Aspirin	Phenacetin	Salicylamide	Acetaminophen	Caffeine	Other
Nebs Tablets and Liquid (Eaton)	—	—	—	325 mg/tablet 120 mg/5 ml	—	alcohol, 7% (liquid)
Neocylate (Central Pharmacal)	—	—	—	—	—	potassium salicylate, 280 mg aminobenzoic acid, 250 mg
Nilain (A.V.P.)	325 mg	—	—	162.5 mg	32.5 mg	—
Nilprin 7½ (A.V.P.)	—	—	—	486 mg	—	—
Pabirin (Dorsey)	300 mg	—	—	—	—	aminobenzoic acid, 300 mg aluminum hydroxide gel, dried, 100 mg
PAC (Upjohn)	228 mg	163 mg	—	—	32 mg	—
Panodynes Analgesic (Keystone)	260 mg	—	64.8 mg	64.8 mg	16.2 mg	—
Percogesic (Endo)	—	—	—	325 mg	—	phenyltoloxamine citrate, 30 mg
Persistin (Fisons)	160 mg	—	—	—	—	salicylsalicylic acid, 485 mg
S-A-C (Lannett)	—	—	230 mg	150 mg	30 mg	—
Sal-Fayne Capsules (Smith, Miller & Patch)	228 mg	166 mg	—	—	32 mg	—
Salicionyl (Upjohn)	—	—	—	—	—	sodium bicarbonate, 1.3 g/180 ml sodium salicylate, 650 mg/180 ml citrates, tartrates, and malates of sodium and potassium
Sine-Aid (Johnson & Johnson)	325 mg	—	—	—	—	phenylpropanolamine hydrochloride, 25 mg
Sinu-Lets (Columbia Medical)	—	150 mg	—	150 mg	—	phenylpropanolamine hydrochloride, 25 mg phenyltoloxamine citrate, 22 mg
SK-APAP Tablets and Elixir (Smith Kline & French)	—	—	—	325 mg/tablet 120 mg/5 ml	—	alcohol, 8% (elixir)
S.P.C. (North American)	—	130 mg	195 mg	—	16.25 mg	—
Stanback Tablets and Powder (Stanback)	324 mg/tablet 648 mg (powder)	—	97 mg/tablet 194 mg (powder)	—	16 mg/tablet 32 mg (powder)	—
Stanco (Stanback)	325 mg	—	—	—	—	—
St. Joseph Aspirin (Plough)	325 mg	—	—	—	—	—
St. Joseph Aspirin for Children Chewable Tablets (Plough)	81 mg	—	—	—	—	—
St. Joseph Fever Reducer for Children Drops and Elixir (Plough)	—	—	—	60 mg/0.6 ml (drops) 120 mg/5 ml (elixir)	—	alcohol, 9.5% (drops), 7% (elixir)
Strascogesic (Pennwalt)	—	—	200 mg	300 mg	—	microcrystalline cellulose, 102.7 mg alcohol, 0.03 ml

Product[a] (manufacturer)	Aspirin	Phenacetin	Salicylamide	Acetaminophen	Caffeine	Other
Tempra Syrup, Tablets, and Drops (Mead Johnson)	—	—	—	120 mg/5 ml (syrup) 325 mg/tablet 60 mg/0.6 ml (drops)	—	alcohol, 10% (syrup and drops)
Tenol (North American)	—	—	—	325 mg	—	—
Trigesic (Squibb)	230 mg	—	—	125 mg	30 mg	—
Tylaprin Elixir (Cenci)	—	—	—	120 mg/5 ml	—	alcohol, 7%
Tylenol Extra Strength (McNeil)	—	—	—	500 mg	—	—
Tylenol Tablets, Chewable Tablets, Drops, and Liquid (McNeil)	—	—	—	325 mg/tablet 80 mg/chewable tablet 60 mg/0.6 ml (drops) 120 mg/5 ml (liquid)	—	alcohol, 7% (drops and liquid)
Uracel (North American)	—	—	—	—	—	sodium salicylate, 324 mg
Valadol Tablets and Liquid (Squibb)	—	—	—	325 mg/tablet 120 mg/5 ml	—	alcohol, 9% (liquid)
Valorin (Otis Clapp)	—	—	—	NS[b]	—	—
Vanquish Caplet (Glenbrook)	227 mg	—	—	194 mg	33 mg	magnesium hydroxide, 50 mg aluminum hydroxide gel, dried, 25 mg
Zarumin (J. B. Williams)	—	—	260 mg	—	—	potassium salicylate, 228 mg

[a] Tablet unless specified otherwise.
[b] Quantity not specified.

Nutritional Supplement, Mineral, and Vitamin Products

Marianne Ivey

Questions to ask the patient

What are your age and weight?

Do you regularly participate in sports?

Do you suffer from any chronic illnesses (e.g., diabetes)?

Are you currently taking any medication (prescription or OTC)?

Are you menstruating now?

Do you eat meats, vegetables, dairy products, and grain products every day?

Why are you requesting a nutritional supplement/vitamin/mineral? What are your symptoms? Have they appeared suddenly or gradually?

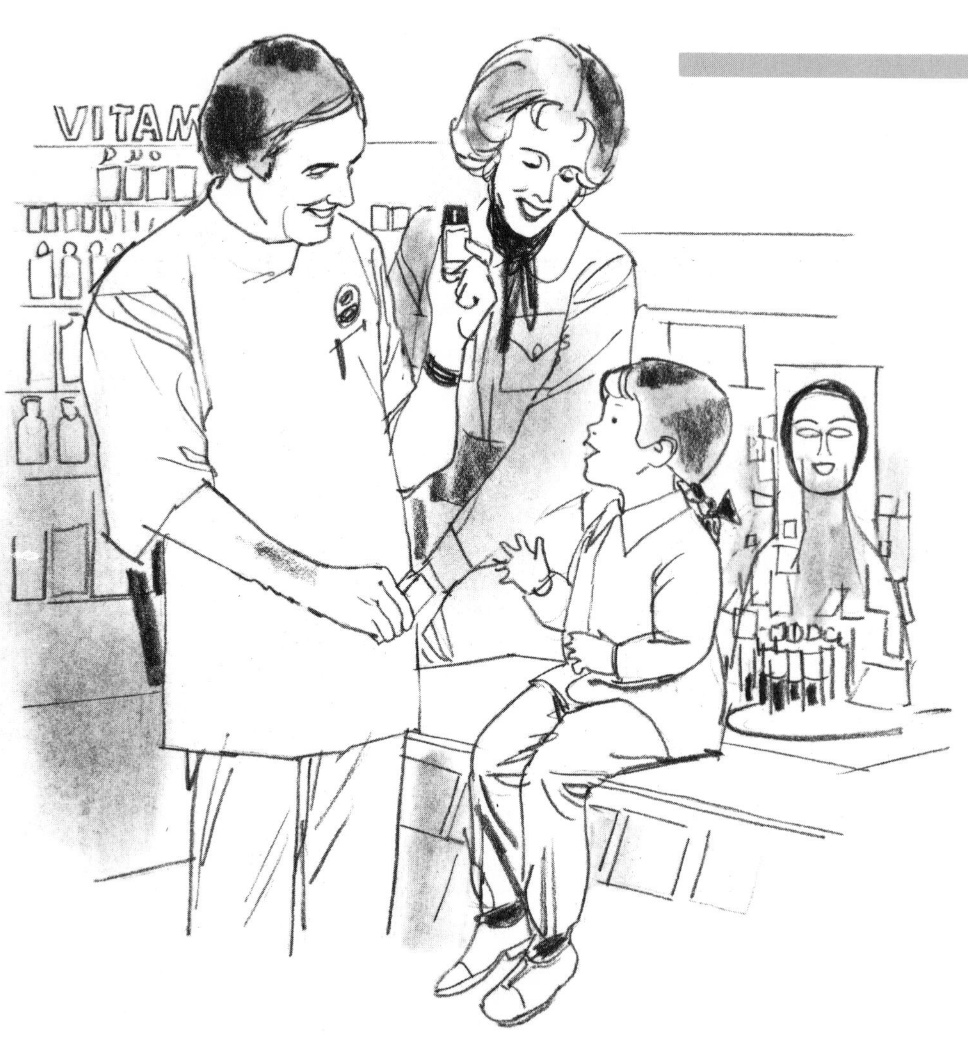

CHAPTER 11

American consumers are convinced that they need more and better nutrients than their diets provide—they spend $350 million a year on vitamin products and $300 to $500 million a year on health foods.[1 2] The health science professions frequently have associated health with nutrition. Actually, there is much to learn about adequate nutrition, and much that has been learned has not been communicated effectively to the general public. In many cases, the average American diet does not need supplementation.[3] Exceptions are described in the sections on iron and folic acid. Misconceptions about the value of supplementation were shown in a survey in which 75 percent of those interviewed believed that supplemental vitamins furnish energy.[4]

Marketing practices may further confuse the issue. The label "organic" is misleading because all foods are organic. Organically grown foods are those which are grown without the use of agricultural chemicals and are processed without chemicals or additives. However, no laws exist that enforce the label, "organically grown," to comply with the definition. There is no evidence that organically grown food is more nutritious than foods grown using chemical fertilizers.[5]

Frequently, "natural" vitamins are supplemented with the synthetic vitamin. For example, the amount of ascorbic acid acquired from rose hips (the fleshy fruit of a rose) is relatively small, and synthetic ascorbic acid is added to prevent an unreasonable tablet size.[6] However, this addition is not indicated on the label, and the price of such products often is considerably higher than for the synthetic, equally effective vitamin.

The pharmacist as a public adviser should be aware that one of the greatest dangers of food fads is that they are sometimes used in place of sound medical care. The false hope of superior health or freedom from disease may attract individuals with cancer, heart disease, arthritis, or other serious illnesses, and the pharmacist should be aware of the therapeutic value, if any, of these fads.

The Food and Drug Administration has issued bans against several claims and statements regarding food and food supplements. Claims cannot be made that foods or diet supplements alone can prevent, cure, or treat illness or that ingredients such as rutin, inositol, bioflavonoids, and aminobenzoic acid have nutritional value. Another FDA rule requires that all nutrients (caloric, protein, carbohydrate, fat) as well as the percentage of the recommended daily dietary allowance (RDA) of vitamins and minerals be listed on the container of all food shipped interstate. Also, it has been proposed that products containing more than 50 percent of the RDA of certain ingredients must be called dietary supplements rather than foods; those containing more than 150 percent of the RDA of a nutrient must be classified and labeled as drugs. Further guidelines for nutritional advice may come from the FDA OTC Panel on Vitamin, Mineral, and Hematinic Drug Products, but the Panel's final report has not yet been published.

Recommended daily allowances were developed by the Food and Nutrition Board of the National Academy of Sciences–National Research Council (Table 1). They have replaced the minimum daily requirement (MDR). The values of the RDA's should be interpreted as goals at which to aim in providing nutritional needs—they are not absolute nutritional standards or recommendations for an ideal diet nor are they required for all individuals. The RDA is not designed to meet the needs of ill patients nor does it account for the nutrients lost in cooking and other handling procedures. The individual RDA depends on age, sex, body size, and activity level of an individual as well as environmental conditions and whether a person is pregnant or lactating or is ill.

Nutritional supplements

Guidelines for determining nutritional status

Usually, the patient's diagnosis of any self-treated condition is made on subjective evidence. The pharmacist's concern and appropriate questions can educate the patient by serving as a model for self-evaluation of a suspected condition.

The assessment of nutritional status is very difficult. Clinical impressions about nutrition are often erroneous because the stages between the well-nourished and the poorly nourished states are not well defined. Only when emaciation from disease, economic circumstances, or climatic conditions are obvious are clinical impressions reliable.

There are guidelines, however, by which the pharmacist can gain a more objective impression of the nutritional status of a patient. They involve knowing the population groups who are most frequently poorly nourished, exercising good observation skills, and knowing questions to ask which may yield helpful information. The groups in the U.S. who are frequently undernourished are infants, preschool children, lactating or pregnant women, and the elderly. School children, factory workers, businessmen, and farmers are less likely to be poorly nourished.

The pharmacist may observe a person's physical condition in order to help guide in diet supplementation. The texture, amount, and appearance of the hair can suggest nutritional status. The eyes, particularly the conjunctiva, can indicate vitamin A and iron deficiencies, and the mouth may show stomatitis, glossitis, hypertrophic or pale gums, or mucous membranes. The number and general condition of the teeth may reflect the patient's choice of food. Visible goiter, the color and texture of the skin, the presence of edema, and obesity or thinness relative to bone structure may also be indications of malnutrition.

The more specific the information from the patient, the more helpful the pharmacist can be in determining the need for nutritional supplementation. Questions regarding foods that generally are not included in the diet may give the pharmacist more information. Previous treatment for similar symptoms may also be important.

Nutritional deficiencies cannot always be corrected at the pharmacy level. Although nutritional deficiencies can lead to disease, disease can lead to nutritional deficiencies. It is the pharmacist's responsibility to refer patients with a suspected serious illness to a physician for a definitive assessment. Guidelines for the clinical appraisal of nutritional status include evaluation of:

- ☐ Medical and dietary history
- ☐ Growth, development, and fitness
- ☐ Signs consistent with deficiencies
- ☐ Biochemical assessment.

The self-treated nutritional deficiencies seldom are severe conditions [e.g., ascorbic acid deficiency (scurvy), niacin deficiency (pellagra), protein deficiency (kwashiorkor)], but rather, milder forms of malnutrition.

Protein and calorie (energy) deficiency

In developing nations, protein-calorie malnutrition (PCM) is fairly common. In the U.S., it is quite uncommon, except in certain disease states; in fact, an excess intake of protein and energy is more common. The RDA for protein is 44 to 56 g for adults, and for energy it is 1,800 to 3,000 cal. In most cases, excess protein intake (to as much as 300 g) does not lead to disease conditions. Excess calorie intake leads to the condition of being overweight and to obesity, which is the degree of overweight that prevents the body from functioning normally.

Etiology. In developing nations, PCM may be caused by a shortage of food supply or by inadequate information and understanding of nutrition or disease. Kwashiorkor is a protein deficiency; marasmus is caused by the inadequacy of all nutrients. In the U.S., PCM is more commonly caused by conditions such as Crohn's disease; malabsorption syndromes; short bowel syndromes caused by surgery, trauma, or radiation; severe burns; jaw fractures; neoplastic diseases; and renal disease. In some very active people—athletes, dancers, manual laborers—protein and calorie intake may not be adequate to meet their needs. However, in the U.S., high activity levels are very infrequent for much of the population.

Treatment. Several products are available for use as dietary supplements or tube-feedings (oral, nasogastric, or gastrostomy tubes). The pharmacist's role regarding these products may be more as a consultant to other health professionals, less as a primary therapist for the self-treating patient. The pharmacist should first establish why the patient believes a dietary supplement, vitamin-mineral supplement, tonic, or health food is needed. Loss of weight or failure to gain weight in a highly active, otherwise healthy individual may safely indicate the recommendation of a product with a high concentration of protein and calories. Patients with a history of weight loss without apparent cause should be referred to a physician. The concern is the possibility of neoplastic disease for which expedient referral of the patient to a qualified practitioner or diagnostic clinic may be crucial.

Supplementary and complete formula products

Supplementary formula products are used as dietary adjuncts to a regular diet; they should not be used as the sole dietary product because they are not nutritionally complete. Some (Mull-Soy and Nutramigen) are milk-free and can be used by individuals who have milk allergy disease. (See Chapter 12 for additional information.) One product (Controlyte) is restricted in its protein content and in electrolytes. It is appropriate for people with acute or chronic renal failure, where the diet must be carefully controlled. Many supplementary formula products can be combined with special recipes to make desserts, malts, shakes, etc. that still maintain the controlled intake.

Complete formulas can be used orally or as tube-feedings, and they may be used as the sole dietary intake if the patient's electrolytes are monitored.[7] They can also be used as supplementation to a regular diet. The complete formulas contain various ingredients that make them appropriate for special needs. Several (Instant Breakfast, Sustacal, and Meritene) are milk-based; others (Compleat-B and Gerber Meat Base Formula) have a mixed-food base. A third type has a chemical, not a natural, food as a base for proteins and carbohydrates. This type supplies the protein in the form of crystalline amino acids or protein hydrolysate (the carbohydrate in the form of oligosaccharide or disaccharide) and the vitamins and minerals as the individual chemicals. These formulas are also called "elemental diets." Examples of chemically defined products are Vivonex and Jejunal. Some complete supplementary products (Precision LR, Flexical, and Portagen) are only partly chemically defined. The differences in their formulation make the products appropriate for different needs.

Nearly all of the chemically defined diets have a very low fat content and contain electrolytes, minerals, trace elements, and water-soluble and fat-soluble vitamins. All of the chemically based products require little or no digestion, are absorbed by a small part of the intestine, and have a low residue. The low residue reduces the number and

Table 1. Recommended Daily Dietary Allowances

	Age, years	Weight, lbs.	Height, in.	Energy, kcal	Protein, g	Vitamin A activity RE[b]	Vitamin A activity IU[c]	Vitamin D, IU	Vitamin E Activity,[d] IU	Ascorbic acid, mg	Folic acid,[e] μg	Niacin, mg[f]	Riboflavin, mg	Thiamine, mg	Vitamin B6,[g] mg	Vitamin B12,[h] μg	Calcium, mg	Phosphorus, mg	Iodine, μg	Iron, mg	Magnesium, mg	Zinc, mg
Children	1-3	28	34	1,300	23	400	2,000	400	7	40	100	9	0.8	0.7	0.6	1.0	800	800	60	15	150	10
	4-6	44	44	1,800	30	500	2,500	400	9	40	200	12	1.1	0.9	0.9	1.5	800	800	80	10	200	10
	7-10	66	54	2,100	36	700	3,300	400	10	40	300	16	1.2	1.2	1.2	2.0	800	800	110	10	250	10
Males	11-14	97	63	2,800	44	1,000	5,000	400	12	45	400	18	1.5	1.4	1.6	3.0	1,200	1,200	130	18	350	15
	15-18	134	69	3,000	54	1,000	5,000	400	15	45	400	20	1.8	1.5	2.0	3.0	1,200	1,200	150	18	400	15
	19-22	147	69	3,000	54	1,000	5,000	400	15	45	400	20	1.8	1.5	2.0	3.0	800	800	140	10	350	15
	23-50	154	69	2,700	56	1,000	5,000		15	45	400	18	1.6	1.4	2.0	3.0	800	800	130	10	350	15
	51+	154	69	2,400	56	1,000	5,000		15	45	400	16	1.5	1.2	2.0	3.0	800	800	110	10	350	15
Females	11-14	97	62	2,400	44	800	4,000	400	12	45	400	16	1.3	1.2	1.6	3.0	1,200	1,200	115	18	300	15
	15-18	119	65	2,100	48	800	4,000	400	12	45	400	14	1.4	1.1	2.0	3.0	1,200	1,200	115	18	300	15
	19-22	128	65	2,100	46	800	4,000	400	12	45	400	14	1.4	1.1	2.0	3.0	800	800	100	18	300	15
	23-50	128	65	2,000	46	800	4,000		12	45	400	13	1.2	1.0	2.0	3.0	800	800	100	18	300	15
	51+	128	65	1,800	46	800	4,000		12	45	400	12	1.1	1.0	2.0	3.0	800	800	80	10	300	15
Pregnant				+300	+30	1,000	5,000	400	15	60	800	+2	+0.3	+0.3	2.5	4.0	1,200	1,200	125	18[i]	450	20
Lactating				+300	+20	1,200	6,000	400	15	80	600	+4	+0.5	+0.3	2.5	4.0	1,200	1,200	150	18	450	25

[a] Excerpted from Food and Nutrition Board, National Academy of Sciences — National Research Council Recommended Daily Dietary Allowances, Revised 1974. The allowances are intended to provide for individual variations among most normal persons as they live in the U.S. under usual environmental stresses. Diets should be based on a variety of common foods in order to provide other nutrients for which human requirements have been less well defined.

[b] Retinol equivalents.

[c] All intakes are assumed to be half as retinol and half as β-carotene when calculated from international units (IU). As retinol equivalents, three-fourths are as retinol and one-fourth as β-carotene.

[d] Total vitamin E activity, estimated to be 80 percent as tocopherol and 20 percent other tocopherols.

[e] The folic acid allowances refer to dietary sources as determined by *Lactobacillus casei* assay. Pure forms of folic acid may be effective in doses less than one-fourth of the recommended dietary allowance.

[f] Although allowances are expressed as niacin, it is recognized that on the average 1 mg of niacin is derived from each 60 mg of dietary tryptophan.

[g] Pyridoxine hydrochloride.

[h] Cyanocobalamin.

[i] This increased requirement cannot be met by ordinary diets; therefore, the use of supplemental iron is recommended.

volume of the stools, making these products appropriate for patients with ileostomies or colostomies who wish to decrease fecal output. The low-residue products may also be appropriate for patients with brain damage from strokes, congenital defects, retardation, or for the aged who have stool incontinence. More commonly, they are used in postoperative care, in GI diseases, and in neoplastic disease where tissue breakdown is extensive.

Formulation and dosage. Supplementary and complete formulas are available in several forms. Some are powders that must be diluted with water or milk, some are liquids that must be further diluted, and some are ready-to-use liquids. The extent of dilution is based on the amount of nutrients needed and the amount that can be tolerated. Most often, adults will not tolerate preparations of more than 25 percent weight/volume (w/v), which generally delivers 1.0 cal/ml, and infants, 12 percent w/v, which generally delivers 0.5 cal/ml. (Infants should be started on a concentration of 7 to 7.5 percent w/v, increasing to 12 percent over 4 or 5 days.) For children over 10 months, 15 percent w/v may be initiated, with gradual increases to 25 percent. Higher concentrations can cause diarrhea because the sugar in the preparations acts as an osmotic diarrheal.

If the preparations are taken orally, 100 to 150 ml should be ingested at one time. Over the course of a day, 2,000 ml (about 2 qt) of most preparations provides about 2,000 cal. If the product is tube-fed, 40 to 60 ml/hour can be given initially. The container should be kept cold to avoid bacterial growth, and all prepared products remaining after 24 hours should be discarded. The tubing should be rinsed three times a day with sterile water. If diarrhea, nausea, or distention occurs, the diet should be withheld for 24 hours then gradually resumed. In elderly or unconscious patients or patients who recently have had surgery, elevation of the head of the bed is advisable during administration of the preparation to avoid aspiration.

Storage. Many of the formulas are relatively new, and complete indications for use and instructions on storage, preparation, and use are not available. In terms of storage of products as they come from the manufacturer, pharmacists should take care not to store them in areas with temperatures higher than 75° F (23.8° C) and should check expiration dates before dispensing.

Cautions. All formulas are excellent media for bacterial growth and should be prepared each day and refrigerated until used. If they become bacterially contaminated, they may cause diarrhea. Diarrhea can also occur from the osmolar load of the carbohydrate, especially simple sugars, or from fat intolerance (however, some elemental diets are fat-free).

Patients must be monitored for biochemical abnormalities of electrolyte values and to ensure adequate nutrition and hydration. Urine and blood glucose concentrations should be measured; diabetics may require increased doses of insulin. Edema may be precipitated or aggravated in patients with PCM or cardiac, renal, or hepatic disease because of the relatively high sodium content of the chemically defined diets. Frequently, hospital dieticians prepare formulas so that the electrolytes can be tailored to the individual patient.

Summary

Although dietary products can be obtained without a prescription, they are complex agents with specific indications. Medical assessment must precede their use. The pharmacist should review dilution, the technique of preparation, storage, and administration of these products with the patient and should offer to discuss with the patient unusual effects, such as diarrhea, that possibly can be caused by the formulas. An antidiarrheal may be indicated or merely a change in the administration or storage process of the product. The pharmacist should not be reluctant to consult a dietician or physician (especially a gastroenterologist, oncologist, or surgeon, who often deals with nutrition problems) concerning nutritional supplementation and should refer patients when necessary.

Minerals

Iron

Iron-deficiency anemia is a widespread problem. Although it causes few deaths, it contributes to the poor health and suboptimal performance of many people. Milder iron deficiencies which do not lead to anemia but which are probably very common no doubt present clinical manifestations, but they are less often recognizable. Iron plays an important role in oxygen and electron transport. In the body, it is either functional or it is stored. Functional iron is found in hemoglobin, myoglobin, heme enzymes, and cofactor and transport iron. The rest is stored in the form of ferritin and hemosiderin. Ferritin is a micelle of ferric hydroxyphosphate surrounded by 24 identical protein units.[8] Hemosiderin consists of aggregated ferritin molecules and additional components.[9] The storage sites of ferritin and hemosiderin are the liver, spleen, and bone marrow.

Normally, adult males have about 50 mg of iron/kg; females have about 35 mg/kg.[10] Hemoglobin is about 0.34 percent iron. Normal hemoglobin in adult males is about 16 to 18 g/100 ml of blood; in adult females, it is 12 to 14 g/100 ml. The RDA for iron is between 10 and 18 mg for all adults.

About 10 percent of oral iron in food or as an iron supplement is absorbed. In an iron-deficient patient, about 20 percent is absorbed. Ingested iron is solubilized in gastric juice and is reduced to the ferrous form. It is then chelated to substances such as ascorbic acid, sugars, and amino acids. These chelates have a low molecular weight and can be solubilized and absorbed before they reach the alkaline media of the distal portion of the small intestine where precipitation occurs. Iron is probably passively absorbed into the mucosal layer, then actively transferred to transferrin and used in the bone marrow for incorporation into red blood cells or incorporated into all of the other body cells. Some of the transferrin iron is stored in the spleen, liver, and bone marrow. Iron is released from the body by the flaking of skin cells; in the urine, sweat, and feces; and by hemorrhagic loss such as menstruation.

Etiology of iron deficiency. Iron deficiency can result from inadequate diet, malabsorption, pregnancy and lactation, or blood loss. Because the amount of normal excretion of iron through the urine, feces, and skin is very small, iron deficiency caused by poor diet or malabsorption may develop very slowly and manifest itself only after a period of years. Unless it is proven otherwise, the development of iron deficiency in an adult male or postmenopausal female is caused by blood loss. Blood loss can occur with conditions such as hiatus hernia, peptic ulcers, esophageal varices, diverticulitis, intestinal parasites (especially hookworm), regional enteritis, and ulcerative colitis. The pharmacist should be aware of the possibility of these serious illnesses.

Blood loss may also occur from drug ingestion. Many drugs directly irritate the gastric mucosa or have an indirect effect on the GI tract. These drugs include the salicylates, nonsalicylate analgesics (e.g., indomethacin and phenylbutazone), reserpine, steroids, and most drugs used in the treatment of neoplasms, such as fluorouracil, mithramycin, and dactinomycin.

Menstrual blood losses may contribute to iron deficiency. Normally, the blood lost during a menstrual period is 60 to 80 ml; in 95 percent of women, this represents about 1.4 mg or less of iron lost.[11] Normal loss in addition to menstrual loss of iron indicates a total daily iron need of 7 to 23 mg. Average U.S. diets contain about 5 to 7 mg of iron/1,000 cal, and women on restricted diets may need supplemental iron. Some women who consider their menses normal actually lose between 100 and 200 ml of blood per period. To make up this loss would require as much as 40 mg/day of iron in the diet (about 10 percent of food iron is absorbed). Clearly, for these women supplemental iron is desirable.

Another source of blood loss is through donation of blood. A donation is usually about 500 ml of blood. If the hemoglobin is normal, about 250 mg of iron is lost.

Iron deficiency may be caused by not eating enough animal protein and cereal food made with iron-fortified flour. Clay eating (geophagia) leads to iron deficiency by the chelation or precipitation of iron in the gut.[12] This disorder, called pica, is practiced by children and women, especially in lower income groups. Chronic diarrhea commonly leads to iron deficiency. Achlorhydria and partial or total gastrectomy cause decreased absorption of iron.

Signs and symptoms. Early symptoms of iron deficiency frequently are vague and are related to other disease states. Easy fatigability, weakness, and lassitude cannot easily be related to iron deficiency. Often, patients without obvious symptoms have iron-deficiency anemia, discovered during a routine medical examination. Other symptoms of anemia include pallor, dyspnea upon exertion, palpitation, and a feeling of exhaustion. Coldness and numbness of extremities may be reported.

Patient consultation. The pharmacist can ascertain the cause of the patient's disease by consulting the medication record. The patient might have been treated for ulcers or hemorrhoids, conditions which could cause blood loss. Checking the medication record for previous use of drugs such as phenylbutazone, reserpine, or warfarin might lead to another suspicion for blood loss. Medications, such as aspirin, which could cause blood loss, are bought without a prescription and often are not included on a medication record. In these cases, the pharmacist must question the patient. A patient who indicates blood loss should be referred to a physician. In any indication of blood loss, time is very important. Abnormal blood loss may be indicated by:

- ☐ Vomiting blood
- ☐ Bright red blood in the stool or dark, tarry stools
- ☐ Large clots or an abnormally large flow (200 ml or more) during the menstrual period
- ☐ Cloudy or pink/red appearance of the urine (ruling out dyes in drugs which may cause urine discoloration).

Blood loss, particularly through the stool, is not always obvious to the patient. Before suggesting self-treatment, the pharmacist must consider the patient's medication history and overall appearance.

Other questions may be asked for indications of iron deficiency: Do you eat balanced meals on a regular basis? Do you have cravings for clay or ice?[13] Have you given blood recently? The pharmacist should ascertain the chronicity of the patient's problem and whether medical care has been sought. Depending on the answers, the pharmacist might suggest iron supplementation with self-monitoring to check for improvement. Generally, iron supplementation should be considered when food intake is restricted or when the patient is pregnant, lactating, or menstruating.

Treatment. If iron supplementation can safely be suggested, the pharmacist must determine which iron product is best. The choice of an iron preparation should be based on how well it is absorbed, how well it is tolerated in therapeutic doses, and price. Because ferrous salts are more soluble than ferric salts, it seems reasonable to choose an iron product of the ferrous group. Ferrous sulfate has been the standard against which other salts of iron—ferrous succinate, ferrous lactate, ferrous fumarate, ferrous glycine sulfate, ferrous glutamate, and ferrous gluconate—have been compared. All are absorbed about as well as ferrous sulfate. Ferrous citrate, ferrous tartrate, ferrous pyrophosphate, and some ferric salts are not absorbed as well.[14]

Ferrous salts have been given in combination with ascorbic acid. At a ratio of 200 mg of ascorbic acid to 30 mg of elemental iron, the increased amount of iron absorbed validated this practice.[14] Some experts feel that the cost of the iron-ascorbic acid combination does not warrant its use for the moderate increase in iron absorption.[15] If cost is a factor, this author suggests the use of ascorbic acid tablets, not in a combination product. This type of therapy is probably more appropriate for people with iron-store deficiencies in addition to plasma deficiencies.

In a 320-mg hydrated ferrous sulfate tablet, 20 percent (about 60 mg) is elemental iron. In patients who have iron deficiencies, 20 percent of the elemental iron is absorbed. If three tablets a day are taken, 36 mg of iron is absorbed; if four tablets are taken, 48 mg is absorbed. Thirty-six to forty-eight mg of iron is enough to support maximum incorporation into red blood cells (0.3 g hemoglobin/100 ml of blood).

Enteric-coated or delayed-release iron preparations are not pharmacologically advantageous. Because progressively less iron is absorbed as it moves from the duodenum to the ileum, these products decrease the overall iron absorption by delaying the time of release. These products generally are more expensive than other iron preparations, and no advantage (except, perhaps, patient compliance) is derived from their use.

All iron products tend to irritate the GI mucosa. The symptoms are nausea, GI pain, and diarrhea and can be decreased by decreasing the dosage. They are also decreased by using other ferrous salts such as succinate, lactate, gluconate, or fumarate or by giving iron with meals. Although giving iron with food is less irritating, food decreases the amount of iron absorbed by 40 to 50 percent.[14] Periodically, physicians recommend iron with instructions for between-meal dosing. It is advantageous for absorption if the patient is able to tolerate the iron taken in this manner. If nausea or diarrhea is a problem, the pharmacist should be consulted; it usually is preferable to suggest taking the iron with food or decreasing the number of tablets than to stop taking the supplement entirely.

Constipation, a frequent side effect of iron therapy, has prompted the formulation of medications that contain iron and a stool softener. If iron and a stool softener do, in fact, prevent constipation, such a preparation is indicated. However, not all patients become constipated with iron therapy. In one study, adverse effects of iron were believed to be psychological.[16] Therefore, pharmacists might consider deemphasizing side effects when discussing iron therapy with patients.

Another observation with iron therapy is that stools become black and tarry. Usually, this effect is caused by unabsorbed iron, but it can also be caused by occult blood, if the patient has indicated GI bleeding in the past. If the stools do not darken during iron therapy, it may be that the iron tablet did not break up.

Monitoring. Iron-deficiency anemia is diagnosed by a physician or in a diagnostic clinic, based on tests such as hemoglobin, hematocrit, serum iron, and iron-binding capacity. In order to monitor the effect of iron therapy, the pharmacist and physician can inquire about the patient's own perception of well-being. The physician usually uses the hemoglobin to measure the effect of iron therapy. The pharmacist might remind the patient who has a prescription for iron to have a blood test to check for the appropriate response in 1 to 2 months. Usually, hemoglobin is corrected in this time; correction of plasma iron takes 3 to 4 months.

Drug interactions. Iron chelates with many substances. Its interaction with antacids is therapeutically significant.[17] The mechanism is probably related to the relative alkalinization of the stomach contents. Therefore, the chelate of iron with the antacid (e.g., magnesium trisilicate) is even more insoluble in the alkaline medium. Iron appears to chelate with several of the tetracyclines, resulting in decreased tetracycline absorption.[18] The manufacturers of allopurinol recommend that iron and allopurinol not be given together. In animals, allopurinol may increase hepatic uptake of iron; however, this effect has not been shown in humans.

Directions to the patient. Most healthy patients who self-medicate should probably not be taking more than one iron tablet per day. The usual dose for iron deficiency is one to four tablets a day. The iron should be taken between meals, or in cases of gastric pain or irritation, with food. Patients should be cautioned that the stool may darken from the iron. If antacids or tetracyclines are taken, iron should be taken at a separate time. One month of therapy is probably reasonable for self-medication with iron. If the patient has no response after this period, a physician should be consulted.

Iron toxicity. Accidental poisoning with iron occurs most frequently in children. The sugar-coated, brown iron tablets look like chocolate and attract children. About 50 percent of iron poisoning cases are fatal. As few as 15 tablets of 0.3 g of ferrous sulfate have been lethal, but the ingestion of as many as 70 tablets has been followed by recovery. The outcome depends on the speed of appropriate treatment.

The symptoms of acute iron poisoning are reflected by several organ systems. Because iron salts in large doses are corrosive to the gastric mucosa, pain, vomiting (the vomitus may contain blood and particles of the iron tablets), and diarrhea occur (ribbons of mucosa may be seen in the watery diarrhea).[19] These symptoms can lead to electrolyte imbalances and shock. In later phases of what may seem like recovery, pneumonitis (if the vomitus is aspirated) and acidosis may occur and cardiovascular collapse may ensue. Autopsies frequently show liver damage, and there may be pyloric stenosis. Renal damage usually does not occur.

The treatment for iron overdose can be started at home by giving milk and inducing vomiting immediately. The remainder of the therapy should be carried out in an appropriately equipped hospital. It includes gastric lavage, the administration of deferoxamine mesylate (5 to 10 g), and supportive care such as oxygen, antibiotics, etc., as the condition requires.

A more insidious kind of iron toxicity can occur during prolonged therapy with iron. In the treatment of refractory anemia, oral iron may be excessively absorbed, leading to iron overload. Alcoholic patients also become iron overloaded. Wine contains iron, and alcohol increases the absorption of ferric iron. Patients with chronic liver disease and chronic pancreatic disease absorb more iron than normal from the gut. Iron overload can also occur when individuals who do not need iron take it for prolonged periods. The pharmacist should be aware of this and discourage the use of iron when there is no evidence to indicate its need.

Calcium

Calcium is a major component of bones and teeth. It is necessary for the clotting of blood and the integrity of many cells, especially those of the neuromuscular system. The present RDA of calcium for adults is 800 to 1,200 mg and 240 to 800 mg for infants and children. (The methods of calculating these values are being reviewed.) The small intestine controls the amount of calcium absorbed. Thus, patients taking relatively low amounts of calcium absorb more, and some taking large amounts excrete more as fecal calcium. Calcium requirements also appear to increase as the consumption of protein increases.[20 21]

A dietary deficiency disease caused by insufficient calcium intake is not known. The major pathologic conditions which may lead to depletion of skeletal minerals are the malabsorption syndromes and uremia. In uremic patients, the kidney is unable to convert vitamin D to its most active form; thus, calcium absorption is impaired when adaptation mechanisms cannot compensate for low calcium intake. Various disturbances, including neuromuscular irritability, may occur and may progress to tetany or major seizures. Other manifestations include osteomalacia and bone deformities. Therapy consists of 4 to 12 g of calcium daily and patients require monitoring. Serum calcium should be maintained between 9 and 11 mEq per 1,000 ml of blood. Urine calcium levels are not an accurate reflection of serum calcium levels.

Calcium can be toxic. Large amounts taken as dietary supplementation or as antacids can lead to high levels of calcium in the urine and renal stones. The latter may result in renal damage.

The most common calcium salts available without a prescription are calcium carbonate, calcium gluconate, and calcium lactate. Of these, calcium carbonate is preferred because it provides more elemental calcium per given weight of calcium salt.

Trace elements

Zinc. The 1974 RDA for zinc is 15 mg for adults (more for pregnant and lactating women) and 3 to 10 mg for infants and children. Zinc is necessary for wound healing, and impairment of taste and smell acuity can be improved with zinc supplementation.[22 23] Poor appetite and poor growth may occur in children with low zinc intake. Zinc supplementation is most important for people with chronic wounds and with wounds following surgery and trauma. Patients on chemically defined diets as a sole nutritional source must be observed for zinc deficiency. Zinc and copper seem to have a relationship, and in some patients, administration of copper increases the zinc level.[24] Some OTC multiple vitamins contain zinc.

Copper. Copper is needed to maintain adequate blood cell production. It also seems required for the use of iron. Intake of 2 to 5 mg daily is adequate to prevent copper deficiencies. Copper deficiency states are rare except in patients whose sole nutritional intake is a chemically defined source, e.g., patients fed intravenously on total parenteral nutrition.[25]

Others. Fluorine, iodine, and chromium are needed in humans and are generally available through the diet. Other species need cobalt, manganese, molybdenum, selenium, nickel, tin, vanadium, and silicon.[26] Further observations in humans on long-term, chemically defined diets may indicate that these elements also are essential to good health.

Some OTC protein products (Gevral Protein, Meritene, and Sustagen) contain trace minerals such as magnesium, zinc, manganese, copper, and iodide. These same trace metals are also commonly found in multiple vitamin and mineral combinations. Some of the trace metals (e.g., zinc, manganese, and copper) are available as single-entity products.

Vitamins

Fat-soluble vitamins

Vitamin A. Vitamin A is needed to prevent night blindness and xerosis (drying) of the conjunctiva, the first symptoms of vitamin A deficiency. Drying of the epithelium on other sites of the body, nerve lesions, and increased pressure in the cerebrospinal fluid also may occur. Pregnant women must have an adequate vitamin A intake to avoid malformation of the fetus. Vitamin A is consumed as preformed vitamin A from animal sources and as carotenoids, of which the most active is carotene, from plant sources. Particularly good sources are kidney, milk products, eggs, fish liver oil, bear liver, and palm oil. If skim milk is used, it should be fortified with vitamin A or supplemented in another way. The term "vitamin A" designates several biologically active compounds. Vitamins A (retinol) and A_2 (3-dehydroretinol) are alcohols. Retinol is the major naturally occurring form. Because the vitamin is fat soluble, it is stored in the body, mainly in the liver. Deficiencies rarely occur in well-nourished populations, and when they do occur, they develop slowly. Serum levels usually remain normal until the liver reserve becomes very small.

There are several etiologies of vitamin A deficiency. Before 1968, there was an epidemic of vitamin A deficiency in Brazil due to the provision of skim milk to Brazilian children without a supplementary vitamin A capsule. The skim milk was the sole diet. Diseases such as cancer, tuberculosis, pneumonia, chronic nephritis, urinary tract infections, and prostatic diseases may cause massive excretion of vitamin A.[27] Those in which there is fat malabsorption, such as GI diseases of sprue, obstructive jaundice, cystic fibrosis, and cirrhosis of the liver, can also cause very low or absent vitamin A stores. In the U.S., vitamin A deficiency occurs more frequently because of diseases of fat malabsorption than because of malnutrition.

The signs and symptoms of vitamin A deficiency related to the eye are drying, wrinkling, and hazing of the cornea. Lack of tears may be caused by obstruction of the tear duct. Bitot spots (small patches of bubbles that resemble tiny drops of meringue) may appear. The conjunctiva may look dry and opaque, and photophobia may occur. The cornea may become ulcerous, and infection may then destroy it. If this occurs, there may be loss of vision. This process occurs more rapidly in children than in adults.

The most recent revision of the RDA for vitamin A uses a new unit of measurement—retinol equivalents (RE). It incorporates vitamin A and its provitamin, carotene.[28] The RDA for adult males is 5,000 International Units (IU), or 1,000 RE. For adult females, it is 4,000 IU (800 RE); pregnant women need 1,000 RE, and lactating women, 1,200 RE. Doses of vitamin A for infants on unfortified or skim milk formulas should be 1,500 IU daily. Patients with corneal lesions due to hypovitaminosis A should take 25,000 to 50,000 IU daily of a water-dispersible, vitamin A preparation. The FDA has ruled that products containing more than 10,000 IU of vitamin A per dose may be sold on prescription only. The duration of therapy should be assessed by clinical evaluation.

If the pharmacist establishes that the patient has poor dietary habits (e.g., the patient is an alcoholic), an OTC multiple vitamin that contains the RDA of vitamin A should be recommended. The incidence of hypervitaminosis has been increasing, particularly among food faddists. Doses as low as 18,500 IU of vitamin A given to infants between 3 and 6 months old for 1 to 3 months have been toxic.[29] Toxicity usually occurs at 20 to 30 times the RDA (20,000 to 30,000 RE; 100,000 to 150,000 IU). Fatigue, malaise, and lethargy are the common signs. Abdominal upset, bone and joint pain, throbbing headaches, insomnia, restlessness, night sweats, loss of body hair, brittle nails, exophthalmus, rough and scaly skin, peripheral edema, and mouth fissures also are common. Constipation, menstrual irregularity, and emotional liability have been reported in some cases.[30] Single doses of 2,000,000 IU (400,000 RE) may precipitate acute toxicity 4 to 8 hours after ingestion. Headache is predominant, but it may be accompanied by diplopia, nausea, vomiting, vertigo, or drowsiness.[31] Treatment consists of the discontinuance of ingestion of the vitamin A. The prognosis is good.

The systemic use of vitamin A for the treatment of acne, prevention of infection, and its topical use in wound healing is not warranted by clinical evidence. A topical product incorporating retinoic acid has shown positive clinical response in the treatment of mild to moderately severe acne.

Regarding vitamin A, it is the author's opinion that the pharmacist should provide patients advice about supplementation to avoid deficiency (if the diet is not adequate); discourage excessive dosage; and refer patients who seem to have clinical vitamin A deficiency to a physician. This latter point is made because of the speed of disastrous consequences and because diagnosis, treatment, and follow-up require laboratory assessment.

Vitamin D. Vitamin D is an oil-soluble vitamin. It is a collective name for several structurally similar chemicals and their metabolites—ergocalciferol (vitamin D_2) is derived from ergosterol, cholecalciferol (vitamin D_3) is derived from cholesterol, and dihydrotachysterol (vitamin D_1) is a synthetic reduction product of vitamin D_2. Some very active metabolites of vitamin D_3 have been identified. One metabolite, 25-hydroxycholecalciferol, is formed in the liver, carried on protein to the kidneys, and further converted to several more active metabolites of which the most active is 1,25-dihydroxycholecalciferol (1,25-DHCC).[32] Vitamin D is needed to stimulate calcium absorption from the small intestine and to mobilize bone calcium. It is closely involved with parathyroid hormone, phosphate, and calcitonin in the homeostasis of serum calcium.

Vitamin D has properties of both hormones and vitamins. If there is sufficient exposure to sunlight, sterol in the skin is irradiated, and vitamin D is synthesized. If sun exposure is not sufficient, it is necessary to obtain vitamin D from the diet. If an adequate amount of vitamin D is not consumed or is not activated by sunlight, rickets, tetany, or osteomalacia may occur. Although diets in the U.S. rarely are deficient in vitamin D to the extent that rickets occurs, vitamin D deficiencies caused by renal disease (the kidney is less capable of forming 1,25-DHCC), malabsorption syndromes, short bowel syndromes due to many causes, hypoparathyroid disease, chronic use of anticonvulsants, and familial hypophosphatemia are common.

Food sources of vitamin D are fish liver oils and irradiated yeast. Many foods are fortified with vitamin D, particularly milk products and cereals. The RDA for vitamin D is 400 IU for infants and adults, including pregnant and lactating women. The FDA has ruled that doses of vitamin D above 400 IU must be available on prescription only.

The signs and symptoms of vitamin D deficiency diseases are reflected as calcium abnormalities, specifically, those involved with the formation of bone. As serum calcium and inorganic phosphate decrease, compensatory mechanisms attempt to increase the calcium. Parathyroid hormone secretion increases, which may lead to secondary hyperparathyroidism. If physiologic mechanisms fail to make the appropriate adjustments in levels of calcium and phosphorus, rickets or osteomalacia develops. Rickets is a failure of mineralization of bone matrix. The epiphyseal plate may widen due to failure of calcification. As a result, rickets is manifested by soft bones and deformed joints. The diagnosis is made radiologically by observing the bone deformities.

Large doses of vitamin D are prescribed for rickets. For children, 1,000 to 4,000 IU per dose is given; for adults with osteodystrophy of renal disease, it is 50,000 to 5,000,000 IU. Smaller doses will be given when 1,25-DHCC becomes available.

The monitoring procedure for therapy, regardless of the particular vitamin D entity used, is extremely important. Urine and blood calcium levels must be checked to avoid hypercalcemia. Because phosphate binds with calcium and may be deposited in soft tissue such as brain, eyes, heart, and kidney, phosphate in the serum also must be regulated.

Concurrent drug therapy must be closely monitored. Phosphate in drugs that are used chronically, such as certain laxatives, may lower the calcium level and contribute to a vitamin D deficiency. Very often, patients who have vitamin D deficiency caused by renal problems are receiving antacid therapy. The pharmacist should point out to patients with renal problems that antacids should be chosen for the specific ingredients they contain, e.g., aluminum antacids may be chosen because they bind phosphates, and magnesium antacids avoided because of their toxicity in renal disease. A calcium antacid may be used to help increase serum calcium levels.

Vitamin D is toxic when taken in large doses for long periods. Hypervitaminosis D can occur with 4,000 IU per day. Doses of 50,000 to 100,000 IU daily are dangerous to adults and children. Doses of 1,380 to 2,370 IU have not been shown to be detrimental to children, but doses over 1,000 IU are not advisable.[33,34]

The signs and symptoms of hypervitaminosis D are anorexia, nausea, weakness, weight loss, polyuria, constipation, vague aches, stiffness, soft tissue calcification, nephrocalcinosis, hypertension, anemia, hypercalcemia, acidosis, irreversible renal failure, and death. The pharmacist should check the medication profile for a possible cause of the problem. For example, if a patient complained of bone pain and stiffness and the medication record showed therapy with vitamin D, the pharmacist might suspect hypervitaminosis. If a recent blood test has not been taken to measure serum calcium, a physician should be consulted.

Most people obtain the RDA of vitamin D in dietary sources and by exposure to sunlight. If a patient asks for a vitamin D supplement and the pharmacist determines that the need is based on poor dietary intake or indoor confinement, a multiple vitamin supplement may be recommended. Patients who request therapeutic doses of vitamin D should be referred to a physician when the pharmacist ascertains that a need exists.

Liquid preparations that contain vitamin D should be measured carefully, particularly when given to infants. Patients using prescription vitamin D products should be encouraged to see a physician regularly. The vitamin D product of choice—1,25-DHCC metabolite—is not yet available commercially. Presently, vitamins D_2 and D_3 probably are interchangeable. Dihydrotachysterol may be the drug of choice in renal disease and hypoparathyroidism because it is active in its present state and needs no further metabolism for vitamin D activity.

Vitamin E. Vitamin E is the most potent of the eight natural alcohol compounds called tocopherols; specifically, it includes alpha tocopherol and salts. The American diet now includes more soybean products, which have a considerable amount of γ-tocopherol. Although γ-tocopherol is less potent, it may contribute as much as 20 percent of the ingested vitamin E. Future revisions of the RDA may list vitamin E as a tocopherol equivalent.

Vitamin E has become an extremely controversial nutrient in the last few years through claims for its therapeutic effect as a drug. As a nutrient in humans, vitamin E seems necessary in preventing problems involving the musculature and the nervous and vascular systems. Many of its effects found in animals, particularly the induction of fertility, have not been shown in humans.

The RDA for adults is 12 to 15 IU daily and less for infants (4 IU) and children. It is dependent on the amount of polyunsaturated fatty acids (PUFA) consumed. The need for vitamin E increases as PUFA consumption increases. The ratio is 0.4 to 0.5 mg of vitamin E per gram of PUFA consumed. Foods high in PUFA also have a high content of vitamin E. The richest natural sources of vitamin E are vegetable oils, particularly safflower oil. Nuts and cereals also contain vitamin E. The refining process of oils and cereals may greatly diminish the content of vitamin E.

Vitamin E deficiency rarely occurs. Reported cases involved premature infants fed commercial formulas that contained relatively low ratios of vitamin E to PUFA and adults and children with fat malabsorption diseases (sprue, cystic fibrosis, pancreatitis, biliary cirrhosis, and idiopathic conditions). In infants, the signs and symptoms were edema, anemia, reticulocytosis, and thrombocytosis.[35] The cause was low vitamin E levels in the serum of the infants. Signs and symptoms in adults included decreased red blood cell survival time and muscle lesions. With vitamin E deficiency, the excretion of creatine in the urine may be very high and enzymes reflecting muscle damage may be increased in the plasma.

The therapeutic dosage of vitamin E for infants is 75 to 100 IU daily. In adults the dose of vitamin E required to return blood levels of tocopherol to normal was

60 to 80 IU of vitamin E daily for several weeks.[36] However, higher doses have been used.

It is unlikely that the pharmacist sees distinguishable vitamin E deficiency in the pharmacy. Infants with edema should be referred to a physician because edema can be a symptom of heart disease, renal disease, or other serious diseases and its cause cannot be distinguished without laboratory tests.

Patients with intermittent claudication and angina pectoris show improvement with daily doses of 400 to 3,200 IU of vitamin E.[37, 38] More studies are needed, particularly with angina, because the beneficial effects were small and not statistically significant. Clinical trials have failed to show that vitamin E protects against miscarriages, sterility, menopausal abnormalities, muscular dystrophies, cystic fibrosis, ulcers, or diabetes. As part of the antioxidant theory of vitamin E, it has been suggested that large doses retard the aging process. This theory suggests that aging is a buildup of cellular components that have been destroyed by their exposure to oxygen, cosmic rays, or pollution. Vitamin E as an antioxidant is claimed to protect against this reaction. The theory has not been proved or disproved clinically, and research continues in this area.

Vitamin E has been ingested in large quantities without apparent pharmacologic toxicity. Thus, long-term use at high doses cannot be discouraged from the basis of toxicology. The pharmacist's role in advising on vitamin E is one of advising patients that:

- ☐ The average American diet adequately protects against vitamin E deficiency.
- ☐ The FDA requires that all infant formulas contain adequate amounts of vitamin E. Human and cow's milk contain enough vitamin E to protect against vitamin E deficiency in infants.
- ☐ High doses of vitamin E are a waste of money.
- ☐ Attempting to self-treat a potentially serious symptom such as chest pain with vitamin E only delays proper medical treatment.

If vitamin E has been prescribed, iron should not be taken at the same time. Studies with supplementation of infant formulas containing iron and vitamin E show that blood tocopherol levels do not increase.[39]

Water-soluble vitamins

Ascorbic acid (vitamin C). As a nutrient, ascorbic acid is necessary to prevent scurvy. Humans and a few other species must consume ascorbic acid because it is not produced by the body. Today, scurvy is rare and develops only when psychiatric illness, alcoholism, age, GI disease, food fads, or ignorance cause inadequate nutritional consumption; infants who are fed artificial formulas without vitamin supplements also may develop scurvy. In adults, scurvy occurs 4 to 5 months after all ascorbic acid consumption is stopped.

Ascorbic acid is involved in the formation of connective tissue, osteoid, and dentin. A deficiency causes impairment of wound healing and reopening of old wounds. Early manifestations include anorexia, weakness, neurasthenia, and joint and muscle aches. Another early sign is prominent hair follicles on the thighs and buttocks due to plugging with keratin. The hair is coiled in the hair follicle and looks like a corkscrew, or it may be fragmented after it erupts. Bleeding abnormalities, such as hemorrhaging in the skin, muscles, joints, GI mucosa, and major organs also occur. The gingiva of the teeth become swollen, hemorrhagic, infected, sometimes necrotic and, if untreated, the teeth fall out. Death may occur suddenly in untreated scurvy. In infants with ascorbic acid deficiency, growth and development are retarded, skin and gum hemorrhaging occur, bone development is impaired, and anemia may develop.

Because only 10 mg of ascorbic acid a day prevents scurvy and a normal diet containing fresh fruits and vegetables contains many times more than this, pharmacists rarely are confronted with symptoms of ascorbic acid deficiency. The most common early symptom of the deficiency is prominent hair follicles. Rough skin probably will be a problem, most often in winter, when fresh fruits and vegetables are not as plentiful. The pharmacist should find out the sites of the roughness and appearance of the hairs. If answers to questions indicate a deficiency, the pharmacist should determine if more serious signs and symptoms exist, such as easy bruisability, spontaneous petechiae, or purpura (blood spots just under the skin). If they do not exist and if the patient does not take a multiple vitamin product or an ascorbic acid supplement, a multiple vitamin product can be recommended. Most of these products contain 40 mg or more of ascorbic acid per dose.

Because the 1974 RDA for ascorbic acid in adults is 45 mg, the pharmacist can also recommend daily dosing (e.g., a 50-mg tablet) with ascorbic acid. If the patient is already taking a daily vitamin supplement, additional vitamin C probably is not helpful. If hemorrhagic signs are present, the pharmacist should refer the patient to a physician because many serious diseases can cause similar problems, the diagnosis for which cannot be determined in a pharmacy.

In the treatment of severely scorbutic patients, 300 mg of ascorbic acid daily for 5 days is recommended to build up the body store, followed by a daily allowance of 45 mg in the food or by a supplement in addition to food.[40] Infants who do not have vitamin C supplements in their formula should receive 35 to 50 mg daily; those who are breast-fed receive a sufficient amount.

Doses of ascorbic acid recommended for prevention (1 to 4 g daily) and treatment (as much as 15 g daily) of the common cold are pharmacologic doses. Since Pauling's[41, 42] writings on ascorbic acid and the common cold, much literature has appeared. The question of the efficacy of ascorbic acid has been reviewed by the Department of Drugs of the American Medical Association, and the studies indicate that there is "little convincing evidence to support claims of clinically important efficacy."[43] The results of one study showing a positive correlation between ascorbic acid in high doses and amelioration of the symptoms of colds was nonreproducible by the same investigators.[44, 45]

Megadoses of ascorbic acid may be harmful. There are indications of increased danger of developing urinary tract stones, interference with the completion of a normal pregnancy (with doses of 6 g daily for 3 days), diarrhea (with doses of 1 g or more daily), and a rebound phenomenon in infants born of mothers who had taken 400 mg of ascorbic acid daily before delivering (these infants required more than the usual amount of ascorbic acid to prevent scurvy).[46-49] However, more clinical evidence is needed to confirm these observations.

Drug interactions can occur with ascorbic acid. The most frequent ones occur with warfarin sodium or dicumarol. The clinical evidence is sketchy, however, and the pharmacist, aware of the concurrent administration of either of these drugs with ascorbic acid, should discuss the possible interaction with the patient and the physician and suggest that prothrombin times be measured regularly. Because ascorbic acid acidifies the urine, other drug interactions can occur. Ascorbic acid is used to acidify the urine of patients taking methenamine compounds. The acid converts the compounds to formaldehyde to produce their antibacterial activity. Patients with spine injuries and neurogenic bladders often take ascorbic acid to prevent urinary tract infections. Ascorbic acid forms a soluble chelate with iron to improve the absorption of the iron. Acidic drugs (e.g., salicylates) are resorbed to a greater extent in the renal tubules with acidified urine.[50] Basic drugs (e.g., tricyclic antidepressants and the amphetamines) are excreted more rapidly in acidified urine and therefore, their effect is antagonized.[51-53]

Urine glucose tests are affected by large quantities of ascorbic acid in the urine. The Tes-Tape and Clinistix tests may read falsely negative, and Clinitest tablets and Benedict's solution may be falsely positive.[54 55] The pharmacist can instruct the patient on the procedure to modify the technique to avoid the interaction with the tape method. Tes-Tape can be dipped in the urine and the color correlation made at the moving front of the liquid on the tape, where different diffusion rates allow the glucose to chromatographically separate from the ascorbic acid on the tape.

The pharmacist should ascertain whether the patient is diabetic or uses other medications whose effects are antagonized or increased by ascorbic acid. It is the author's opinion that the unproven efficacy, possible adverse effects, and interactions do not lend themselves to the recommendation of doses of ascorbic acid larger than the RDA.

The question of stability of ascorbic acid tablets is controversial. One study showed poor stability and recommended that ascorbic acid tablets be stored in a refrigerator. Other investigators suggest that tablets stored under normal conditions retain 95-percent potency for more than 5 years.[56] Presently, it seems reasonable to store the tablets in a tightly covered container at room temperature.

There are many sizes of ascorbic acid tablets and concentrations of liquids available. They are available as ascorbic acid and sodium ascorbate. The latter is the soluble salt for parenteral use.

Thiamine hydrochloride (vitamin B_1). Thiamine is a coenzyme in several enzyme-catalyzed reactions in humans. Several of these reactions are important in providing energy. The RDA for thiamine is 1.0 to 1.5 mg for adults, 0.7 to 1.2 mg for children, and 0.3 to 0.5 mg for infants. The amount needed increases with the increased consumption of calories. The most familiar natural source of thiamine is the hull of rice grains. Other good sources are pork, beef, fresh peas, and beans. It was in animals and humans whose diets largely consisted of polished rice that thiamine deficiency disease (beriberi) was first observed. Today, beriberi caused by nutritional deficiency rarely occurs in the western world, unless it is precipitated by economic or medical pathology. Thiamine deficiency is most common in alcoholics, whose nutrition is severely or entirely neglected.

Signs and symptoms of thiamine hydrochloride deficiency are evident in 12 to 14 days after thiamine intake is stopped. The abnormalities center in the cardiovascular and neurological systems. The deficiency causes cardiac failure possibly accompanied by edema, tachycardia upon only minimal exertion, enlarged heart, and electrocardiograph abnormalities. The patient may have pain in the precordial or epigastric area. Neuromuscular symptoms are paresthesia of the extremities of maximal use, weakness, and atrophy. An acute form of thiamine hydrochloride deficiency occurs in alcoholics and other patients who have been vomiting for extended periods. The neurological signs (Wernicke's encephalopathy) are particularly evident. Nystagmus occurs when the patient is asked to gaze up and down along a vertical plane or from side to side along a horizontal plane. Administration of glucose solutions without the administration of thiamine may precipitate symptoms that range from mild confusion to coma. Death is common if treatment is withheld. Damage to the cerebral cortex may occur in patients who survive and can lead to Korsakoff's psychosis. The symptoms of the psychosis are impaired retentive memory and cognitive function; the patient commonly confabulates when given a piece of information or when asked a question.

Beriberi may develop in infants whose mothers are on a polished rice diet and in the Orient in regions where thiamine hydrochloride supplements are not used. The signs and symptoms of infantile beriberi also are neurological. Aphonia, or silent crying, may occur, and the signs of meningitis may be mimicked. Death will ensue if treatment is not initiated with thiamine.

The dosage of thiamine for the treatment of the symptoms of heart failure caused by this deficiency is 5 to 10 mg three times daily. At this dose the failure is rapidly corrected, but the neurological signs correct much more slowly. The dosage of thiamine for neurological deficits is between 30 and 100 mg given parenterally for less than a week or until an oral diet can be started.

The pharmacist may wish to recommend multiple vitamin supplements to patients known to have poor dietary habits due to alcoholism.

The toxicity of thiamine is relatively mild. The oral dosage must exceed 200 to 300 mg before toxicity occurs. Most of the excess dose, i.e., more than 2 to 3 mg, is excreted in the urine. After parenteral administration, symptoms of itching, tingling, and pain may be noticed. There have been rare reports of anaphylactic reactions occurring after parenteral injections.

Thiamine is available as an elixir, an injectable solution, a powder, and a tablet. If it is mixed in a solution, the solution should be acidic.

Riboflavin (vitamin B_2). Riboflavin is a constituent of two coenzymes that are essential to oxidative enzyme systems involved in electron transport. Cellular growth cannot occur without riboflavin. The RDA for riboflavin is 1.1 to 1.8 mg for adults (more for pregnant and lactating women); for children, it ranges from 0.8 to 1.2 mg; and for infants, it is 0.4 to 0.6 mg. It appears that the need for riboflavin increases during periods of increased cell growth, e.g., during pregnancy and wound healing. Natural sources of riboflavin are eggs, meat, milk, fish, and liver.

Riboflavin deficiency caused by inadequate nutrition is rare and is found among the poor and in alcoholics. It usually accompanies other vitamin deficiencies. The signs and symptoms of riboflavin deficiency are angular stomatitis, cheilosis, and sore throat. Those of later stages of the deficiency are seborrheic dermatitis of the face and generalized dermatitis. Photophobia may occur, and the eyes may itch and burn. The utilization of folic acid may be dependent on riboflavin; thus, anemia may accompany riboflavin deficiency. The signs and symptoms of riboflavin deficiency may be indicative of other very serious conditions, such as blood dyscrasia.

A complete dietary history should be obtained from the patient. In some cases, a therapeutic trial of riboflavin may be carried out before diagnosis is made. The therapeutic dose is 10 mg orally. Larger doses are not harmful but provide no additional benefit. The patient should be monitored to assess improvement of symptoms.

Riboflavin is not very soluble. If its absorption is a problem, 25 mg of the soluble riboflavin salt may be given intramuscularly. Riboflavin is also given intravenously as a component of injectable multivitamins, but the dosage is relatively low (about 10 mg per dose). Intravenous doses of 50 mg of riboflavin can decrease pulse rates in adults. Excess riboflavin is excreted in the urine. It has a yellow fluorescence.

Most OTC multiple vitamin products contain between 1 and 5 mg of riboflavin per dose; some products contain as much as 10 mg.

Niacin (nicotinic acid). Niacin and niacinamide are constituents of the coenzymes, nicotinamide adenine dinucleotide (NAD) and nicotinamide adenine dinucleotide phosphate (NADP). These enzymes are electron transfer agents, i.e., they accept or donate hydrogen in the respiratory mechanism of all body cells. Niacin results from the biological transformation of the amino acid, tryptophan, and is converted to niacinamide. Both niacin and niacinamide are effective in treating niacin deficiency (pellagra). Niacinamide produces less flushing than niacin but is not effective in lowering lipoproteins, whereas niacin in high doses is effective.

The RDA for niacin is 12 to 20 mg for adults. More is needed during physiological stress (pregnancy, lactation, burns, hyperthyroidism, etc.). The RDA is somewhat dependent on caloric intake—1,000 cal provide 4.4 mg of niacin. Foods rich in niacin and/or tryptophan are beef, cow's milk, and whole eggs.

Pellagra is rare, occurring most frequently in alcoholics, the elderly, and individuals on bizarre diets. It also occurs in areas where much corn is eaten because, although corn contains enough niacin to prevent pellagra, the niacin is bound to indigestible constituents, making it unavailable. The main systems affected are the nervous system, the skin, and the GI tract. Symptoms affecting the nervous system are peripheral neuropathy, myclopathy, and encephalopathy. Mania may occur, and seizures and coma precede death. Before the cause was discovered, many psychiatric admissions were due to the symptoms of niacin deficiency. There is a characteristic rash in niacin-deficient patients. Skin over the face and on pressure points may be thickened and hyperpigmented, may appear as a severe burn, and may become secondarily infected. The entire GI tract is affected, including angular fissures around the mouth, atrophy of the epithelium of the tongue, and hypertrophy of the papillae. Inflammation of the small intestine may also occur and is associated with episodes of bleeding and/or diarrhea. A summary of the symptoms of niacin deficiency in the various systems is called the 3 D's—diarrhea, dementia, and dermatitis.

The diagnosis is clear if all systems are affected. However, if the skin is unaffected, the diagnosis is much more difficult. A complete dietary history with subsequent calculation of the consumption of niacin may point to the disease. Treatment involves the ingestion of 300 to 500 mg of niacinamide daily in divided doses. Because other nutritional deficiencies often are present, the therapy should include the other B vitamins, vitamin A, and iron.

The use of niacin in much higher doses has been used for other therapeutic purposes such as lowering lipids in the blood. Its side effects at these dosages prevent it from being the drug of choice. Niacinamide is ineffective as a lipid-lowering agent. Niacin is also used for patients with peripheral vascular disease, but the clinical results of its use in these patients are varied. Dosages suggested by the manufacturer are 150 mg per day in divided doses. Niacin and niacinamide, in doses of as much as 3,000 mg daily, have been used in megavitamin therapy for schizophrenia. Most controlled studies do not show significantly different results when compared with placebo.[57]

High dosages of niacin cause significant and potentially life-threatening side effects. Because of the effects on the GI tract, high doses of niacin are contraindicated in patients with gastritis or peptic ulcer. Niacin can release histamine, and its use in patients with asthma should be undertaken carefully. It also can impair liver function, causing cholestatic jaundice and can disturb glucose tolerance and cause hyperuricemia. If niacin and niacinamide are used in high doses, laboratory parameters, suggested by the potential side effects, should be followed.

Niacin and niacinamide are available as tablets of many strengths, as injectable powders, and as elixirs (50 mg/0.5 ml). Doses of niacin in supplemental products usually are 10 to 20 mg; products containing 20 mg usually are used as prenatal vitamins. Products containing 100 mg of niacinamide are classified by the FDA as drugs rather than as dietary supplements. They are available without a prescription.

Pyridoxine hydrochloride (vitamin B_6). Pyridoxine hydrochloride, pyridoxal hydrochloride, and pyridoxamine are all equally effective in nutrition. Pyridoxine hydrochloride is the form most frequently used in vitamins. The RDA is 1.6 to 2 mg for adults and 0.3 to 1.2 mg for infants and children; for pregnant and lactating women, it is 2.5 mg. Foods rich in pyridoxine hydrochloride are meats, cereals, lentils, nuts, and some fruits and vegetables such as bananas, avocados, and potatoes. Cooking destroys some of the vitamin. The average U.S. diet provides the RDA; certain restricted diets and haphazard diets do not. Artificial infant formulas are required to contain pyridoxine hydrochloride.

The symptoms of pyridoxine hydrochloride deficiency in infants are convulsive disorders and irritability. Treatment with pyridoxine hydrochloride (e.g., 2 mg daily for infants) brings the encephalogram back to normal. Symptoms in adults whose diets are deficient in pyridoxine hydrochloride or who have been given a pyridoxine hydrochloride antagonist are indistinguishable from those of niacin and riboflavin deficiencies. They include pellagra-like dermatitis, oral lesions, peripheral neuropathy, and dulling of mentation. Other conditions or circumstances may also be related to pyridoxine hydrochloride requirements. Treatment of sideroblastic anemia requires 50 to 200 mg daily of pyridoxine hydrochloride to aid in the production of hemoglobin and erythrocytes. Because these amounts are more than physiological requirements, the anemia is not a nutritional deficiency.

Several drugs affect pyridoxine hydrochloride utilization. Isoniazid and cycloserine (antitubercular drugs) seem to antagonize pyridoxine hydrochloride. Perioral numbness resulting from peripheral neuropathy is a clinical manifestation of this antagonism, occurring most frequently in patients with poor diets. Psychotic behavior or seizures, both produced by cycloserine, can be prevented with increased intake of pyridoxine hydrochloride. To overcome the antagonism, 50 mg of pyridoxine hydrochloride daily with isoniazid and as much as 200 mg daily with cycloserine should be used. Penicillamine may bind with pyridoxine hydrochloride causing pyridoxine hydrochloride-responsive neurotoxicity. Estrogen seems to increase significantly the amount of tryptophan excreted in the urine. Thus, women taking oral contraceptives have shown increased tryptophan metabolite excretion.[58-60] Pyridoxine hydrochloride corrects this abnormality. A multivitamin product has been formulated that contains more than 10 times the RDA of pyridoxine hydrochloride. It also contains 0.1 mg of folic acid and vitamin E, both of which are depleted with the use of contraceptive steroids.[61] Pyridoxine hydrochloride can act as an antagonist to the pharmacologic action of levodopa, a drug used in treating parkinsonism. Because it facilitates the transformation of levodopa to dopamine before the former can cross into the CNS, pyridoxine hydrochloride should be avoided by patients taking levodopa. However, it may be useful for patients who have taken an overdose of levodopa. The pharmacist should inform patients taking levodopa of the effects of pyridoxine hydrochloride. A vitamin product that does not contain pyridoxine hydrochloride has been formulated for parkinsonian patients taking levodopa. A carbidopa and levodopa combination product is not affected by the concurrent administration of pyridoxine hydrochloride. Pyridoxine hydrochloride is available as a tablet in varying strengths and as an injectable solution (50 mg/ml and 100 mg/ml).

Cyanocobalamin (vitamin B_{12}). Cyanocobalamin is involved with folic acid in many body cell activities, and it is necessary for the incorporation of folic acid into cells. It also is involved in fat and carbohydrate metabolism as a constituent of a coenzyme system. The RDA for cyanocobalamin is 3 μg for adults; for infants and children, it ranges from 0.3 to 2 μg. More is needed by pregnant and lactating women because of the drain of cyanocobalamin by the fetus and by the production of milk. Cyanocobalamin is produced almost exclusively by microorganisms; hence, its presence in animal protein. It may also be found in the root nodules of legumes because of the presence of organisms.

Cyanocobalamin deficiency may be caused by inadequate ingestion, absorption, utilization, or increased requirement or excretion of this vitamin.[62] Vegetarian diets may need supplementation with cyanocobalamin. Because cyanocobalamin is so well conserved by the body through enterohepatic cycling, it requires decades for the deficiency to develop. In patients whose deficiency is related to malabsorption, the reabsorption phase of the enterohepatic cycle is affected, and the deficiency occurs in 3 to 6 years. In healthy individuals who have not restricted their diets, adequate cyanocobalamin levels are maintained by the body. Some people lack the glycoprotein (intrinsic factor) necessary for the absorption of cyanocobalamin, resulting in pernicious anemia.

Because cyanocobalamin is important in cell production, the signs and symptoms of a deficiency are manifested in organ systems with rapidly duplicating cells. Thus, an effect on the hematopoietic system results in anemia. The GI tract is also affected, with glossitis and epithelial changes occurring along the entire tract. Because of the importance of cyanocobalamin in the production of myelin, deficiency states cause many neurological symptoms and signs, such as paresthesia (manifested as tingling and numbness in the hands and feet), progressing to unsteadiness, poor muscular coordination, mental slowness, confusion, agitation, optic atrophy, hallucinations, and overt psychosis. Surgical removal of portions of the stomach and small intestine often result in cyanocobalamin deficiency. Regional enteritis, tropical sprue, idiopathic steatorrhea, and celiac disease impair the absorption of cyanocobalamin.

Certain drugs may cause poor absorption of cyanocobalamin. Neomycin reduces the absorption, and malabsorption is increased if colchicine is also a part of therapy.[63,64]

Treatment of cyanocobalamin deficiency did involve the administration of crude liver extracts orally and parenterally. Because crystalline cyanocobalamin is now readily available, this is the preferred form. Treatment of pernicious anemia or permanent gastric or ileal damage with cyanocobalamin is lifelong.

Cyanocobalamin is available in tablet and injectable dosage forms. Oral forms can be used if the deficiency is nutritionally based; intramuscular or subcutaneous administration is necessary for deficiencies caused by malabsorption. Hydroxycobalamin is a long-acting form equal in hematopoietic effect to cyanocobalamin. Because it is bound to blood proteins, it remains in the body for a longer period. However, this advantage is not great enough to justify the cost and pain of injecting it. There are a few OTC products that contain more than 1.5 times the RDA of cyanocobalamin. These products are no longer classified as dietary supplements but as drugs. Cyanocobalamin has no therapeutic value beyond that of correcting cyanocobalamin deficiencies, unless its placebo effect is considered. The deficiency can be corrected with 1 μg of oral cyanocobalamin daily or 100 μg given parenterally each month. Doses larger than needed do not cause toxicity because excretion through the urine occurs when tissue and plasma binding sites are saturated.

Folic acid. In its function in the body, folic acid (pteroylglutamic acid) is closely related to cyanocobalamin. Folates must be enzymatically converted before they can be absorbed and, in the body, folate coenzymes are involved in the transfer of one-carbon units in the synthesis of protein. The RDA for folic acid is 400 μg for adults and 50 to 300 μg for infants and children, depending on age. During pregnancy, 800 μg is required and during lactation, 600 μg.

The folate content of food is subject to destruction depending on how it is processed. Canning, long exposure to heat, and refining destroy 50 to 100 percent of the folates. Generally, foods richest in folates are fresh green vegetables. Yeast and liver and other organ meats also contain folates.

The requirement for folic acid is related to metabolic rate and cell turnover. Thus, increased amounts of folic acid are needed during pregnancy (especially with twin or multiple fetuses); during infections; in hemolytic anemias and blood loss where red blood cell production attempts to meet the increased need; in infancy; and in cases of increased metabolic rates such as in hyperthyroidism. Rheumatoid arthritis, perhaps because of the proliferation of synovial membranes or the possible salicylate-induced blood loss, also increases folate requirements. Certain hematopoietic malignancies also cause an increased need for folic acid.

It is fairly easy for individuals to become folate deficient, particularly if fresh vegetables and fruits are not eaten. The symptoms of deficiency are much the same as those of cyanocobalamin deficiency—sore mouth, diarrhea, and CNS symptoms such as irritability and forgetfulness. A common sign of folic acid deficiency is megaloblastic anemia.

The causes of folic acid deficiency are similar to those of B vitamin deficiencies. Nutritionally, the diet must include foods that need little cooking because folates are heat labile. Alcoholics frequently have folic acid deficiency as do individuals with malabsorption diseases. Conditions that cause rapid cell turnover may induce potentially life-threatening folic acid deficiency.

Several drugs taken chronically may increase the need for folic acid. Phenytoin and possibly other related anticonvulsants may cause an inhibition of folic acid absorption, leading to megaloblastic anemia.[65] This problem is further complicated by the fact that folic acid supplementation may decrease serum phenytoin levels, decreasing seizure control.[66] With this in mind, when dispensing folic acid to patients whose medication record indicates concurrent use of phenytoin, the pharmacist should ask if seizure activity is controlled. Another possible drug interaction occurs with oral contraceptive drugs, which may cause folic acid deficiencies.[67] This effect is extremely rare and probably is not a significant side effect.[68-70] Trimethoprim may act as a folic acid antagonist in humans. Megaloblastic anemia may be precipitated in patients who had a relatively low folate level at the onset of trimethoprim therapy; short-term therapy, however, does not lead to megaloblastic anemia. Pyrimethamine, which is related to trimethoprim, in large doses may induce megaloblastic anemia. Folinic acid may be administered to reverse the anemia because the mechanism of pyrimethamine's folic acid antagonism is inhibition of the production of active tetrahydrofolate.[71] Methotrexate also causes folic acid antagonism.

Folic acid given without cyanocobalamin to patients with pernicious anemia can correct the anemia but has no effect on the damage to the nervous system. The symptoms of the damage include incoordination, impaired sense of position, and a spectrum of mental disturbances. Because of this effect of folic acid, OTC vitamin preparations are not permitted to contain more than 0.4 mg of folic acid; vitamins for pregnant or lactating women can contain as much as 0.8 mg.[72] The inclusion of cyanocobalamin in the oral preparation is, of course, not helpful if the patient has pernicious anemia. Cyanocobalamin must be given parenterally to these patients, who must be monitored carefully.

The dose of folic acid for correction of a deficiency is usually 100 μg (0.1 mg). If the deficiency occurs with conditions that may increase the folate requirement or suppress the formation of red blood cells (e.g., pregnancy, hypermetabolic states, alcoholism, hemolytic anemia, etc.), the dose is 0.5 to 1 mg. Doses larger than 1 mg are excreted in the urine and, except in some life-threatening hematologic diseases, are not beneficial. Maintenance therapy for deficiencies can be stopped after 1 to 4 months if the diet contains at least one fresh fruit or vegetable daily.[73] For chronic malabsorption diseases, folic acid may be required for a long period, and parenteral doses are needed in severe cases. The toxicity of folic acid is nearly nonexistent because of its water solubility and water excretion—15 mg can be given daily without toxic effect.

Pantothenic acid. Pantothenic acid is a precursor to coenzyme A, a product active in many biological reactions in the body. Although its RDA has not been established, it is contained in many foods which makes it easily available. Intake of 5 to 10 mg daily of pantothenic acid satisfies the need. Pantothenic acid deficiency is very hard to detect. In malabsorption syndromes, it is difficult to separate pantothenic acid deficiency symptoms from many other ones. Pantothenic acid has been withheld experimentally, and the resulting symptoms are abdominal pain, vomiting, and cramps. Later, muscle tenderness, weakness, paresthesia, and insomnia occur. Administration of large doses of pantothenic acid reverse these symptoms.

Pantothenic acid is not known to have any therapeutic use. It frequently is incorporated into oral multiple vitamin preparations. As much as 20 g has been administered, and the toxicity is minimal, appearing as diarrhea.

Biotin. Although biotin is one of the B-complex vitamins, the RDA has not yet been established. Biotin is widely distributed in animal tissue and appears necessary for the formation of protein from amino acids. In rats, biotin also seems necessary for the appropriate utilization of glucose, and some of its effects are similar to those of insulin. In humans, biotin is synthesized by gut flora. Serum levels of biotin in normal subjects are 213 to 404 ng/ml. Biotin deficiency in humans can be caused by the ingestion of a large number of egg whites. Egg whites contain avidin, a protein that inactivates biotin; this inactivation causes a dermatitis, a grayish color of the skin, anorexia, anemia, hypercholesterolemia, and lassitude.[74] In pregnant women, biotin blood levels decrease as gestation progresses.

In rats, a combination of oxytetracycline and succinylsulfathiazole inhibited the intestinal synthesis of biotin. A similar effect might be expected in humans after using gut-sterilizing antibiotics, but it has not been reported.

Biotin has been incorporated into several multiple vitamin preparations. It has been used therapeutically in infants and children to treat seborrheic dermatitis and proprionicacidemia. There was slight improvement in muscle tone with oral doses (5 mg for 5 days).[75]

Bioflavonoids. The term "bioflavonoids" has been used to designate flavones and flavonols. Bioflavonoids were called vitamin P ("P" for permeability), but this designation is no longer used because no vitamin activity has been documented. This group of agents includes rutin and hesperidin, which have stimulated controversy in the medical literature. The controversy stems from their proposed use in the treatment of vascular bleeding disorders such as vascular purpura, retinal hemorrhages, cerebrovascular accidents, and lymphedema. Deficiency states have not been induced or discovered in humans or animals. There appears to be no clinical use for the agents. Studies involving rutin as a pharmacologic entity continue, particularly in Europe.[76,77]

Choline. Choline is a precursor of acetylcholine, which is an important donator of a methyl group used in the formation of other substances. It may be formed from methionine by the donation of a methyl group from the methionine. Choline is a component of several phospholipids. No choline deficiency disease in humans has been reported. Rats, hamsters, dogs, chickens, and pigs develop choline deficiency diseases including fatty liver, cirrhosis, anemia, renal lesions, and hypertension. These findings have been the basis for treating alcoholics with choline, although the literature reports no therapeutic value. Although choline is found in egg yolks, cereal, fish, and meat, it is also synthesized in the body; therefore, it is doubtful that it is a vitamin. Choline is available as a tablet, powder, syrup, and in combination with other nutritional ingredients. Its stated use is the decrease of fatty liver.

Inositol. Inositol is a sugar found in large amounts in muscle and brain tissues. It is widely distributed in nature and is synthesized in the body, but its biologic value and metabolism are unknown. In cell culture, inositol appears necessary for amino acid transport and for the movement of potassium and sodium. As a sugar, it is approximately one-third as effective as glucose in correcting diabetic ketosis. Inositol is available as a tablet, powder, and syrup. Its value in human nutrition has not been documented.

References

1. Editorial, *Chem. Eng. News,* **51,** 9(1973).
2. B. Wolnak, *Food Drug Cosmet. Law J.,* **27,** 453(1972).
3. D. Coldsmith, *Mod. Med.,* **43,** 121(1975).
4. *A Study of Health Practices and Opinions.* Final Report. Conducted for FDA, HEW. Contract Number FDA 66-193, June 1972, and FDA Talk Paper, October 6, 1972.
5. Editorial, *Nutr. Rev., Suppl.,* **32,** 53(1974).
6. A. Kamil, *J. Nutr.,* **4,** 92(1972).
7. R. M. Kark, *J. Am. Diet Assoc.,* **64,** 476 (1974).
8. R. R. Crichton, *N. Engl. J. Med.,* **284,** 1413(1971).
9. T. H. Bothwell and C. A. Finch, "Iron Metabolism," Little, Brown, Boston, Mass., 1962.
10. Committee on Iron Deficiency, *J. Am. Med. Assoc.,* **203,** 407(1968).
11. L. Hallberg *et al.,* "Iron Deficiency Pathogenesis, Clinical Aspects, Therapy," Academic Press, New York, N.Y., p. 169.
12. V. Minnich *et al., Am. J. Clin. Nutr.,* **21,** 78(1968).
13. W. H. Crosby, *J. Am. Med. Assoc.,* **235,** 2765(1976).
14. H. Brise and L. Hallberg, *Acta Med. Scand., Suppl.* **376,** 23(1962).
15. C. V. Moore, in "Modern Nutrition in Health and Disease: Dietotherapy," 5th rev., R. S. Goodheart and M. E. Shils, Eds., Lea and Febiger, Philadelphia, Pa., 1973, p. 316.
16. D. N. S. Kerr and L. S. P. Davidson, *Lancet,* **2,** 489(1958).
17. G. J. L. Hall and A. E. Davis, *Med. J. Aust.,* **2,** 95(1969).
18. P. J. Neuvonen *et al., Br. Med. J.,* **4,** 532(1970).
19. M. N. Gleason *et al.,* "Clinical Toxicology of Commercial Products," 3d ed., Williams and Wilkins, Baltimore, Md., 1969, p. 108.
20. S. Margen and D. H. Calloway, *Fed. Proc.,* **26,** 629(1967).
21. R. M. Walker and H. M. Linkswiler, *J. Nutr.,* **102,** 1297(1972).
22. C. F. Mills, "Trace Element Metabolism in Animals," Livingstone, Edinburgh, Scotland, 1970, p. 75.
23. H. H. Sandstead, *Am. J. Clin. Nutr.,* **26,** 1251(1973).
24. R. W. Vilter, *N. Engl. J. Med.,* **291,** 188(1974).
25. M. F. Ivey *et al., Am. J. Hosp. Pharm.,* **32,** 1032(1975).
26. W. Mertz, *J. Am. Diet Assoc.,* **64,** 163(1974).
27. T. Moore, "Vitamin A," Elsevier, Amsterdam, The Netherlands, 1957, p. 355.
28. J. Bieri, *J. Am. Diet Assoc.,* **64,** 171(1974).
29. National Academy of Sciences National Research Council, Food and Nutrition Board, *Recommended Dietary Allowances,* Publ. 1694, 7th ed., Washington, D. C., 1968.
30. "Modern Nutrition in Health and Disease: Dietotherapy," 5th rev., R. S. Goodheart and M. E. Shils, Eds., Lea and Febiger, Philadelphia, Pa., 1973, p. 152.
31. "Harrison's Principles of Internal Medicine," M. M. Wintrobe *et al.,* Eds., McGraw-Hill, New York, N.Y., 1974, p. 439.
32. J. Myrtle and A. Norman, *Science,* **171,** 79(1971).
33. S. Fomon *et al., J. Nutr.,* **89,** 345(1966).
34. D. Fraser and R. Slater, *Pediatr. Clin. North Am.,* **May, 1958,** p. 417.
35. J. Ritchie *et al., N. Engl. J. Med.,* **279,** 1185(1968).
36. M. Horwitt, *Am. J. Clin. Nutr.,* **8,** 451(1960).
37. J. T. B. Williams *et al., Surg. Gynecol. Obstet.,* **662,** 132(1971).
38. T. W. Anderson, *Can. Med. Assoc. J.,* **10,** 40(1974).
39. L. A. Barness *et al., Am. J. Clin. Nutr.,* **21,** 40(1968).
40. "Modern Nutrition in Health and Disease: Dietotherapy," 5th rev., R. S. Goodheart and M. E. Shils, Eds., Lea and Febiger, Philadelphia, Pa., 1973, p. 253.
41. L. Pauling, *Proc. Nat. Acad. Sci. (U.S.A.),* **67,** 1643(1970).
42. L. Pauling, *Am. J. Clin. Nutr.,* **24,** 1294(1971).
43. M. Dykes and P. Meier, *J. Am. Med. Assoc.,* **231,** 1073(1973).
44. T. Anderson *et al., Can. Med. Assoc. J.,* **107,** 503(1972).
45. T. Anderson *et al., Can. Med. Assoc. J.,* **111,** 31(1974).
46. M. Briggs *et al., Lancet,* **2,** 201(1973).
47. E. Samborskaja and T. Ferdman, *Nutr. Abstr. Rev.,* **37,** 73(1967).
48. G. A. Goldsmith, *J. Am. Med. Assoc.,* **216,** 337(1971).
49. W. A. Cochrane, *Can. Med. Assoc. J.,* **93,** 893(1965).
50. G. Levy and J. Leonards, *J. Am. Med. Assoc.,* **217,** 81(1971).
51. F. Sjoquist, *Clin. Pharmacol. Ther.,* **10,** 826(1969).
52. L. Gram *et al., Clin. Pharmacol. Ther.,* **12,** 239(1971).
53. M. Rowland, *J. Pharm. Sci.,* **58,** 508(1969).
54. J. Feldman *et al., Diabetes,* **19,** 337(1970).
55. J. Mayson *et al., Am. J. Clin. Pathol.,* **58,** 297(1972).
56. Apharmacy Weekly, **14(34),** 2(1975).
57. T. Ban, *Can. Psychiatr. Assoc. J.,* **16,** 413(1971).
58. M. Baumblatt and F. Winston, *Lancet,* **1,** 832(1970).
59. A. Lubby *et al., Lancet,* **2,** 1083(1970).
60. A. Lubby *et al., Am. J. Clin. Nutr.,* **24,** 684(1971).
61. T. Necheles and L. Snyder, *N. Engl. J. Med.,* **282,** 858(1970).
62. "Modern Nutrition in Health and Disease: Dietotherapy," 5th rev., R. S. Goodheart and M. E. Shils, Eds., Lea and Febiger, Philadelphia, Pa., 1973, p. 225.
63. W. Faloon and R. Chodos, *Gastroenterology,* **56,** 1251(1969).
64. E. Jacobson *et al., Am. J. Med.,* **28,** 524(1960).
65. C. Gerson, *Gastroenterology,* **63,** 246(1972).
66. H. Kutt *et al., Arch. Neurol. (Chicago),* **14,** 489(1966).
67. T. Necheles and L. Snyder, *N. Engl. J. Med.,* **282,** 858(1970).
68. N. Elgee, *Ann. Intern. Med.,* **72,** 409(1970).
69. R. Swerdloff *et al., West. J. Med.,* **122,** 22(1975).
70. A. Bingel and P. Benoit, *J. Pharm. Sci.,* **62(2),** 179(1973).
71. "The Pharmacological Basis of Therapeutics," 5th ed., L. S. Goodman and A. Gilman, Eds., Macmillan, New York, N.Y., 1975, p. 1058.
72. *Fed. Regist.,* **41(203),** 46172(1976).
73. "Modern Nutrition in Health and Disease: Dietotherapy," 5th rev., R. S. Goodheart and M. E. Shils, Eds., Lea and Febiger, Philadelphia, Pa., 1973, p. 242.
74. V. Sydenstricker *et al., J. Am. Med. Assoc.,* **118,** 1199(1942).
75. N. Barnes *et al., Lancet,* **2,** 244(1970).
76. E. Földi-Börcsok and M. Földi, *Am. J. Clin. Nutr.,* **26,** 185(1973).
77. R. Eastham *et al., Br. Med. J.,* **4,** 491(1972).

Products 11 MULTIPLE VITAMIN

Product * (manufacturer)	Vitamin A, IU	Vitamin D, IU	Vitamin E, IU	Ascorbic acid (C), mg	Thiamine (B_1), mg	Riboflavin (B_2), mg	Niacin
Abdec Baby Drops [a] (Parke-Davis)	5,000 [b]	400	—	50	1.0 [c]	1.2	10 [d]
Abdec Kapseals (Parke-Davis)	10,000	400	5	75	5.0 [f]	3.0	25 [d]
Abdol c Minerals (Parke-Davis)	5,000 [b]	400	—	50	2.5 [f]	2.5	20 [d]
Abdol c Vitamin C (Parke-Davis)	5,000	400	—	50	2.5 [f]	2.5	20 [d]
A.C.N. (Person & Covey)	25,000 [b]	—	—	250	—	—	25 [d]
Adabee (Robins)	10,000	—	—	250 [e]	15.0 [f]	10.0	50 [d]
Adabee c Minerals (Robins)	10,000	—	—	250 [e]	15.0 [f]	10.0	50 [d]
ADC Drops [a] (Parke-Davis)	5,000 [b]	400	—	50	—	—	—
Allbee-T (Robins)	—	—	—	500	15.0 [f]	10.0	100
Allbee with C (Robins)	—	—	—	300	15.0 [f]	10.0	50 [d]
Aprisac (North American)	—	—	5	—	—	—	—
AVP Natal (A.V.P.)	5,000	—	—	100	—	—	—
B-C-Bid Capsules (Geriatric Pharm)	—	—	—	300	15.0 [f]	10.0	50 [d]
B-Complex Capsules (North American)	—	—	—	—	1.5 [c]	2.0	10 [d]
B Complex Tablets (Squibb)	—	—	—	—	0.64	0.66	8.1
B Complex with Vitamin C (Squibb)	—	—	—	300	10.0	10.0	100
Beta-Vite Liquid [n] (North American)	—	—	—	—	10.0 [c]	—	—
Beta-Vite w/Iron Liquid [n] (North American)	—	—	—	—	10.0 [c]	—	—
Bewon Elixir [n] (Wyeth)	—	—	—	—	0.25 [c]	—	—
B Nutron (Nion)	—	—	—	—	2.0	3.0	10 [d]
Brewers Yeast (North American)	—	—	—	—	0.06	0.02	0.15
Calcicaps (Nion)	—	400	—	—	—	—	—
Calcicaps with Iron (Nion)	—	400	—	—	—	—	—
Calcidin (Abbott)	—	—	—	—	—	—	—
Calcium, Phosphate, and Vitamin D (Squibb)	—	180	—	—	—	—	—
Calciwafers (Nion)	—	—	66.7	—	—	—	—
Cal-Prenal (North American)	4,000 [q]	400	—	50	2.0 [c]	2.0	10 [d]
C-B Vone Capsules (USV)	—	—	—	250	15.0 [f]	10.0	75 [d]
Cebēfortis (Upjohn)	—	—	—	150	5.0 [f]	5.0	50 [d]
Cebētinic (Upjohn)	—	—	—	25	2.0 [f]	2.0	10 [d]
Cecon Solution [a] (Abbott)	—	—	—	60	—	—	—
Cevi-Bid (Geriatric Pharm)	—	—	—	500	—	—	—
Ce-Vi-Sol Drops [a] (Mead Johnson)	—	—	—	35	—	—	—
Cherri-B Liquid [a] (North American)	—	—	—	—	1.5 [c]	0.3	6 [d]
Chew-E (North American)	—	—	200	—	—	—	—

Cyanocobalamin (B_{12}), μg	Folic acid, μg	Pantothenic acid, mg	Iron, mg	Calcium, mg	Phosphorus, mg	Magnesium, mg	Other
—	—	5.0 [e]	—	—	—	—	—
2.0 [g]	—	5.0	—	—	—	—	—
1.0 [g]	100	2.5 [i]	15 [j]	44 [k]	34 [k]	1.0 [j]	potassium, 5.0 mg [j] manganese, 1.0 mg [j] zinc, 0.5 mg [j] others [z]
1.0 [g]	—	5.0 [i]	—	—	—	—	—
—	—	—	—	—	—	—	hesperidin, 50 mg
—	—	—	—	—	—	—	—
—	—	—	15	103	80	—	—
—	—	—	—	—	—	—	—
5.0	—	25.0 [i]	—	—	—	—	desiccated liver, 150 mg
—	—	10.0 [i]	—	—	—	—	—
—	—	—	75 [o]	58 [k]	45 [k]	—	manganese, 2.5 mg [j] zinc, 0.1 mg [j] copper, 0.1 mg [j]
—	—	—	66 [m]	—	—	—	purified veal bone ash, 500 mg
5.0	—	—	—	—	—	—	—
—	—	1.0 [i]	—	—	—	—	dried yeast, 100 mg desiccated liver, 70 mg
1.0	—	—	—	—	—	—	—
4.0	—	20.0 [i]	—	—	—	—	—
25.0	—	—	—	—	—	—	—
25.0	—	—	75 [o]	—	—	—	—
—	—	—	—	—	—	—	—
1.0 [g]	20	0.2 [i]	8 [p]	—	—	—	brewers yeast, 150 mg manganese sodium citrate, 16 mg
—	—	0.05	—	—	—	—	—
—	—	—	—	750	360	—	—
—	—	—	46 [p]	750	360	—	—
—	—	—	—	—	—	—	iodine and calcium iodate, 60, 150, and 300 mg lime
—	—	—	—	192	96	—	—
—	—	—	—	171.1 [k] 35.3 [p]	136.7 [k]	—	—
2.0 [r]	100	—	50 [m]	230	—	—	iodine, 150 μg [l]
5.0	—	7.5 [h]	—	—	—	—	choline bitartrate, 52 mg desiccated liver, 50 mg
2.0	—	10.0 [i]	—	—	—	—	—
5.0	—	—	38 [p]	—	—	—	—
—	—	—	—	—	—	—	—
—	—	—	—	—	—	—	—
—	—	—	—	—	—	—	alcohol, 5%
—	—	0.12 [h]	—	—	—	—	—
—	—	—	—	—	—	—	—

Product * (manufacturer)	Vitamin A, IU	Vitamin D, IU	Vitamin E, IU	Ascorbic acid (C), mg	Thiamine (B_1), mg	Riboflavin (B_2), mg	Niacin, mg
Chew-Vite (North American)	5,000	400	—	50	3.0	2.5	20 [d]
Chocks (Miles)	5,000	400	15	60	1.5	1.7	20
Chocks-Bugs Bunny (Miles)	5,000	400	15	60	1.5	1.7	20
Chocks-Bugs Bunny Plus Iron (Miles)	5,000	400	15	60	1.5	1.7	20
Chocks Plus Iron (Miles)	5,000	400	15	60	1.5	1.7	20
Cod Liver Oil Concentrate Capsules (Schering)	10,000	400	—	—	—	—	—
Cod Liver Oil Concentrate Tablets (Schering)	4,000	200	—	—	—	—	—
Cod Liver Oil Tablets with Vitamin C (Schering)	4,000	200	—	50	—	—	—
Combex Kapseals (Parke-Davis)	—	—	—	—	10.0 [f]	10.0	10 [d]
Combex Kapseals c Vitamin C (Parke-Davis)	—	—	—	50	10.0 [f]	10.0	10 [d]
Dayalets (Abbott)	5,000	400	30	60	1.5 [c]	1.7	20 [d]
Dayalets plus Iron (Abbott)	5,000	400	30	60	1.5 [c]	1.7	20 [d]
De-Cal (North American)	—	125	—	—	—	—	—
Di-Calcium Phosphate Capsules (North American)	—	333	—	—	—	—	—
Dical-D (Abbott)	—	132 200	—	—	—	—	—
Dical-D with Vitamin C Capsules (Abbott)	—	132	—	15	—	—	—
Duo-CVP Capsules (USV)	—	—	—	—	—	—	—
Dura-C 500 Graduals (Amfre-Grant)	—	—	—	500	—	—	—
Engran-HP (Squibb)	8,000	400	30	60	1.7	2.0	20
Epsilan-M (Warren-Teed)	—	—	100	—	—	—	—
Feminaid (Nion)	5,000	400	10	200	2.0	3.0	15 [d]
Feminins (Mead Johnson)	5,000	400	10	200	1.5 [c]	3.0	15
Femiron with Vitamins (J. B. Williams)	5,000	400	—	60	1.5	1.7	20 [d]
Ferritrinsic (Upjohn)	—	—	—	50	2.0 [f]	2.0	10 [d]
Ferrolip Plus (Flint)	—	—	—	50	2.5 [f]	1.0	5 [d]
Filibon Capsules (Lederle)	4,000 [q]	400	—	50 [i]	3.0	2.0	10 [d]
Filibon OT Tablets (Lederle)	4,000 [q]	400	—	50 [i]	3.0	2.0	10 [d]
Flintstones (Miles)	5,000	400	15	60	1.5	1.7	20
Flintstones Plus Iron (Miles)	5,000	400	15	60	1.5	1.7	20
Ganatrex [a] (Merrell-National)	5,000 [b]	400	30	60	1.5 [c]	1.7	20 [d]
Geralix Liquid [y] (North American)	—	—	—	—	3.3 [c]	1.7	—
Geriamic (North American)	—	—	—	75	15.0 [c]	5.0	30 [d]
Gerilets (Abbott)	5,000	400	45	90 [e]	2.25 [c]	2.6	30 [d]

oxine chloride mg	Cyanocobalamin (B_{12}), µg	Folic acid, µg	Pantothenic acid, mg	Iron, mg	Calcium, mg	Phosphorus, mg	Magnesium, mg	Other
	1.0 [r]	—	—	—	—	—	—	—
	6.0	400	—	—	—	—	—	—
	6.0	400	—	—	—	—	—	—
	6.0	400	—	18	—	—	—	—
	6.0	400	—	18	—	—	—	—
	—	—	—	—	—	—	—	—
	—	—	—	—	—	—	—	—
	—	—	—	—	—	—	—	—
	1.0 [g]	—	6.0 [h]	—	—	—	—	liver concentrate, 380 mg
	1.0 [g]	—	6.0 [h]	—	—	—	—	liver concentrate, 340 mg
	6.0	400	—	—	—	—	—	—
	6.0	400	—	18	—	—	—	—
	—	—	—	—	250	—	—	—
	—	—	—	—	75 [k] 14 [p]	58 [k]	—	—
	—	—	—	—	147 [k] 295 [k]	114 [k] 228 [k]	—	—
	—	—	—	—	147 [k]	114 [k]	—	—
	—	—	—	—	—	—	—	citrus bioflavonoid compound, 200 mg
	—	—	—		—	—	—	—
	8.0	800	—	18	650	—	100	iodine, 150 µg
	—	—	—	—	—	—	—	—
	10.0	100	10.0	18	126	—	—	zinc, 10.0 mg potassium, 10.0 mg
	10.0	100	10.0	18	—	—	—	zinc, 10.0 mg
	5.0	100	10.0 [i]	20 [m]	—	—	—	—
	—	33	—	60 [j]	—	—	—	intrinase, ⅓ NF XI unit desiccated liver, 100 mg
	10.0	—	—	28 [s]	—	—	—	—
	2.0	—	—	30 [m]	230 [t]	—	0.15 [u]	potassium, 0.835 mg [j] manganese, 0.05 mg [u] iodine, 10 µg [l] others [z]
	2.0	—	—	30 [m]	230 [t]	—	0.15 [u]	potassium, 0.835 mg [j] dioctyl sodium sulfosuccinate, 100 mg iodine, 10 µg [l] others [z]
	6.0	400	—	—	—	—	—	—
	6.0	400	—	18	—	—	—	—
	6.0	—	—	—	—	—	—	alcohol, 15% invert sugar
	—	—	—	—	33 [w]	—	0.33	alcohol, 15% choline bitartrate, 100 mg inositol, 100 mg others [z]
	3.0	—	2.0 [i]	50	—	—	—	brewers yeast, 50 mg choline bitartrate, 25 mg methionine, 25 mg inositol, 20 mg
	9.0	400	—	27	—	—	—	biotin, 0.45 mg

Product * (manufacturer)	Vitamin A, IU	Vitamin D, IU	Vitamin E, IU	Ascorbic acid (C), mg	Thiamine (B_1), mg	Riboflavin (B_2), mg	Niacin, mg
Geriplex (Parke-Davis)	5,000 [q]	—	5	50 [e]	5.0 [f]	5.0	15 [d]
Geriplex-FS Kapseals (Parke-Davis)	5,000 [q]	—	5	50 [e]	5.0 [f]	5.0	15 [d]
Geriplex-FS Liquid [x] (Parke-Davis)	—	—	—	—	1.2 [c]	1.7 [k]	15 [d]
Geritinic (Geriatric Pharmaceutical)	—	—	—	—	1.0 [c]	1.0	10 [d]
Geritol Junior Liquid [n] (J. B. Williams)	8,000 [b]	400	—	—	5.0	5.0	100 [d]
Geritol Junior Tablets (J. B. Williams)	5,000	100	—	30	2.5	2.5	20 [d]
Geritol Liquid [n] (J. B. Williams)	—	—	—	—	5.0	5.0	100 [d]
Geritol Tablets (J. B. Williams)	—	—	—	75	5.0	5.0	30 [d]
Gerix Elixir [x] (Abbott)	—	—	—	—	6.0 [c]	6.0	200 [d]
Gerizyme [y] (Upjohn)	—	—	—	—	3.3 [c]	3.3	33.3 [d]
Gevrabon [x] (Lederle)	—	—	—	—	5.0	2.5	50 [d]
Gevral T Capsules (Lederle)	10,000 [q]	400	5	150	10	10	100 [d]
Gevrite (Lederle)	5,000 [b]	—	—	75	1.3	1.8	18 [d]
Golden Bounty B Complex with Vitamin C (Squibb)	—	—	—	100	4.0	4.8	4.67
Golden Bounty Multivitamin Supplement with Iron (Squibb)	5,000	400	30	60	1.5	1.7	20
Hi-Bee W/C Capsules (North American)	—	—	—	300	15.0 [f]	10.0	50 [d]
Iberet (Abbott)	—	—	—	150 [e]	6.0 [c]	6.0	30 [d]
Iberet-500 (Abbott)	—	—	—	500 [e]	6.0 [c]	6.0	30 [d]
Iberet Oral Solution [n] (Abbott)	—	—	—	37.5	1.5 [c]	1.5	7.5 [d]
Iberet-500 Oral Solution [n] (Abbott)	—	—	—	75	0.9 [c]	0.9	4.5 [d]
Iberol (Abbott)	—	—	—	75 [e]	3.0 [c]	3.0	15 [d]
Incremin with Iron Syrup [n] (Lederle)	—	—	—	—	10.0 [c]	—	—
K-Forte Potassium Supplement with Vitamin C Chewable (O'Connor)	—	—	—	10	—	—	—
Lederplex Capsules (Lederle)	—	—	—	—	2.0	2.0	10 [d]
Lederplex Liquid [n] (Lederle)	—	—	—	—	2.5	2.5	12.5 [d]

xine chloride ng	Cyanocobalamin (B_{12}), μg	Folic acid, μg	Pantothenic acid, mg	Iron, mg	Calcium, mg	Phosphorus, mg	Magnesium, mg	Other
	2.0 [g]	—	—	30 [j]	59 [k]	46 [k]	—	aspergillus oryzae enzymes, 162.5 mg choline dihydrogen citrate, 20 mg others [z]
	2.0 [g]	—	—	30 [j]	59 [k]	46 [k]	—	aspergillus oryzae enzymes, 162.5 mg dioctyl sodium sulfosuccinate, 100 mg others [z]
	5.0 [g]	—	—	15 [v]	—	—	—	poloxamer 188, 200 mg alcohol, 18%
	3.0	—	—	35 [v]	10 [w]	8 [w]	1.0 [j]	yeast concentrate, 125 mg potassium, 1.0 mg [j] iodine, 20 μg [l] others [z]
	3.0	—	4.0 [h]	15 [v]	—	—	—	—
	2.5	—	2.0 [i]	25 [j]	—	—	—	—
	3.0	—	4.0 [h]	15 [v]	—	—	—	methionine, 100 mg choline bitartrate, 100 mg
	3.0	—	2.0 [i]	10 [j]	—	—	—	—
	6.0	—	—	15	—	—	—	choline, 200 mg inositol, 200 mg betaine hydrochloride, 100 mg
	3.3	—	3.3 [h]	5 [p]	100 [w]	—	3.5 [j]	inositol, 100 mg potassium, 10.0 mg [j] alcohol, 18% others [z]
	1.0	—	10.0	20	—	—	2.0	potassium, 10 mg alcohol, 18% iodine, 100 μg [l] others [z]
	5.0	—	5.0 [i]	15 [m]	107 [k]	82 [k]	6.0 [u]	potassium, 5.0 mg [j] zinc, 1.5 mg [u] iodine, 150 μg [l] others [z]
	—	—	—	10 [m]	230 [t]	—	—	dioctyl sodium sulfosuccinate, 100 mg
	25.0 [r]	—	—	—	—	—	—	—
	6.0	400	—	18	—	—	—	—
	—	—	10.0 [i]	—	—	—	—	—
	25.0	—	10.0 [i]	105	—	—	—	—
	25.0	—	10.0 [i]	105	—	—	—	—
	6.25	—	2.5 [h]	26	—	—	—	—
	3.8	—	1.5 [h]	16	—	—	—	—
	12.5	—	3.0 [i]	105	—	—	—	—
	25.0	—	—	30 [o]	—	—	—	sorbitol, 3.5 g lysine monohydrochloride, 300 mg
	—	—	—	—	—	—	—	potassium, 39 mg[p] (also citrate and chloride)
	1.0	3.0 [i]	—	—	—	—	—	liver fraction and desiccated liver, 340 mg choline, 20 mg inositol, 10 mg
	6.25	—	2.5 [h]	—	—	—	—	liver fraction and desiccated liver, 590 mg choline, 25 mg inositol, 5 mg

Product * (manufacturer)	Vitamin A, IU	Vitamin D, IU	Vitamin E, IU	Ascorbic acid (C), mg	Thiamine (B_1), mg	Riboflavin (B_2), mg	Niacin, m
Lederplex Tablets (Lederle)	—	—	—	—	2.0	2.0	10 [d]
Lipoflavonoid Capsules (Smith, Miller & Patch)	—	—	—	100	0.33 [c]	0.33	3.33 [d]
Lipotriad Capsules (Smith, Miller & Patch)	—	—	—	—	0.33 [c]	0.33	3.33 [d]
Lipotriad Liquid [n] (Smith, Miller & Patch)	—	—	—	—	1.0 [c]	1.0	10 [d]
Liquid Geritonic [n] (Geriatric Pharmaceutical)	5,000	400	—	60	3.0 [f]	3.0	10 [d]
Livitamin Capsules (Beecham Labs)	—	—	—	100	3.0 [f]	3.0	10 [d]
Livitamin Chewable (Beecham Labs)	—	—	—	100 [i]	3.0 [f]	3.0	10 [d]
Livitamin Liquid [y] (Beecham Labs)	—	—	—	—	3.0 [c]	3.0	10 [d]
Lofenalac (Mead Johnson)	1,600	400	10	52	0.5	0.6	8.0
Lufa Capsules (USV)	—	—	8	—	2.0 [f]	2.0	5.0 [d]
Methisdrol Capsules (USV)	—	—	—	—	3.0 [f]	3.0	10 [d]
Mol-Iron Panhemic Chronosules (Schering)	—	—	—	150	6.0 [f]	6.0	30 [d]
Monster Vitamins (Bristol-Myers)	3,500	400	—	60	0.8	1.3	14 [d]
Monster Vitamins & Iron (Bristol-Myers)	3,500	400	—	60	0.8	1.3	14 [d]
Mucoplex (Stuart)	—	—	—	—	—	1.5	—
Multicebrin (Lilly)	5,000	500	2.5	56	1.5 [c]	2.0	6
Multiple Vitamins (North American)	5,000	400	—	50	3.0 [f]	2.5	20 [d]
Multiple Vitamins with Iron (North American)	5,000	400	—	50	2.0 [f]	2.5	20 [d]
Multivitamin Supplement with Iron (Fisons)	5,000 [b]	—	30	60 [e]	1.5 [f]	1.7	20 [d]
Mulvidren Softabs (Stuart)	4,000	400	—	25 56 [e]	2.0 [f]	2.0	10 [d]
M.V.M. Liquid (Amfre-Grant)	10,000	400	4.5	150	6.0 [c]	3.0	60 [d]
Myadec Tablets and Capsules (Parke-Davis)	10,000	400	30	250	10.0 [f]	10.0	100 [d]
Nap Tabs (North American)	—	—	—	150	5.0 [c]	5.0	50 [d]
Natabec (Parke-Davis)	4,000 [q]	400	—	50	3.0 [f]	2.0	10 [d]
Natabec F.A. (Parke-Davis)	4,000 [q]	400	—	50	3.0 [f]	2.0	10 [d]
Natalins Tablets (Mead Johnson)	8,000	400	30	90	1.7	2.0	20
Natural Grapefruit Extract with Vitamins C and E Chewable (O'Connor)	—	—	30	60	—	—	—

doxine rochloride , mg	Cyanocobalamin (B_{12}), µg	Folic acid, µg	Pantothenic acid, mg	Iron, mg	Calcium, mg	Phosphorus, mg	Magnesium, mg	Other
	1.0	—	3.0 [i]	—	—	—	—	liver fraction and desiccated liver, 250 mg choline, 50 mg inositol, 25 mg
3	1.67	—	0.33 [i]	—	—	—	—	choline bitartrate, 233 mg lemon–bioflavonoid complex, 100 mg
3	1.67	—	0.33 [i]	—	—	—	—	choline bitartrate, 233.3 mg
	5.0	—	1.0 [i]	—	—	—	—	sugar free
	5.0	—	1.0 [i]	63 [j]	—	—	—	aminoacetic acid, 30 mg potassium, 30 mg [q] choline bitartrate, 30 mg others [z]
	5.0	—	2.0 [i]	33 [m]	—	—	—	desiccated liver, 150 mg copper, 0.66 mg [j]
	5.0	—	2.0 [i]	17 [m]	—	—	—	copper, 0.33 mg [u]
	5.0	—	2.0 [h]	36	—	—	—	liver fraction 1, 500 mg copper, 0.66 mg [j]
	2.0	100	3.0	12	600	450	70	potassium, 650 mg zinc, 4.0 mg iodine, 45 µg others [z]
	2.0	—	—	—	—	—	—	unsaturated fatty acids, 423 mg choline bitartrate, 233 mg desiccated liver, 87 mg methionine, 66 mg
	2.0 [r]	—	2.0 [h]	—	—	—	—	choline bitartrate, 240 mg methionine, 110 mg inositol, 83 mg others [z]
	25.0	—	—	390 [j]	—	—	—	—
	2.5	50	5.0	—	—	—	—	—
	2.5	50	5.0	12 [m]	—	—	—	—
	5.0	—	—	—	—	—	—	liver fraction A, 375 mg liver fraction 2, 375 mg
	1.8	—	—	—	—	—	—	—
	1.0	—	1.0 [i]	—	—	—	—	—
	1.0	—	1.0	15 [m]	—	—	—	—
	6.0	400	—	18 [m]	—	—	—	—
	3.0	—	3.0 [i]	—	—	—	—	saccharin calcium, 1.6 mg
	—	—	6.0 [i]	—	38	29	6.0	potassium, 5.0 mg manganese, 1.0 mg
	5.0 [g]	—	—	20 [j]	—	—	25 [j]	copper, 2.0 mg [j] zinc, 1.5 mg [j] manganese, 1.0 mg [j] iodine, 150 µg [l]
	12.5 [r]	—	25.0 [r]	30 [m]	—	—	—	choline bitartrate, 50 mg inositol, 50 mg aminobenzoic acid, 15 mg biotin, 12.5 µg
	5.0 [g]	—	—	55 [j]	600 [t]	—	—	—
	5.0 [g]	100	—	55 [j]	600 [t]	—	—	—
	8.0	800	—	45	200	—	100	iodine, 150 µg
	—	—	—	—	—	—	—	natural grapefruit extract, 100 mg

Product * (manufacturer)	Vitamin A, IU	Vitamin D, IU	Vitamin E, IU	Ascorbic acid (C), mg	Thiamine (B_1), mg	Riboflavin (B_2), mg	Niacin, mg
Natural Theratab (North American)	10,000 [b]	400	25	150	25.0 [c]	25.0	100 [d]
Neo-Calglucon [n] (Dorsey)	—	—	—	—	—	—	—
Neofol B-12 (Nion)	—	—	—	—	—	—	—
Norimex Capsules (North American)	—	—	—	—	0.183 [f]	0.170	0.895 [d]
Norimex-Plus Capsules (North American)	3,333	133	—	25	1.67 [f]	0.83	6.67 [d]
Obron-6 (Pfipharmecs)	5,000	400	—	50	3.09	2.0	20
One-A-Day (Miles)	5,000	400	15	60	1.5	1.7	20
One-A-Day Plus Iron (Miles)	5,000	400	15	60	1.5	1.7	20
One-A-Day Vitamins Plus Minerals (Miles)	5,000	400	15	50	1.5	1.7	20
Optilets-500 (Abbott)	10,000	400	30	500 [e]	15.0 [c]	10.0	100 [d]
Optilets-M-500 (Abbott)	10,000	400	30	500 [e]	15.0 [c]	10.0	100 [d]
Orexin Softabs (Stuart)	—	—	—	—	10.0 [f]	—	—
Ostrex Tonic Tablets (Commerce)	—	—	—	—	5.0 [c]	—	—
Paladac [n] (Parke-Davis)	5,000	400	—	50	3.0 [c]	3.0 [k]	20 [d]
Paladac c Minerals (Parke-Davis)	4,000 [q]	400	10	50 [e]	3.0 [f]	3.0	20 [d]
Peritinic (Lederle)	—	—	—	200	7.5	7.5	30 [d]
Poly-Vi-Sol (Mead Johnson)	2,500	400	15	60	1.05	1.2	13.5
Poly-Vi-Sol with Iron (Mead Johnson)	2,500	400	15	60	1.05	1.2	13.5
Probec (Stuart)	—	—	—	250	15.0 [f]	10.0	50 [d]
Probec-T (Stuart)	—	—	—	600	15.0 [f]	10.0	100 [d]
Ray-D (Nion)	—	400	—	—	1.0 [f]	2.0	10
Roeribec (Pfipharmecs)	—	—	—	500	10.0	10.0	100 [d]
Simron Plus (Merrell-National)	—	—	—	50	—	—	—
Spancap C Capsules (North American)	—	—	—	500	—	—	—
S.S.S. Tonic [y] (S.S.S.)	—	—	—	—	1.7	0.8	0.7 [d]
Stresscaps Capsules (Lederle)	—	—	—	300	10.0	10.0	100 [d]
Stresstabs 600 (Lederle)	—	—	30	600	15.0	15.0	100 [d]
Stuart Formula (Stuart)	5,000 [b]	400	15	60	1.5 [f]	1.7	20 [d]
Stuart Formula Liquid [n] (Stuart)	3,333 [b]	333	0.1	—	1.33 [c]	1.33	10 [d]
Stuart Hematinic (Stuart)	—	—	—	25	1.7 [f]	1.7	25 [d]
Stuart Hematinic Liquid [n] (Stuart)	—	—	—	—	1.7 [c]	1.7	10 [d]

...oxine ...chloride ...mg	Cyanocobalamin (B_{12}), µg	Folic acid, µg	Pantothenic acid, mg	Iron, mg	Calcium, mg	Phosphorus, mg	Magnesium, mg	Other
	100.0	100	50.0 [i]	50 [p]	—	—	7.2 [p]	inositol, 250 mg choline bitartrate, 150 mg zinc, 0.18 mg others [z]
	—	—	—	—	115	—	—	formic acid, 19.0 mg butylparaben, 0.6 mg
	10.0 [r]	100	—	—	—	—	—	brewers yeast
...0	—	—	—	—	—	—	—	dried yeast, 368 mg lysine monohydrochloride, 15.6 mg desiccated liver, 5.0 mg
...7	—	—	—	3	29	22	—	protein hydrolysate, 215 mg choline, 100 mg inositol, 20 mg others [z]
	2.0	—	0.92	35	—	—	15	potassium, 1.7 mg zinc, 0.4 mg manganese, 0.33 mg
	6.0	400	—	—	—	—	—	—
	6.0	400	—	18	—	—	—	—
	6.0	400	10.0	18	100	100	100	zinc, 15 mg copper, 2.0 mg iodine, 150 µg
	12.0	—	20.0 [i]	—	—	—	—	—
	12.0	—	20.0 [i]	20	—	—	80	copper, 2.0 mg zinc, 1.5 mg manganese, 1 mg iodine, 150 µg
	25.0	—	—	—	—	—	—	saccharin calcium, 0.3 mg
	—	—	—	84 [j]	750	375	—	copper, 0.061 mg
	5.0 [g]	—	5.0 [e]	—	—	—	—	—
	5.0 [g]	—	5.0 [i]	5 [k]	23 [k]	17 [k]	1.0 [u]	potassium, 2.5 mg [j] iodine, 50 µg [l]
	50.0	50	15.0	100 [m]	—	—	—	dioctyl sodium sulfosuccinate, 100 mg
	4.5	300	—	—	—	—	—	—
	4.5	300	—	12	—	—	—	—
	3.0	—	10.0 [i]	—	—	—	—	—
	5.0	—	20.0 [i]	—	—	—	—	—
	—	—	—	—	375	300	—	iodine (kelp), 100 µg brewers yeast
	4.0	—	20.0 [i]	—	—	—	—	—
	3.33	100	—	11 [p]	—	—	—	polysorbate 20, 400 mg
	—	—	—	—	—	—	—	—
	0.2	—	—	15 [v]	—	—	—	—
	4.0	—	20.0 [i]	—	—	—	—	—
	12.0	—	20.0 [i]	—	—	—	—	—
	6.0	400	—	18	160	125	100	iodine, 150 µg
	—	—	1.43 [h]	5 [j]	—	—	—	manganese, 0.33 mg [j]
	2.0	—	1.7 [i]	22 [m]	—	—	—	—
	—	—	1.43 [h]	22 [p]	—	—	—	liver fraction, 1.54 mg

Product * (manufacturer)	Vitamin A, IU	Vitamin D, IU	Vitamin E, IU	Ascorbic acid (C), mg	Thiamine (B_1), mg	Riboflavin (B_2), mg	Niacin, m
Stuartinic (Stuart)	—	—	—	300 225 [e]	6.0 [f]	6.0	20 [d]
Stuart Prenatal Formula (Stuart)	8,000 [q]	400	30	60	1.7 [f]	2.0	20 [d]
Super Calcicaps (Nion)	—	133	—	—	—	—	—
Super D Cod Liver Oil [n] (Upjohn)	4,000	400	—	—	—	—	—
Super D Perles [n] (Upjohn)	10,000	400	—	—	—	—	—
Super Plenamins (Rexall)	8,000	400	1.8	56	2.3 [c]	2.35	18
Surbex (Abbott)	—	—	—	—	6.0 [c]	6.0	30 [d]
Surbex-T (Abbott)	—	—	—	500 [e]	15.0 [c]	10.0	100 [d]
Surbex with C (Abbott)	—	—	—	250 [e]	6.0 [c]	6.0	30 [d]
Taka-Combex Kapseals (Parke-Davis)	—	—	—	30	10.0 [f]	10.0	10 [d]
Tega-C Caps (Ortega)	—	—	—	500	—	—	—
Tega-C Syrup [n] (Ortega)	—	—	—	500	—	—	—
Tega-E Caps (Ortega)	—	—	400 1,000	—	—	—	—
Thera-Combex Kapseals (Parke-Davis)	—	—	—	250	25.0 [f]	15.0	100 [d]
Thera-Combex H-P Kapseals (Parke-Davis)	—	—	—	500	25.0 [f]	15.0	100 [d]
Theragran (Squibb)	10,000	400	15	200	10.0	10.0	100 [d]
Theragran Liquid [n] (Squibb)	10,000	400	—	200	10.0	10.0	100 [d]
Theragran-M (Squibb)	10,000	400	15	200	10.0	10.0	100 [d]
Therapeutic Vitamins (North American)	1,000 [b]	400	15	200	10.0 [f]	10.0	100 [d]
Thera-Spancap (North American)	10,000	400	—	150	6.0 [f]	6.0	60 [d]
Theron (Stuart)	10,000 [q]	400	—	34 299 [e]	15.0 [f]	10.0	100 [d]
Tonebec (A.V.P.)	—	—	—	300	15.0 [f]	10.0	5 [d]
Tri-Vi-Sol Chewable (Mead Johnson)	2,500	400	—	60	—	—	—
Tri-Vi-Sol Drops [a] (Mead Johnson)	900	240	—	21	—	—	—
Tri-Vi-Sol with Iron Drops [a] (Mead Johnson)	1,500	400	—	35	—	—	—
Unicap (Upjohn)	5,000	400	5	45	2.8 [c]	3.2	36
Unicap Chewable (Upjohn)	4,000	400	—	75	2.0 [f]	2.0	18 [d]
Unicap Therapeutic (Upjohn)	5,000	400	30	300	10.0 [f]	10.0	100 [d]
Vastran (Wallace)	—	—	—	100	10.0 [c]	5.0	50
Venthera (Amfre-Grant)	10,000	400	50	200	12.5 [c]	12.5	100 [d]
Vi-Aqua (USV)	5,000	400	0.5	37.5	4.7	4.7	18
Vicon (Meyer)	2,000	—	25	75	5.0 [f]	2.5	12.5 [d]
Vicon-C (Meyer)	—	—	—	300	20.0 [f]	10.0	100 [d]
Vicon Forte (Meyer)	12,500 [q]	—	50	150	10.0 [f]	5.0	25 [d]

…oxine …chloride …mg	Cyanocobalamin (B_{12}), µg	Folic acid, µg	Pantothenic acid, mg	Iron, mg	Calcium, mg	Phosphorus, mg	Magnesium, mg	Other
	25.0	—	10.0 [i]	100 [m]	—	—	—	—
	8.0	800	—	60 [m]	200 [j]	—	100 [u]	iodine, 150 µg [l]
	—	—	—	—	334	41.7	—	—
	—	—	—	—	—	—	—	—
	—	—	—	—	—	—	—	—
	1.5	—	—	—	—	—	—	—
	5.0	—	10.0 [i]	—	—	—	—	—
	10.0	—	20.0 [i]	—	—	—	—	—
	5.0	—	10.0 [i]	—	—	—	—	—
	1.0 [g]	—	6.0 [h]	—	—	—	—	liver concentrate, 340 mg aspergillus oryzae enzymes, 162.5 mg
	—	—	—	—	—	—	—	—
	—	—	—	—	—	—	—	—
	—	—	—	—	—	—	—	—
	5.0 [g]	—	20.0 [h]	—	—	—	—	aspergillus oryzae enzymes, 162.5 mg
	5.0 [g]	—	20.0 [h]	—	—	—	—	—
	5.0	—	20.0 [i]	—	—	—	—	—
	5.0	—	20.0 [h]	—	—	—	—	—
	5.0	—	20.0 [i]	12	—	—	65	copper, 2.0 mg zinc, 1.5 mg manganese, 1.0 mg iodine, 150 µg
	5.0 [r]	—	20.0 [i]	—	—	—	—	—
	6.0 [r]	—	6.0 [i]	—	—	—	—	—
	5.0	—	20.0 [i]	15 [m]	100 [j]	—	—	zinc, 1.5 mg [j] manganese, 1.0 mg [j]
	—	—	10.0 [i]	—	—	—	—	—
	—	—	—	—	—	—	—	—
	—	—	—	—	—	—	—	—
	—	—	—	10	—	—	—	—
	—	—	—	—	—	—	—	—
	2.0	—	5.0 [i]	—	—	—	—	—
	4.0	—	20.0 [i]	10 [j]	50 [t]	—	6.0 [j]	potassium, 5.0 mg [j] copper, 1.0 mg [j] manganese, 1.0 mg [j] iodine, 150 µg [l]
	2.0	—	5.0 [i]	—	—	—	—	—
	10.0	—	20.0 [i]	15 [m]	105	80	6.0	potassium, 5.0 mg zinc, 1.5 mg iodine, 150 µg others [z]
	0.5	—	10.0 [i]	—	—	—	—	—
	—	—	5.0 [i]	—	—	—	35 [u]	zinc, 10 mg [u] manganese chloride, 2 mg
	—	—	20.0 [i]	—	—	—	70 [j]	zinc, 80 mg [j]
	—	—	10.0 [i]	—	—	—	70 [j]	zinc, 80 mg [j] manganese chloride, 4 mg

Product * (manufacturer)	Vitamin A, IU	Vitamin D, IU	Vitamin E, IU	Ascorbic acid (C), mg	Thiamine (B_1), mg	Riboflavin (B_2), mg	Niacin, m
Vicon Plus (Meyer)	4,000 [q]	—	50	150	10.0 [f]	5.0	25 [d]
Vigran (Squibb)	5,000	400	30	60	1.5	1.7	20
Vigran Chewable (Squibb)	2,500	10	10	40	0.7	0.8	9
Vigran plus Iron (Squibb)	5,000	400	30	60	1.5	1.7	20
Vi-Magna (Lederle)	5,000	400	—	56	2.8 [c]	2.8	18
Vio-Bec (Rowell)	—	—	—	500	25.0 [f]	25.0	100 [d]
Vi-Penta Infant Drops [a] (Roche)	5,000	400	2	50	—	—	—
Vi-Penta Multivitamin Drops [a] (Roche)	5,000 [b]	400	2	50	1.0 [c]	1.0	10 [d]
Vi-Syneral Basic Vitamin Drops [a] (Fisons)	5,000	400	5	60	—	—	—
Vi-Syneral One-Caps (Fisons)	5,000 [b]	—	30	60 [e]	1.5 [f]	1.7	20 [d]
Vitagett (North American)	5,000 [b]	400	3	50	3.0 [f]	2.5	20 [d]
Vita-Kaps Tablets (Abbott)	5,000	400	—	50 [e]	3.0 [c]	2.5	20 [d]
Vita-Kaps-M Tablets (Abbott)	5,000	400	—	50 [e]	3.0 [c]	2.5	20 [d]
Vitamin-Mineral Capsules (North American)	5,000 [b]	400	—	50 [e]	3.0 [f]	2.5	20 [d]
Viterra (Pfipharmecs)	5,000	400	3.7	50	3.1	3.0	25
Viterra 100% RDA (Pfipharmecs)	5,000	400	30	60	1.5	1.7	20
Viterra 100% RDA Plus Iron (Pfipharmecs)	5,000	400	30	60	1.5	1.7	20
Viterra Therapeutic (Pfipharmecs)	10,000	400	5	150	10.3	10.0	100.8
Vi-Zac (Meyer)	5,000	—	50	500	—	—	—
VM Preparation [x] (Roberts)	—	—	—	—	3.0 [c]	2.0	20 [d]
Zincaps (Ortega)	—	—	—	—	—	—	—
Zymacep Capsules (Upjohn)	5,000	400	—	100	5.0 [c]	5.0	30 [d]
Zymadrops [a] (Upjohn)	2,000	400	—	50	1.0 [c]	1.0	10 [d]
Zymalixir Syrup [n] (Upjohn)	—	—	—	—	1.0 [c]	1.0	8.0 [d]
Zymasyrup [n] (Upjohn)	5,000	400	—	60	1.0 [c]	1.0	10 [d]
Zymatinic Drops [a] (Upjohn)	—	—	—	—	0.6 [c]	0.6	4.8 [d]

doxine ochloride mg	Cyanocobalamin (B_{12}), µg	Folic acid, µg	Pantothenic acid, mg	Iron, mg	Calcium, mg	Phosphorus, mg	Magnesium, mg	Other
	—	—	10.0 [i]	—	—	—	70 [j]	zinc, 80 mg [j] manganese chloride, 4 mg
	6.0	400	—	—	—	—	—	—
	3.0	200	—	—	—	—	—	—
	6.0	400	—	27	—	—	—	—
	0.5	—	1.0 [i]	—	—	—	—	—
	—	—	40.0 [i]	—	—	—	—	—
	—	—	—	—	—	—	—	—
	—	—	10.0 [h]	—	—	—	—	biotin, 30 µg
	—	—	—	—	—	—	—	—
	6.0	400	—	18 [j]	—	—	—	—
	2.5	—	5.0 [i]	13 [j]	215 [k]	166 [k]	7.5 [j]	potassium, 5.0 mg [j] manganese, 1.5 mg [j] zinc, 1.4 mg [j]
	2.0	—	5.0 [i]	—	—	—	—	—
	2.0	—	5.0 [i]	10	—	—	5.0	zinc, 1.5 mg copper, 1.0 mg manganese, 1.0 mg iodine, 150 µg
	2.0	—	2.0 [i]	13 [j]	46 [k]	35 [k]	1.0 [j]	potassium, 5.0 mg [j] manganese, 1.5 mg [j] zinc, 1.4 mg [j]
	2.0	—	4.6	10	110	40	5.0	zinc, 1.2 mg copper, 1.0 mg manganese, 1.0 mg iodine, 150 µg
	6.0	400	—	—	—	—	—	—
	6.0	400	—	18	—	—	—	—
	5.0	—	4.6	10	50	—	5.0	zinc, 1.2 mg copper, 1.0 mg manganese, 1.0 mg iodine, 150 µg
	—	—	—	—	—	—	—	zinc, 80 mg [j]
	—	—	—	50	94	94	—	manganese, 2 mg
	—	—	—	—	—	—	—	zinc, 25 mg [j]
	4.0	—	10.0 [i]	—	—	—	—	—
	—	—	3.0 [h]	—	—	—	—	—
	2.0	—	—	15 [p]	—	—	—	liver concentrate, 65 mg alcohol, 1.5%
	3.0	—	3.0 [h]	—	—	—	—	alcohol, 2%
	0.6	—	—	5 [p]	—	—	—	liver concentrate, 39 mg alcohol, 1.5%

amin formulations change frequently; efore, the product label should be sulted before dispensing.
uantities given are per 0.6 ml.
lmitate.
drochloride.
acinamide.
dium salt.
ononitrate.
ystalline.

[h] Panthenol.
[i] Calcium salt.
[j] Sulfate.
[k] Phosphate.
[l] Potassium iodide.
[m] Fumarate.
[n] Quantities given are per 5 ml.
[o] Pyrophosphate.
[p] Gluconate.
[q] Acetate.

[r] Concentrate.
[s] Ferrocholinate.
[t] Carbonate.
[u] Oxide.
[v] Ammonium citrate.
[w] Glycerophosphate.
[x] Quantities given are per 30 ml.
[y] Quantities given are per 15 ml.
[z] Also contains other vitamins and/or minerals.

Products 11 FOOD SUPPLEMENT

Product (manufacturer)	Dosage form[a]	Calories	Protein, g	Carbo-hydrate, g	Fat, g	Vitamins, minerals	Indicated use
Casec (Mead Johnson)	powder, 1 tbsp	17	4.0	trace	0.1	various[b c]	sodium restriction cholesterol restriction
Citrotein (Doyle)	powder, 35.4 g	127	7.67	23.3	0.33	various[b c]	supplementary nourishment
Compleat-B (Doyle)	liquid, 400 ml/can	400	16	48	16	various[b c]	tube feeding
Controlyte (Doyle)	powder, 120 g	280	trace	40	13.4	sodium, 8.4 mg potassium, 2.2 mg calcium, 2.2 mg phosphorus, 4.5 mg	protein restriction electrolyte restriction high caloric requirement tube feeding
Flexical (Mead Johnson)	powder	250	5.6	38.1	8.5	various[b c]	supplementary nourishment tube feeding
Gevral Protein (Lederle)	powder, 26 g	97.8	15.6	6.3	0.52	various[b c]	supplementary nourishment
Instant Breakfast (various)	powder, 3.66 g	130	8.0	23	1.0	various[b c]	supplementary nourishment
Isocal (Mead Johnson)	liquid, 240 ml	250	8.1	31.2	10.5	various[b c]	supplementary nourishment tube feeding
Lolactene (Doyle)	powder, 60 g	227	15	30	5.3	various[b c]	lactose restriction supplementary nourishment tube feeding
Meritene (Doyle)	powder, 34.2 g liquid, 300 ml/can	277 (powder) 300 (liquid)	18	31 (powder) 34.5 (liquid)	9 (powder) 10 (liquid)	various[b c]	supplementary nourishment tube feeding
Nutrament (Drackett)	powder, 60 g liquid, 375 ml/can	360	23.5	50	9	various[b c]	supplementary nourishment
Nutri-1000 (Syntex)	liquid, 300 ml/can	313	10.1	3.3	16	various[b c]	supplementary nourishment tube feeding
Precision High Nitrogen Diet (Doyle)	powder, 87.9 g	300	12.5	62	0.14	various[b c]	high protein requirement
Precision Isotonic Diet (Doyle)	powder, 61.8 g	250	7.5	37.5	7.8	various[b c]	food intolerance tube feeding
Precision LR Diet (Doyle)	powder, 90 g	316	7.5	71	0.23	various[b c]	supplementary nourishment
Precision Moderate Nitrogen Diet (Doyle)	powder, 82.5 g	333	10.8	50	10.3	various[b c]	supplementary nourishment
Prototabs (North American)	tablet	—	0.25[d]	—	—	—	amino acid deficiency

Product (manufacturer)	Dosage form[a]	Calories	Protein, g	Carbo-hydrate, g	Fat, g	Vitamins, minerals	Indicated use
Stuart Amino Acids and B₁₂ (Stuart)	tablet	—	0.6[d]	—	—	cyanocobalamin, 1 μg	amino acid deficiency
Stuart Amino Acids Powder (Stuart)	powder	—	amino acids[d]	—	—	—	amino acid deficiency
Sustacal (Mead Johnson)	liquid, 360 ml	360	21.7	49.6	8.3	various[b c]	supplementary nourishment tube feeding
Sustagen (Mead Johnson)	liquid, 240 ml	390	23.5	3.5	66.5	various[b c]	supplementary nourishment tube feeding
Vivonex (Eaton)	powder, 80 g	300	6.125	69	0.435	various[b c]	supplementary nourishment tube feeding
Vivonex High Nitrogen (Eaton)	powder, 80 g	300	12.5	63.3	0.261	various[b c]	enteral hyperalimentation tube feeding

[a] One serving. Powder must be added to liquid as package directs.
[b] Includes vitamins A, D, E, ascorbic acid, thiamine, riboflavin, niacin, pyridoxine hydrochloride, cyanocobalamin, and/or various other substances having vitamin activity.
[c] Includes iron, calcium, phosphorus, iodine, magnesium, copper, zinc, potassium, sodium, and manganese.
[d] Amino acids, including leucine, lysine, phenylalanine, threonine, methionine, arginine, isoleucine, valine, histidine, tryptophan, and/or others.

Products 11 HEMATINIC

Product (manufacturer)	Iron	Vitamins	Other
Arne Timesules (Haag)	ferrous sulfate, 150 mg	—	—
Cefera (Haag)	ferrous fumarate, 200 mg	ascorbic acid, 100 mg	—
Chel-Iron Liquid and Tablets (Kinney)	ferrocholinate, 417 mg/5 ml 330 mg/tablet	—	—
Chel-Iron Pediatric Drops (Kinney)	ferrocholinate, 208 mg/ml	—	—
C-Ron (Rowell)	ferrous fumarate, 200 mg	ascorbic acid, 100 mg	—
C-Ron Forte (Rowell)	ferrous fumarate, 200 mg	ascorbic acid, 600 mg	—
Dical-D with Iron Capsules (Abbott)	10 mg	ergocalciferol, 132 IU	dibasic calcium phosphate, 500 mg
Femiron (J. B. Williams)	ferrous fumarate, 20 mg	—	—
Feosol Spansules and Tablets (Smith Kline & French)	ferrous sulfate, 167 mg/spansule 200 mg/tablet	—	—

Product (manufacturer)	Iron	Vitamins	Other
Ferancee (Stuart)	elemental, 67 mg (as ferrous fumarate)	sodium ascorbate, 114 mg ascorbic acid, 49 mg	—
Ferancee-HP (Stuart)	ferrous fumarate, 330 mg	ascorbic acid, 350 mg sodium ascorbate, 283 mg	—
Fergon Capsules and Tablets (Breon)	ferrous gluconate, 435 mg/capsule 320 mg/tablet	—	—
Fergon c C Caplets (Breon)	ferrous gluconate, 450 mg	ascorbic acid, 200 mg	—
Fer-In-Sol Drops, Syrup, and Capsules (Mead Johnson)	ferrous sulfate, 75 mg/0.6 ml 150 mg/5 ml 190 mg/capsule	—	—
Fermalox Tablets (Rorer)	ferrous sulfate, 200 mg	—	magnesium hydroxide, 100 mg aluminum hydroxide gel, dried, 100 mg
Fero-Grad-500 Tablets (Abbott)	105 mg	sodium ascorbate, 500 mg	—
Fero-Gradumet Tablets (Abbott)	105 mg	—	—
Ferrated Liver Concentrate Capsules (Fougera)	ferrous sulfate, 233 mg	niacinamide, 5 mg riboflavin, 1 mg thiamine hydrochloride, 0.5 mg	liver concentrate, 455 mg
Ferrobid (Meyer)	ferrous fumarate, 225 mg	ascorbic acid, 100 mg	copper sulfate, 8 mg
Ferrolip Tablets and Syrup (Flint)	ferrocholinate, 333 mg/tablet 417 mg/5 ml	—	—
Ferro-mandets (Lederle)	ferrous fumarate, 60 mg	ascorbic acid, 50 mg	—
Ferronord (Cooper)	ferroglycine sulfate complex	—	—
Ferro-Sequels (Lederle)	ferrous fumarate, 150 mg	—	dioctyl sodium sulfosuccinate, 100 mg
Fuma Drops (North American)	ferrous fumarate, 100 mg/5 ml	—	cherry flavor
Fumaral Elixir and Spancaps (North American)	ferrous sulfate, 325 mg/10 ml ferrous fumarate, 330 mg/ capsule	ascorbic acid, 200 mg/capsule	alcohol, 5% (elixir)
Hytinic Capsules and Elixir (Hyrex)	elemental, 150 mg/capsule 100 mg/5 ml (as polysaccharide–iron complex)	—	—
Iron with Vitamin C (Squibb)	50 mg	sodium ascorbate, 25 mg	—
Ionized Yeast (Glenbrook)	ferrous sulfate, 341 mg/ 6 tablets	thiamine, 2.25 mg/6 tablets	—
Laud-Iron (Amfre-Grant)	ferrous fumarate, 324 mg and 100 mg/5 ml	—	—
Laud-Iron Plus Chewing Tablets (Amfre-Grant)	ferrous fumarate, 100 mg	cyanocobalamin, 5 μg	—
L-Glutavite Capsules and Powder (Cooper)	16%	—	monosodium L-glutamate

Product (manufacturer)	Iron	Vitamins	Other
Mol-Iron Liquid and Tablets (Schering)	ferrous sulfate, 195 mg/4 ml 195 and 390 mg/tablet	—	alcohol, 4.75% /4 ml
Mol-Iron with Vitamin C (Schering)	ferrous sulfate, 195 and 390 mg	ascorbic acid, 75 and 150 mg	—
Niferex Elixir, Capsules, and Tablets (Central Pharmacal)	elemental, 100 mg/5 ml 150 mg/capsule 50 mg/tablet (as polysaccharide–iron complex)	—	alcohol, 10% (elixir)
Niferex with Vitamin C Tablets (Central Pharmacal)	elemental, 50 mg (as polysaccharide–iron complex)	sodium ascorbate, 168.75 mg ascorbic acid, 100 mg	—
Recoup Tablets (Lederle)	ferrous fumarate, 150 mg	ascorbic acid, 300 mg	dioctyl sodium sulfosuccinate, 50 mg
Simron Capsules (Merrell-National)	ferrous gluconate, 85 mg	—	polysorbate 20, 400 mg
Toleron Suspension and Tablets (Mallinckrodt)	ferrous fumarate, 100 mg/5 ml 200 mg/tablet	—	—
Tri-Tinic Capsules (North American)	ferrous fumarate, 110 mg	ascorbic acid, 75 mg folic acid, 0.5 mg cyanocobalamin, 7.5 μg	liver-stomach concentrate, 240 mg
Vitron-C (Fisons)	ferrous fumarate, 200 mg	ascorbic acid, 125 mg	—

Infant Formula Products

Kenneth J. Bender
Michael W. McKenzie
A. Jeanece Seals

Questions to ask the patient

What is the child's age and weight?

Is the child under a physician's care?

Has your pediatrician recommended a formula?

Is the child allergic to milk? Are there other dietary restrictions?

Is diarrhea a problem? If so, what is the frequency? Does the child have fever, dry skin, or loss of appetite?

Do you understand the directions for mixing the formula? Repeat them in your own words.

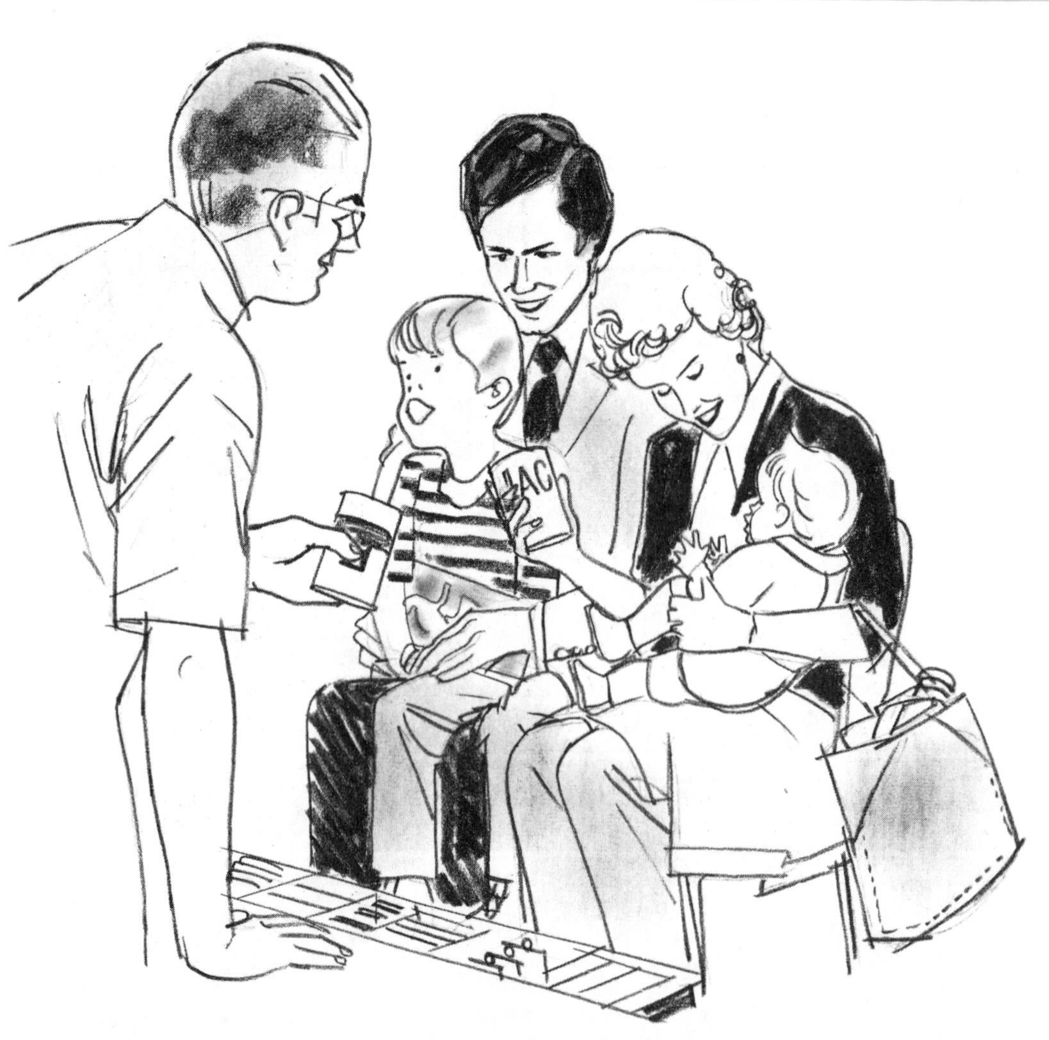

CHAPTER 12

Interest in nutrition by health professionals and the American public has been rising. The growing interest may have been signaled by the 1969 White House Conference on Food, Nutrition, and Health. Dr. Richard Fuisz noted the 1970's to be "a time when the importance of nutrition in infancy will be resurrected." [1]

Figures from 1971 indicate that sales of infant formulas were about $202 million, evenly divided between the ready-to-feed liquids and preparations that require mixing. Of those requiring mixing, powders that must be reconstituted were less popular than the concentrates that must be diluted. Pharmacies and groceries were the major distributors of infant formulas, although about 6 percent were distributed by nutrition and infant care centers. The special or therapeutic formulas (including soy base) made up about $30 million of the total sales in 1971, and pharmacies distributed 80 percent of these.[2]

Milk, alone or in a mixture, is an infant's most important food. Early commercial formulas did not provide an adequate substitute for breast milk. They were high in carbohydrates and were often linked with bacterial infections because of poor sanitation. However, in the last 30 years, there has been a considerable increase in formula feeding of infants. The main factors responsible for this increase are technical advances in producing sanitary formulas and the change in women's attitudes toward breast-feeding. The frequency of breast-feeding during the newborn period decreased from about 65 percent in the 1940's to 25 percent in 1958.[3] Although there appears to be a growing trend to breast-feed among middle- and upper-income mothers, the proportion of infants who are breast fed at the age of 1 month remains constant—about 20 percent.[4]

The composition of commercial infant formulas is in accordance with guidelines generated from extensive assessment of infant nutritional needs. Formula variation provides the opportunity to select a product which is acceptable to a particular infant and satisfies special nutritional requirements. These variations, however, have produced differences in palatability, digestibility, and convenience of administration. The pharmacist should be able to evaluate indications and advise on the selection and preparation of infant formulas.

Nutritional requirements of the infant

The growth rate of infants from birth to 1 year is faster than at any other time. Infants are expected to double their birth weight at 6 months and to triple it at 1 year. Because of this rapid growth rate, the nutritional adequacy of an infant's diet is very important.

Three basic nutrition principles should be considered when evaluating an infant formula: it should be adequate, but not excessive, in all the essential nutrients; it should be readily digestible; and it should have a reasonable distribution of calories derived from protein, fat, and carbohydrate. Metabolic studies by Fomon [5] suggest that 7 to 16 percent of the calories should be derived from protein, 30 to 55 percent from fat, and 35 to 65 percent from carbohydrate. Human milk provides 7 percent, 55 percent, and 38 percent of its calories from protein, fat, and carbohydrate, respectively; corresponding figures for whole cow's milk are 20, 50, and 30 percent.

Caloric allowance

The metabolic calorie [large calorie or kilocalorie (Kcal)] is the amount of heat required to raise the temperature of 1,000 g of water 1° C. The Recommended Daily Dietary Allowance (RDA), as established by the National Academy of Sciences/National Research Council, is 117 cal/kg/day for infants from birth to 6 months, and 108 cal/kg/day from 6 months to 1 year (Table 1). A full-term, full-weight infant should have no difficulty in consuming enough of a standard diluted formula (20 cal/oz) to meet these needs. A premature or low birth weight infant has a higher caloric need and may require as much as 130 cal/kg/day.[6]

Protein allowance

The RDA for protein is 2.2 g of protein/kg from birth to 6 months and 2.0 g from 6 months to 1 year. Low birth weight infants may have a higher protein requirement. It is important that the source of protein contains the eight essential amino acids—isoleucine, leucine, lysine, methionine, phenylalanine, threonine, tryptophan, and valine. There is evidence that histidine is essential for the newborn.[7] Both human and cow's milk contain histidine in quantities exceeding estimated infant requirements of 26 mg/100 cal and can be fed to newborns until the body begins to synthesize histidine (2 to 3 months after birth). Tyrosine and cystine, as well as histidine, may initially be essential for the premature infant.[7,8]

Carbohydrate allowance

Although there is no RDA for carbohydrates, a human infant efficiently uses 35 to 65 percent of the total calories from a carbohydrate source.[5] Most of the sources of carbohydrates used in infant formulas are monosaccharides or disaccharides, which are more easily digested and absorbed by the infant than polysaccharides (starch). Lactose, the "milk sugar" disaccharide, is the most common carbohydrate in an infant's diet. It is hydrolyzed by acids and the enzyme lactase to glucose and galactose. Disaccharide hydrolysis in a newborn may be incomplete, and because lactase activity develops late in fetal life, a premature infant is especially prone to lactose intolerance during the first weeks after birth.[9]

Fat allowance

A normal caloric distribution in an infant's diet derives 30 to 55 percent of the calories from dietary fat.[5] Diets that supply more calories from fat may cause ketosis because ketone bodies are formed from excess free fatty acids.[10] Fat is an efficient source of calories because of its high caloric density. It contains 9 cal/g compared with 4 cal/g for protein and carbohydrate. Fat in a diet increases palatability and enhances the absorption of lipid-soluble vitamins.

Fat also supplies essential fatty acids that are not synthesized in the human body. Linoleic and arachidonic acids enable optimum use of caloric intake and proper skin composition; four other fatty acids also are essential.[11] Because all are precursors of the prostaglandins, the manifestations of fatty acid deficiency may be the result of impaired prostaglandin synthesis. The actions of the prostaglandins appear to be related to cyclic adenosine monophosphate (cAMP) and range from mediating inflammatory response and hormone control to transporting water and electrolytes.

The digestibility of the fat source is important. Medium-chain fatty acids (8 to 10 carbons) that are unsaturated (have double bonds) are most easily absorbed. Monounsaturated fatty acids have one double bond; polyunsaturated fatty acids are dienoic, trienoic, or tetraenoic, depending on the number of double bonds. Linoleic acid represents the bulk of polyunsaturated fatty acids in infant formulas.

Table 1. Infant Allowance[a]

	Age, years	
	0.0-0.5	0.5-1.0
Weight, lbs	14	20
Height, in	24	28
Energy, kcal	kg × 117	kg × 108
Protein, g	kg × 2.2	kg × 2.0
Vitamin A activity		
RE[b]	420[c]	400
IU	1,400	2,000
Vitamin D activity, IU	400	400
Vitamin E activity, IU[d]	4	5
Ascorbic acid, mg	35	35
Folic acid, μg[e]	50	50
Niacin, mg[f]	5	8
Riboflavin, mg	0.4	0.6
Thiamine, mg	0.3	0.5
Vitamin B_6, mg[g]	0.3	0.4
Vitamin B_{12}, μg[b]	0.3	0.3
Calcium, mg	360	540
Phosphorus, mg	240	400
Iodine, μg	35	45
Iron, mg	10	15
Magnesium, mg	60	70
Zinc, mg	3	5

[a] Excerpted from Food and Nutrition Board, National Academy of Sciences—National Research Council Recommended Daily Dietary Allowances, Revised 1974.

[b] Retinol equivalents.

[c] Assumed to be all as retinol in milk during the first 6 months of life. All subsequent intakes are assumed to be one-half as retinol and one-half as β-carotene when calculated from international units. As retinol equivalents, three-fourths are as retinol and one-fourth as β-carotene.

[d] Total vitamin E activity, estimated to be 80 percent as α-tocopherol and 20 percent other tocopherols. See text for proportionate amounts of polyunsaturated fatty acids required.

[e] The folic acid allowances refer to dietary sources as determined by *Lactobacillus casei* assay. Pure forms of folic acid may be effective in doses less than one-fourth of the RDA.

[f] Although allowances are expressed as niacin, it is recognized that on the average 1 mg of niacin is derived from each 60 mg of dietary tryptophan.

[g] Pyridoxine hydrochloride.

[b] Cyanocobalamin.

Vitamin and mineral allowances

Although certain infants may need vitamin supplementation in their diets (Table 2), indiscriminate vitamin supplementation, especially with lipid-soluble vitamins A and D (ergocalciferol), is potentially hazardous. (See Chapter 11 for a complete discussion of vitamins.)

Iron deficiency anemia is the most prevalent nutritional deficiency in infants. As a result, the American Academy of Pediatrics Committee on Nutrition recommended the use of iron-fortified formula in the first year of life.[12] The RDA for iron is 10 mg; 32 oz of iron-fortified commercial formula meet the requirement.

Premature infants on restricted diets may need vitamin E supplementation. Hemolytic anemia has been reported in premature infants who have received formulas with high levels of polyunsaturated fatty acids without vitamin E supplementation.[13] In order to avoid hemolytic anemia in premature infants, Dicks-Bushnell and Davis [14] recommend that the ratio of vitamin E intake to polyunsaturated fatty acids (E/PUFA) not be less than 0.4, where E/PUFA is:

$$\frac{\text{Vitamin E per unit volume (IU of } \alpha\text{-tocopherol)}}{\text{PUFA per unit volume (grams of linoleic and arachidonic)}}$$

The American Academy of Pediatrics Committee on Nutrition is considering a minimal allowance for E/PUFA in all formulas. Desai *et al.*[15] noted that E/PUFA values may be misleading when calculations are based on the total tocopherols of a commercial formula. Formulas that incorporate vegetable oils include large amounts of less active forms of tocopherols such as β, γ, and δ. The E/PUFA values in Table 2 for formulas used in premature infants are based on the international units of active α-tocopherol.

High levels of iron intake (8 mg/kg or more) have also been found to contribute to hemolytic anemia in premature infants, possibly by interfering with the intestinal absorption of vitamin E in the infant.[16] For this reason, the premature infant should not receive iron in excess of the levels recommended by the Committee on Nutrition.

It generally is agreed that fluoride supplementation of 0.5 mg/day (irrespective of the infant's milk or formula) increases tooth resistance to dental caries when the quantity of fluoride in the water supply is less than 1.0 mg/liter.[17] Fluoride intake in excess of approximately 0.5 mg daily by the infant is unnecessary, and excessive intake will result in fluorosis and mottled tooth enamel.

Content of milk and formulas

A formulation may be altered by the manufacturer in response to changes in availability of ingredients or modifications in recommended allowances. For example, the carbohydrate source for Lofenalac was changed from a combination of maltose, sucrose, dextrins, and arrowroot starch to corn syrup and tapioca starch when arrowroot starch became unavailable. The fat source of Similac was modified by adding soy oil to the combination of corn and coconut oils in response to the decreased availability and rising cost of corn oil. Current ingredients and quantities then may only be obtained by direct communications to the manufacturer. Texts rapidly become outdated and even product labels may reflect old formulations until their supply is depleted and new labels are printed.

Human milk vs. cow's milk

Human milk is the standard against which all other formulas can be compared. Obviously, it is more effective than cow's milk in meeting the nutritional requirements of the human infant. The differences in composition reflect the individual needs of the human infant and the calf. Although certain conditions in the infant may necessitate the use of therapeutic formulas, human milk is the most appropriate diet for the majority of infants. When human milk is not chosen, it is often because of the mother's desire not to breast-feed.

One problem associated with human milk is created by a substance secreted by some women, $3\alpha,20\beta$-pregnanediol, which seems to increase the incidence and severity of hyperbilirubinemia in infants by inhibiting glucuronide formation. This substance does not pose a significant drawback to breast-feeding, and an interruption of breast milk for 1 to 2 days is usually enough to reverse the infant's raised bilirubin.

Another potential problem in using human milk arises when the mother is taking medication. Drugs that are excreted in human milk may have undesirable effects on the infant.[18] Drugs also have been reported to alter breast milk composition. Barsivala and Virkar,[19] for example, reported changes in milk protein, fat, and calcium content in women taking combination-type oral contraceptives. Although these contraceptive agents are not specifically contraindicated for nursing mothers, the infant should be observed for adverse effects. Also, lactation is diminished by progesterone-estrogen combinations if taken prior to the establishment of adequate milk secretion, i.e., 3 to 4 weeks postpartum.[20]

Cow's milk has about three times the amount of ash and protein normally found in human milk (Fig. 1). This difference reflects the calf's larger growth rate and proportionate demand for protein and minerals. The urea formed from protein nitrogen combines with the mineral residue (ash) to create a higher renal solute load for the infant using cow's milk. Although cow's milk is usually diluted with water and carbohydrates, the load of solutes requiring renal excretion generally remains greater than the load from human milk.

Cow's milk not only has a higher percentage of protein than human milk, but the protein differs in composition. The difference in protein composition alters digestibility and may create a milk "sensitivity" where the infant has difficulty in digesting a milk-base formula. Compared with human milk, cow's milk has a high proportion of casein protein (crude protein mixture of α-, β-, γ-, and κ-caseins) to lactalbumin protein (primarily α-lactoglobulin but includes α-lactalbumin). Casein is relatively insoluble and occurs in milk as a "tough" curd; lactalbumin is highly soluble and occurs in milk as whey. The large amount of curd in cow's milk slows gastric emptying time and may cause GI distress. Heating cow's milk reduces the curd tension. Milk sensitivity differs from milk allergy in that sensitivity may be relieved by altering the ratio of casein and lactalbumin, but an allergic reaction necessitates the elimination of all animal milk protein. Although heating cow's milk may increase digestibility by reducing curd tension, it will not alter its antigen activity in allergic infants.

The fat in cow's milk differs from that in human milk in two ways. The triglycerides in cow's milk contain primarily short- and long-chain fatty acids (e.g., butyric, caproic). Human milk fat includes medium-chain fatty acids (e.g., capric, lauric) but not the short-chain group. In addition, human milk contains more monounsaturated fatty acids, and cow's milk butterfat primarily consists of saturated fatty acids. Commercial milk-base formulas incorporate the highly digestible, unsaturated, medium-chain triglycerides (MCT) by replacing butterfat with vegetable oil and special MCT oils.

The percentage of carbohydrates in cow's milk is smaller than in human milk, and carbohydrate supplementation is often necessary. Lactose, the carbohydrate source in both cow's and human milk, is absorbed into the brush-border of the small intestine and cleaved by the disaccharidase into galactose and glucose which are then absorbed actively against concentration gradients.

Cow's milk and human milk differ in absolute and proportionate amounts of calcium and phosphorus. The effect of this difference on calcium absorption is not clear because of the interrelation of additional factors such as

Table 2. Desirable Supplementation for Milk and Milk Substitutes[a]

Formulas	E/PUFA[b]	Iron	Vitamin D	Niacin	Ascorbic acid	Folic acid	Pyridoxine[c]	Vitamin E	Thiamine	Fluoride[d]
For full-term infants										
Human milk		+	+	*	**		±		±	+
Cow's milk (fortified)		+		+	+					+
Goat's milk (unfortified)		+	+	+	+	+	±			+
Standard commercial: Iron fortified										+
Not iron fortified		+								+
For premature infants										
Human milk (see above)	0.5 [e]									+
Pregestimil	3.33[f]	+								+
Premature Formula	0.31[f]	+						+		+
Similac PM 60/40	0.53[g]	+								+
SMA Improved (30 cal/oz)	1.3 [e]	+								+

[a] Desirable supplementation determined from formula content and recommended daily allowance (RDA) when respective formula is infant's only nutrient source. The length of time in which the infant receives the unsupplemented formula may determine clinical significance. Formulas generally have adequate levels of riboflavin and cyanocobalamin.
[b] Supplementation desired for premature infant with products whose ratio of vitamin E to polyunsaturated fatty acids (E/PUFA) is less than 0.4.
[c] Desirable supplementation of pyridoxine determined from RDA and the following values listed in S. Fomon, "Infant Nutrition," 2d ed., Saunders, Philadelphia, Pa., 1974, pp. 363, 372: human milk, 0.1 mg/liter; goat's milk, 0.07 mg/liter. [d] Desirable supplementation of 0.5 mg/day when fluoride concentration of water supply is less than 1 mg/liter. From S. H. Y. Wei, in "Infant Nutrition," 2d ed., Saunders, Philadelphia, Pa., 1974, p. 351.
[e] E/PUFA value obtained from Wyeth Laboratories (personal communication).
[f] E/PUFA value obtained from Mead Johnson Laboratories (personal communication). [g] E/PUFA value obtained from Ross Laboratories (personal communication).
+ indicates commonly accepted indication for supplementation. *Although human milk appears deficient in niacin as recommended in the RDA, it contains sufficient tryptophan to provide an adequate amount of niacin equivalent. **Ascorbic acid supplementation may be required if mother does not have adequate intake. ± indicates that a value falls below RDA, but that supplementation is generally not necessary because additions to diet are made before deficiencies become evident.

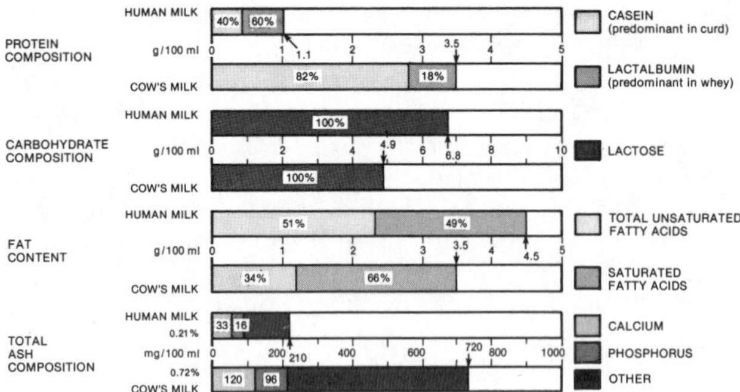

Figure 1. Comparison of human and cow's milk.

vitamin D, fat absorption, and active transport. For the premature infant, a low phosphorus intake is required to minimize renal solute load.

Goat's milk

Goat's milk is not widely used, but it is generally accepted as nutritionally adequate. It contains primarily medium- and short-chain fatty acids and may be more readily digested than cow's milk. Because goat's milk is deficient in folates, supplementation of approximately 50 μg of folate (as folic acid) daily should be given to prevent megaloblastic anemia in infants fed only with goat's milk.

Standard formula

Calories. In normal dilution, most formulas provide 20 cal/oz, approximating the caloric content of human and cow's milk. The caloric recommendations are traditionally based on comparison studies of varied concentrations fed *ad libitum* to normal infants. These studies show that, although infants in the first 41 days do not consume enough dilute formula to obtain their required calories, they exceed the acceptable caloric intake when given formulas of higher caloric concentration.[21] Advantages and disadvantages of high caloric intake in infancy are debated, because the increased weight gain may be proportionate to the gain in body length. Most nutritionists agree, however, that the incidence of overfed and overweight infants is higher than underfed infants.

Protein. Evaporated cow's milk supplies two-thirds of the calories of most standard formulas; about 15 percent of these calories are derived from casein protein. This protein source can be altered to produce a ratio of lactalbumin and casein resembling human milk. Through electrodialysis or ion exchange processes, the protein components can then be demineralized and additions made to produce the average concentrations found in human milk.

Variations in protein source have been developed because of milk allergy. Soy is the most frequently used alternative protein source; others include beef heart and hydrolysates of casein. The hydrolysates are enzymatic breakdown products with reduced antigenicity. As measured by weight gain in rats, beef heart is about 80 percent as efficient as casein; soy, about 70 percent; and hydrolysates of casein are roughly equivalent to casein in efficiency.[22] Serum albumin levels obtained from infants are used as a more direct measurement of satisfactory protein nutritional status.[23]

Fat. To obtain an easily digestible fat source, most commercial formulas have replaced butterfat with vegetable oil. Digestibility of vegetable oil is increased with a high proportion of unsaturated fatty acids and is decreased with a large amount of long-chain fatty acids. Corn and soy oils are easier to digest than coconut oil, which has a relatively high number of long-chain, saturated fatty acids. Commercial formulas have been produced from which about 85 percent of the fat is absorbed—the absorption rate of fat in human milk.[24]

Carbohydrates. Carbohydrates supply 40 percent of the calories of most standard formulas. If more than 50 percent of the calories are derived from carbohydrates, an infant's ability to hydrolyze disaccharides may be compromised. The increased passage of disaccharides in the feces creates an osmotic gradient in the colon which results in loose, watery, characteristically acidic stools. The excess lactose in the ileocecal region is fermented by bacteria to produce carbon dioxide and lactic acid. This process irritates the colon and may cause diarrhea, resulting in dehydration and electrolyte imbalance.

Formulas that contain sucrose and corn syrup as carbohydrate sources have a sweeter taste than those that contain lactose. Although there are differences in response to the sweeter formulas (female infants are more responsive than males; newborns who weigh more than 3,540 g at birth are more responsive than those who have a lower birth weight), the consequences of long-term use of the sweeter formulas and the criteria with which to select an optimum carbohydrate source are not yet known.[25]

Electrolytes and minerals. The amount of sodium, potassium, and chloride in standard formulas is calculated on the basis of the relatively high obligatory losses of the infant and the smaller amount required for growth. If fluid retention is a concern, a product with a low sodium content should be considered. Commercial therapeutic formulas with no nutritional value, such as Pedialyte and Lytren, have been developed to replace electrolytes and are used in cases of diarrhea or vomiting. Because of the critical nature of electrolyte imbalance and dehydration associated with infant diarrhea and vomiting, oral electrolyte replacements should be used cautiously as temporary treatment for conditions which may require intravenous therapy and inpatient monitoring.

The amount of calcium and phosphorus needed to replace an infant's obligatory loss is less than that required for growth. In milk and milk-base formulas, much of the available phosphorus is released from the slowly digested casein and may not be available during calcium absorption.[26] This "bound" phosphorus alters the calcium-to-phosphorus ratio and enhances absorption of calcium. If a formula combines this effect with a well-absorbed fat mixture and an adequate supply of vitamin D, optimum calcium absorption is achieved.

Iron and vitamins. Supplementing certain infant diets with vitamins and iron may be required (see Table 2). For example, supplementary iron and vitamin D are required by infants on human milk or unfortified cow's milk. Only about 40 percent of the infant formulas are iron-fortified. Wet-packed cereals, e.g., strained baby food, which are often assumed to be sources of iron, often contain the iron in a biologically unavailable form, such as sodium ferric pyrophosphate.[27]

Ascorbic acid supplementation is necessary with cow's milk but unnecessary with human milk from a well-nourished woman. Supplementing ascorbic acid with commercially prepared strained foods often is difficult because of losses of the vitamin during processing. Strained fruits are inadequate as sources for ascorbic acid except for those whose juices are fortified with ascorbic acid or strained bananas, to which ascorbic acid is added to prevent color change.

Indications for therapeutic formulas

Milk allergy

Most therapeutic formulas provide a protein substitute for milk proteins. Food allergy may appear in infants because the immature digestive and metabolic processes may not be completely effective in converting dietary proteins into nonantigenic amino acids. Estimates of 1 percent of the infant population being allergic to cow's milk (as measured by rash, wheezing, etc.) may be conservative because syndromes such as failure to thrive, anemia, and recurrent infections have been linked to serum antigen-antibody reactions to milk protein.

The formulas that include water-soluble soy isolates (Isomil, Neo-Mull-Soy, ProSobee, Nursoy) are whiter and more palatable than soy-base formulas that derive their protein from soy flour (Mull-Soy). Some "hypoallergenic" formulas incorporate enzymatic hydrolysates of casein (Nutramigen, Pregestimil). Meat Base Formula derives its substitute for milk protein from beef heart and may require carbohydrate supplementation.

Fat restrictions

Fat and protein composition can be altered to achieve a "humanized" formula which is more easily digested. The fat in these formulas is made up of triglycerides of mainly medium-chain fatty acids. The digestibility of medium-chain triglyceride oil closely approximates that of human milk fat. MCT oil ensures acceptance by infants who will not tolerate long- or short-chain fatty acids. It can be combined with a fat source, such as corn oil, to provide lecithin phospholipids.

Conditions which may necessitate a low or moderate intake of fat include cystic fibrosis and celiac disease. The latter is characterized by an intolerance of the gluten protein of wheat and rye and by the transient inability to absorb fat and starch. Formulas with a moderate amount of MCT oil are helpful in these conditions because their fat is more easily assimilated than butterfat (Pregestimil, 2.8 g MCT/100 ml; Portagen, 3.1 g MCT/100 ml). Soy-base formulas are not recommended for cystic fibrosis patients because of the reported hypoproteinemic edema resulting from their use in this condition.[28]

Caloric and carbohydrate deficiencies

Low birth weight infants (less than 2 kg at 3 weeks) or premature infants (born before 37 weeks from the first day of the last menstrual period) need a higher caloric concentration in their formula than full-term infants because of increased caloric need and decreased ability to consume an adequate volume of formula. The commercial preparations that provide the required higher caloric concentrations and are used in the hospital setting for these infants are Premature Formula and specifically concentrated SMA-Improved and Similac PM 60/40 (80 cal/100 ml).

Disaccharidase deficiency may occur as a congenital defect or secondary to cystic fibrosis or celiac disease. The absence of disaccharidase leads to malabsorption and acidic diarrhea. In these cases, the formula CHO-Free which has no carbohydrates may be given temporarily. Formulas without the suspect disaccharide (Lactose Free) may then be tried to reestablish the infant's diet.

In cases of galactosemia, a relatively rare disorder which may result from either a deficiency of galactose 1-phosphate uridyl transferase or from a deficiency of galactokinase, it is necessary to eliminate dietary lactose. This enables the body to convert glucose only to the amount of galactose it requires. Dietary lactose may be essentially eliminated by using soy isolates or Nutramigen, which contains only 16 mg/67 cal of lactose (equivalent to 8 mg galactose) as a contaminant of its casein protein, or Meat Base Formula, which has only trace amounts of galactose from the heart muscle protein. Galactosemia from an inborn enzyme deficiency is characterized in untreated infants by failure to thrive, liver disease, cataracts, and mental retardation.

Congenital heart disease

Infants with congenital heart disease often require a formula with an increased caloric concentration because they may tire in feeding before a volume with sufficient nutrients has been consumed. In addition, an excessive renal load must be avoided.

Lonalac, a sodium-free formula, may be used to limit sodium intake but may only be used for a short time before sodium must be supplemented. This formula presents a renal solute load that is slightly less than that of whole cow's milk, and caution is required in view of the limited liquid-volume intake which is characteristic of the heart patient.

Phenylketonuria

Phenylketonuria results from the failure of phenylalanine to be converted to tyrosine in the body. The accumulation of phenylalanine alters brain development and leads to mental retardation. Phenylalanine restriction is the only indication for Lofenalac, which may be used to eliminate dietary phenylalanine. Phenylalanine, an essential amino acid, must then be supplied in monitored quantities and is often done so with formulas that have a predominance of whey protein and, therefore, contain much less phenylalanine than casein.

Excessive phenylalanine restriction which brings blood levels below 2 mg/100 ml has resulted in retarded bone growth, vacuolization of bone marrow cells, megaloblastic anemia, hypoglycemia, and death.[29] Lofenalac, like other therapeutic formulas, should be used only as directed and indicated. Indiscriminate use of therapeutic formulas or arbitrary interchanging of therapeutic formulas with standard formulas must be avoided.

Formula and bottle preparation

Preparation of infant formulas requires careful aseptic technique, and the directions should be adequately explained to parents to ensure satisfactory nutrition for their infant. There are three forms of infant formulas—ready-to-feed, concentrated liquid, and concentrated powder. The latter two require the addition of water or, to add calories, a water-carbohydrate solution such as water-dextrose or water-honey. Failure to properly dilute a concentrated formula could result in a hypertonic solution that could precipitate diarrhea and dehydration. In an extreme case, overconcentrated formula produced renal failure, disseminated intravascular coagulation, gangrene of the legs, and coma.[30]

Equal amounts of water and concentrated liquid formula provide the necessary 20 cal/fl oz. The powdered formula requires one packed, level measure of powder (1 tbsp)/2 oz of water, or 8 fl oz/qt. For special dilutions of therapeutic formulas and other modified formulas, the directions on the products should be followed.

Infants are highly susceptible to infections because of insufficient antibody formation and decreased material antibody titer. Until an infant can produce adequate antibodies, it is especially important to clean all equipment used in formula preparation. Bottles, nipples, can opener, funnel, caps, and other equipment should be washed with hot, soapy water and rinsed thoroughly with hot, running water (water should be squeezed through the holes in the nipples) (Table 3).

Formula may be prepared for individual feedings or for a 24-hour supply, the latter being the most advantageous and efficient procedure for milk, water, and carbohydrate mixtures. Formula can be prepared to prevent bacterial contamination by terminal heating and by aseptic technique.[31 32] Although the terminal heating method has been recommended as the most effective, there are some special formulas, e.g., CHO-Free liquid and Meat Base Formula, which should not be terminally heated because the procedure may cause separation of the ingredients and make feeding difficult. The terminal heating method is more convenient than aseptic technique for preparing a day's supply.

The commercially sterilized liquid formulas and bacteriologically safe powdered formulas may be prepared more conveniently in single bottles. A day's supply of bottles may be prepared in advance and the formula added at feeding time. This eliminates the need for refrigeration of bottled formula and prefeeding warming.

The terminal heating method can allow bacterial growth during storage if instructions are not followed or bottles are not thoroughly cleaned of milk film.[33] However, evaporated milk formula carefully prepared just prior to feeding in bottles cleaned with hot tapwater is bacteriologically safe.[34] Milk formulas mixed at feeding time in "unsterilized" but clean bottles showed a definite bacteriologic advantage over the stored formula in homes

Table 3. Formula Preparation

Terminal heating[a]	Aseptic[a]	Single-bottle (for supplementing the diet of breast-fed infant or when traveling)[c]
Rinse the bottle and nipple with cool water immediately after the feeding. Wash the day's supply of bottles, nipples, and caps with hot, soapy water and rinse well.	Rinse the bottle and nipple with cool water immediately after the feeding. Wash the day's supply of bottles, nipples, and caps with hot, soapy water and rinse well.	Rinse the bottle and nipple with cool water immediately after the feeding. Wash the day's supply of bottles, nipples, and caps with hot, soapy water and rinse well.
Rinse the outside of the formula can and shake the contents well. Open the can with a clean can opener, mix the formula with water, or water-carbohydrate solution if prescribed, and pour the solution into bottles. Attach the nipples and cover them loosely with caps.	Boil the bottles, nipples, caps, cap opener, and mixing utensils for 5 min in a deep cooking utensil with enough water to cover each item. Remove the items with tongs and place the bottles on a clean towel or rack.	For formulas that require water, pour into each bottle the amount of water needed to prepare the feeding. Attach the nipples and cover them loosely with caps. Place the bottles on a rack in a deep cooking utensil containing 2 to 3 inches of water. Bring water to a boil, cover, and allow it to boil gently for 25 min. Remove the cooking utensil from the stove, allow it to cool, and tighten the caps and bottles. The bottles may be left inside the cooking utensil until they are needed.
Place the bottles on a rack in the deep cooking utensil containing 2 to 3 inches of water. Heat water to boiling and allow it to boil gently for 25 min while covered before removing from the stove.	While the equipment is being cleaned, boil some water in a covered saucepan or tea kettle for 5 min (slightly more water than the prescribed amount should be used to allow for evaporation).	For formulas that need no water, boil the bottles, nipples, caps, and can opener for 5 min. Put the nipples and caps on the bottles with aseptic care.
After the sides of the cooking utensil have cooled enough to be touched comfortably, remove the lid and the formula bottles. (Leaving the utensil closed for this period is recommended to prevent formation of milk film on bottles and clogging of nipples.)[b]	Remove the boiled water from the stove, allow it to cool, and measure the required amount.	At feeding time, remove the cap and nipple aseptically. Add the appropriate amount of formula and replace the nipple. With the powdered formula, also replace the cap, and shake the bottle vigorously to mix.
Warm the bottle of formula to the desired temperature before feeding.	Rinse, shake the can well, and add the commercially processed formula or evaporated milk and carbohydrate mixture to the boiled water and stir with a clean spoon. (If bottled milk or other unsterilized milk is used, it should be boiled with the water. Evaporated milk, carbohydrate modifiers, and commercially processed formulas usually are not boiled.)	Feed the infant while formula is at room temperature.
	Pour the formula into bottles and attach the nipples and caps with aseptic care. Store them in the refrigerator. Formula should be used within 24 hr.	
	Warm the bottle of formula to the desired temperature before feeding.	

[a]"Handbook of Infant Formulas," 6th ed., J. B. Roerig, Division of Pfizer, New York, N.Y., 1969, p. 86.

[b]H. K. Silver, *Pediatrics*, **20**, 997(1957).

[c]"Handbook of Infant Formulas," 6th ed., J. B. Roerig, Division of Pfizer, New York, N. Y., 1969, p. 88.

where sanitary conditions were poor and instructions for terminal heating and formula storage were not properly followed.[35]

Common problems with formulas

Infants are particularly susceptible to dehydration because of their high metabolic rate and ratio of surface area to weight and height. Depletion of fluid volume by diarrhea can quickly (within 24 hours) produce severe dehydration with fluid electrolyte imbalance, shock, and possibly result in death. A common etiology of diarrhea in infants is improper dilution of concentrated liquid or powder formula and, therefore, care must be taken to ensure proper formula preparation.

If diarrhea is a problem, the severity, frequency of stools, duration, and how the infant formula is prepared should be ascertained. If the diarrhea is serious (many more stools per day than the normal range of one to five) or has continued for several days, or if the infant is clinically sick (fever, lethargy, anorexia, irritability, dry skin), the infant should be referred immediately to a physician for appropriate care.

Medical care will be directed at identifying the cause of the diarrhea as well as correcting the physiological imbalances. Reducing fat intake, using MCT sources, or temporarily eliminating lactose may be helpful in determining if the diarrhea is diet related.

Mild diarrhea of short duration may resolve without medical measures, but the infant should be closely observed. Because improper digestion of the infant's formula may initiate diarrhea and because continuation of a formula while diarrhea persists may yield only marginal absorption of nutrients, a temporary (24-hour) discontinuation of usual foods may be helpful. The benefit of Lytren or Pedialyte for short-term management of electrolyte loss has been questioned. These solutions should not be used when parenteral rehydration is required or to provide nutritional value.

Indiscriminate vitamin supplementation can lead to hypervitaminosis. An infant should not receive vitamin supplementation if an iron-fortified standard formula is used unless it has been prescribed to correct a deficiency.

Feeding formula to the infant

Complaints about an infant's rejection of a formula may in some cases be resolved by examining the specific feeding problem. "Spitting up" is often caused by improper burping, feeding a large amount too quickly, or lying the infant face down too soon after feeding. During feeding, the infant should be held at a 45° angle with the head nestled in the curve of the arm. If the infant finishes a bottle and still seems hungry, another bottle should be offered. Infants should be burped at each feeding for 10 to 15 minutes after every 2 to 3 oz of formula by placing them over the shoulder or on the lap and patting them on the back to bring up swallowed air. Many infants are chronic "spitters" of formula; if they are growing and gaining weight, there is no reason to be concerned.

Larger nipple holes may be required to aid feeding. They can be enlarged with a hot needle or cross-cut nipples may be used.

Guidelines for product selection

Recommendations for the type of infant formula and its method of preparation must take into consideration the parents' ability to follow directions, their attitudes and preferences, and the sanitary conditions and refrigeration facilities available. Instruction in aseptic technique may include a step-by-step emphasis on the importance of sanitary conditions. For example, the top of the infant formula container should be thoroughly cleaned before opening, either by rinsing the top with hot tapwater or by dipping it in boiling water for about 15 seconds before it is opened. Partially used formula cans should be kept covered, placed in the refrigerator, and stored no longer than 48 hours.

For many parents, cost may be a critical factor in the selection of an infant formula. The concentrated formula preparations are less expensive than the ready-to-feed; powdered preparations range between the two. Convenience is also a consideration. The powder and concentrated liquid formulas require more manipulative functions in preparation and more attention to aseptic technique. A formula that is well-tolerated by the infant, convenient to prepare by the parents, and within the family budget should be used.

References

1. R. Fuisz, in "Infant Nutrition," Medcom, New York, N.Y., 1972, p. 3.
2. Ross Laboratories, Supplement to *Chain Store Age Super Markets,* **S3**, Sept., 1972.
3. S. Fomon, "Infant Nutrition," 2d ed., Saunders, Philadelphia, Pa., 1974, p. 7.
4. P. S. Berman, *Report of Market Research Data,* Ross Laboratories, Columbus, Ohio (Jan., 1974).
5. S. Fomon, in "Infant Nutrition," Medcom, New York, N.Y., 1972, p. 31.
6. L. A. Barness, in "Infant Nutrition," Medcom, New York, N.Y., 1972, p. 29.
7. S. Fomon, in "Infant Nutrition," Medcom, New York, N.Y., 1972, p. 121.
8. G. Gaull *et al., Pediatr. Res.,* **6,** 538(1972).
9. S. Fomon, in "Infant Nutrition," Medcom, New York, N.Y., 1972, p. 194.
10. S. Fomon, in "Infant Nutrition," Medcom, New York, N.Y., 1972, p. 31.
11. H. Schlenk, *Fed. Proc.,* **31,** 1430(1972).
12. Committee Statement, Committee on Nutrition, American Academy of Pediatrics, Iron-Fortified Formulas, Newsletter Supplement (Dec. 15, 1970).
13. S. A. Hashim and R. H. Asfour, *Am. J. Clin. Nutr.,* **21,** 7(1968).
14. M. W. Dicks-Bushnell and R. C. Davis, *Am. J. Clin. Nutr.,* **20,** 262(1967).
15. I. D. Desai *et al., Nutr. Rep. Int.,* **6,** 83(1972).
16. L. A. Barness, in "Infant Nutrition," Medcom, New York, N.Y., 1972, p. 28.
17. S. H. Y. Wei, in "Infant Nutrition," 2d ed., Saunders, Philadelphia, Pa., 1974, p. 351.
18. *Med. Lett. Drugs Ther.,* **16,** 25(1974).
19. V. M. Barsivala and K. D. Virkar, *Contraception,* **7,** 307(April, 1973).
20. C. S. Catz and G. P. Giacoia, *Pediatr. Clin. North Am.,* **19,** 151(1972).
21. S. Fomon, in "Infant Nutrition," Medcom, New York, N.Y., 1972, p. 27.
22. S. Fomon, "Infant Nutrition," Saunders, Philadelphia, Pa., 1967, p. 59.
23. S. Fomon, "Infant Nutrition," 2d ed., Saunders, Philadelphia, Pa., 1974, p. 128.
24. Wyeth Laboratories, "First After Mother's Milk," Wyeth Laboratories, Philadelphia, Pa., 1971, p. 6.
25. R. E. Nisbett and S. B. Gurwitz, *J. Comp. Physiol. Psychol.,* **73,** 215(1970).
26. A. White *et al.,* "Principles of Biochemistry," 4th ed., McGraw-Hill, New York, N.Y., 1968, p. 888.
27. S. Fomon, "Infant Nutrition," 2d ed., Saunders, Philadelphia, Pa., 1974, p. 300.
28. P. A. di Sant'Agnese in "Current Pediatric Therapy," S. S. Gellis and B. M. Kagan, Eds., Saunders, Philadelphia, Pa., 1973, p. 234.
29. "Amino Acid Metabolism and Genetic Variation," W. L. Nyhan, Ed., McGraw-Hill, New York, N.Y., 1967, pp. 6-63.
30. C. A. L. Abrams *et al., J. Am. Med. Assoc.,* **232,** 1136(1975).
31. W. A. Silverman *et al., Pediatrics,* **28,** 675(1961).
32. H. K. Silver, *Pediatrics,* **20,** 998(1957).
33. H. K. Silver, *Pediatrics,* **20,** 997(1957).
34. C. C. Fischer and M. A. Whiteman, *J. Pediatr.,* **55,** 118(1959).
35. V. C. Vaughn *et al., J. Pediatr.,* **61,** 547(1962).

Product[a] (manufacturer)	Calories per 30 ml	Calories per 100 ml	Protein, g/100 ml	Fat, g/100 ml	Carbohydrate, g/100 ml	Sodium, mEq/100 ml	Potassium, mEq/100 ml	Chloride, mEq/100 ml	Calcium, mg/100 ml	Phosphorus, mg/100 ml
STANDARD FORMULAS										
Breast milk	22	75	1.1	4.5	6.8	0.7	1.3	1.1	33.6	16.0
Cow's milk, whole, fortified	21	69	3.5	3.5	4.9	2.5	3.6	2.7	120.0	96.0
Evaporated milk, diluted 1:1, fortified	21	69	3.5	4.0	4.9	2.8	3.9	3.2	134.6	102.5
Goat's milk, fresh	21	69	3.6	4.0	4.6	1.4	4.6	4.5	128.0	104.9
Bremil (Syntex)	20	66	1.5	3.5	7.0	1.3	2.2	1.3	62.0	41.3
Enfamil (Mead Johnson)	20	66	1.5	3.7	7.0	1.1	1.8	1.1	55.0	43.0
Enfamil with Iron (Mead Johnson)	20	66	1.5	3.7	7.0	1.1	1.8	1.1	55.0	43.0
Similac (Ross)	20	66	1.8	3.6	7.0	1.3	2.3	1.8	69.9	49.2
Similac with Iron (Ross)	20	66	1.8	3.6	7.0	1.3	2.3	1.8	69.9	49.2
SMA Improved (Wyeth)	20	66	1.5	3.5	6.8	0.7	1.4	1.0	44.0	33.0
THERAPEUTIC FORMULAS										
Milk Allergy										
Isomil (Ross)	20	66	2.0	3.6	6.8	1.4	1.8	1.5	69.9	50.2
Meat Base Formula (1:1½ dilution) (Gerber)	17	56	2.8	3.2	4.0	0.8	0.9	0.7	97.5	65.0
Mull-Soy (Syntex)	20	66	3.1	3.6	5.2	1.6	4.0	1.6	120.0	78.2
Neo-Mull-Soy (Syntex)	20	66	1.8	3.5	6.4	1.7	2.5	0.6	84.0	41.0
Nursoy (Wyeth)	20	66	1.5	3.5	6.8	0.7	2.1	1.0	44.0	33.0
Nutramigen (Mead Johnson)	20	66	2.2	2.6	8.6	1.3	2.6	2.3	88.7	62.5
Pro-Sobee (Mead Johnson)	20	66	2.5	3.4	6.8	2.1	2.2	0.7	94.0	65.0
Soyalac (Loma Linda)	20	66	2.1	4.0	5.8	1.4	2.3	1.0	40.6	35.6
Electrolyte Imbalance										
Lytren (Mead Johnson)	8	26	none	none	6.6	2.5	2.5	3.0	7.9	8.6
Pedialyte (Ross)	6	20	none	none	5.0	3.0	2.0	3.0	7.9	none
Middle Chain Triglyceride Requirement										
Portagen (Mead Johnson)	20	66	2.3	3.1	7.4	1.7	2.6	2.0	67.0	53.0
Carbohydrate and/or Fat Restriction										
CHO-Free Formula Base (Syntex)	12	40	1.8	3.5	0.02	1.6	2.2	0.6	87.0	66.9
Pregestimil (Mead Johnson)	20	66	2.2	2.8	8.8	1.9	2.3	2.2	90.0	70.0
Skim milk, fortified, market average	11	36	3.6	trace	5.3	2.3	3.6	3.0	122.7	98.0
High Protein and/or Caloric Requirement										
Premature Formula (Mead Johnson)	24	81	2.8	3.7	9.1	2.0	3.2	2.3	93.4	72.1
Probana (Mead Johnson)	20	66	4.2	2.2	7.9	2.5	2.9	2.8	110.7	85.[illegible]
Renal Solute Restriction										
Breast Milk (see above)										
Similac PM 60/40 (Ross)	20	66	1.5	3.4	7.2	0.6	1.4	1.2	32.0	16.5
Sodium Restriction										
Lonalac (Mead Johnson)	20	66	3.4	3.5	4.8	0.1	2.6	1.7	113.2	103.3
Phenylketonuria										
Lofenalac (Mead Johnson) (Rx)	20	66	2.5	2.7	8.5	1.9	2.5	2.2	90.0	62.5

[a] Values are based on ready-to-use strength and were obtained with cooperation of the Dietary Service, Shands Hospital, Gainesville, Florida, and manufacturers cited.

n, g/ 0 ml	Type of carbohydrate	Source of protein	Type of fat	Vit. A, IU/ liter	Vit. D, IU/ liter	Thiamine, mg/liter	Niacin[b] (equivalent), mg/liter	Ascorbic acid, mg/liter
.15	lactose	human milk	human milk fat	2,400	5	0.16	3.5	8
.05	lactose	cow's milk	butterfat	1,850	400	0.29	1.0	10
.05	lactose	cow's milk	butterfat	1,850	400	0.20	1.0	7
.1	lactose	goat's milk	goat's milk fat	2,074	24	0.40	1.9	15
ce	sucrose, lactose	cow's milk	corn, peanut, soy, coconut oils	2,500	400	0.40	6.0	50
ce	lactose	cow's milk	corn, oleo, coconut oils	1,600	400	0.40	7.5	52
.2	lactose	cow's milk	corn, oleo, coconut oils	1,600	400	0.40	7.5	52
ce	lactose	cow's milk	soy, coconut, corn oils	2,500	400	0.65	7.0	55
.2	lactose	cow's milk	soy, coconut, corn oils	2,500	400	0.65	7.0	55
.3	lactose	demineralized whey	safflower oil (blend)	2,500	400	0.67	9.5	55
.2	sucrose, malto-dextrins	soy isolate	soy, corn, coconut oils	2,500	400	0.40	9.0	47
.5	sucrose, modified tapioca starch	beef heart	sesame, beef fat	1,500	400	0.50	10.0	50
.5	sucrose, inverted sucrose	soy	soy oil	2,000	400	0.53	9.5	42
.8	sucrose	soy isolate	soy oil	2,000	400	0.50	7.0	50
.2	sucrose, corn syrup	soy isolate	safflower oil (blend)	2,500	400	0.67	9.5	55
.2	sucrose, arrowroot starch	hydrolyzed casein	corn, MCT oils	2,000	400	0.60	8.0	52
.2	corn syrup solids	soy isolate	soy oil	2,000	400	0.60	8.0	52
.0	sucrose, dextrose, maltose, dextrins	soy	soy oil	2,000	400	0.36	0.8	30
ne	dextrose, maltose, dextrins	none	none	none	none	none	none	none
ne	glucose	none	none	none	none	none	none	none
.2	sucrose, malto-dextrose	casein	corn, MCT oils	2,667	267	1.00	12.0	53
.8	none	soy	soy oil	2,000	400	0.50	7.0	52
.2	glucose, tapioca starch	hydrolyzed casein	corn, MCT oils	2,000	400	0.60	8.0	52
ce	lactose	cow's milk	none	4,167	400	0.40	trace	19
ce	lactose, sucrose	cow's milk	corn oil	1,500	400	0.30	4.7	50
ce	dextrose, lactose	cow's milk	butterfat, corn oil	5,000	1,000	0.60	8.0	52
.26	lactose	demineralized whey, hydrolyzed casein	corn, coconut oil	2,500	400	0.65	7.3	55
ce	lactose	casein	coconut oil	960	none	0.42	0.8	none
.2	corn syrup, tapioca starch	hydrolyzed casein	corn oil	2,000	400	0.60	8.0	52

ee Table 1 for explanation of niacin equivalent.

Weight Control Products

Glenn D. Appelt

Questions to ask the patient

What is your age, height, and weight?
How long have you had a weight problem?
Have you consulted a physician about the problem?
Are you following a diet?
Which diet preparations have you used previously?
Were they effective?
Are you being treated for any chronic disease such as high blood pressure or diabetes?
What medication are you currently taking?

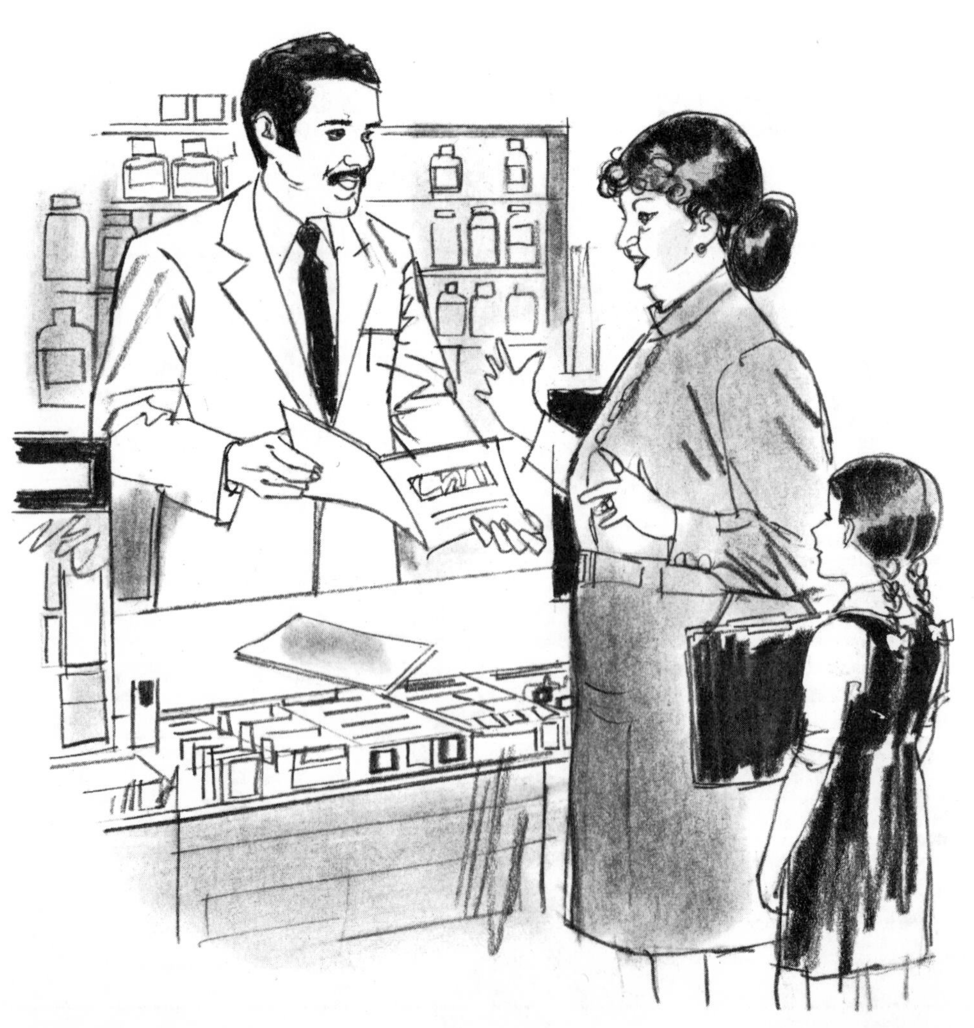

CHAPTER 13

Obesity is the pathological accumulation of fat in excess of that needed for the normal functioning of the body.[1] From a practical viewpoint, obesity may be defined as that physical state where body weight in relation to height is more than 20 percent above the ideal (Table 1).[2] The cause of obesity is caloric intake exceeding caloric expenditure. Although "obesity" is often associated with "overweight," the latter is not in itself a good index for obesity. Athletes, for example, may be overweight but not obese. Daily caloric allowances for persons with moderate physical activity vary with age and sex.[3] Values for males (weight, 154 lb; height, 5 ft 10 in) in a temperate climate range from 3,200 cal at age 25 to 2,550 cal at age 65. Corresponding figures for females (weight, 128 lb; height, 5 ft 4 in) are 2,300 and 1,800 cal. The values for women increase slightly (300 cal) during pregnancy and significantly (1,000 cal) during lactation.

It takes 3,500 excess cal to result in 1 lb of fat. The majority of obesity cases involve overeating, particularly of carbohydrates or fats. The calories ingested beyond those necessary for normal energy requirements are mostly deposited and stored as fat. Because the lack of enough food is rarely a problem in the U.S., Americans are required to make the decision of how much and what type of food to consume. Apparently, many are unwilling to make wise choices; obesity is a chronic American affliction. Some estimates are that 35 percent of Americans are overweight by accepted standards.[4]

Etiology of obesity

The question of why individuals ingest more calories than they expend is a complex one. The answer may be related to physiological, genetic, environmental, or psychological factors. Endocrine disorders, a possible physiological factor, are apparently rarely involved in obesity. Obesity may be the result of an anatomic or a biochemical lesion in the feeding centers of the brain, although this is not proven in humans.[5] Another theory suggests that in the obese person, there is a deficiency of an enzyme responsible for the oxidation of α-glycerophosphate, resulting in increased use of this substrate for the synthesis of triglycerides.[6] A recent hypothesis holds that prostaglandins are involved in the development of obesity through an effect of lipogenesis.[7] Overproduction of prostaglandins in the adipose cells may result in an increase in fat tissue.

Miller *et al.*[8] believe that thin and obese people differ in the degree of thermogenesis after ingestion of food. Overeating in nonobese subjects causes an increase of heat production which tends to dissipate the excess calories. In obese subjects, the thermal dissipation of energy is less pronounced, resulting in the storage of fat. The thermogenesis theory has been expanded to include a description of a specialized form of fat tissue (brown fat) which functions in thermogenesis. The role of brown fat is unclear, but it appears to favor increased hydrolysis of triglycerides.[9]

The Hirsch hypothesis relates infantile obesity to an excess of fat cells during infancy which predisposes the individual to obesity later in life.[10] Obese patients not only have larger than normal fat cells but also an increased number of these cells. Apparently, as people lose weight on a low calorie diet, the size of each fat cell decreases but the total number of fat cells remains the same; when people return to increased weight levels, the fat cells return to their original size. Angel[11] believes that obesity in children of "hyperplastic obesity" is the result of new fat cells, whereas "adult onset obesity" represents an expansion of fat cells already present. Some experiments suggest that the earlier the onset of obesity, the greater the number of fat cells.[12] After the age of 20, obesity is almost exclusively caused by the expansion of existent cells. Accordingly, an overweight child or adolescent may be more susceptible to obesity as an adult.

A child who has one obese parent has a 40-percent chance of being obese; if both parents are obese, there is an 80-percent possibility.[13] These data suggest a direct genetic component, and although it has not been proved in human obesity, animal studies indicate this relationship.[14] In experimental animals, genetic transmission of obesity is associated with modification of organ size and composition.[15 16] Human data suggest fundamental relationships between body build and obesity.[17 18] These studies reveal that obese women differ from nonobese women in a morphological characteristic other than the degree of adiposity. Obese women were more endomorphic than nonobese women, i.e., ("abdomen mass overshadows thoracic bulk; all regions are notable for softness and roundness; and the hands and feet are relatively small.")

An example of environmental influence on obesity is the widespread advertising of food products. Occupational, economic, and sociocultural factors may also be considered in the broad environmental sense. It now appears that socioeconomic status and related social factors are important in the development of obesity. Obesity is seven times more common among women of low socioeconomic groups than among those of high groups.[19] The mental health indexes of the obese subjects in the low socioeconomic group reflected "immaturity," "rigidity," and "suspiciousness" when compared to those of individuals of average weight in the same group. A defect in impulse control might be suspected by the high "immaturity" rating. Obesity was more prevalent in lower socioeconomic status young females than upper socioeconomic status young females.[20] Another study confirmed the greater incidence of obesity among women of low socioeconomic status and found a similar but less marked trend in men. In addition, suggestive relationships between ethnic and religious factors and obesity were found for both sexes.[21]

Obesity has a psychogenic component in 90 percent of the cases.[22] Although the psychological aspect of caloric excess is usually exemplified by compulsive overeating replacing other gratifications, other factors are involved. Stunkard[23] has reported on the relationship of obesity to physical activity and emotions. Decreased physical activity may play a role in the development and maintenance of obesity. This involves the aspect of caloric expenditure rather than caloric ingestion, and stresses the idea of caloric disequilibrium in the consideration of obesity. Mental depression may not be a purely incidental occurrence in obese people but rather one of the main reasons for the obesity.[23] Another psychological aberration in obese patients is the disturbance in body image where one's body is viewed as "grotesque and loathsome." [24]

Appetite control

The hypothalamus apparently contains centers which are intimately involved in the process of food ingestion. Studies in rats show a "satiety center" and an "appetite center" located in the hypothalamic region.[25] Destruction of the satiety center leads to marked overeating with subsequent obesity; conversely, the obliteration of the appetite center results in emaciation. These results indicate that there may be a feedback inhibition of the appetite center by impulses from the satiety center after the ingestion of food. The glucostatic hypothesis of appetite regulation states that hunger is related to the degree that glucose is used by cells called "glucostats." [26] When glucose utilization by glucostats in the satiety center is low, the inhibitory effect on the appetite center is reduced, favoring eating behavior. Conversely, when glucose utilization is high, the appetite center is inhibited and the desire for food intake is reduced.

The hypothalamus contains high concentrations of noradrenergic terminals.[27] A discrete fiber system that supplies the hypothalamus with most of its noradrenergic terminals is called the "ventral noradrenergic bundle." Destruction of the noradrenergic terminals in the hypothalamus or damage of the ventral noradrenergic bundle results in obesity in animals.[28] It is suggested that this noradrenergic bundle normally mediates satiety and that it may serve as a substrate for amphetamine-induced loss of appetite.[29]

The interpretation of visual and chemical stimuli related to food occurs in the cerebral cortex, and acceptance or rejection of the sight, aroma, or taste of foods involves this area of the CNS. Hoebel[30] has suggested that an obese person responds differently from people of normal weight to the appearance, taste, and sight of food. Research involving the trigeminal nerve, a pathway relaying sensory input from the oral cavity to the hypothalamus, indicates a possible role of this system in food intake. The trigeminal circuit is a system of oral touch, and the excessive nibbling common to obese individuals may be due to a greater sensitivity to this stimulus in these persons.[31]

Role of obesity in other conditions

Studies of life insurance records show a significant association between early mortality and obesity. Cardiovascular diseases account for the majority of this early mortality.[32] There is evidence that sustained hypertension is more common in overweight people, although the correlation between blood pressure and adiposity is weak.[33] Vascular change and cerebral vascular disease have been associated with obesity.[34 35]

The relationship between obesity and diabetes mellitus is clear cut.[32] An early study revealed that 85 percent of those over 40 who developed diabetes mellitus were overweight.[36] Glucose intolerance commonly occurs with obesity, and relative insulin resistance is noted in obese subjects.[37 38] The hyperinsulinemia that occurs in obesity is related to the increase in body fat.[39] Weight reduction results in an improvement in glucose tolerance in the obese diabetic and a reduction in the hyperinsulinemia in both nondiabetic and diabetic obese persons.[40 41] The severity of diabetes mellitus and the need for medication can often be decreased by weight reduction.

Hyperostosis of the spine (formation of bony bridges between the vertebrae) has been associated with hyperglycemia and obesity, although these factors are at least partly independent of each other.[42] Excess obesity may contribute to respiratory stress. Obesity alters pulmonary function resulting in plethora reduction of lung volume, hypercapnia, and pulmonary hypertension.[43] The description by Charles Dickens of Joe (the fat boy) in *The Pickwick Papers* reveals a person with marked obesity and somnolence. Burwell *et al.*[44] believe this to be the first description of this condition in the literature and called it a "Pickwickian syndrome." A person so described is obese, exhibits narcoleptic behavior, and has an excessive appetite.

Varicose veins and back trouble may be directly related to excess weight.

Signs and symptoms of obesity

Common patient complaints regarding obesity are often cosmetic, involving a desire to obtain the "slim look." Remarks such as "I can't tie my shoes without getting out of breath" indicate actual physical discomfort. The obese patient may complain of persistent backache and varicose veins.

Because obesity may be caused by the inactivity resulting from mental depression, patients who remain obese after prolonged self-medication with OTC obesity control products should be referred to a physician.[20] It is conceivable that a psychogenic component involving inactivity due to depression or a compulsive anxiety reaction related to repeated "snacking" may be involved in such cases. It is important for the pharmacist to emphasize that weight loss will not occur unless caloric disequilibrium is corrected. Chronic use of OTC drugs to correct obesity may indicate a more severe underlying problem.

Treatment

Diets in the 800 to 1,000 cal/day range are frequently used in weight reduction programs. Total fasting or semistarvation is sometimes proposed as a means of weight reduction in grossly obese persons.[45 46] Starvation, either total or partial, depletes the body of lean tissue and essential electrolytes in addition to fat.[47] The ketosis and ketoacidosis of a fasting state reflect a metabolic alteration. If total fasting is employed as a means of treating obesity, hospitalization is recommended in order to better treat mood changes or alteration of physiologic functions such as cardiac arrhythmias.[48] "Crash" diets involving 500 cal daily for 4 to 8 weeks have recently been implicated in loss of scalp hair.[49] This apparently reflects the trauma of semistarvation.

Group therapy and behavior modification are sometimes effective in the treatment of obesity. Groups such as TOPS (Take Off Pounds Sensibly) have been successful in the treatment of obesity.[50] The group pressure resulting from praise or criticism apparently is an effective deterrence to overeating for many persons. Behavior modification involving the consideration of eating as a "pure" activity and a slower pace of eating may be beneficial. In addition, a "diet diary" and using a "unit dose" concept of foods may prove helpful in a weight reduction program. Psychotherapeutic approaches also show promise in obesity control.[51]

In refractory cases of gross obesity, intestinal bypass operations have been performed.[52] This type of procedure is probably the most hazardous measure used to treat extreme obesity.

Drug treatment of obesity is of limited value.[53] Amphetamines have been prescribed for obesity. Amphetamine and related drugs are thought to suppress appetite by an effect on the appetite centers in the hypothalamus.[54] Tolerance develops to the appetite suppressant activity of amphetamine, making long-term use undesirable. Because overeating seems to be primarily controlled by psychological behavioral factors, overeating will occur as soon as the anorexogenic effects disappear. Amphetamine and related drugs have the potential for abuse and dependence. It is apparent that they have only limited value for short-term use in obesity control and only as an adjunct to dietary control.

Human chorionic gonadotropin has been used by some clinicians in the treatment of obesity. The effectiveness of this hormone in the treatment of obesity has not been established.[37]

OTC obesity control products are represented by phenylpropanolamine (a drug that may act similarly to amphetamine), benzocaine (a local anesthetic), and methylcellulose (a bulk producer). It is reasonable to expect weight loss in an individual who takes OTC weight reduction drugs or other substances such as carbohydrate dietary aids, if the calorie intake is reduced so that caloric expenditure is greater. Whether the agent is pharmacologically active or a placebo, if it allows the patient to accomplish this, weight will be lost. Dietary aids such as carbohydrate "candy" type foods and low caloric, nutritionally balanced liquids are not considered drugs but are available as adjuncts in a weight reduction program. In addition, synthetic sweeteners such as saccharin may be valuable in reducing excess consumption of sugar, lowering caloric intake.

In summary, dietary management through proper guidance and patient motivation are of prime importance in any weight reduction program. The first few months of a weight reduction program seem to be the most successful. This may due to the willingness of the patients to subject themselves to self-discipline.

Table 1. Desirable Weights for Men and Women According to Height and Frame, Ages 25 and Over[a]

Height (in shoes)[b]	Weight in pounds (in indoor clothing) Small frame	Medium frame	Large frame
Men			
5 ft 2 in	112–120	118–129	126–141
5 ft 3 in	115–123	121–133	129–144
5 ft 4 in	118–126	124–136	132–148
5 ft 5 in	121–129	127–139	135–152
5 ft 6 in	124–133	130–143	138–156
5 ft 7 in	128–137	134–147	142–161
5 ft 8 in	132–141	138–152	147–166
5 ft 9 in	136–145	142–156	151–170
5 ft 10 in	140–150	146–160	155–174
5 ft 11 in	144–154	150–165	159–179
6 ft 0 in	148–158	154–170	164–184
6 ft 1 in	152–162	158–175	168–189
6 ft 2 in	156–167	162–180	173–194
6 ft 3 in	160–171	167–185	177–199
6 ft 4 in	164–175	172–190	182–204
Women			
4 ft 10 in	92–98	96–107	104–119
4 ft 11 in	94–101	98–110	106–122
5 ft 0 in	96–104	101–113	109–124
5 ft 1 in	99–107	104–116	112–128
5 ft 2 in	102–110	107–119	115–131
5 ft 3 in	105–113	110–122	118–134
5 ft 4 in	108–116	113–126	121–138
5 ft 5 in	111–119	116–130	125–142
5 ft 6 in	114–123	120–135	129–146
5 ft 7 in	118–127	124–139	133–150
5 ft 8 in	122–131	128–143	137–154
5 ft 9 in	126–135	132–147	141–158
5 ft 10 in	130–140	136–151	145–163
5 ft 11 in	134–144	140–155	149–168
6 ft 0 in	138–148	144–159	153–174

[a] Prepared by the Metropolitan Life Insurance Company. Derived primarily from data of the Build and Blood Pressure Study, 1959.
[b] Based on 1-inch heels for men and 2-inch heels for women.

Ingredients in OTC products

Phenylpropanolamine. Phenylpropanolamine is a sympathomimetic agent which is chemically and pharmacologically related to ephedrine and amphetamine. It acts indirectly and has prominent peripheral adrenergic effects and weak central stimulant actions.[55] In the past, a controversy has existed as to the effectiveness of phenylpropanolamine as an anorexogenic agent.[56] Early animal studies indicated its usefulness in diminishing food intake in animals.[57,58] Later clinical studies indicated a possible appetite suppressant activity of the drug. Hoebel *et al.* [59,60] conducted double-blind studies with volunteer human subjects who were concerned about their weight. Results from one experiment indicated that phenylpropanolamine (25 mg), taken 30 minutes before lunch, reduced intake of a liquid diet.[59] In another study, volunteers reported a significant reduction in the size of supper and the number of snacks when taking phenylpropanolamine (25 mg).[60] A double-blind, clinical evaluation of a phenylpropanolamine/caffeine/vitamin combination showed a significantly greater weight loss as compared to a placebo when used over a 4-week period by patients on a 1,200-cal diet.[61]

All authorities, however, do not agree on the effectiveness of phenylpropanolamine as an anorexogenic agent. The *AMA Drug Evaluations* states that "This agent is probably ineffective in the dose provided (25 mg)." [62] A basic pharmacology textbook states that the drug is ineffective as an appetite suppressant.[63] In addition, no mention of its use in obesity is made in a standard pharmacy reference.[55]

Amphetamine and related prescription drugs apparently depress appetite by stimulating the satiety center in the ventromedial nucleus of the hypothalamus. This may occur indirectly on the frontal lobes of the cortex.[64] Although the effects of phenylpropanolamine on the cardiovascular system and CNS are not as strong as those of amphetamine, there is the possibility of side effects, particularly if the recommended dosage is exceeded. Phenylpropanolamine may produce several untoward effects, including nervousness, restlessness, insomnia, headache, nausea, tachycardia, palpitation, and excessive rise in blood pressure.[55] Various adverse reactions of the cardiovascular system have been reported, and the label on products containing phenylpropanolamine warns against exceeding the dosage regimen of 25 mg three times a day.[65-69] Phenylpropanolamine dosage information from the minutes of the FDA OTC Panel on Cold, Cough, Allergy, Bronchodilator, and Antiasthmatic Drugs may be pertinent, although the Panel was not reviewing anoretics as such.[70] In doses of as much as 50 mg every 3 hours, side effects such as nervousness, insomnia, motor restlessness, and nausea can occur, although the incidence is equal to or slightly greater than with a placebo. A dose of 25 to 50 mg every 4 hours, not to exceed 150 mg in 24 hours, was found to be safe. Because phenylpropanolamine is an adrenergic substance, it may elevate blood sugar levels and produce cardiac stimulation. For these reasons, the labels on products containing this drug warn that individuals who have diabetes mellitus, heart disease, hypertension, or thyroid disease should seek medical advice before taking the drug.

Many drug interactions with adrenergic agents are theoretically possible, but clinically, phenylpropanolamine has only been implicated in interactions with monoamine oxidase inhibitors.[71-73] Severe hypertensive episodes may be more likely when preparations containing phenylpropanolamine in a free form, rather than in slow-release form, are ingested by patients taking monoamine oxidase inhibitors concurrently.[72 73] There is one report of a positive phentolamine pheochromocytoma test in hypertension induced by phenylpropanolamine.[74] Reserpine and guanethidine may interfere with actions of phenylpropanolamine.[55] Some OTC products contain caffeine and phenylpropanolamine; the possibility of an additive effect with these two cardiac stimulants should be considered.[67]

Bulk producers. Typical examples of bulk producers are methylcellulose, carboxymethylcellulose, psyllium mucilloid, agar, and karaya gum. It has been suggested that the bulk-producing activity produces a sense of fullness, reducing the desire to eat. The usefulness of the bulk-forming agents as appetite suppressants in the control of obesity has not been established.[75] A radiographic study shows that a methylcellulose mass is almost entirely gone from the stomach in 30 minutes. In addition, there is an increase in intestinal peristalsis following the rapid gastric emptying.[76] Neither bulk production by methylcellulose nor gastric transport rate increase offers a mechanism to produce satiety. No experimental evidence exists to support an appetite suppressant claim. These bulk-producing substances have been approved for dietary use by the FDA.[77] It is assumed that the benefit of bulk producers in obesity control would be related to reduction of calorie intake, irrespective of the ingestion of the bulk producer. It would appear that the bulk producers are no more effective than a low-calorie, high-residue diet in a weight reduction program. The laxative effect of bulk producers may not always be desirable. There is some danger of esophageal obstruction with methylcellulose wafers, and it is recommended that generous amounts of water accompany the ingestion of the bulk producers to minimize this danger.[75] Drugs with anticholinergic properties reduce bowel motility, and concurrent use of these drugs with bulk producers may be hazardous because they may produce blockage.

Benzocaine. The incorporation of benzocaine in a preparation designed for weight control was suggested in 1958 by Plotz.[78] A preparation containing benzocaine and methylcellulose in wafers of chewing gum was tried for 10 weeks in 50 patients who were 12 to 102 lb overweight. The patients were instructed to chew one or two wafers, followed by drinking a glass of water, just before meals. They were also placed on diets of reduced calorie intake, and directed to chew the gum every 4 hours if there was a strong desire to eat. Ninety percent of the overweight individuals experienced weight loss. However, the study was not controlled, and the weight loss could have been caused by the benzocaine, the methylcellulose, or the diet itself. The dose of benzocaine used was small, and any marked degree of numbness in the oral cavity was questionable. It is conceivable that subtle effects on taste sensitivity or modification of taste occur, and that perceived analgesia or numbness is not necessary for possible appetite suppressant activity. It has already been suggested that obese persons may be more sensitive to taste stimuli.[31]

Constant snacking is characteristic of the "oral syndrome" in many obese persons. A nontraditional appetite control plan using benzocaine, glucose, caffeine, and vitamins in a hard candy form has been tried.[78] The subjects ingested the candies when they had the desire to snack and before and after meals. The purpose of the approach was to keep the patients orally active while elevating their blood glucose levels. The influence of benzocaine was considered to be a requisite for "meaningful losses" in this study.

Capsules or tablets containing benzocaine are designed to be swallowed and hence, the drug does not come into contact with the oral cavity. Any appetite suppression would depend upon an effect on the GI mucosa. There are no conclusive clinical data in the literature to support such an activity.

Although they are rare, cyanotic reactions have been reported following the administration of benzocaine.[79] Reports of methemoglobinemia in infants also are in the literature.[80-83] These reactions refer mainly to infants and therefore, are not specifically relevant to the use of the drug in the noninfant obese population. It is important, however, to be aware that this potential for benzocaine toxicity exists. A fatal anaphylactic reaction occurred in an adult a few minutes after the ingestion of a throat lozenge containing benzocaine.[84] Conceivably, obese persons may take preparations containing benzocaine over long periods, possibly exposing themselves to the consequences of sensitivity induced by the drug. Also, there are no conclusive data to support the appetite suppression effect of benzocaine.

Other products

Glucose. The claim has been made that preparations containing glucose and vitamins elevate blood glucose levels when taken before meals or at snack time, so that the satiety center exerts an inhibitory influence on the appetite center. This assertion, however, is questionable. A clinical study reported that a glucose load (50 g) taken 20 minutes before lunch depressed caloric intake relative to control load at lunch ($P<0.01$).[85] It is suggested that reactions to the oral qualities of the glucose load constitute the principal factor in the first 20 minutes rather than GI or postabsorptive effects on satiety. However, the efficacy of glucose in long-term weight control programs has not been established.

Low-calorie, nutritionally balanced foods. The "canned diet" products are considered substitutes for the usual diet. One product typical of this group supplies 70 g of protein daily, an amount which the manufacturer states "is the recommended daily dietary allowance of protein for normal adults." It also contains 20 g of fat and 110 g of carbohydrate in a daily ration. Powder, granule, and liquid forms are now available, and these products are also formulated into cookies and soups.

These dietary foods are low in sodium. Weight loss in the first 2 weeks is probably caused, in part, by loss of water from the tissues. Whether a loss of weight over a short period is significant with regard to the effective long-term treatment of obesity is somewhat questionable.

The pharmacist should be aware that products that substitute 900 cal daily for the usual diet are usually effective in reducing weight. Moreover, it appears that any diet of 900 cal which supplies adequate protein and lower carbohydrate and fat intake would result in weight loss in an obese patient.

Artificial sweeteners. Sucrose overuse is common. A sucrose substitute, saccharin, contains no calories and may allow for significant calorie reduction in certain patients. Saccharin is about 400 times more potent than sucrose as a sweetener. It produces a bitter taste in some individuals, and it is not heat stable; nevertheless, it is the most popular artificial sweetener, especially since the prohibition of the nonregulated use of cyclamates. Saccharin may have considerable importance in reducing caloric intake for some persons. For instance, if saccharin is used to sweeten a cup of coffee instead of 1 tsp of sugar, 33 cal are removed from the diet. In 1972, bladder tumors were discovered in rats fed saccharin *in utero* and throughout life. The FDA then removed saccharin from the list of food additives generally recognized as safe. Saccharin is presently permitted in products labeled specifically as diet foods or beverages. It may accumulate in fetal tissues and should not be used during pregnancy.[86]

Aspartame is a synthetic dipeptide about 180 times as sweet as sugar. The manufacturer has suspended marketing of aspartame after a metabolite of aspartame was reported to produce uterine polyps in rats. If, after further evaluation, aspartame becomes available, the FDA will require the following label warning: "Phenylketonurics: contains phenylalanine." Women with homozygous phenylketonuria (PKU) who were treated with low-phenylalanine diets and are now at childbearing age may not be aware of the disease.[87] Phenylalanine blood levels of over 12 mg percent during pregnancy increase the risk of fetal abnormalities.

Sugar alcohols such as sorbitol and mannitol have been used as sugar substitutes. The ingestion of sufficient amounts of dietetic candies containing sorbitol may result in an osmotic catharsis in small children.[88]

Dosage forms

OTC products for obesity control are available as liquids, powders, granules, tablets, capsules, sustained-release capsules, wafers, cookies, soups, chewing gum, and candy preparations. If candy cubes, wafers, or chewing gum are substituted for high calorie desserts or "snacks," the confectionogenic nature of the dosage form may offer a psychologic aid to the patients, as compared to a standard tablet or capsule. The ingestion of large quantities of diet candy would, of course, contribute significantly to calorie intake.

Guidelines for product selection

It is of paramount importance that the pharmacist advise the patient of the importance of a diet plan or program. Weight cannot be lost without a concerted effort to change life style and maintain it. An appreciation of the caloric value of food types should be conveyed to the patient in order that the diet be carried out appropriately. An OTC obesity control product should be considered as an adjunct to this planned weight reduction program. Vitamins are sometimes added to OTC obesity control products on the assumption that dieting individuals may not have an adequate vitamin intake. This may be justified in individual cases but cannot be applied to all patients. Caffeine is included in some preparations, probably in an effort to allay fatigue, a factor which may lead to an impulsive desire to eat.

Summary

The effectiveness of a weight reduction program depends largely on the education of the patient and the acceptance of the regimen necessary to achieve long-term weight control. A patient should recognize the many facets of a successful weight reduction program, including motivation, physical activity, reduced caloric intake, and possibly a pharmacologic "crutch" such as an OTC drug. The role of the pharmacist is to supply pertinent information regarding these matters.

References

1. R. S. Goodhart and M. E. Shils, "Modern Nutrition in Health and Disease," Lea and Febiger, Philadelphia, Pa., 1973, p. 625.
2. Metropolitan Life Insurance Company Statistical Bulletin, **47**, 1(1966).
3. M. G. Wohl, "Modern Nutrition in Health and Disease," Lea and Febiger, Philadelphia, Pa., 1960, p. 532.
4. M. G. Wagner, *J. Am. Diet. Assoc.*, **57**, 311(1970).
5. J. Mayer, *Annu. Rev. Med.*, **14**, 111(1963).
6. D. J. Galton, *Br. Med. J.*, **2**, 1498(1966).
7. P. B. Curtis-Prior, *Lancet*, **1**, 897(1975).
8. D. S. Miller *et al.*, *Am. J. Clin. Nutr.*, **20**, 1223(1967).
9. R. E. Smith and B. A. Horowitz, *Physiol. Rev.*, **49**, 330(1969).
10. J. Hirsch and J. L. Knittle, *Fed. Proc.*, **29**, 1516(1970).
11. A. Angel, *Can. Med. Assoc. J.*, **110**, 540(1974).
12. L. B. Salans *et al.*, *J. Clin. Invest.*, **52**, 929(1973).
13. S. R. Williams, "Nutrition and Diet Therapy," Mosby, St. Louis, Mo., 1967, p. 477.
14. J. Mayer, *Bull. N.Y. Acad. Med.*, **36**, 323(1960).
15. K. J. Carpenter and J. Mayer, *Am. J. Physiol.*, **193**, 449(1958).
16. N. B. Marshall *et al.*, *Am. J. Physiol.*, **189**, 342(1957).
17. C. C. Seltzer and J. Mayer, *J. Am. Med. Assoc.*, **189**, 667(1964).
18. C. C. Seltzer and J. Mayer, *J. Am. Diet. Assoc.*, **55**, 454(1969).
19. M. E. Moore *et al.*, *J. Am. Med. Assoc.*, **181**, 962(1962).
20. A. Stunkard *et al.*, *J. Am. Med. Assoc.*, **221**, 579(1972).
21. P. B. Goldblatt *et al.*, *J. Am. Med. Assoc.*, **192**, 97(1965).
22. "Drugs of Choice 1972-1973," W. Modell, Ed., Mosby, St. Louis, Mo., 1972, p. 285.
23. A. Stunkard, *Psychosom. Med.*, **20**, 366(1958).
24. A. Stunkard and M. Mendelson, *J. Am. Diet. Assoc.*, **38**, 328(1961).
25. A. W. Hetherington and S. W. Ransom, *Am. J. Physiol.*, **136**, 609(1942).
26. J. Mayer, *Ann. N.Y. Acad. Sci.*, **63**, 15(1955).
27. V. Vngorstedt, *Acta Physiol. Scand. Suppl.*, **365**, 1(1971).
28. J. E. Ahlskog and B. G. Hoebel, *Science*, **182**, 166(1973).
29. R. M. Gold, *Science*, **182**, 488(1973).
30. B. G. Hoebel, *Annu. Rev. Physiol.*, **33**, 533(1971).
31. H. P. Ziegler, *Psychology Today*, Aug. 1975, p. 62.
32. H. H. Marks, *Metabolism*, **6**, 417(1957).
33. G. V. Mann, *N. Engl. J. Med.*, **291**, 178(1974).
34. S. L. Wilens, *Arch. Intern. Med.*, **79**, 120(1947).
35. S. Heyden *et al.*, *Arch. Intern. Med.*, **128**, 956(1971).
36. G. F. Baker, "Clinic and Metropolitan Life Insurance Co.: Diabetes in the 1940's," New York Metropolitan Life Insurance Co. Press, 1940.
37. G. V. Mann, *N. Engl. J. Med.*, **291**, 226(1974).
38. S. M. Genuth, *Ann. Intern. Med.*, **79**, 812(1973).
39. A. Z. El-Khodary *et al.*, *Metabolism*, **21**, 641(1972).
40. J. H. Karam *et al.*, *Lancet*, **1**, 286(1965).
41. R. S. Yalow *et al.*, *Ann. N.Y. Acad. Sci.*, **131**, 357(1965).
42. H. Julkunen *et al.*, *Ann. Rheu. Dis.*, **30**, 605(1971).
43. R. H. L. Wilson and N. L. Wilson, *J. Am. Diet. Assoc.*, **55**, 465(1969).
44. C. S. Burwell *et al.*, *Am. J. Med.*, **21**, 811(1956).
45. W. L. Bloom, *Metabolism*, **8**, 214(1959).
46. S. M. Genuth *et al.*, *J. Am. Med. Assoc.*, **230**, 987(1974).
47. R. E. Bolinger *et al.*, *Arch. Intern. Med.*, **118**, 3(1966).
48. I. C. Gilliand, *Postgrad. Med. J.*, **44**, 58(1968).
49. R. B. Odum and D. K. Goette, *J. Am. Med. Assoc.*, **235**, 476(1976).
50. A. Stunkard *et al.*, *Arch. Intern. Med.*, **125**, 1067(1970).
51. A. Stunkard *et al.*, *Arch. Gen. Psychiatry*, **26**, 391(1972).
52. H. F. Conn, "Current Therapy," Saunders, Philadelphia, Pa., 1975, p. 406.
53. *FDA Drug Bull.*, December, 1972.

54. S. Cole, *Psychol. Bull.*, **79**, 13(1973).
55. "Remington's Pharmaceutical Sciences," 15th ed., A. Osol *et al.*, Eds., Mack Publishing, Easton, Pa., 1975, p. 820.
56. H. I. Silverman, *Am. J. Pharm.*, **135**, 45(1963).
57. M. L. Tainter, *J. Nutr.*, **27**, 89(1944).
58. A. Epstein, *Comp. Physiol. Psychol.*, **52**, 37(1959).
59. B. G. Hoebel *et al.*, *Obesity/Bariatric Med.*, **4**, 192(1975).
60. B. G. Hoebel, *Obesity/Bariatric Med.*, **4**, 200(1975).
61. S. I. Griboff *et al.*, *Curr. Ther. Res.*, **17**, 535(1975).
62. "AMA Drug Evaluations," 2d ed., Publishing Sciences Group, Acton, Mass., 1973, p. 370.
63. A. Goth, "Medical Pharmacology," 7th ed., Mosby, St. Louis, Mo., 1974, p. 110.
64. W. C. Bowman *et al.*, "Textbook of Pharmacology," Blackwell Scientific Publications, Oxford, England, 1968, p. 332.
65. P. R. Salmon, *Br. Med. J.*, **1**, 193(1965).
66. S. R. Shapiro, *N. Engl. J. Med.*, **280**, 1363(1969).
67. R. B. Peterson and L. A. Vasquez, *J. Am. Med. Assoc.*, **223**, 324(1973).
68. S. Ostern and W. H. Dodson, *J. Am. Med. Assoc.*, **194**, 472(1965).
69. P. H. Livingston, *J. Am. Med. Assoc.*, **196**, 1159(1966).
70. Summary Minutes of OTC/FDA Panel on Cold, Cough, Allergy, Bronchodilator, and Antiasthmatic Drugs, June 19-20, 1973, Food and Drug Administration, Bureau of Drugs, Washington, D. C., 1973.
71. C. M. Tonks and A. T. Lloyd, *Br. Med. J.*, **1**, 589(1965).
72. A. M. S. Mason and R. M. Buckle, *Br. Med. J.*, **1**, 875(1969).
73. M. F. Cuthbert *et al.*, *Br. Med. J.*, **1**, 404(1969).
74. F. C. Duvernoy, *N. Engl. J. Med.*, **280**, 877(1969).
75. "The Pharmacological Basis of Therapeutics," 5th ed., L. S. Goodman and A. Gilman, Eds., Macmillan, New York, N.Y., 1975, p. 979.
76. E. J. Drenick, *J. Am. Med. Assoc.*, **234**, 271(1975).
77. D. C. Fletcher, *J. Am. Med. Assoc.*, **230**, 901(1974).
78. C. W. McLure and C. A. Brusch, *J. Am. Med., Women's Assoc.*, **28**, 239(1973).
79. B. M. Bernstein, *Rev. Gastroenterol.*, **17**, 123(1950).
80. H. de C. Peterson, *N. Engl. J. Med.*, **263**, 454(1960).
81. N. Goluboff and D. J. MacFadyen, *J. Pediatr.*, **47**, 22(1955).
82. J. A. Wolff, *Pediatrics*, **20**, 915(1957).
83. N. Goluboff, *Pediatrics*, **21**, 340(1958).
84. D. J. Hesch, *J. Am. Med. Assoc.*, **172**, 62(1960).
85. D. A. Booth *et al.*, *Nature*, **228**, 1104(1970).
86. *The Medical Letter*, **17**, 61(1975).
87. R. Koch, *N. Engl. J. Med.*, **292**, 596(1975).
88. J. R. Gryboski, *N. Engl. J. Med.*, **275**, 718(1966).

Products **13** APPETITE SUPPRESSANT

Product (manufacturer)	**Phenylpropanolamine hydrochloride**	**Bulk producer**	**Other**
Anorexin Capsules (Thompson)	25 mg	carboxymethylcellulose sodium, 50 mg	caffeine, 100 mg; vitamin A, 1667 IU; vitamin D, 133 IU; thiamine, 1 mg; riboflavin, 1 mg; pyridoxine hydrochloride, 0.33 mg; cyanocobalamin, 0.33 μg; ascorbic acid, 20 mg; niacinamide, 7 mg; calcium pantothenate, 0.33 mg
Appedrine Tablets (Thompson)	25 mg	carboxymethylcellulose sodium, 50 mg	caffeine, 100 mg; vitamin A, 1667 IU; vitamin D, 133 IU; thiamine, 1 mg; riboflavin, 1 mg; pyridoxine hydrochloride, 0.33 mg; cyanocobalamin, 0.33 μg; ascorbic acid, 20 mg; niacinamide, 7 mg; calcium pantothenate, 0.33 mg
Dexatrim Capsules (Thompson)	50 mg	—	caffeine, 200 mg
Diet-Trim Tablets (Pharmex)	NS[a]	carboxymethylcellulose	benzocaine
Grapefruit Diet Plan with Diadax Tablets (O'Connor)	10 mg	—	natural grapefruit extract, 16.6 mg; ascorbic acid, 10 mg; vitamin E, 3.6 mg
Grapefruit Diet Plan with Diadax Vitamin Fortified Continuous Action Capsules (O'Connor)	30 mg	—	natural grapefruit extract, 50 mg; ascorbic acid, 30 mg; vitamin E, 11 mg
Nature's Trim Plan with Diadax Tablets (O'Connor)	75 mg	—	lecithin, 125 mg; cider vinegar, 25 mg; pyridoxine hydrochloride, 21 mg; iodine (kelp), 0.15 mg
Odrinex Tablets (Fox)	25 mg	methylcellulose, 50 mg	caffeine, 50 mg
Prolamine Capsules (Thompson)	35 mg	—	caffeine, 140 mg
Spantrol Capsules (North American)	75 mg	carboxymethylcellulose sodium, 135 mg	caffeine (anhydrous), 150 mg; benzocaine, 9 mg; ascorbic acid, 30 mg; thiamine hydrochloride, 1 mg; riboflavin, 1.2 mg; niacinamide, 10 mg; pyridoxine hydrochloride, 1 mg; iron, 10 mg
Vita-Slim Capsules (Thompson)	50 mg	—	vitamin A, 2500 IU; vitamin E, 15 IU; ascorbic acid, 30 mg; folic acid, 0.2 mg; thiamine, 0.75 mg; riboflavin, 0.85 mg; niacinamide, 10 mg; pyridoxine hydrochloride, 10 mg; cyanocobalamin, 3 μg; calcium pantothenate, 5 mg; iron, 9 mg; lecithin, 300 mg; kelp, 75 μg

[a] Quantity not specified.

Product (manufacturer)	Dosage form	Calories supplied	Essential composition
BULK PRODUCERS			
Dex-A-Diet Plan Formula (O'Connor)	capsule	NS[a]	carboxymethylcellulose sodium, 200 mg; vitamins; minerals
Diet-Aid (Rexall)	tablet	NS[a]	alginic acid, 200 mg; carboxymethylcellulose sodium, 100 mg; sodium bicarbonate, 70 mg
Instant Mix Metamucil (Searle)	powder in single dose packets	3/packet	psyllium mucilloid, 3.7 g; citric acid; sodium bicarbonate (equiv. to 250 mg sodium)
Melozets (Calgon)	wafer	30	methylcellulose, flour, sugar
Metamucil (Searle)	powder	14/tsp	psyllium mucilloid, 50%; dextrose, 50%
Reducets (Columbia Medical)	capsule	0	benzocaine, 5 mg; methylcellulose, 100 mg; multivitamins; minerals
ARTIFICIAL SWEETENERS			
Ril-Sweet (Plough)	liquid	0	saccharin sodium, 3.3%
Sucaryl Sodium (Abbott)	tablet solution	0	saccharin sodium, 5 mg/tablet, 0.8% (solution)
Sweeta (Squibb)	tablet liquid	0	saccharin, 15 mg/tablet, 14 mg/2 drops
LOW CALORIE FOODS			
Dietene (Doyle)	powder	353/100 g powder	nonfat dry milk, sugar, milk protein, cocoa, magnesium sulfate, carrageenan, artificial flavor, lecithin, polysorbate 80, zinc sulfate, malt, vitamins
Metrecal (Drackett)	cookie	25	flour, sugars, milk protein concentrate, vegetable shortening, yeast, vitamins, minerals
Slender (Carnation)	liquid powder to be mixed with milk	225/can 165 mixed with 6 oz skim milk 225 mixed with 6 oz whole milk	nonfat dry milk, sucrose, vegetable oil, artificial flavors, vitamins, minerals
LOW CALORIE CANDY			
Ayds (Campana)	candy cube	25/cube	corn syrup, vegetable oils, sweetened condensed whole milk, vitamins, minerals
Dex-A-Diet (O'Connor)	chewable tablet	4–5	glucose, vitamins
Slim-Line Candy (Thompson)	caramel	21/piece	benzocaine, 8 mg; methylcellulose, 45 mg; corn glucose syrup; sweetened condensed skim milk; sugar; dried sweet whey; corn syrup solids; hardened coconut oil; cocoa; chocolate; salt; glyceryl monostearate; soya lecithin; natural and artificial flavoring
Slim-Line Candy (Thompson)	hard candy	21/piece	benzocaine, 8 mg; methylcellulose, 45 mg; sugar; corn glucose syrup; citric acid; natural and artificial flavoring
Slim-Mint (Thompson)	chewing gum	6/piece	benzocaine, 8 mg; essential oils, 3350 ppm; methylcellulose, 45 mg; sugars, 1.45 g

[a] Quantity not specified.

Sleep Aid and Sedative Products

James P. Caro

Questions to ask the patient

How long has insomnia been a problem? Do you have difficulty sleeping every night or only occasionally?

Is the problem related to falling asleep or remaining asleep?

Can you relate the insomnia to a cause such as a change in work shifts, anxiety, or pain?

Do you use tranquilizers or sleeping pills?

Do you drink coffee or alcohol?

Do you have any chronic diseases?

Have you used sleep-aid products? Which ones? Were they effective?

Are you under the care of a physician?

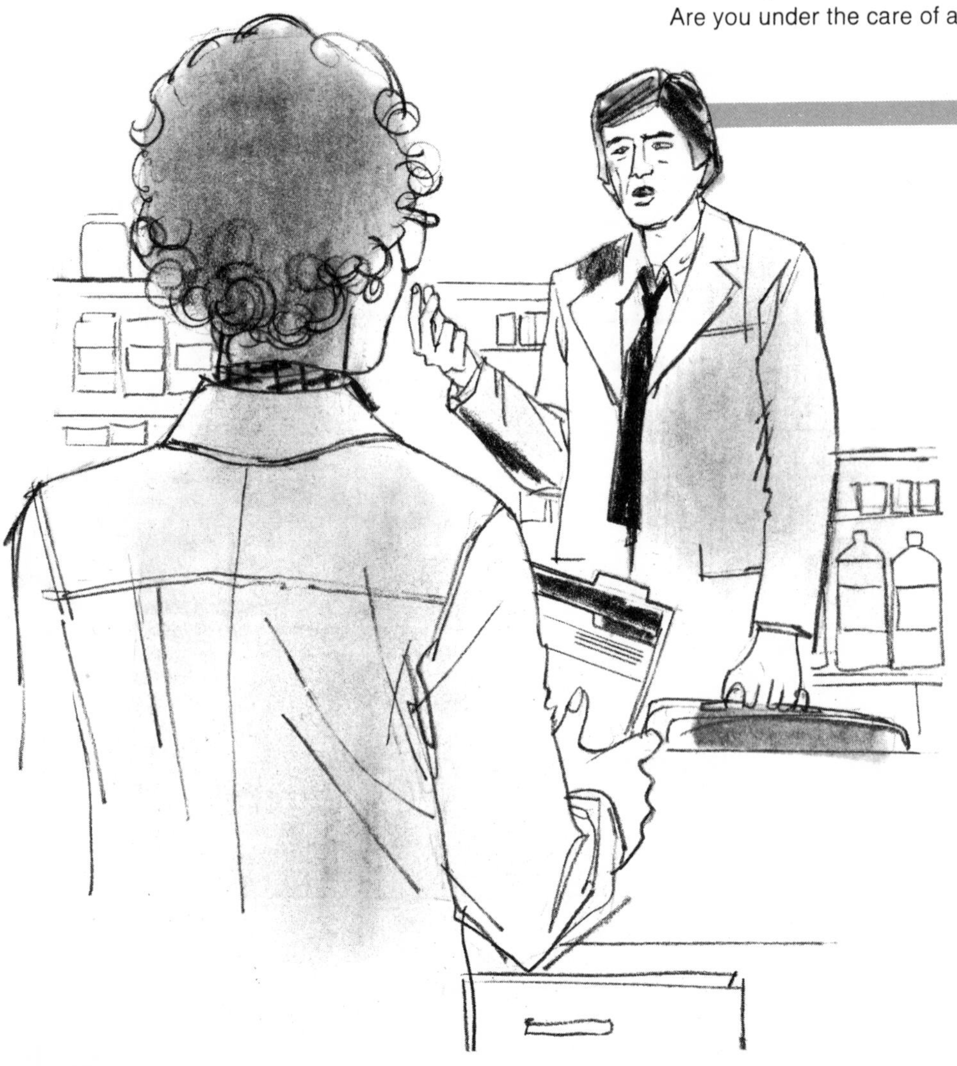

CHAPTER 14

Although many nonprescription preparations are heavily promoted as providing "safe and restful sleep" or relief from "simple nervous tension," claims for the safety and efficacy of these products are unsubstantiated. Many of these products contain drugs found in prescription medications (e.g., bromides, antihistamines, scopolamine) but in much lower doses, and it is assumed that these lower doses minimize the untoward effects of these agents. Unfortunately, the sedative effects are also minimal because, in most cases, sedation is only a secondary (or side) effect rather than the primary pharmacologic effect of the drug. In addition, the sedative effect of these agents is subject to considerable personal variation; some individuals may even experience a paradoxical state of excitement. The low efficacy of these preparations may pose an additional hazard because individuals who do not experience sedation at normal doses may exceed the recommended dose and suffer toxic effects.

Considering the widespread use of OTC sedatives without medical supervision, the need to ensure that they are used appropriately and safely is essential. Preliminary reports from the FDA OTC Panel on Sedatives, Tranquilizers and Sleep Aids question the safety and efficacy of many products on the market.[1]

Physiology of sleep

The sites and mechanisms of action of sleep-inducing drugs are largely unknown. Neurophysiological investigations have yielded many theories concerning the influence of brain structures on consciousness and have provided some insight into the complex feedback systems that control consciousness. It is now known that the brain stem coordinates the activity of these systems.

The brain stem contains the reticular activating system (RAS) which monitors and selectively limits all sensory input to the brain. Although the RAS responds to stimuli by arousing the brain, the cerebral cortex discriminates between stimuli even during sleep. For this reason, only selected stimuli will produce arousal from sleep.[2]

Sleep is characterized by a diminution of activity in the ascending and descending RAS pathways. This process of reticular deactivation occurs by a passive limitation of sensory input (e.g., sleeping in a dark, quiet room) and by active influence from the cerebral cortex, medulla, and possibly other structures.[3]

Sleep is classified into rapid eye movement (REM) and non- rapid eye movement (non-REM) stages (Fig. 1). Non-REM sleep is subdivided into stages I through IV, according to increasing depth of sleep. In young adults, REM sleep constitutes about 25 percent of a night's sleep. During REM sleep, the body is physiologically more active than in non-REM stages. In young adults, there is an initial awake period (sleep latency) followed by a rapid progression through stages I-IV of non-REM. This sequence is then reversed, followed by the first REM period. This initial sequence of non-REM sleep (REM latency) lasts about 70 minutes. The first REM period is very short and is followed by another cycle. In each successive cycle, less time is spent in stage IV and more time is spent in the other stages, including REM. In the elderly, both sleep latency and REM latency are increased, stage IV may be decreased or absent, and awakenings are more frequent.[4]

Etiology of insomnia

The occasional inability to attain restful sleep is a common problem. It is estimated that about 50 percent of the population experiences insomnia at some time, and 33 percent voices it as an ongoing complaint.[5] Although insomnia is usually transient and self-limiting, it may be of sufficient duration or severity to interfere with an individual's functioning during the waking hours. Severe or chronic insomnia may be a symptom of serious psychological or physical illness.

Insomnia can be classified as either difficulty in falling asleep or difficulty in remaining asleep.[6] Difficulty in falling asleep may be caused by:

☐ *Situational stress and anxiety.* These are usually acute and transient. They include anything that may cause worry or excitement. Situational stress and anxiety are probably the most frequent causes of insomnia in young people.

☐ *Pain or physical discomfort.* Examples are headache and dental pain.

☐ *Change in daily rhythm.* For example, a change in work shifts or "jet lag."

Difficulty in remaining asleep may be caused by:

☐ *Age.* Elderly individuals are prone to early or frequent awakening because sleep cycles change with age.

☐ *Depression.* Some types of depression are associated with awakenings during the night or early morning. If anxiety occurs with depression, the patient may complain of difficulty in falling and remaining asleep.

☐ *Physical conditions with noctural exacerbation.* Autonomic nervous system bursts during REM sleep precipitate angina attacks, vascular headaches, and duodenal ulcer distress which disturb sleep. Asthma, epilepsy, and lumbosacral and cervical disk disease have also been implicated in sleep disturbances.

☐ *Endocrine abnormalities.* Hypo- and hyperthyroidism as well as other endocrine disorders disturb sleep patterns, but the mechanism is unknown.

☐ *Sleep apnea.* This sleep disturbance is most common in men over 40 and is manifested by loud, irregular snoring. In this syndrome, respiration actually stops for periods of 20 to 90 seconds many times during the night. The patient may be unaware of irregular respiration and complain only of feeling tired during the day. Researchers believe that sleep apnea is caused by a defect in CNS respiratory control which, in some cases, is complicated by an anatomic upper airway obstruction.

☐ *Nocturnal myoclonus.* This syndrome consists of recurrent, rhythmic movement of one or both legs.

The patient may not awaken fully and so may be unaware of this phenomenon.

Drugs may cause sleep disturbances. Certain anorexic preparations (prescription and OTC) containing CNS stimulants, caffeine, and aminophylline may cause nervousness and prevent sleep in some individuals. Drugs that cause sleep disturbances by suppressing REM or stage IV sleep are listed in Table 1. Abrupt withdrawal of a REM suppressant after chronic use precipitates a compensatory rebound of REM sleep. This rebound is associated with disturbances in sleep patterns and accompanying nightmares. REM rebound may also occur as a patient develops tolerance to a REM suppressing hypnotic. Deprivation of stage IV sleep results in symptoms which suggest a depressive and hypochondriacal reaction.[7]

Ingredients in OTC products

Bromides. Bromides were first used for their CNS depressant effect in the mid-1880's for the treatment of epilepsy. They are no longer prescribed as anticonvulsants because excess sedation accompanies the therapeutic effect and because therapeutic blood levels are close to those producing toxicity.

The therapeutic and toxic effects of bromides result from a displacement of chloride ion by bromide ion in body fluids. The presence of bromide in the CNS produces a nonspecific, reversible depression.[8] Bromide is slowly excreted by the kidneys; it has a half-life of approximately 12 days. The long half-life constitutes the greatest hazard of bromides because continuous use can result in an accumulation of the drug and subsequent toxicity. One study indicates that daily ingestion of 16.5 mEq of bromide (maximum recommended OTC dose) can theoretically produce intoxication in about 8 days in an average adult.[9] Children and patients with renal insufficiency are even more susceptible to toxic effects.

The side effects associated with bromides are headache, vertigo, GI disturbances, and a rash similar in appearance to acne (bromoderma nodosa).

Acute bromide intoxication is rare because ingestion of toxic doses irritates the GI tract and causes vomiting. Chronic bromide intoxication (bromism) is more likely. The symptoms of bromide poisoning are bromide rash, confusion, irritability, tremor, anorexia, weight loss, ataxia, stupor, and coma. Treatment is aimed at increasing bromide excretion by administering sodium chloride (P.O. or I.V.) and water. The use of diuretics will also increase bromide excretion.[10]

Bromides are contraindicated in children, pregnant or lactating women, and patients with impaired renal function. Bromides may enhance the effect of other CNS depressants; therefore, concurrent use of these agents should be avoided.

Bromide compounds are unsuitable as sleep aids or sedatives because single doses produce no effect and continuous use poses a high risk of toxicity.[1] Therefore, bromides are no longer used in OTC sleep aid and sedative products.

Scopolamine. Scopolamine is an anticholinergic agent which differs from atropine in that it lacks a CNS stimulant effect. Scopolamine acts as a hypnotic by depressing the cerebral cortex, especially the motor areas.[11] It suppresses spontaneous electrical activity as well as the arousal response to photostimulation.[12] In animals, scopolamine antagonizes the EEG response produced by stimulation of the reticular formation and hypothalamus.[13] These findings indicate that scopolamine suppresses the brain structures responsible for maintaining consciousness.

Scopolamine is readily absorbed from the GI tract. Therapeutic doses (0.6 mg oral or parenteral) produce drowsiness, euphoria, fatigue, and dreamless sleep.[14] In some individuals, therapeutic doses cause excitement, restlessness and delirium; this excitement occurs most commonly when severe pain is present.

Scopolamine may disrupt the sleep cycle by decreasing REM time. When scopolamine is discontinued after several days of use, a rebound in REM occurs. This effect may result in nightmares, insomnia, and a feeling of having slept badly.[3] Although the dose of scopolamine in OTC preparations is probably insufficient to produce "REM rebound," patients who use these preparations chronically or who exceed the recommended dosage may experience this effect.

Scopolamine is also used as a preanesthetic medication for its sedative and antisecretory action. In obstetrics, it is combined with narcotics to produce a state of amnesia and partial analgesia ("twilight sleep"). Although scopolamine is effective in the prevention of motion sickness, it has been replaced by newer agents (e.g., dimenhydrinate) with fewer side effects.

The most common side effect of scopolamine is dryness of the mouth and throat. Other effects such as blurred vision, photophobia, and urinary retention are uncommon at the dosage provided in OTC preparations.

Infants and young children are particularly susceptible to the toxic effects of belladonna alkaloids. The fatal dose of scopolamine in children may be as low as 10 mg.[15] The symptoms of poisoning are delirium, tachycardia, fever, and hot, dry, flushed skin. In severe cases, respiratory depression and coma may result.

Treatment of oral scopolamine poisoning consists of delaying and preventing absorption of the drug by administering milk or activated charcoal, followed by inducing emesis, and counteracting the central and peripheral effects with physostigmine. In addition, general measures such as reducing fever, controlling convulsions, and maintaining urinary output are used.

Scopolamine is available for nonprescription use as the aminoxide hydrobromide salt. Theoretically, the use of this salt minimizes toxic effects and provides sustained action because the aminoxide hydrobromide is slowly metabolized to the parent base. The advantages of this compound over others have not been proved conclusively.[1] The amount of scopolamine in OTC products ranges from 0.1 to 0.5 mg per dose. Scopolamine alone is ineffective as a sleep aid at these doses. However, it may enhance sedation produced by other components of OTC products.

Table 1. Drugs Which Alter Sleep Stages[a]

Drugs decreasing REM sleep	Drugs decreasing Stage IV sleep
Alcohol	Amphetamines
Amphetamines	Barbiturates
Barbiturates	Benzodiazepines
Diphenhydramine	Chloral hydrate
Ethchlorvynol	Glutethimide
Glutethimide	Reserpine
Methyprylon	
Narcotics	
Scopolamine	
Tricyclic antidepressants	

[a]Adapted from G. Fass, *Am. J. Nursing*, **71**, 2316(1971).

Scopolamine should not be used in children under 12 or in patients with narrow-angle glaucoma, coronary insufficiency, or prostatic hypertrophy. This agent should be used cautiously with other drugs possessing anticholinergic activity (e.g., other belladonna alkaloids, phenothiazines, tricyclic antidepressants, and antihistamines) and CNS depressants because concurrent use may result in the enhancement of the anticholinergic action or the CNS depression.

Antihistamines. Antihistamines can produce both stimulation and depression of the CNS. Although drowsiness usually results from therapeutic doses, excitation is a symptom of intoxication. The mechanisms by which antihistamines exert their CNS effects are unclear, but similarities between the actions of antihistamines and scopolamine suggest that an antagonism of acetylcholine in the CNS is common to both.[16] The CNS depressant action of antihistamines is unpredictable because individuals vary in sensitivity to this effect and tolerance develops with continued use.

The efficacy of antihistamines as sleep aids is questionable. The results of one study indicate that 50 mg of methapyrilene is no more effective than placebo.[17] The FDA Panel has recommended an additional testing period of 3 years due to a lack of data on the safety and efficacy of these products.[1]

Side effects of antihistamines include drowsiness, dizziness, tinnitus, blurred vision, GI disturbances, and dryness of the mouth and throat. Antihistamines may also cause CNS stimulation, resulting in nervousness and insom-

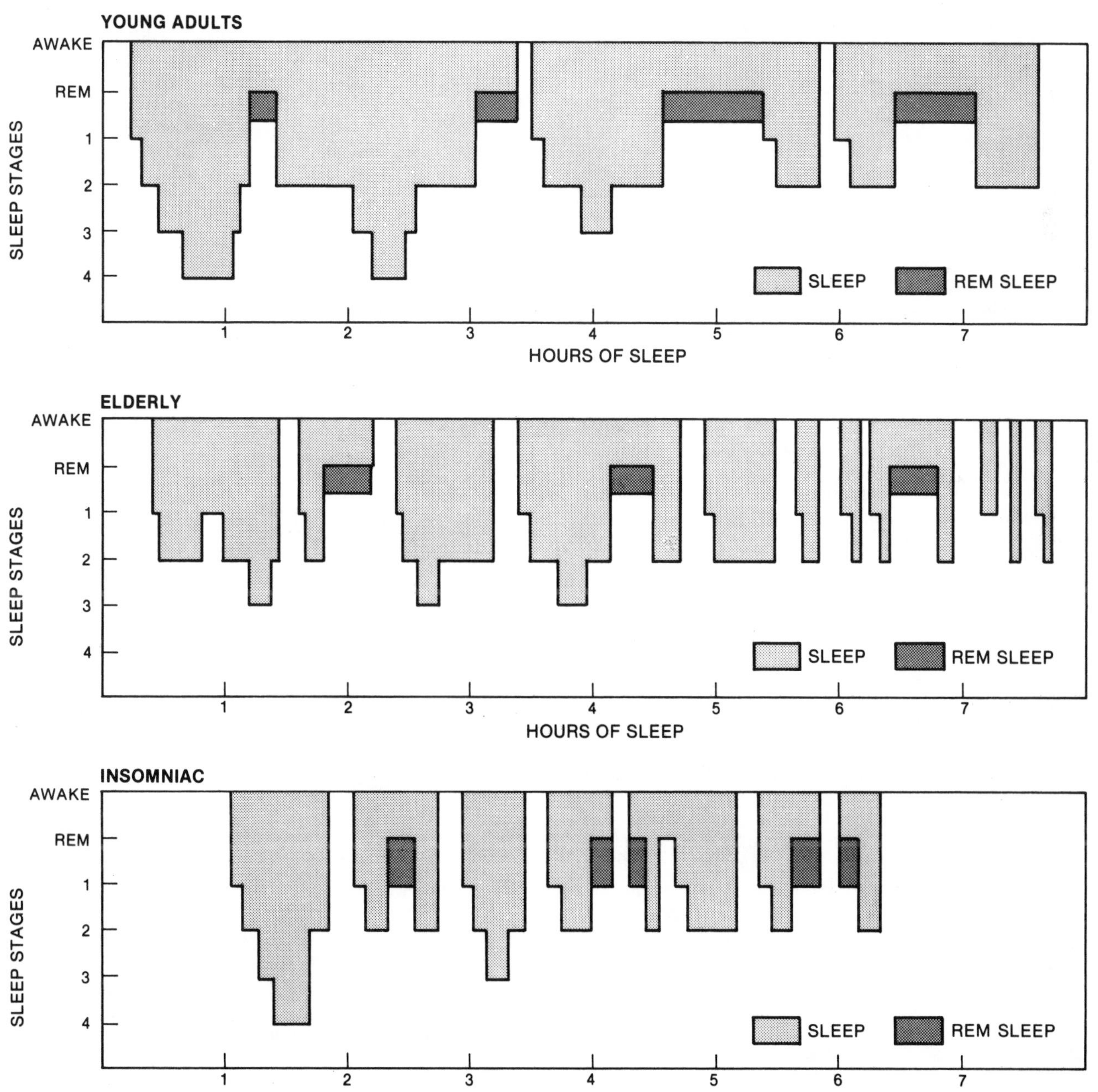

Figure 1. Hours of sleep and sleep stages in young adults, the elderly, and insomniacs. Adapted from J. A. Brandner, Ed., *Patient Care*, Vol. X, No. 3, 113 (1976).

nia. However, this effect is uncommon, occurring primarily in children.

Although the antihistamines have a wide margin of safety, potential poisoning with these agents should not be discounted if an acute overdose is taken, especially in combination with alcohol. The symptoms observed with intoxication result from the CNS effects—the pupils become fixed and dilated, fever may be present, and excitement, hallucinations, and convulsions occur. In severe cases, these symptoms are followed by coma and cardiorespiratory collapse. Treatment consists of preventing absorption of the drug, emesis, and supportive measures such as assisting ventilation and controlling convulsions.

The antihistamines commonly used in OTC sleep aid products are methapyrilene and pyrilamine, alone or in combination. The dosage ranges from 10 to 50 mg per dose.

Antihistamines have produced teratogenic effects in animals and, therefore, should be avoided by pregnant women. High doses may precipitate convulsions and should be used with caution in epileptics. The CNS depressant effect of antihistamines is enhanced by alcohol and other CNS depressant drugs.

Salicylates and salicylamide. Salicylates are included in sleep aid products primarily to relieve minor pain which may hinder sleep. Salicylamide is not metabolized to salicylate in the body. However, it has analgesic, antipyretic, and anti-inflammatory effects similar to those of salicylates. Although salicylamide also has sedative properties, the doses contained in OTC preparations (200 to 400 mg) are probably insufficient to produce sedation.[18] In addition, the results of one study indicate the bioavailability of salicylamide is poor because it is relatively insoluble and rapidly inactivated in the GI tract and liver.[19]

The side effects most commonly associated with salicylates are those involving the GI tract. Salicylates cause GI distress, bleeding, and may aggravate symptoms of peptic ulcer.

The toxic dose of any salicylate is 0.4 to 0.5 g/kg. The symptoms of intoxication include hyperpnea, lethargy, vomiting, tinnitus, and dizziness. In severe cases, subsequent alterations of acid-base balance occur, and coma and respiratory failure may result. Treatment consists of preventing absorption, controlling convulsions, and assisting respiration. In severe cases, the urine can be alkalinized to increase salicylate excretion.[20]

Salicylates are present in OTC sleep aid products as various salts, in doses ranging from 80 to 200 mg. Salicylamide is included in doses of 200 to 400 mg.

Salicylates should not be used by pregnant women or by patients with GI ulcers or allergy to salicylates. Salicylates potentiate the action of oral anticoagulants and methotrexate, and concurrent use of these drugs may result in serious toxic effects. Salicylates antagonize the uricosuric effect of sulfinpyrazone and probenecid and cause additive ulcerogenic effects on the gastric mucosa when used concurrently with alcohol or with corticosteroids.[21]

Adjunctive measures for relieving insomnia

In addition to advising patients on the proper use of OTC sleep aid preparations, the pharmacist can recommend nondrug measures which may help relieve insomnia. These include:

- ☐ Abstaining from beverages containing caffeine
- ☐ Avoiding heavy meals several hours before bedtime
- ☐ Avoiding naps during the day
- ☐ Performing light exercise before bedtime
- ☐ Designating a specific time for sleep
- ☐ Relaxing by engaging in positive activities such as reading in bed, watching TV, or listening to relaxing music
- ☐ Minimizing external stimuli which might disturb sleep, such as using dark shades over the windows to keep out light and ear plugs to keep out noise

Summary

Insomnia is usually a transient, self-limiting condition caused by stress or change of location or schedule. Patients who request OTC sleep aid or sedative products should be informed that these products are only for occasional use at recommended dosages. Bromide and scopolamine preparations should not be recommended because they are ineffective at recommended doses and higher doses may precipitate toxicity. The antihistamines are the most satisfactory ingredients of OTC sleep aid and sedative products. The FDA OTC Panel has recommended additional testing of these agents at doses greater than those presently used and is considering the introduction of diphenhydramine as an OTC sleep aid. The use of an antihistamine product along with nondrug measures is probably the most rational advice a pharmacist can give a patient suffering from insomnia. Patients using any OTC sleep aid or sedative product should be cautioned that their ability to drive or operate hazardous machinery may be impaired and that concurrent use of these products with alcohol or other CNS depressants will intensify the CNS depression.

References

1. *Fed. Regist.* Part II (Dec. 8, 1975), p. 57297.
2. "The Anatomy of Sleep," Roche Laboratories, Nutley, N.J., 1966, pp. 39-59.
3. "The Nature of Sleep," G. E. W. Wolstenholme and M. O'Connor, Eds., Little Brown, Boston, Mass., 1961, pp. 86-102.
4. K. L. Melmon and H. F. Morrelli, "Clinical Pharmacology–Basic Principles in Therapeutics," 1st ed., Macmillan, New York, N.Y., 1972, pp. 482-490.
5. J. Moriarity, *Dis. Nerv. Syst.*, **36**, 279(1975).
6. C. C. Brown *et al.*, *Patient Care*, **10**, 98(1976).
7. G. Fass, *Am. J. Nursing*, **71**, 2316(1971).
8. "The Pharmacological Basis of Therapeutics," 5th ed., L. S. Goodman and A. Gilman, Eds., Macmillan, New York, N.Y., 1975, p. 121.
9. G. Torosian *et al.*, *Am. J. Hosp. Pharm.*, **30**, 716(1973).
10. R. H. Dreisbach, "Handbook of Poisoning," 8th ed., Lange Medical Publications, Los Altos, Calif., 1974, p. 297.
11. "Martindale: The Extra Pharmacopoeia," 26th ed., N. W. Blacow, Ed., The Pharmaceutical Press, London, England, 1972, p. 295.
12. A. M. Ostfeld and A. Arugete, *J. Pharmacol. Exp. Ther.*, **137**, 133(1962).
13. K. A. Exley *et al.*, *Br. J. Pharmacol.*, **13**, 485(1958).
14. "The Pharmacological Basis of Therapeutics," 5th ed., L. S. Goodman and A. Gilman, Eds., Macmillan, New York, N.Y., 1975, p. 517.
15. R. H. Dreisbach, "Handbook of Poisoning," 8th ed., Lange Medical Publications, Los Altos, Calif., 1974, p. 305.
16. R. H. Dreisbach, "Handbook of Poisoning," 8th ed., Lange Medical Publications, Los Altos, Calif., 1974, pp. 606-608.
17. G. Teutsch *et al.*, *Clin. Pharmacol. Ther.*, **17**, 195(1975).
18. "The Pharmacological Basis of Therapeutics," 5th ed., L. S. Goodman and A. Gilman, Eds., Macmillan, New York, N.Y., 1975, p. 348.
19. L. Flekenstein *et al.*, *Clin. Pharmacol. Ther.*, **19**, 451(1976).
20. R. H. Dreisbach, "Handbook of Poisoning," 8th ed., Lange Medical Publications, Los Altos, Calif., 1974, pp. 258-262.
21. "Evaluations of Drug Interactions," 2d ed., American Pharmaceutical Association, Washington, D. C., 1976.

Product (manufacturer)	Scopolamine	Antihistamine	Analgesic
Compoz Tablets (Jeffrey Martin)	—	methapyrilene hydrochloride, 15 mg pyrilamine maleate, 10 mg	—
Dormin Capsules (Dormin)	—	methapyrilene hydrochloride, 25 mg	—
Nervine Capsule-Shaped Tablets (Miles)	—	methapyrilene hydrochloride, 25 mg	—
Nervine Effervescent Tablets (Miles)	—	methapyrilene fumarate, equivalent to 25 mg of hydrochloride	—
Nervine Liquid (Miles)	—	methapyrilene fumarate, equivalent to 25 mg of hydrochloride/5 ml	—
Nite Rest Capsules (Amer. Pharm.)	aminoxide hydrobromide, 0.25 mg	methapyrilene hydrochloride, 50 mg	—
Nytol Capsules and Tablets (Block)	—	methapyrilene hydrochloride, 50 mg/capsule 25 mg/tablet	salicylamide, 380 mg/capsule 200 mg/tablet
Quiet World Tablets (Whitehall)	hydrobromide, 0.083 mg	methapyrilene hydrochloride, 16.67 mg	aspirin, 227.5 mg acetaminophen, 162.5 mg
Relax-U-Caps (Columbia Medical)	—	methapyrilene hydrochloride, 25 mg	—
Sedacaps (Vitarine)	—	methapyrilene hydrochloride, 25 mg	—
Seedate Capsules (Amer. Pharm.)	aminoxide hydrobromide, 0.125 mg	methapyrilene hydrochloride, 25 mg	—
Sleep-Eze Tablets (Whitehall)	hydrobromide, 0.125 mg	methapyrilene hydrochloride, 25 mg	—
Sleepinal Capsules (Thompson)	—	methapyrilene hydrochloride, 50 mg	—
Sominex Tablets and Capsules (J. B. Williams)	aminoxide hydrobromide, 0.25 mg/tablet 0.5 mg/capsule	methapyrilene hydrochloride, 25 mg/tablet 50 mg/capsule	salicylamide, 200 mg/tablet and capsule
Somnicaps (Amer. Pharm.)	—	methapyrilene hydrochloride, 25 mg	—
Tranquil Capsules (North American)	—	methapyrilene fumarate, 25 mg	sodium salicylate, 25 mg acetaminophen, 25 mg
Tranquim Capsules (Thompson)	—	methapyrilene hydrochloride, 50 mg	—

Stimulant Products

Charles A. Walker

Questions to ask the patient

How long do you intend to use a stimulant product?

Are you a regular coffee drinker?

Have you ever experienced unpleasant reactions to coffee?

Which stimulant products have you used before? How well did they work?

Are you presently being treated for a condition that requires the use of other drugs?

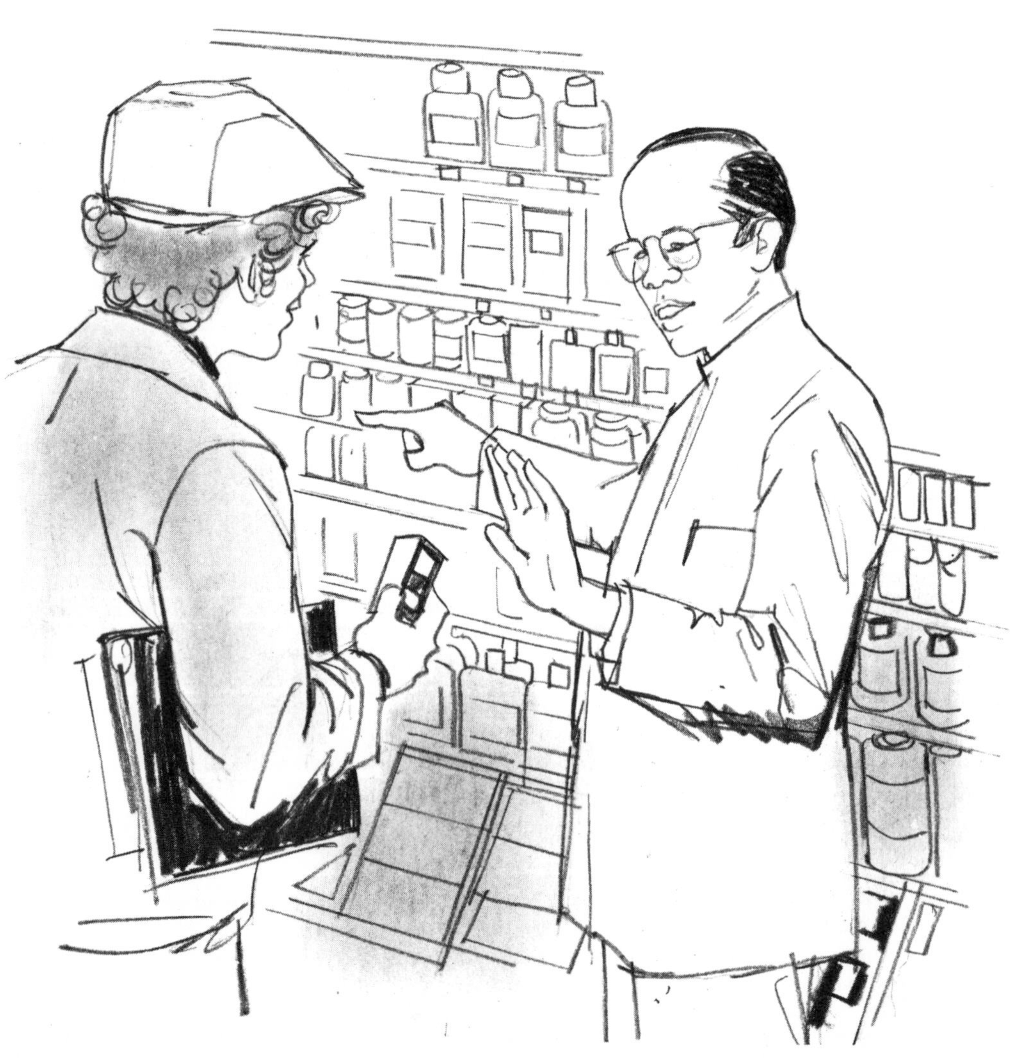

CHAPTER 15

Most OTC stimulants used today contain caffeine (1,3,7-trimethylxanthine) as the active component and are classified as "stay-awake aids." The related dimethylxanthines, theophylline and theobromine (Fig. 1), are not used therapeutically as stimulants. Many nonalcoholic beverages are made from plant products that contain xanthines. Coffee, tea, and cola soft drinks contain concentrations of caffeine that can affect the CNS. Coffee beans and tea leaves contain 1 to 2 percent caffeine, cocoa and tea contain theobromine, and tea also contains theophylline. The average cup of coffee contains 100 to 150 mg of caffeine.[1] The amount varies depending on the method of extraction (Table 1). Only traces of caffeine are found in cocoa. Federal standards of identity for soda water beverages allow for the addition of not more than 0.02 percent of caffeine by weight.

More than 25 OTC analgesic products contain as much as 64 mg of caffeine per dose. Caffeine is considered a relatively safe substance when administered orally in doses of less than 200 mg.[2]

Approximately 7 million kg of caffeine are consumed yearly in the U.S. Caffeine is most commonly used by the public to induce wakefulness and to relieve the sense of boredom and fatigue associated with performing tedious work for extended periods. For example, it is used to prevent "highway hypnosis" encountered during long periods of continuous driving. Caffeine is also inappropriately used to combat symptoms of hangover and to antagonize the depressant properties of alcohol and other sedatives.

Effects of caffeine on the nervous system

Indications for the use of stimulants are drowsiness and fatigue. In a study on driver performance, it was found that caffeine can improve alertness, but contradictory evidence exists on the sobering effect of caffeine. Mental activity was improved by caffeine in tests that involved simple arithmetic, typing, and decoding, especially in long sessions, when fatigue and boredom are possible factors.[2]

Improvement of skeletal muscle tone is a fundamental property of caffeine that is useful in combating fatigue.[3] This effect is produced mainly by CNS stimulation and, in part, by a direct action on the voluntary musculature. It is difficult to separate the central from the peripheral influences, but the central effects probably are the more important and pronounced.

In humans, the physiological consequences of various doses of caffeine have been studied. Small doses (50 to 200 mg) stimulate cerebrocortical areas associated with conscious mental processes (Fig. 2)—ideas become clearer, thoughts flow more easily and rapidly, and fatigue and drowsiness decrease.[3] A few incidents have been reported where continuity of thought is difficult, impressions are so rapid that attention is distracted, and a greater effort is required to limit thoughts to a single subject.[4] Doses larger than 250 mg often cause insomnia, restlessness, irritability, nervousness, tremor, headaches and, in rare cases, a mild form of delirium manifested as perceived noises and flashes of light. Goldstein *et al.*[5] investigated the objective and subjective effects of caffeine. One double-blind study evaluated the effects of placebo vs. caffeine (150 or 300 mg) on objective performance and mood. The results of this study indicate that, although caffeine produces a subjective feeling of increased alertness and physical activity, objective performance requiring alertness and psychomotor coordination is not improved.

Injected doses of caffeine larger than 250 mg stimulate vagal respiratory and vasomotor areas of the medulla oblongata.[4] Caffeine is therapeutically effective in treating drug-induced depression of the medullary respiratory center. Doses of more than 10 g ingested orally are required to induce convulsions.[3] In cases of oral overdosage, the stomach should be emptied by inducing emesis or by using gastric lavage. Depressants, such as barbiturates, have been used to control caffeine-induced convulsions.

Effects of caffeine on the cardiovascular system

Xanthines may directly stimulate the myocardium, promoting an increase in cardiac force, rate, and output.[6] These cardiac effects may be masked, however, because xanthines, especially caffeine in large doses, also stimulate the medullary vagal nuclei and tend to reflexly produce a decrease in heart rate. Large doses (more than 250 mg) may induce cardiac irregularities attributed to the direct effects of caffeine on the myocardium.[3] Experimentally, caffeine has been shown to stimulate the synthesis and release of norepinephrine in the brain and the release of epinephrine from the adrenal medulla.[3] However, the evidence does not implicate the involvement of these amines in cardiovascular problems (due to caffeine intake) of human patients.

In humans, caffeine does not cause a consistent decrease in systemic mean blood pressure despite a decrease in peripheral resistance. Generally, with moderate doses of caffeine, blood pressure is maintained by increased cardiac output. However, large intravenous doses of caffeine have been shown to cause a transient fall in blood pressure due to medullary vagal nuclei stimulation, which also can result in bradycardia and a slight decrease in cardiac output.[3]

Xanthine compounds have been shown to cause marked vasoconstriction of cerebral blood vessels. The property has been reported to be a mechanism of action in the relief of hypertensive headache by caffeine.[4]

In an investigation regarding the effect of 140 mg of caffeine in tea on hemodynamic measurements in patients with cardiac disease, there was a significant rise in the cardiac index, stroke index, oxygen consumption, and minute ventilation.[7] A small but significant increase in brachial arterial pressure and ventricular filling pressure also occurred. No arrhythmias were seen in any of the patients as a result of the oral ingestion of tea.

There have been conflicting reports of positive correlation between coronary artery disease and coffee consumption. One study compared the histories of 700 heart attack patients with the histories of 13,000 other patients.[8] Patients who drank as many as 5 cups of coffee per day had a 50 percent greater risk of heart attack than those who abstained; patients who drank 6 or more cups per day had a 100 percent greater risk of heart attack than abstainers. These results have been disputed by other studies that failed to show a correlation between coffee consumption, serum lipids, serum cholesterol, and coronary disease.[9,10]

Other effects of caffeine

"Caffeinism" is the syndrome associated with excessive caffeine intake. The ingestion of more than 1,000 mg of caffeine daily (about 10 cups of coffee) can produce symptoms similar to those of anxiety neurosis. The CNS symptoms related to excessive stimulation include nervousness, irritability, agitation, headache, tachypnea, tremulousness, and muscle twitches. Sensory disturbances such as hyperesthesia, tinnitus, and visual hallucinations may occur. Insomnia may be a consequence of caffeinism and characterized by a delay in sleep onset or by frequent awakenings.

The effects of regular coffee, decaffeinated coffee, and caffeine on gastric acid secretion and lower esophageal sphincter pressure have been investigated in healthy subjects.[11] The results of this study suggest that regular and decaffeinated coffee are more potent stimulants of gastric acid secretion than caffeine, that decaffeination diminishes the acid secretory potency of coffee only minimally, and that regular and decaffeinated coffee increase lower esophageal sphincter pressure, whereas caffeine alone has only a minimal effect. These results indicate that clinical recommendations based on the known GI effect of caffeine may bear little relation to the actual observed action of regular or decaffeinated coffee.[11] They suggest that the effects of caffeine alone may not be similar to the effects of beverages in which caffeine is present. However, decaffeination does not necessarily completely remove undesirable effects of caffeinated beverages.

The value of caffeine in mixtures for relief of headache and other pain is questionable except in the treatment of vascular headache. In one study caffeine in combination with aspirin was no more effective than aspirin alone for headache.[12] Caffeine generally is believed to play a minor role in the toxic effects from excessive use of analgesic mixtures.[13,14] Caffeine taken with analgesics may, by its stimulant properties, enhance the mood of a person when pain is accompanied by minor depression.

Because caffeine has a hyperglycemic effect, it may elevate blood glucose levels and produce high readings for serum uric acid when the Bittner (1963) assay is used.[15] Caffeine or its metabolites interfere in vanillylmandelic acid (4-hydroxy-3-methoxymandelic acid, VMA) determination. The test is used for detection of elevated adrenal or sympathetic catecholamine levels as seen in pheochromocytoma or neuroblastoma. An increase in urine levels of catecholamines may be detected following caffeine ingestion.[15]

Figure 3 shows the human metabolism of caffeine, after which approximately two-thirds of the drug is excreted in the urine as monomethylxanthine or dimethyluric acid.

Table 1. Caffeine Content of Beverages[a]

Beverage	Approximate amount of caffeine per unit
Brewed coffee	100–150 mg/cup
Cola drinks	40–60 mg/glass
Decaffeinated coffee	2–4 mg/cup
Instant coffee	86–99 mg/cup
Tea	60–75 mg/cup

[a]Adapted from J. F. Greden, *Am. J. Psychiatr.*, **131 (10)**, 1090 (1974).

Although coffee and preparations containing caffeine are often prohibited in individuals suffering from gout, this prohibition may not be justified.[3] Uric acid is not formed following caffeine ingestion, and the methylxanthines and methyluric acids which do appear as metabolites do not provoke attacks of gout. Therefore, it is doubtful that therapeutic doses of caffeine aggravate the disease.

In a study of the use of caffeine in hyperkinetic children, it was concluded that caffeine may have a place in the therapeutic management of children with minimal brain dysfunction syndrome and consequent hyperkinetic impulse syndrome.[16]

A mild degree of tolerance and physical dependence occur with caffeine ingestion. Irritability, nervousness, and headache were reported in habitual coffee users (5 or more cups per day), following withdrawal from the beverage.[17] Although these symptoms do not prove actual caffeine physical dependence, they might indicate psychological dependence. Another study conducted to determine tolerance to caffeine on healthy subjects provided some information on physiological changes associated with chronic caffeine administration.[18] In this study, it was established that 150 mg of caffeine taken at bedtime reduces pulse rate significantly in non-coffee-drinkers but not in those who habitually consume caffeinated beverages. The study also indicated that caffeine administration (150 mg) to non-coffee-drinkers delays the onset of sleep and modifies sleeping patterns. On the other hand, chronic coffee drinkers show no symptoms of bradycardia or insomnia.[18] Although results indicate possible physical changes in coffee drinkers, it is the general opinion that caffeine tolerance in chronic users occurs because of increased metabolism.

The chronic use of caffeine may produce a degree of tolerance to insomnia and a decrease in the mental alertness produced by caffeine, i.e., a decrease in the ability of caffeine to act as a stimulant.[19]

Potential interactions

Caffeine can interact with other drugs. It was observed in experimental animals that isoniazid and meprobamate potentiate the caffeine effect.[20,21] Meprobamate can increase caffeine concentration in the brain by 55 percent and can decrease it in the liver and kidney.[22] It is important for the pharmacist to be cognizant of these possible interactions of caffeine in patients taking these specific medications.

Caffeine toxicity

Fatal caffeine poisoning is extremely rare. Death has been reported in only a few cases following intravenous injection or oral administration . In adults, the lethal intravenous dose of caffeine was reported to be 3.2 g; reported oral lethal doses range from 18 to 50 g.[23] The route of administration influences the severity of toxic manifestations. Peak blood levels occur within 2 hours after oral administration. [24] The average half-life is 3 to 3.5 hours.[25] Children are very susceptible to caffeine toxicity. Caffeine-containing drugs should be kept out of the reach of children.

The suggested treatment for caffeine overdosage includes:

☐ Ingestion of an aluminum hydroxide gel as an antacid and protective agent against GI irritation

☐ Oxygen inhalation

☐ Short-acting barbiturates injected cautiously to control neuromuscular irritability and convulsions

- ☐ Intravenous fluids to combat dehydration
- ☐ Antibiotics for complicating infections
- ☐ Evacuation

Renal irritation and nephrotoxicity can occur following chronic abuse of analgesic drug mixtures that contain caffeine. One study reported a significant number of renal tubular cells and red blood cells in the urine of 10 healthy volunteers following the ingestion of 1.2 g of caffeine per day for 5 days.[16]

Summary

The pharmacist should advise caffeine product users of the possible side effects and dangers of overconsumption of these compounds. Because of the possible interactions of caffeine with other drugs, the intake of caffeine should be reduced during the treatment of specific diseases, especially cardiovascular, psychological, or renal problems. The use of analgesic combinations that contain caffeine is not advisable for patients with rheumatoid arthritis or other conditions that require large doses (10 to 30 tablets daily) of medication because, in these amounts, there is danger of caffeine toxicity. Caffeine consumption should be avoided prior to blood or urine analysis.

The pharmacist should caution against the overuse of caffeine. Habitual overuse can lead to sleep deprivation. CNS stimulants can facilitate the ability to ignore sensation of tiredness, but they do not replenish depleted energy. Continuous use of coffee or caffeine tablets does not allay emotional fatigue. Neither coffee nor caffeine tablets taken after consumption of alcohol induce sobriety, but the degree of CNS depression is lessened and somnolence is diminished or eliminated. In other words, a person may still be inebriated but will not feel sleepy.

References

1. I. B. Syed, *Bulletin of I.M.A.*, vol. 6, 1975.
2. J. R. Dipalma, "Drill's Pharmacology in Medicine," 4th ed., McGraw-Hill, New York, N.Y., 1971, p. 537.
3. "The Pharmacological Basis of Therapeutics," 5th ed., L. S. Goodman and A. Gilman, Eds., Macmillan, New York, N.Y., 1975, p. 368.
4. "The Pharmacological Principles of Medical Practice," 7th ed., J. C. Krantz and C. J. Carr, Eds., Williams and Wilkins, Baltimore, Md., 1969, pp. 256-260.
5. A. Goldstein *et al.*, *J. Pharmacol. Exp. Ther.*, **150**, 146(1965).
6. I. Starr *et al.*, *J. Clin. Invest.*, **16**, 799(1937).
7. L. Gould *et al.*, *J. Clin. Pharmacol.*, **13(11, 12)**, 469-473(1973).
8. H. Jick *et al.*, *Lancet*, **2**, 1278(1972).
9. S. Heyden, *Z. Ernaehrung*, **9**, 388(1969).
10. J. A. Little *et al.*, *Lancet*, **1**, 732(1966).
11. S. Cohen and G. H. Booth, *N. Engl. J. Med.*, **293**, 897-899(1975).
12. C. G. Moertel *et al.*, *J. Am. Med. Assoc.*, **229**, 55(1974).
13. L. J. Cass and W. S. Fredrik, *Curr. Ther. Res. Clin. Exp.*, **4**, 583(1962).
14. M. Grotto *et al.*, *Arch. Int. Pharmacodyn. Ther.*, **155**, 365(1965).
15. F. H. Meyers *et al.*, "Review of Medical Pharmacology," 4th ed., Lange Medical Publications, Los Altos, Calif., 1974, p. 678.
16. R. C. Schnackenber, *Am. J. Psychiatry*, **130**, 796(1973).
17. R. H. Dreisbach and C. Pfeiffer, *J. Lab. Clin. Med.*, **28**, 1212(1942).
18. T. Colton *et al.*, *Clin. Pharmacol. Ther.*, **9**, 31(1968).
19. K. H. Pieper, *Arzneim. Forsch.*, **13**, 585(1963).
20. E. M. Boyd, *Toxicol. Appl. Pharmacol.*, **1**, 258(1959).
21. H. Besson and A. Debay, *Ann. Pharm. Fr.*, **22**, 345(1964).
22. M. Inselvini and H. Casier, *Arch. Int. Pharmacodyn. Ther.*, **122**, 163(1959).
23. R. H. Cheney, *J. Pharmacol. Exp. Ther.*, **53**, 304(1935).
24. J. Axelrod and J. Reichenthal, *J. Pharmacol. Exp. Ther.*, **107**, 519(1953).
25. C. Landis, in "Problems of Addiction and Habituation," vol. 13, P. H. Hoch and J. Zubin, Eds., Grune and Stratton, New York, N.Y., pp. 37-48.

Products 15 STIMULANT

Product (manufacturer)	Caffeine	Other
Amostat Tablets (North American)	100 mg	—
Caffedrine Capsules (Thompson)	250 mg	—
Double-E Alertness Capsules (Keystone)	180 mg	thiamine hydrochloride, 5 mg
Nodoz Tablets (Bristol-Myers)	100 mg	—
Prolamine Capsules (Thompson)	140 mg	phenylpropanolamine hydrochloride, 35 mg
Quick-Pep Tablets (Thompson)	150 mg	niacin, 10 mg thiamine mononitrate, 3 mg
Tirend Tablets (Norcliff-Thayer)	100 mg	—
Verb T.D. Capsules (Amer. Pharm.)	200 mg	—
Vivarin Tablets (J. B. Williams)	200 mg	dextrose, 150 mg
Wakoz (Jeffrey Martin)	200 mg	—

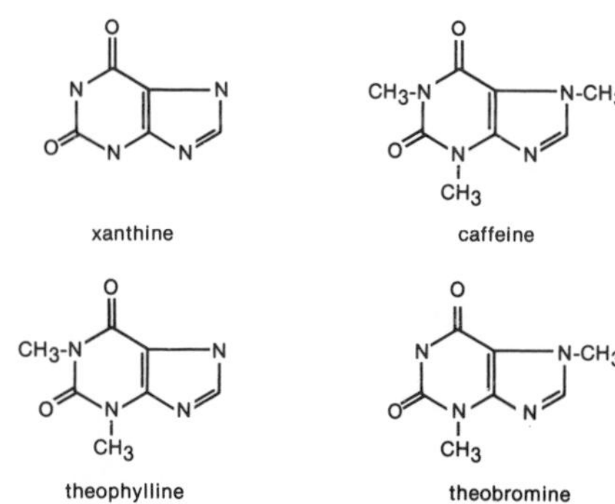

Figure 1.
Structure of methylated xanthines.

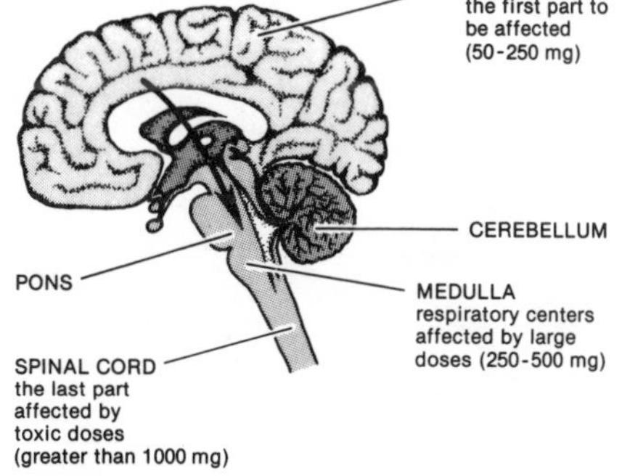

Figure 2.
The site of action of caffeine in the central nervous system. (The arrow indicates the progression of the effect.)

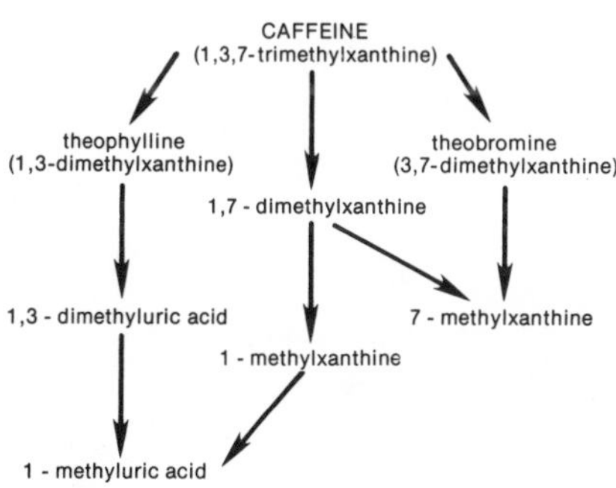

Figure 3.
Caffeine metabolism in humans.

Menstrual Products

Keith W. Reichmann

Questions to ask the patient

How many days until your next period?

What contraceptive measures (if any) do you use?

How do the present symptoms vary from those of your normal cycle (flow, duration, intensity)?

Are you under the care of a physician?

Do you have discharging between your periods? Is the discharge accompanied by pain, itching, pus, or foul odor?

Have you had these symptoms before? What treatment was used? Was it helpful?

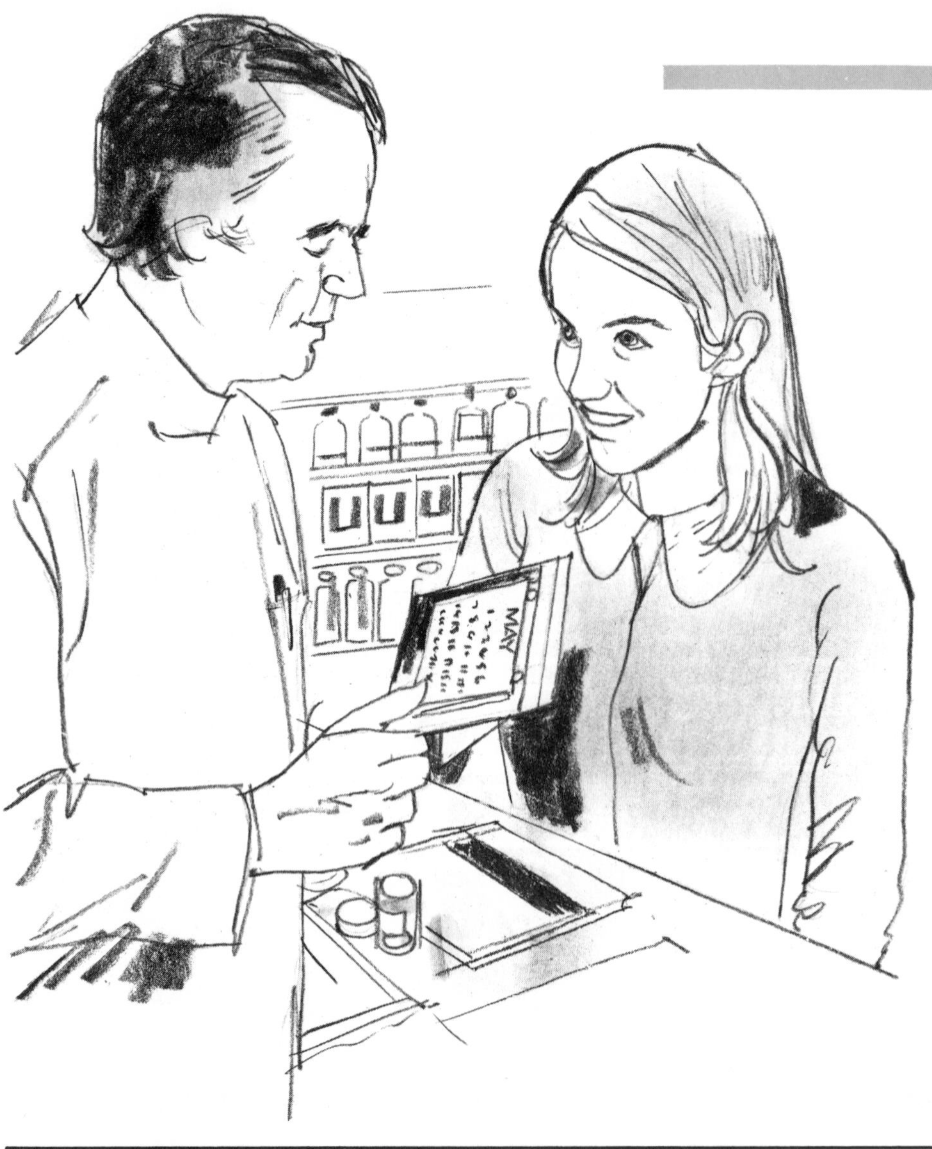

CHAPTER 16

Menstruation is a natural sequence in the reproductive cycle of women. It is the cyclic bleeding from the uterus through the vagina that, in most cases, occurs regularly during the reproductive life of women. Between the ages of 11 and 15, most girls experience menarche, or the beginning of menstruation. Menses, or monthly flow, occurs on a fairly regular basis for the next 35 to 40 years. The time from the onset of one normal menstrual period to the onset of the next one is the menstrual cycle. The average menstrual cycle is 28 to 35 days, and menses lasts for an average of 4 to 7 days.[1 2] The normal length and amount of flow of the cycle vary with each woman.

Menopause is the cessation of the menstrual cycle. Climacteric, often called the "change of life," is the period during which ovarian activity gradually decreases and finally ceases. This usually occurs between the ages of 45 and 55 years. The terms "menopause" and "climacteric" frequently are used interchangeably. At menopause, the uterus, vagina, and vulva decrease in size. The patient may experience "hot flashes" (warm sensations that begin on the trunk and spread to the face) accompanied by redness and sweating. Other menopausal symptoms include irritability, nervousness, fatigability, and headaches. Only a minority of women experiences these symptoms, and most have no complaints attributable to menopause.[3 4]

Physiology of the menstrual cycle

Hormonal control

Menstruation is regulated by the hypothalamus, the anterior pituitary, and the ovaries. The hypothalamus, located at the base of the cerebral cortex, regulates many body functions. It secretes follicle stimulating hormone (FSH) releasing factor, luteinizing hormone (LH) releasing factor, and luteotropic hormone (LTH, also called prolactin) inhibiting factor, which in turn regulate the secretion of FSH, LH, and LTH by the anterior pituitary. These hormones are important in the control of the female reproductive cycle.

The FSH produced stimulates the growth and development of the primordial follicles of the ovaries.[1 5 6] Some of the follicles develop during each menstrual cycle, but usually only one develops completely enough to rupture and release a mature ovum (ovulation). In a 28-day cycle, ovulation usually occurs on about the 14th day of the cycle. LH from the anterior pituitary acts synergistically with FSH to stimulate follicular maturation. Immediately before ovulation, there is a greatly increased secretion of both hormones (Fig. 1).

As the follicle matures, it secretes estrogens which suppress the production of FSH. Although the level of LH also decreases rapidly after ovulation, LH stimulates the ruptured follicle to become the corpus luteum. The corpus luteum secretes large amounts of estrogen and progesterone, which further suppress the production of FSH; progesterone also decreases the production of LH. The estrogens secreted by the maturing follicle stimulate the endometrium of the uterus to proliferate. After ovulation, however, the rapid proliferation ceases. Under the influence of estrogens and progesterone secreted by the corpus luteum, functional differentiation of the endometrium occurs.[6] The endometrium is now rich with blood vessels and glycogen-filled glands and is prepared to receive the ovum which has been progressing downward from the ovary through the fallopian tube. If the ovum has become fertilized, it may become implanted in the endometrium, and intrauterine pregnancy begins.

If implantation does not occur, the corpus luteum begins to regress about 12 days after ovulation, is reabsorbed by the ovarian tissue, and ceases the production of estrogens and progesterone which are needed to maintain the endometrium. The blood vessels of the endometrium constrict, causing local ischemia, rupture of the vessels, and the sloughing of the upper two-thirds of the endometrium.[2] Thus, menstruation begins.

Menstrual flow

The amount of menstrual flow, or discharge, varies between 60 and 250 ml [7] among individuals. Heavier flow may warrant medical attention. The flow is normally heaviest on the second day of menses. The discharge is dark red and consists of blood, cervical mucus, disintegrated vaginal epithelium, and the secretions of vulval sebaceous glands as well as bacteria. The amount of actual blood loss during an entire menstrual period is approximately 30 to 130 ml.[1 8 9] It has been suggested that menstrual blood does not clot because it lacks fibrinogen and prothrombin.[10] It has also been speculated that menstrual blood does clot, but the clots are dissolved *in utero* by fibrinolytic enzymes.[11]

Problem signs and symptoms

Discomfort usually accompanies menstruation, although the symptoms and intensity vary. The etiology of the symptoms is complex and is not fully understood; hormonal changes during the cycle are responsible for some of the complaints.

Dysmenorrhea

Dysmenorrhea is pain at the time of menstruation for which no organic cause can be found.[12] It may occur shortly after the menarche (primary dysmenorrhea) or later in life (secondary dysmenorrhea).

In one report, 50 percent of young women experienced dysmenorrhea, but only 17 percent considered the discomfort worthy of complaint.[13] More recently it was found that 45 percent of teenage girls complained of dysmenorrhea.[13]

Dysmenhorrhea is characterized by lower abdominal cramping accompanied by headache, backache, nausea, and sometimes vomiting. Most women suffer discomfort for several hours on the first day of menstruation but rarely are incapacitated.

The etiology of primary dysmenorrhea is unknown,

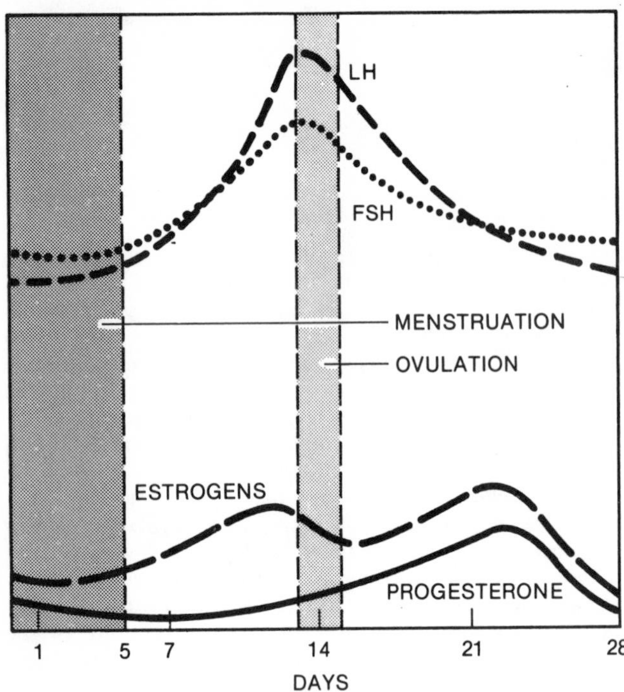

Figure 1. Hormonal fluctuation during the menstrual cycle. (FSH—follicle stimulating hormone; LH—luteinizing hormone.)

but it is generally associated with a degree of hormonal imbalance. A possible explanation involves prostaglandin production by the endometrium.[14] Under the influence of progesterone, the secretory endometrium synthesizes prostaglandin $F_{2\alpha}$ (dinoprost), a neurohormone which causes contraction of smooth muscles. The prostaglandin is released when the endometrium breaks down at menstruation, and the action on uterine muscle and vasculature causes contraction and associated pain. It is felt that if an excessive amount is released into the circulation, the systemic effects characteristically associated with dysmenorrhea, e.g., diarrhea, nausea, flushing, and syncope, occur. Dysmenorrhea is usually relieved after delivery of a full-term fetus. Secondary dysmenorrhea can be a symptom of a more serious condition, such as endometriosis, uterine hypoplasia, pelvic inflammation disease, pelvic neoplasm, or retroversion of the uterus.[7 15] It may also be a result of constipation, poor posture, or exposure to cold. Dysmenorrhea can be aggravated by emotional factors.

Dalton[16] described congestive and spasmodic (secondary) dysmenorrhea. Congestive dysmenorrhea is caused by fluid retention and is characterized by a dull, aching pain in the lower abdomen and other symptoms of premenstrual tension. Spasmodic dysmenorrhea is "spasms of acute colicky pains" occurring about every 20 minutes.

Other problems

The high level of estrogen prior to menstruation may cause weight gain through the retention of sodium and water. The fluid is retained extracellularly, and edema can occur in the ankles, hands, breasts, face, and abdomen. As much as 10 lb may be gained, and some clothes and even dentures may not fit well.[9 17]

About 50 percent of women experience a degree of premenstrual tension, especially in their 30's and 40's. Premenstrual tension is characterized by nervousness, irritability, depression, headache, abdominal distention, nausea, vomiting, diarrhea and/or constipation, fatigue, breast tenderness, and generalized edema. The fluid retention responsible for weight gain may also cause many of these symptoms. Some of the psychological symptoms such as insomnia, agitation, anxiety, and depression may be caused by sodium retention and potassium depletion, and fatigue and sweating may be attributed to decreased blood sugar levels.[18] Symptoms may occur 7 to 10 days before menstruation, disappearing with the onset of menses.[7 15 17] The degree of premenstrual tension varies. Some women may exhibit no symptoms. The amount of premenstrual discomfort correlates well with a woman's general response to stress.[10] Women in high school and college scored 3 to 5 percent lower on examinations taken just prior to or during menses than at other times in their menstrual cycle.[19]

Lower abdominal pain at the time of ovulation (mittelschmerz) may be mild or acute and usually lasts for only a few hours. It is not experienced by all women or during every cycle. The etiology of the pain is unknown but may be the result of irritation to the lining of the pelvic cavity caused by occasional ovarian or intra-abdominal bleeding at the time of ovulation.[9]

Amenorrhea is the absence (not postmenopausal) of menses. It may be permanent or temporary and can be caused by an alteration of hormonal balance (including that caused by oral contraceptives), anemia, an altered emotional state, overwork, or a change in environment. The most common cause is pregnancy. Amenorrhea is a frequent result of other pathological conditions such as tuberculosis, diabetes mellitus, nephritis, obesity, malnutrition, and syphilis.[1] Hypomenorrhea is a diminished amount of flow or a shortened duration of menstruation. Hypermenorrhea, or menorrhagia, is abnormally profuse or prolonged menstruation. It may be caused by glandular imbalance or delayed repair of the endometrium.[1 7 15 20] Metrorrhagia is uterine bleeding that occurs at a time other than the menstrual period. The bleeding may be prolonged, but it is not always excessive. It is caused by many conditions, including lesions of the cervix or endometrium and neoplasms of the uterus or ovaries, and should always be investigated.[1 15] The "spotting" that some women experience is a mild form of metrorrhagia.

Acne is often worse premenstrually or at the time of menstruation. This is when the level of estrogens is the lowest, but the role of estrogens in acne is unknown. It has been suggested that estrogens make sebaceous gland secretions more fluid and inhibit the formation of "blackheads" and other lesions that are characteristic of acne.[21] Other studies indicate that estrogens decrease the size of sebaceous glands and/or the production of androgen, which stimulates the sebaceous glands.[3 22]

Treating menstrual discomfort

Although the discomfort associated with menstruation is common and may not be serious, the patient should be referred to a physician, especially if the symptoms are new or unusual. Symptoms of amenorrhea, hypermenorrhea, metrorrhagia, and severe pain or nausea must be evaluated by a physician to determine if they are indicative of a more serious condition.

The pharmacist should recommend periodic examination of individuals using OTC medication regularly. If a physician has been consulted about the present symptom, it is important to find out when, what type of medication or treatment was recommended, and if the recommendations were followed. If self-medication is appropriate, it is important to determine which, if any, nonprescription remedies were tried previously (and with what results), other diseases or conditions that might exhibit similar symptoms, other medications being taken, and when the symptoms (pain or bleeding) occurred in relation to a normal cycle.

Some women decrease their sodium and fluid intake during the last half of their cycle. The decrease in sodium is probably safer and more beneficial than restricted fluid intake in reducing the expected edema. Symptomatic relief of pain and cramping can sometimes be obtained by application of heat to the abdomen or use of the knee-chest position.

Ingredients in OTC products

Analgesics, diuretics, and antihistamines are the usual nonprescription medications used for discomfort associated with menstruation.

Analgesics. Analgesics are more useful in relieving headache and muscle pain than deep, visceral pain. They are well absorbed from the GI tract and are widely distributed in the body. The effectiveness of aspirin and acetaminophen as analgesics is nearly the same. If the only symptom described is pain, it is appropriate to recommend and less expensive to use plain aspirin, acetaminophen, or aspirin, phenacetin, and caffeine than one of the combination OTC menstrual products. The recommended dosage for single-entity analgesics is 300 to 600 mg of aspirin or acetaminophen every 4 to 6 hours not to exceed 2,400 mg in 24 hours. These products are relatively nontoxic, unless they are used regularly for more than 10 days or in massive doses.

Acute salicylate poisoning is common, especially in children. As with all other drug products, menstrual products should be kept out of the reach of children.

Allergic reactions to the analgesics are infrequent but are slightly more common with the salicylates than with phenacetin or acetaminophen. The GI irritation produced by the salicylates can be minimized by ingesting food, milk, or an antacid with the medication.

Self-medication with analgesics, particularly the salicylates, should be discouraged in certain conditions. The salicylates are contraindicated with anticoagulants or uricosuric agents, and they should not be used in cases of active peptic ulcers. (See Chapter 10 for a discussion of internal analgesics.)

Diuretics. Although the effectiveness of OTC diuretics is doubtful, they are often found in menstrual products. Prescription diuretics, such as hydrochlorothiazide (50 to 100 mg/day), often help relieve premenstrual tension, although their exact mechanism is unknown.

One of the most commonly used OTC premenstrual diuretics is pamabrom, a xanthine diuretic which probably acts directly on renal tubules. It increases sodium excretion without producing significant potassium loss. Pamabrom has received favorable reports. Unfortunately, the reports are old and based on poorly controlled studies.[11, 23] It is claimed that pamabrom relieves the fluid retention that causes weight gain and premenstrual tension without the need for further diuretic treatment or potassium supplementation. It does not deplete body fluids below the normal body balance. Intake should not exceed 200 mg/day.[24]

Caffeine is also a xanthine derivative that inhibits the renal reabsorption of sodium and water, thus promoting diuresis. It is usually considered to be free of toxicity in the amount usually used in premenstrual products (30 mg), but in higher doses (100 mg), it is a CNS stimulant.

Ammonium chloride is a short-term diuretic. It is an acid-forming salt which has limited value as a diuretic. It promotes the loss of extracellular electrolytes and water for 1 to 2 days. The effective dose is 4 to 8 g/day, but no available OTC product provides or recommends this dose. It should not be used in cases of decreased renal function.[25-27]

Antihistamines. Antihistamines are used for their sedative side effects which possibly help relieve the nervousness and irritability associated with premenstrual tension. Their usefulness is questionable, however, because of the low dosage. The amount contained in menstrual products is one-eighth to one-half the usual recommended dose for this effect.[28, 29] The antihistamine most frequently used in menstrual products is pyrilamine maleate. Methapyrilene fumarate and phenindamine tartrate are also used. Even in the low dosages in menstrual products, the antihistamines may cause drowsiness.

Miscellaneous. Other ingredients are found in various menstrual products, but their value is questionable. Homatropine methylbromide is found in subtherapeutic dosages. Even at these doses, however, patients with glaucoma should not use products containing homatropine. One product contains cinnamedrine hydrochloride, an antispasmodic intended to relieve the cramping associated with menstruation. Although the manufacturer claims that the product is effective, the real value of cinnamedrine has not been established.[30]

Guidelines for product selection

After discussing the extent of the problem with the patient, the pharmacist can help in product selection. In this discussion the pharmacist has learned of the severity of the problem and of other pathological conditions or allergies. If a patient profile is maintained, it also can provide information on allergies, potential drug interactions, idiosyncrasies, and medications currently being used.

If the patient experiences only pain, an analgesic can be recommended. If edema and/or tension occur, one of the combination products may be considered, but proof of their efficacy is lacking. The pharmacist must keep in mind that a patient suffering from severe symptoms should be referred to a physician. In most cases, however, the complaints accompanying menstruation can be controlled by OTC products. In the severe cases, the physician will generally prescribe a more potent medication after the cause of the symptoms has been determined.

Current advertising often stresses that women need iron supplementation because of blood loss during menstruation. However, the actual loss of blood during a normal menstrual period is relatively low, and an average diet can easily replace the amount of iron that is lost.[31] If the flow is very heavy or after pregnancy, a physician should be consulted; after the appropriate testing, iron supplements may be prescribed.

Related menstrual products

Feminine napkins and tampons. Taboos and superstitions about menstruation have existed for hundreds of years. Even today, such ideas continue, not only among primitive people. However, knowledge has helped to eliminate most of the superstitions, especially those about feminine napkins and tampons. It is important that misconceptions about menstruation be dispelled. Pharmacists should be prepared and willing to provide this health education. Feminine napkins are available in many shapes and sizes and can be worn by using belts, special panties, or regular panties.[32-34]

Feminine napkins are usually made of gauze packed with cotton and/or cellulose. They are worn over the perineum to absorb the menstrual discharge. Tampons are also made of cotton and are inserted into the vagina to absorb the menstrual discharge before it leaves the vagina.[32]

Young girls who are beginning menstruation and women with a light menstrual flow can use napkins marketed as "mini-pads," "junior," "teenage," or "for light days." "Regular" (for normal flow) and "super" (for heavy flow) napkins are also available. Tampons are less bulky than napkins and offer equal protection without chafing, binding, or irritation. Girls and women who have a light or normal flow can use the regular tampon; the super tampon is available for a heavier flow. Two regular tampons can be used at the same time.

Napkins and tampons create very few problems. Occasionally, internal irritation occurs when using a tampon. This generally is eliminated by frequent changing. When the last tampon is forgotten and not removed, it can cause irritation. Feminine napkins can chafe the inner thigh. Talcum or a medicated powder, frequent changing of napkins, and temporary use of tampons can soothe the skin. Odor caused by the decomposition of blood on the napkin can be reduced by frequent changing. Napkins and tampons should be changed every 3 to 4 hours during heavy flow, less frequently when the flow is lighter.

Cleansing products. Personal hygiene during menstruation is important. Perspiration or products of menstrual flow have no odor unless they are left on the surface of the skin. Therefore, regular bathing or showering is recommended. Towelettes to clean the external genitalia provide more protection than routine cleansing. The value of douching is questionable and is generally not encouraged. If douching is used, it should not be done more than twice a week unless otherwise directed by a physician. (See Chapter 18 on feminine cleansing and deodorant products.)

Summary

Although most women experience discomfort during menstruation, symptoms can generally be controlled by OTC products; women who have severe or unusual symptoms should be referred to a physician. Single-entity analgesics, such as aspirin and acetaminophen, seem to relieve the pain that may accompany ovulation or menstruation. If minor edema and tension occur, a combination product containing a diuretic (pamabrom or caffeine) may be helpful. Pamabrom is probably more effective than caffeine, but the value of diuretics for premenstrual tension is debatable. The value of an antihistamine as a sedative to help relieve irritation and tension is not proven. However, if a product with an antihistamine is recommended, pyrilamine maleate appears to be the agent of choice. Cinnamedrine hydrochloride may give some relief from cramping. Generally, dosages of menstrual products should not exceed two tablets every 6 hours.

Normal personal hygiene should continue during menstruation. Cleanliness and frequent changing of napkins and tampons eliminate nearly all irritation and offensive odor. Unless otherwise advised by a physician, normal activities, such as sports and taking a bath or shower, can continue. They cause no undue stress or harm to the reproductive organs.

References

1. M. M. Bookmiller and G. L. Bowen, "Textbook of Obstetrics and Obstetric Nursing," 4th ed., Saunders, Philadelphia, Pa., 1963, p. 64.
2. E. S. Taylor, "Essentials of Gynecology," 4th ed., Lea and Febiger, Philadelphia, Pa., 1969, p. 69.
3. V. B. Mountcastle, "Medical Physiology," vol. 1, 12th ed., Mosby, St. Louis, Mo., 1968, p. 1015.
4. E. S. Taylor, "Essentials of Gynecology," 4th ed., Lea and Febiger, Philadelphia, Pa., 1969, pp. 484, 493.
5. D. W. Smith *et al.*, "Care of the Adult Patient," 3d ed., Lippincott, Philadelphia, Pa., 1971, p. 879.
6. "Best and Taylor's Physiological Basis of Medical Practice," 9th ed., J. R. Brobeck, Ed., Williams and Wilkins, Baltimore, Md., 1973, pp. 7-102.
7. T. R. Harrison *et al.*, "Principles of Internal Medicine," McGraw-Hill (Blakiston Div.), New York, N.Y., 1966, p. 94.
8. E. S. Taylor, "Essentials of Gynecology," 4th ed., Lea and Febiger, Philadelphia, Pa., 1969, p. 73.
9. E. C. Pierson and W. V. D'Antonio, "Female and Male: Dimensions of Human Sexuality," Lippincott, Philadelphia, Pa., 1974, p. 130.
10. J. L. McCary, "Human Sexuality," 2d ed., Van Nostrand Reinhold, New York, N.Y., 1973, p. 93.
11. C. Huggins *et al., Am. J. Obstet. Gynecol.,* **78,** 46(1943).
12. R. C. Benson, in "Current Medical Diagnosis and Treatment," M. A. Krupp and M. J. Chatton, Eds., Lange Medical Publications, Los Altos, Calif., 1974, p. 407.
13. E. S. Taylor, "Essentials of Gynecology," 4th ed., Lea and Febiger, Philadelphia, Pa., 1969, p. 533.
14. E. R. Novak *et al.*, "Novak's Textbook of Gynecology," 8th ed., Williams and Wilkins, Baltimore, Md., 1970, p. 637.
15. "The Merck Manual," 11th ed., Merck & Co., Rahway, N.J., 1966, p. 659.
16. K. Dalton, "The Menstrual Cycle," Pantheon, New York, N.Y., 1969, p. 39.
17. K. Dalton, "The Menstrual Cycle," Pantheon, New York, N.Y., 1969, p. 56.
18. K. Dalton, "The Menstrual Cycle," Pantheon, New York, N.Y., 1969, p. 62.
19. K. Dalton, *Lancet,* **2,** 1386(Dec. 28, 1968).
20. E. C. Hughes, "Obstetric-Gynecologic Terminology," F. A. Davis, Philadelphia, Pa., 1972, p. 292.
21. W. F. Ganong, "Review of Medical Physiology," 6th ed., Lange Medical Publications, Los Altos, Calif., 1973, p. 333.
22. W. Bickers and M. Woods, *N. Engl. J. Med.,* **245,** 453(Sept. 20, 1951).
23. R. B. Greenblatt, *GP, XI,* 66(March, 1955).
24. Product information provided by Chattem Laboratories, Chattanooga, Tenn.
25. "The Pharmacological Basis of Therapeutics," 4th ed., L. S. Goodman and A. Gilman, Eds., Macmillan, New York, N.Y., 1970, p. 845.
26. "AMA Drug Evaluations," 2d ed., Publishing Sciences Group, Acton, Mass., 1973, p. 75.
27. V. H. Lee and B. Rowles, *J. Am. Pharm. Assoc.,* in press.
28. "The Pharmacological Basis of Therapeutics," 4th ed., L. S. Goodman and A. Gilman, Eds., Macmillan, New York, N.Y., 1970, pp. 642-643.
29. "AMA Drug Evaluations," 2d ed., Publishing Sciences Group, Acton, Mass., 1973, p. 494.
30. Product information provided by Glenbrook Laboratories, New York, N.Y.
31. D. C. Price *et al., Can. Med. Assoc. J.,* **90,** 51(1964).
32. F. Sadik, *J. Am. Pharm. Assoc.,* **NS 12,** 565(1972).
33. Product information provided by Personal Products Co., Milltown, N.J.
34. Product information provided by Kimberly-Clark Corp., Neenah, Wis.

Product[a] (manufacturer)	Analgesic	Diuretic	Antihistamine	Caffeine	Other
Aqua-Ban (Thompson Medical)	—	ammonium chloride, 325 mg	—	100 mg	—
Cardui (Chattem)	salicylamide, 250 mg phenacetin, 125 mg	pamabrom, 25 mg	pyrilamine maleate, 12.5 mg	—	—
Femcaps Capsules (Buffington)	aspirin[b] phenacetin[b]	—	—	citrate[b]	ephedrine sulfate, 8 mg atropine sulfate, 0.03 mg
Femicin (Norcliff-Thayer)	salicylamide, 225 mg acetaminophen, 160 mg	—	pyrilamine maleate, 15 mg	65 mg	homatropine methyl-bromide, 0.5 mg
Flowaway Water 100's (DeWitt)	—	uva ursi extract, 98 mg buchu leaves extract, 24 mg	—	20 mg	potassium nitrate, 171 mg
Fluidex (O'Connor)	—	buchu powdered extract, 65 mg couch grass powdered extract, 65 mg corn silk powdered extract, 32.5 mg hydrangea powdered extract, 32.5 mg	—	—	—
Fluidex-Plus with Diadax (O'Connor)	—	buchu powdered extract, 65 mg couch grass powdered extract, 65 mg corn silk powdered extract, 32.5 mg hydrangea powdered extract, 32.5 mg	—	—	phenylpropanolamine hydrochloride, 25 mg
Humphrey's No. 11 (Humphrey's Pharmacal)	—	—	—	—	cimicifuga, 3X pulsatilla, 3X sepia, 3X
Lydia Pinkham (Smith, Miller & Patch)	—	—	—	—	extract of Jamaica dogwood, pleurisy root, and licorice[b] ferrous sulfate[b]
Lydia Pinkham Vegetable Compound Liquid (Smith, Miller & Patch)	—	—	—	—	extract of Jamaica dogwood, pleurisy root, and licorice[b] alcohol[b]
Midol (Glenbrook)	aspirin, 453.6 mg	—	—	32.4 mg	cinnamedrine, 14.9 mg
Odrinil (Fox)	—	buchu powdered extract 34.4 mg uva ursi powdered extract, 34.4 mg corn silk powdered extract, 34.4 mg juniper powdered extract, 16.2 mg	—	extract, 16.2 mg	—
Pamprin (Chattem)	salicylamide, 250 mg phenacetin, 125 mg	pamabrom, 25 mg	pyrilamine maleate, 12.5 mg	—	—
Pre-Mens Forte (Blair)	—	ammonium chloride, 500 mg	—	100 mg	—
Trendar (Whitehall)	acetaminophen, 240 mg	pamabrom, 50 mg	phenindamine tartrate, 12.5 mg	—	—

[a] Tablet unless specified otherwise.   [b] Quantity not specified.

Contraceptive Methods and Products

James Huff
Luis Hernandez

Questions to ask the patient

Are you currently using a contraceptive method or product? If so, what do you use?

Have you consulted a physician or family planning service?

Do you understand the principles of contraception?

Do you have any problems possibly related to your method/product of contraception, such as irritation, inconvenience, or unusual symptoms?

Do you think you might have VD?

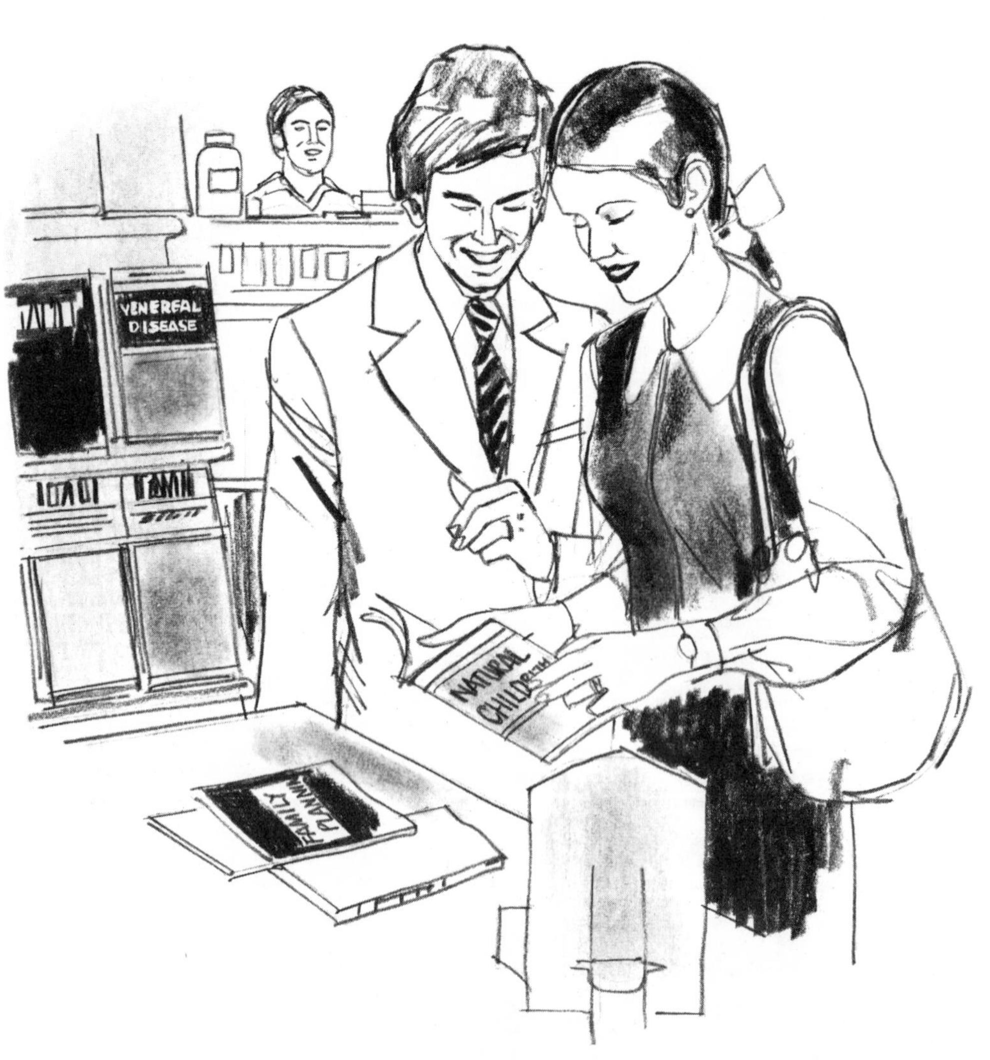

CHAPTER 17

Recent trends to smaller families and the increase in venereal disease suggest that the pharmacist and other health-care practitioners must be able to supply accurate and definitive information on methods of contraception and VD prevention. In addition, with the controversy that surrounds oral contraceptive therapy, OTC contraceptive items represent a viable alternative for many persons.

Pharmacists, who are frequently the first health professionals consulted, should be knowledgeable about the various methods of contraception and should assist their patients in determining which methods or products best suit the patients' needs.

Conception

Conception is the union of an ovum (egg) from the female and a spermatozoon (sperm) from the male, and contraception is the voluntary prevention of conception (impregnation). Anything that blocks any part of the fertilization process in the male or female or that prevents or even delays the union of the sperm with the egg can prevent conception and is called a contraceptive agent, device, or method.

After ovulation, the egg remains fertilizable for about 6 to 24 hours, possibly as long as 48 hours. (See Chapter 16 for a discussion of the female reproductive cycle.) After ejaculation, the sperm retains its ability to fertilize an egg for about 28 to 48 hours, although normal sperm life may be 72 hours in the presence of cervical mucus and as long as 5 or more days under "optimum conditions." In general, for intercourse to result in conception, it must take place within the 4-day period including 2 days before the release of the egg, the day of ovulation, and 1 day after.

The survival time of sperm in a condition in which they can fertilize the egg is a major consideration in preventing conception. Although the sperm may remain active (maximum duration of motility is 48 to 60 hours), they may be beyond the point where they can fertilize an egg, i.e., past the maximum period of sperm viability.[1-4] Sperm remain viable in the vagina for 2.5 hours, in the cervix for perhaps 48 hours, in the cavum uteri for 48 hours, and in the fallopian tube, where they also can fertilize an egg, for a maximum of 48 hours.[1] The time periods are not additive.

The ejaculated sperm of mammals with scrotal testicles lose their fertility because of the abdominal temperature in the female genitalia and the alkaline secretion of the accessory male sex glands with which they are mixed during ejaculation.[5]

Need for information

Contrary to popular belief, many persons in the U.S. do not understand the basic principles of reproduction and conception.[6 7] Family planning services generally are lacking or unused at colleges and universities and, although many elementary and secondary schools attempt to provide sex education and birth control programs, they are frequently inadequate, underfunded, or instituted after sex patterns have been established.[8-13]

Illegitimacy and unwanted pregnancies are frequent occurrences.[14-16] Additionally, the number of gonorrhea cases has been increasing since the mid-1960's at an annual rate of 12 percent.[17]

All this evidence suggests that pharmacists must be able to provide nonjudgmental counseling and recommendations to their patients, particularly young persons and those from lower socioeconomic situations who have limited access to such information.

Prevention of conception

Contraception can be accomplished by preventing semen from entering the vagina or the cervical canal, by preventing follicular development, by preventing attachment of a mature egg to the endometrium, by limiting intercourse to times when a mature egg is not available for fertilization, or by immobilizing sperm that have entered the vaginal canal.

The ideal method should be effective, safe, simple, easy to dispense, inexpensive, reversible, and acceptable. Several methods approach this ideal, but none has achieved it.

Methods of contraception that do not require a prescription include abstinence, coitus interruptus (withdrawal), coitus reservatus, condoms, creams and jellies, douching, foaming tablets, foam, rhythm, sponges, and suppositories. The pharmacist should suggest that the patient consult a physician or a family planning service before selecting a birth control method.

By 1973, 18.6 million of the 26.6 million married couples in the U.S. were using contraception.[18] The choice of the most acceptable method of contraception is a paramount issue. Selection of a contraceptive method is extremely personal and should be individualized. The key to its success is motivation: if it is strong, nearly any contraceptive method will be reasonably successful.[19]

Methods of contraception

Rhythm. The rhythm method is abstinence from sexual relations during the fertile period of the female cycle. Rhythm is one of the least effective methods. However, some couples, especially if the woman has a regular menstrual cycle, find this method satisfactory.

The major, relatively simple techniques for establishing the time of ovulation are the calendar method (Ogino-Knaus), the thermal or temperature method (basal body temperature, BBT), and the cervical mucus method (ovulation method).[20] The calendar method predicts ovulation on the basis of probabilities calculated from a woman's menstrual history; the thermal method detects, whereas the cervical mucus method predicts, ovulation on the basis of specific physiological changes that occur during the menstrual cycle.

If ovulation could be determined accurately, rhythm would undoubtedly become a more acceptable method of contraception. If intercourse were avoided for 2 days prior to ovulation, the day of ovulation, and 1 day after ovulation, theoretically, conception would not occur. These 4 days constitute the fertile (unsafe) phase of the menstrual cycle; the intermenstrual days before and after are the infertile (safe) phase. The alternation of the fertile phase with the preceding and succeeding infertile phases is called the rhythm.[21] Unfortunately, most women differ tremendously in the length of the menstrual cycles, making it nearly impossible to determine precisely when ovulation occurs.[22]

When ovulation begins, a woman's basal body temperature drops slightly, followed by a rise of about 0.5° over 24 to 72 hours. After 2 days of elevated temperature, the safe period begins. The temperature fluctuation and a meticulous graphical record of at least 1 year's menstrual cycles form the basis of predicting ovulation and using the rhythm method. For added safety, intercourse should be avoided a few days before and after the unsafe period, thereby lengthening the period of abstinence.

A thermometer specifically designed to check basal body temperature should be used. It records 96 to 100° F (35.5 to 37.7° C) with 0.1° intervals, allowing detection of small changes in body temperature. Better accuracy is achieved from a rectal recording of 5 minutes as soon as the woman awakens and before getting out of bed.[23] The thermometer should be shaken down the night before and placed at the bedside (to prevent physical exertion upon awakening which causes a rise in temperature). Charts for recording the basal body temperature during the menstrual cycle are available.

For Catholic patients, pharmacists should be aware that the methods of contraception approved by the Catholic church are abstinence and rhythm.[20] The patient should be fully informed of the risks and difficulties inherent in practicing rhythm.

Coitus interruptus (incompletus), or withdrawal. Coitus interruptus involves the removal of the stimulated penis from the vagina and the area of external genitalia before ejaculation. Coitus reservatus differs from coitus interruptus in that penetration takes place in the normal way, but ejaculation is avoided, and the penis remains in the vagina until it becomes flaccid. The problem with both methods is that sperm in the urethral secretions released prior to ejaculation can fertilize the egg.

OTC contraceptive products

Condoms

Contraceptive methods used by males are receiving increased attention.[24-27] The most common methods are coitus interruptus and the use of condoms. Both require control and forethought.

Condoms (sheaths, bags, French letters, prophylactics, protectives, rubbers, scum bags, skins, safes) are among the most widely used, most effective, and practical contraceptives. They are simple to use, harmless, inexpensive, easy to buy, and do not require a physical examination or physician's advice. They are the only relatively effective, easily obtained contraceptive used by males. One significant characteristic of condoms is that their purpose and function are easy to understand: sperm are deposited in the condom and not in the vagina.

Offering dual protection against pregnancy and VD, the condom today is a carefully produced, rigorously tested, and highly effective contraceptive product which is readily available through nonclinical channels.[28-30]

The annual production of condoms in the U.S. is estimated at more than 750 million. Americans spend nearly $150 million a year on condoms, most of which are obtained from pharmacies.[31]

Condoms are made of rubber (or latex) and collagenous tissue (frequently obtained from young lamb cecum). These materials are elastic, strong, and thin. The skin condom, the first type developed, generally is considered a luxury, and rubber condoms are used more frequently.

The psychological and physiological needs of the potential condom buyer and user are met by a wide choice

Table 1. Comparison of Contraceptive Effectiveness[a]

Oral contraceptive									
Combination	*Sequential*	**Intrauterine device**	**Diaphragm and spermicide**	**Condom**	**Rhythm**	**Spermicide**	**Coitus interruptus**	**Douche**	**Reference**
1	2	3	4	6	—[b]	5	7	—	51
1	1	2	2	2	2[c], 4[d]	3[e], 4[f]	4	5	52
1	1	2	5	3	4	6	6	7	53
1	1	—	2	2	4	3[e], 4[g]	4	5	54
1	2	2	3	4	7	6	5	8	55
—	—	—	2	1	4	—	3	5	56
1	1	2	4	5	3	6	—	—	57
1.0	1.3	2.2	3.1	3.3	3.8	4.6	4.8	6.0	Mean[h]

[a] Scale of 1 (best) through 8 (worst) is used.

[b] Dashes indicate that figures for the particular method of contraception were not reported.

[c] Thermometer.

[d] Calendar.

[e] Foam.

[f] Cream, jelly, foaming tablets, suppositories, and sponge with liquid or powder.

[g] Cream or gel, vaginal tablets, suppositories, sponge, and foam.

[h] Average per class indicating rank order.

of styles: opaque, transparent, colored, plain ended, reservoir ended, rippled or pagoda shaped, strictured or contoured, flocked with a rough rubber surface, dry, lubricated with a water-soluble substance or with silicone, and several different sizes.[28] Condom thickness appears better correlated with durability (therefore, effectiveness) than with other dimensions. Condoms usually are thicker toward the closed end.

Although condoms provide a high degree of protection against conception, accidents can happen. When condoms are used correctly, failures may result from tearing or rupture of the condom; this is the major cause of failure, but it is infrequent.[32]

Two techniques help prevent bursting of the condom: if it is plain ended, it should be unrolled on the erect penis with about 0.5 inch of space left at the end to accommodate the ejaculation; if the natural moisture in the woman's genital tract is scant, the outside of the condom should be lubricated to prevent tearing upon insertion.[33] The best lubricant for the nonlubricated condom is a contraceptive cream or jelly. Petroleum jelly, liquid petrolatum, and other oils should not be used because they may cause rubber to deteriorate.

An often overlooked reason for inadvertent impregnation is improper use of the condom, probably from lack of knowledge. First, prior to ejaculation, sperm in the urethral secretions can cause conception. Second, because of loss of erection following ejaculation, semen may leak out the open end of the condom or the condom may slip off while the penis is still in the vagina or upon withdrawal. For best contraceptive effectiveness, the condom must be put on prior to the first insertion of the penis into the vagina and worn throughout coitus. Following ejaculation, the penis should be removed from the vagina before leakage occurs or before the condom can slip off. Accidents can be avoided if the ring (or open end) at the top of the condom is held securely to prevent spillage during withdrawal. As an added protection, the condom can be coated with a vaginal contraceptive (foam, cream, or jelly) in conjunction with the use of a vaginal contraceptive prior to intercourse. This method provides lubrication and a secondary defense against spilled semen.

The reservoir-end condom is less likely to burst because there is ample space to hold the ejaculated semen; the lubricated kind allows easier insertion. The lubricated, reservoir-end condom is the preferred type; however, the user may have reasons for preferring another type.

The condom is an effective mechanical barrier to infection.[34,35] Because it is the only contraceptive that prevents both the contact and the infection, substantially reducing the risk of transmitting gonorrhea and syphilis, its use should be encouraged. Improvement of the product, its packaging, design, and promotion could result in its wider use and decrease unwanted pregnancies and VD.[36]

VD is an epidemic disease caused by *Neisseria gonorrhoeae*.[37-39] In the U.S., 3 million adolescents and young adults are infected at any given time.[17] One million new cases are reported annually, three times more than all other reportable infectious diseases. However, apparently, only one case in eight is reported. The disease is rampant because gonorrhea infection confers little or no immunity against subsequent infections; many affected persons are not inconvenienced by the signs and symptoms and do not seek treatment; and nearly 50 percent have no noticeable symptoms and, thus, are unsuspecting carriers.

Fewer than 6 in 10 pharmacies displayed condoms in 1975.[31] Reasons for not displaying them were fear of community disapproval or pharmacists' personal disapproval.

Table 2. Persons Seeking Advice on Contraception from the Pharmacist

Frequency	Persons seeking advice	
	From male pharmacists	*From female pharmacists*
Male	**Percent**	**Percent**
Often	21	3
Rarely	68	73
Never	11	20
Female		
Often	19	35
Rarely	71	52
Never	10	13

Most pharmacists are not reluctant, however, to show female contraceptive products, and a significant number will not sell contraceptives to unmarried minors.[40] These practices are not conducive to the pharmacist becoming an active member of the health-care team, especially in the area of preventive medicine: 14 or more million Americans have VD, and contraception generally is preferrable to abortion and unwanted pregnancy.

Vaginal contraceptives

There are four basic types of chemical contraceptives used vaginally: creams, jellies, and pastes that usually are squeezed from a tube; suppositories; soluble films; and foams, either in tablet form or pressurized containers.[41] Research is directed toward the identification of vaginal preparations with both contraceptive and prophylactic properties.

Vaginal spermicides. The combination of a diaphragm and chemical spermicide has been used for many years as an effective method of contraception. Vaginal spermicidal preparations designed to be used without a diaphragm or other contraceptive devices are available. Both types contain two components: a spermicidal chemical that actively immobilizes and kills sperm, and an inert base that mechanically guards the cervical os. The base is formulated to promote spreading over the os. Spermicides are inexpensive and harmless and are generally accepted as effective. The nonreactive base of the vaginal spermicides may be an aerosol foam, cream, or jelly. The vaginal spermicides are formulated as foams, creams, jellies, gels, vaginal suppositories, and vaginal tablets.

The choice of cream or jelly depends on individual preference. The cream provides greater lubrication during intercourse. The jelly affords easier removal and dissipation because it is completely water soluble. Foams, on the other hand, do not contribute any appreciable lubrication but have the advantage of being almost totally undetectable during use.

The vaginal spermicidal preparations are not the same as the creams and jellies intended for use with a diaphragm; they generally are more potent and of a different consistency than the agents used with other contraceptive devices. This distinction should be considered carefully when dispensing these products.

The most commonly used spermicidal chemicals are the polyoxyethylated alkylphenols (nonionic surface-active agents). The number of polyoxyethylene groups in the side chain determines spermicidal activity.

Some products are formulated to create a distinctly acid pH in the vaginal tract. A pH below 3.5 is considered spermicidal with increasing effectiveness as the pH decreases. Boric acid and ricinoleic acid are used in vaginal spermicidal products for this purpose. Phenylmercuric acid also is used in these products.

Using a special applicator, the required amount of vaginal spermicide is deposited near the cervix. Coital movements distribute the agent throughout the vagina and over the cervix. The spermicide should be inserted not more than 1 hour, preferably 10 to 30 minutes, before intercourse. One full application of spermicide is enough for only one intercourse; if intercourse is repeated, another dose of the contraceptive must be inserted. Douching should not be attempted for 6 to 8 hours after intercourse. It dilutes or removes the spermicidal agent, without necessarily removing viable sperm.

The vaginal spermicide alone is less effective in preventing pregnancy than the diaphragm-cream technique, which adds a better mechanical barrier. However, the foam, cream, or jelly alone is simpler to use and avoids the medical examination and prescription.

In one study of 2,168 women using the diaphragm and jelly, accidental pregnancies in the first 12 months of use ranged from 1.9 per 100 for women under 18 to 3.0 per 100 for women 30 to 34 years old.[42] These rates compared favorably with those for prescription oral contraceptive agents and the intrauterine device (IUD).

Allergic reactions to spermicides are uncommon, but they are important. If either partner experiences an allergic response to the spermicide, the pharmacist should instruct the person to discontinue use immediately and contact a physician. In some cases, a chemical contraceptive may cause local irritation or soreness. In general, switching to another brand of contraceptive is sufficient to ameliorate the signs and symptoms. If a person does not wish to see a physician, the pharmacist should recommend an alternative product with a different formula.

Aerosol foams. This method of contraception involves the use of an aerosol dispenser to load a vaginal applicator by which the spermicidal foam is inserted before coitus. Prefilled applicators also are available. Basically, the foam is a spermicidal cream, packaged as an aerosol, that foams when it is released. It is one of the most effective and acceptable vaginal contraceptive methods and is considered by many women more esthetically pleasing than vaginal jellies or tablets. Good adherence to the vaginal walls and tenacious covering of the cervical os make the foams one of the best vaginal contraceptives. The foams leak very little during or after intercourse.

The applicator is filled by attaching it to the aerosol container of foam and activating the aerosol valve until the applicator is filled. The applicator is then inserted into the vagina in the same way as the cream and jellies, making certain that placement is well into the vagina before the plunger is depressed to deposit the foam at the cervical os.

The only difference or advantage of the newer, prefilled foams is that the applicator can be filled with foam and be ready to use as long as 7 days prior to insertion. Foam must be inserted and applied no more than 1 hour before sexual intercourse and should remain in the vaginal tract for 8 hours after intercourse. An additional applicatorful should be inserted each time intercourse is repeated. As with all topically applied chemical contraceptives, irritation of the vagina and penis may occur, and, in these cases, the foams should be discontinued immediately.

In one study, a vaginal contraceptive foam was used by nearly 3,000 women for approximately 28,000 cycles with a pregnancy rate of 3.98 per 100 woman-years.[43] The rate is relatively low for a vaginal contraceptive; effectiveness was attributed to patient instruction and motivation as well as frequent contact between patient and clinic staff. The only side effect that caused patients to stop using the foam was irritation to the patient (107 women) or to the patient's partner (17 men).

Suppositories and tablets. Suppositories contain spermicides, usually mercurial compounds, incorporated in a cocoa butter or glycerin base which melts or dissolves at body temperature. After insertion, the user should wait at least 20 minutes before intercourse to allow for melting and distribution of the suppository. This waiting is a disadvantage that, along with variations in melting time, contributes to lower effectiveness.

Foaming tablets, upon coming in contact with the moisture in the vagina, disintegrate and release carbon dioxide, covering the uterine entrance with foam to block the sperm. A tablet should be inserted into the vagina near the cervix from a few minutes to 1 hour before intercourse. To determine if the tablet is fresh, it should be moistened with a drop of water. Then when the bubbling begins, the tablet should be inserted immediately. Foaming tablets should be stored in a dry cool place and should be used within 6 months of purchase. Successful use depends on the presence of adequate fluid in the vagina to produce complete disintegration prior to intercourse. As with the aerosol foam, a new tablet should be inserted before each intercourse.

Suppositories and foaming tablets probably are less protective than the foams, creams, or jellies. However, if they are used regularly, they provide a higher degree of protection than other methods used irregularly.

Sponges. A circular sponge, commercial or homemade, has been used as a barrier-type contraceptive agent. Sponges generally are not available in the U.S. They are 1.2 to 1.9 cm thick and 5 to 7.5 cm in diameter, generally with a string attached. For greater protection, both sides should be coated with a contraceptive agent prior to insertion deep into the vagina. Alone, the sponge is better than nothing.

Douching. To mechanically flood and flush out the vagina (with water alone or with a spermicidal agent) immediately after coitus to remove the semen is an age-old means of attempting to avoid pregnancy. Unfortunately, this after-the-fact method is totally unreliable for conception control. Douching is the least effective of the methods in use and should be discouraged.

The Obstetrics and Gynecology Advisory Committee of the Food and Drug Administration is studying vaginal douches to determine whether they have any contraceptive effect.[44] Advertising for most of these products stresses their use for hygienic purposes, not for contraception.

Presumably, if done quickly and thoroughly, douching washes the semen out of the vagina before the sperm can enter the uterus, and conception will not occur. However, if no other means of contraception is used, douching cannot, even theoretically, be effective—direct cervical insemination can occur prior to douching. Sperm can reach the cervix within 90 seconds of ejaculation. Immediate postcoital tests revealed active spermatozoa in the endocervix within 1.5 to 3 minutes after coitus, and spermatozoa have been recovered from the fallopian tubes 30 minutes after insemination.[45] It is highly improbable that douching will be initiated quickly enough or with proper thoroughness to remove all traces of semen and, therefore, all sperm from the vagina.

This method of contraception is mentioned because it is practiced widely, and a number of commercial douche products are available. No convincing evidence is available that shows that douching with or without added chemicals is an effective contraceptive. Furthermore, plain tapwater is spermicidal, readily available, costs nothing, and is less irritating than chemical solutions.

If anything is used following unprotected coitus, it should be the insertion of a spermicidal foam or cream, not only because it is highly effective but also because it takes less time to load and discharge an applicatorful than it does to douche.

Contraceptive effectiveness

The reliability of a contraceptive method relates directly to the motivation to use it consistently—the most frequent cause of contraceptive failure is failure to use the contraceptive. Any contraceptive method works better than none at all, the most effective being the one that will be used consistently. The effectiveness of a contraceptive method depends on the acceptability and suitability for the needs of a couple at a particular time. Contraceptive failure is often caused by ambivalent feelings about pregnancy.[46]

Sandberg and Jacobs[47] studied the psychological reasons behind undesired pregnancies resulting from misuse or rejection of contraception. They concluded that from "the large number of illegitimate births, legally and illegally induced abortions, and legitimate but undesired pregnancies in this country and abroad," it is obvious "that contraceptive measures are commonly ignored or actively rejected by a substantial proportion of coitally active human beings who consciously deny procreative intent. While many of the reasons for misuse or rejection of contraception are included within the commonly discussed areas of contraceptive knowledgeability, acceptability, availability, cost, religious proscription, etc., innumerable other reasons, principally in the psychological and interpersonal relationship realms, are also operative, consciously and unconsciously, in both partners. . . . Even with the future availability of an 'ideal' contraceptive, it is probable for reasons of psychology rather than technology that social systems which require or allow volitional and individually initiated contraceptive use as the sole method for population control will fail to accomplish that goal."

One report involving a total of 562 women who had applied for or had obtained abortions revealed that the main reasons for unplanned pregnancies were misinformation about the menstrual cycle, the risk of pregnancy, improper use of contraceptives, fear of side effects, and actual method failure.[48] In one group studied, deficiencies in medical management were emphasized—most women were given inadequate information or poor advice from their physicians. Contraceptives used in the other group were rhythm, foam, withdrawal, the pill, diaphragm, IUD, and condom. Lack of understanding of conception and contraception were important factors. Results from both groups indicated that better sex education is needed to reduce the number of unplanned pregnancies ending in abortion. Better education among health-care professionals is also needed not only to increase their knowledge, but also to reduce their inhibitions and to correct their misconceptions.

Theoretical contraceptive effectiveness relies on the assumption that the method is used according to instructions. Actual effectiveness is reduced by inconsistent or incorrect use.[49] Effectiveness in use depends on factors other than biological efficiency, e.g., personal preference, the mores of the social group, availability, cost (initial and long-range), storage, use (ease, frequency, and propensity), timing in relation to intercourse, interference with intercourse, requirements for medical consultation, and side effects. The overall usefulness of a contraceptive method is determined essentially by ability to reduce the probability of conception, by consistency of use, and by continuation of use.[50]

Table 1 shows the rank [from best (oral contraceptives) to worst (douching)] of contraceptive methods in different studies, calculated on the basis of 100 woman-years.[51-57] These rankings are rough but fairly accurate estimations of the true order that would result under ideal test conditions. The newer vaginal spermicides, especially the foam, would probably rank better than the rhythm method. The failure rates are based on actual results. (No distinction was made between failure of the method or failure caused by the carelessness of the patient.) Of 100 women using no contraception, 80 can expect to become pregnant within 1 year; using combined steroids, 0.1; sequential steroids, 5; IUD's, 5; diaphragm, 12; condom, 14; withdrawal, 18; jelly alone, 20; rhythm, 24; and douche, 31.[55,58] If the most popular contraceptive methods could be tested clinically under ideal conditions, the order of effectiveness probably would be: oral contraceptives (combination, sequential) > IUD's > condom and diaphragm with chemical spermicide (more effective in combination than alone) > chemical spermicide alone > rhythm > coitus interruptus > douching.

Toxicity potential

The active ingredients in many spermicidal preparations are potentially toxic if they are ingested in pure form, but the toxic agents are present only in small percentages.[59] Signs and symptoms of toxicity vary depending on the ingredient ingested. The possibility of a child ingesting enough of the toxic agent to manifest overt signs and symptoms of acute toxicity is remote; nevertheless, contraceptive preparations should be kept out of the reach of children.

Family planning and contraception

There is much literature and information available on contraception and family planning techniques, methods, and practices. The *Manual of Family Planning and Contraceptive Practice*[60] presents in detail the methods of population control suggested in hospitals, public health services, and offices of private physicians. Other organizations (see listing) are excellent sources of educational material. These organizations can assist the pharmacist in becoming an information outlet on family planning and birth control. When dispensing a birth control agent, the pharmacist should discuss the available literature on the particular method and be able to supplement the written material by answering individual questions.

Manufacturers of contraceptive products should make available contraceptive displays of all forms of contraceptive devices and products and literature. This approach will promote increased knowledge and use. Condoms, especially, should be displayed. *The Medical Letter* states that "condoms can substantially reduce the risk of transmitting gonorrhea and syphilis and their use should be encouraged."[34,35]

Table 2 shows the lack of rapport between pharmacists and patients in the area of family planning and contraception.[9] The results should motivate pharmacists to reevaluate their present policies. In this survey, 65 to 93 percent of patients purchasing a contraceptive rarely or never ask for advice on contraceptives. The pharmacist must take an active role as a qualified consultant in the area of contraception information.

In a study of low-income women, 55 percent (966) indicated that they needed and wanted to learn more about contraceptives.[61] More than one-third of these women preferred to go to a private doctor for contraceptive supplies; 26 percent to clinics; 16 percent to pharmacies; 6 percent to hospitals; and 11 percent did not know where to go. Again, these results point out the need for accurate information on where contraceptives can be prescribed, which ones are prescription-only and nonprescription, and where they are available.

At the end of 1969, despite a 42 percent growth in family planning services in the U.S. over the previous 18 months, only one in five women estimated to be in need of subsidized family planning help was receiving it.

The first national family planning service resource list identifies about 4,500 facilities in the U.S. and three territories that provided these services: 90 percent offered the pill, IUD, and foam; 75 percent, the condom; and 67 percent, the diaphragm and jelly.[62]

Pharmacists should become more familiar with family planning programs and be able to supply or suggest this information. They must not refuse to offer advice on birth control and contraception to anyone, regardless of the circumstances. To dictate that sex without marriage is wrong not only causes loss of rapport but also prevents or damages the pharmacist's reputation as a reliable, unbiased source of birth control information.

Two opposite viewpoints have been expressed concerning the pharmacist's role in advising on birth control and contraception.[63 64] One advocates a more active role for the pharmacist as a birth control consultant; the other insists that the pharmacist is a poor choice for this very special liaison and ultimately disrupts the necessary intimacy and rapport between physician and patient. Cutright [64] believes "neither married nor unmarried women in the United States are so ignorant that they fail to give correct answers to the questions of where they should go to get effective contraception. They say they should go to a physician, a hospital or Planned Parenthood. These are precisely the right answers. A wrong answer would be 'go to my pharmacist,' or 'ask my mother.' The reason the former are correct and the latter incorrect is that the practice of effective contraception by the female is difficult without the aid of the physician."

Four out of five responding pharmacists in one survey believed that providing contraceptive advice and information should be part of their professional duties.[63] However, only 1 percent displayed condoms on self-service counters, 85 percent required a prescription, and 13 percent did not carry condoms. Fifty-eight percent placed vaginal foams, creams, and jellies on self-service counters, 20 percent sold them on request, 9 percent required a prescription, and 7 percent did not stock them. In this same report, the authors suggest that because pharmacies are distributed widely and "already respond to many consumer needs insofar as services and hours are concerned, a more formal, coordinated effort to enlist the professional involvement of the pharmacist seems in order." Whether or not the pharmacist makes this effort is a moot point; "not to make the attempt, however, will certainly help perpetuate those dismal statistics on unwanted births, illegitimacy, and deadened lives."

FAMILY PLANNING SOURCES OF INFORMATION

☐ Planned Parenthood-World Population (PPWP)
810 Seventh Avenue
New York, N.Y. 10019

Voluntary health agency supported by public contributions, offers a national program of family planning service, referral for voluntary abortion and sterilization, public information, education for marriage, clinical research related to birth control, and patient-level pamphlets (some in Spanish): "Planned Parenthood," "Modern Methods of Birth Control," "The Doctor Talks About Birth Control. A Teen-age Fact Book," "Questions and Answers About Intrauterine Devices (IUD)," "Questions and Answers on Sterilization for Men and Women," "What You Should Know About 'The Pill'," "The Safe Period."

☐ Planned Parenthood Federation of America, Inc.
810 Seventh Avenue
New York, N.Y. 10019

Publishes *Family Planning Perspectives* bimonthly and maintains a Perspectives Reprints list of articles relevant to all aspects of family planning.

☐ International Planned Parenthood Federation
111 Fourth Avenue
New York, N.Y. 10003

Organized for the formation of family planning associations; training of physicians, nurses, health visitors, and social workers in the practical administration of family planning services; the encouragement of research into human reproductive processes and into biological methods of controlling families.

☐ The Population Council
Publications Office
245 Park Avenue
New York, N.Y. 10017

Publishes the monthly *Studies in Family Planning* and the occasional monograph series *Reports on Population/Family Planning* in English, French, and Spanish; the Council endeavors to advance knowledge in the broad field of population by fostering research, training, and technical consultation and assistance in the social and biomedical sciences.

☐ American Medical Association
535 North Dearborn
Chicago, Ill. 60610

☐ American College of Obstetricians and Gynecologists
1 E. Wacker Drive
Chicago, Ill. 60601

☐ Population Planning Associates
105 North Columbia Street
Chapel Hill, N.C. 27514

Offers a mail-order line of American and British condoms and promotes their use by advertising them in newspapers and magazines.

☐ Zero Population Growth
1346 Connecticut Avenue, N.W.
Washington, D. C. 20036

Activities aimed at population education and political action to remove laws that inhibit or restrict individual freedom of choice of medically approved contraception techniques. Seeks to deal actively with the population crisis.

☐ The Alan Guttmacher Institute
515 Madison Avenue
New York, N.Y. 10022

Publishes *Family Planning/Population Reporter* and *Planned Parenthood Washington Memo;* the Institute has prepared a detailed two-volume manual to assist administrators and program officials to develop a statewide approach to planning for family planning programs that will meet federal and state requirements. *Developing Statewide Family Planning Programs: A Planning Handbook* is available for $50 for both volumes from Planning Unit, The Alan Guttmacher Institute, 515 Madison Avenue, New York, N.Y. 10022. It includes worksheets and sample data collection instruments to facilitate a "do-it-yourself" approach.

☐ Population Information Program
Science Communication Division
Department of Medical and Public Affairs
George Washington University
2001 S Street, N.W.
Washington, D. C. 20009

Publishes *Population Reports.*

☐ The Bureau of Community Health Services
Health Services Administration
U.S. Department of Health, Education and Welfare
5600 Fishers Lane
Room 12A-33
Rockville, Md. 20852

Publishes *Family Planning Digest.*

☐ Dr. James Huff
Director
Biomedical Sciences Section
Information Center Complex
P.O. Box X
Building 7509
Oak Ridge National Laboratory
Oak Ridge, Tenn. 37830

A limited number of reprints of a three-part series OTC and prescription-only contraceptives and family planning is available. The articles were authored by Dr. James Huff and Luis Hernandez (*J. Am. Pharm. Assoc.*, **NS14(3), NS14(5),** and **NS14(7),** 1974).

Summary

The pharmacist's role as a health consultant in the area of conception control is significant. The practicing pharmacist is integrally involved in supplying information on all methods of contraception. The specific concerns of the pharmacist are those agents that do not require the services of a physician. Inasmuch as the pharmacist dispenses prescription-only contraceptives, a knowledge of them and of IUD's and surgical techniques is essential.

The personal nature of contraception should be considered and dealt with in a professional way. The more objectively the conception control methods are presented, the easier it is for the patient to make a choice.

Pharmacists should watch for side effects experienced by patients taking oral contraceptives or using vaginal spermicides and should advise immediate physician referral in these cases. The pharmacist also should contact the patient's physician to discuss the untoward reactions.

References

1. W. J. Dignam, in "Birth Control: A Continuing Controversy," Charles C Thomas, Springfield, Ill., 1967, pp. 142-151.
2. G. Pincus, "The Control of Fertility," Academic Press, New York, N.Y., 1965, p. 96.
3. B. J. Duffy and M. J. Wallace, "Biological and Medical Aspects of Contraception," University of Notre Dame Press, Notre Dame, Ind., 1969, pp. 83-85.
4. T. Mann, "The Biochemistry of Semen and of the Male Reproductive Tract," Wiley and Sons, New York, N.Y., 1954, pp. 29, 30.
5. H. Knaus, "Periodic Fertility and Sterility in Woman: A Natural Method of Birth Control," Chicago Medical Book, Chicago, Ill., 1934, p. 32.
6. T. Crist, *Obstet. Gynecol. News,* **5(24),** 16(1970).
7. E. M. Nash and L. M. Louden, *J. Am. Med. Assoc.,* **210(13),** 2365-2369(1969).
8. G. Hollis and K. Lashman, *Fam. Plann. Perspect.,* **6(3),** 173-175(1974).
9. N. N. Wagner *et al., J. Am. Pharm. Assoc.,* **NS10(5),** 258-260(1970).
10. B. N. Fujita *et al., Am. J. Obstet. Gynecol.,* **109(5),** 787-793(1971).
11. N. N. Wagner *et al., Postgrad. Med.,* **46(4),** 68-71(1969).
12. S. O. Gustavus and C. A. Huether, *Fam. Plann. Perspect.,* **7(5),** 203-207(1975).
13. M. L. Finkel and D. J. Finkel, *Fam. Plann. Perspect.,* **7(6),** 256-260(1975).
14. M. Zelnick and J. F. Kanter, *Fam. Plann. Perspect.,* **6(2),** 74-80(1974).
15. J. Sklar and B. Berkov, *Fam. Plann. Perspect.,* **6(2),** 80-90(1974).
16. L. Morris, *Fam. Plann. Perspect.,* **6(2),** 91-97(1974).
17. Editorial, *Sci. Am.,* **234(6),** 50(1976).
18. C. F. Westoff, *Fam. Plann. Perspect.,* **8(2),** 54-57(1976).
19. R. W. Kistner, *J. Am. Med. Assoc.,* **215(7),** 1162(1971).
20. C. Ross and P. T. Piotrow, *Popul. Rep.,* **I(1),** I/1-I/19(1974).
21. J. Rock, in "Manual of Family Planning and Contraceptive Practice," 2d ed., M. S. Calderone, Ed., Williams and Wilkins, Baltimore, Md., 1970.
22. L. Mastroianni, Jr., *Fam. Plann. Perspect.,* **6(4),** 209-212(1974).
23. B. J. Pisani, in "Manual of Family Planning and Contraceptive Practice," 2d ed., M. S. Calderone, Ed., Williams and Wilkins, Baltimore, Md., 1970.
24. "Control of Male Fertility," J. J. Sciarra *et al.,* Eds., Harper and Row, Hagerstown, Md., 1975, 337 pp.
25. "Schering Workshop on Contraception: the Masculine Gender," G. Raspe and S. Bernhard, Eds., Pergamon Press, Oxford, England, 1973, 332 pp.
26. J. S. Lubin, *Playgirl,* **3(9),** 11, 12, 119(1976).

27. P. E. Pothier, National Library of Medicine, literature search no. 75-24, 1-11, 142 citations, Jan., 1973-Nov. 1975.

28. I. A. Dalsimer *et al., Popul. Rep.,* **H(1),** H/1-H/19(1973).

29. J. J. Dumm *et al., Popul. Rep.,* **H(2),** H/21-H/36(1974).

30. "The Condom: Increasing Utilization in the United States," M. H. Redford *et al.,* Eds., San Francisco Press, San Francisco, Calif., 1974, 320 pp.

31. *Fam. Plann. Perspect.,* **8(3),** 134(1976).

32. C. Tietze, "Family-Planning Programs: An International Survey," Basic Books, New York, N.Y., 1969, pp. 183-191.

33. A. F. Guttmacher *et al.,* "Planning Your Family," Macmillan, New York, N.Y., 1964, pp. 41, 42.

34. *Med. Lett. Drugs Ther.,* **13(21),** 85-87(1971).

35. *Med. Lett. Drugs Ther.,* **13(26),** 108(1971).

36. P. D. Harvey, *Fam. Plann. Perspect.,* **4(4),** 27-30(1972).

37. R. Helmer, "The Venus Dilemma," Nash Publishing, Los Angeles, Calif., 1974, 172 pp.

38. R. Stiller, "The Love Bugs: a Natural History of the VD's," Thomas Nelson, Nashville, Tenn., 1974, 158 pp.

39. K. L. Jones *et al.,* "VD," Harper and Row, New York, N.Y., 1973, 116 pp.

40. *Fam. Plann. Dig.,* **1(4),** 1-3(1972).

41. R. Belsky, *Popul. Rep.,* **H(3),** H/37-H/55(1975).

42. M. E. Lane *et al., Fam. Plann. Perspect.,* **8(2),** 81-86(1976).

43. G. S. Bernstein, *Contraception,* **3(1),** 37-43(1971).

44. W. Rinehart, *Popul. Rep.,* **J(9),** J/141-J/154(1976).

45. C. C. Marcus and S. L. Marcus, in "Progress in Infertility," Little, Brown, Boston, Mass., 1968, pp. 21-62.

46. H. Lehfeldt, *Mod. Aspects Hum. Sexual.,* **5(5),** 68-77(1971).

47. E. C. Sandberg and R. I. Jacobs, *Am. J. Obstet. Gynecol.,* **110(2),** 227-242(1971).

48. *Fam. Plann. Perspect.,* **8(2),** 72, 75(1976).

49. C. Tietze, in "Manual of Family Planning and Contraceptive Practice," 2d ed., M. S. Calderone, Ed., Williams and Wilkins, Baltimore, Md., 1970, pp. 268, 269.

50. C. Tietze and S. Lewit, *Fertil. Steril.,* **22(8),** 508-513(1971).

51. D. P. Swartz and R. L. VandeWiele, "Methods of Conception Control." A Programmed Instruction Course, Ortho Pharmaceutical Corp., Raritan, N.J., Frame 219 (Revised 1967).

52. "The Consumers Union Report on Family Planning," Consumers Union of the United States, Inc., Mount Vernon, N.Y., 1966, pp. 65-69.

53. P. R. Ehrlich and A. H. Ehrlich, "Population Resources Environment, Issues in Human Biology," Freeman, San Francisco, Calif., 1970, p. 219.

54. Planned Parenthood Federation of America, "Methods of Contraception in the United States" (pamphlet), Planned Parenthood Federation of America, Inc., New York, N.Y., 1963.

55. G. Pincus, *Science,* **153,** 493-500(1966).

56. International Planned Parenthood Federation, "Medical Handbook, Part I, Contraception," International Planned Parenthood Federation, London, England, 1964, 62 (U.S.A. Metropolitan Areas).

57. International Planned Parenthood Federation, "Medical Handbook, Part I, Contraception," International Planned Parenthood Federation, London, 65 (Selected World Clinical Studies), 1964.

58. P. R. Ehrlich and A. H. Ehrlich, "Population Resources Environment, Issues in Human Biology," Freeman, San Francisco, Calif., 1970, p. 219.

59. R. E. Gosselin *et al.,* "Clinical Toxicology of Commercial Products: Acute Poisoning," 4th ed., Williams and Wilkins, Baltimore, Md., 1976, sec. II, pp. 1-273; sec. V, pp. 1-799.

60. "Manual of Family Planning and Contraceptive Practice," 2d ed., M. S. Calderone, Ed., Williams and Wilkins, Baltimore, Md., 1970.

61. R. J. Wolff and B. Z. Bell, *Stud. Fam. Plann.,* **56,** (August, 1970).

62. *Fam. Plann. Perspect.,* **8(3),** 130-131(1976).

63. M. J. Rumel *et al., Fam. Plann., Perspect.,* **3(4),** 80-82(1971).

64. P. Cutright, *Fam. Plann. Perspect.,* **3(1),** 25-48(1971).

Product (manufacturer)	Dosage form	Spermicide	Other
Anvita (A. O. Schmidt)	cream	phenylmercuric borate, 1:2000	boric acid, aluminum potassium sulfate, thymol, chlorothymol, aromatics, cocoa butter
Crescent Cream (Milex)	cream	glyceryl ricinoleate, 0.36%	sodium lauryl sulfate, 0.6%; 8-hydroxyquinoline sulfate, 0.02%
Crescent Vaginal Jelly (Milex)	gel	glyceryl ricinoleate, 1%	sodium chloride 5%; sodium lauryl sulfate, 0.008%; lactic acid
Dalkon Kit (Robins)	foam	nonoxynol 9	benzethonium chloride
Emko (Emko)	foam	nonoxynol 9, 8%	benzethonium chloride, 0.2%; stearic acid; triethanolamine; glyceryl monostearate; poloxamer 188; polyethylene glycol 600; substituted adamantane; dichlorodifluoromethane; dichlorotetrafluoroethane
Koromex (Holland-Rantos)	foam	nonoxynol 9, 12.5%	propylene glycol, isopropyl alcohol, laureth 4, cetyl alcohol, polyethylene glycol stearate, fragrance, dichlorodifluoromethane, dichlorotetrafluoroethane
Koromex II Cream (Holland-Rantos)	cream	octoxynol, 3.0%	propylene glycol, stearic acid, sorbitan stearate, polysorbate 60, boric acid, fragrance
Koromex II and II-A Jelly (Holland-Rantos)	gel	octoxynol, 1% (II) nonoxynol 9, 2% (II-A)	propylene glycol, cellulose gum, boric acid, sorbitol, starch, simethicone, fragrance
Milex Creme (Milex)	cream	glyceryl ricinoleate, 0.36%	sodium lauryl sulfate, 0.6%; 8-hydroxyquinoline sulfate, 0.02%

Feminine Cleansing and Deodorant Products

Stephen G. Hoag

Questions to ask the patient

Have you noted a discharge?
Have you experienced pain or itching?
Are there any sores in the genital area?
How long has the condition been present?
Do you douche? How frequently?
Have you ever had a reaction to ointments or sprays?
What drugs are you currently taking or using?
To your knowledge, are you pregnant or do you have diabetes?

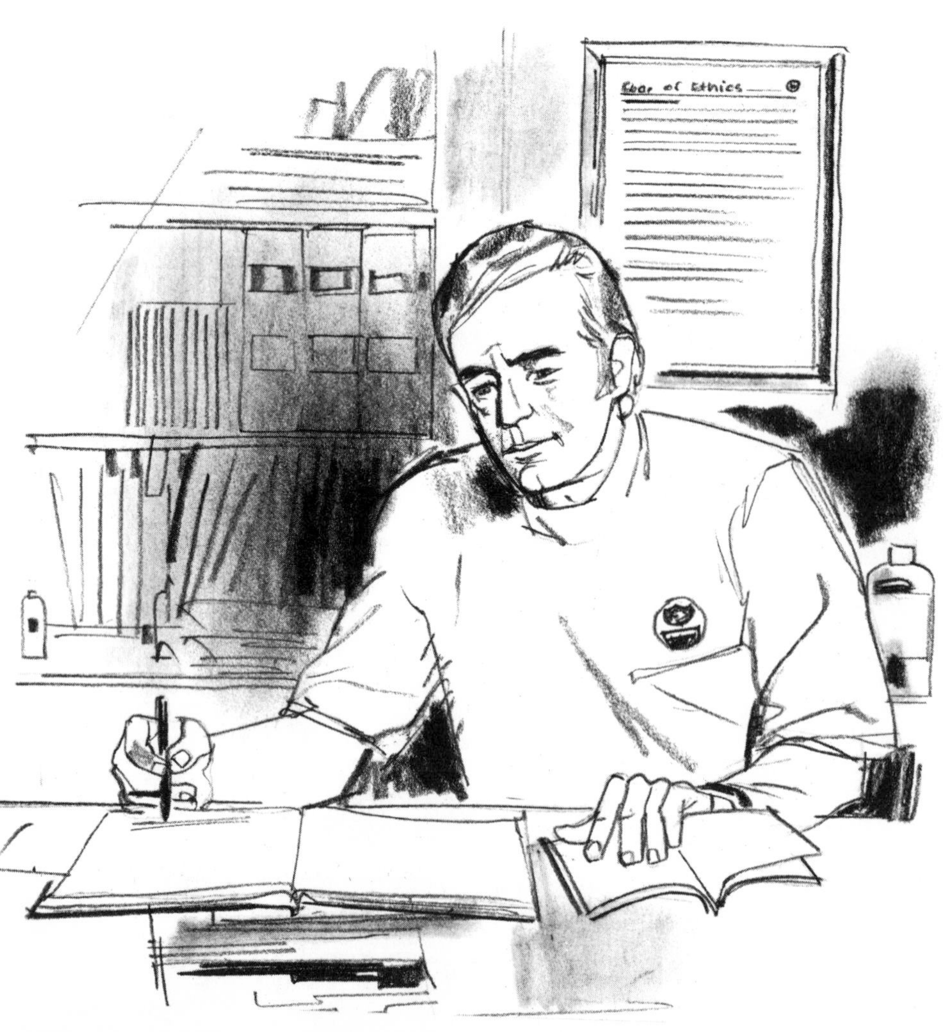

CHAPTER 18

American society today is probably unsurpassed in history in its concern for cleanliness, personal hygiene, and elimination of body odors. Many products are available which are intended to keep us clean and odor free from head to toe. Included in this group of personal toiletry and cosmetic products are douches and feminine deodorant products. Vaginal douche products are not new. Feminine deodorant sprays, on the other hand, are relative newcomers to the field. Carsch[1] calls these aerosol sprays "the most recent marketing phenomenon of the cosmetic industry."

In general, feminine toiletry and cosmetic products are used (appropriately or not) for general cleansing of the vaginal or perineal areas; deodorizing; relief of itching, burning, erythema, and edema; removing secretions or discharge; and psychological reasons, such as producing a soothing and refreshing feeling. Some of these feminine products, such as douches, may also be prescribed by physicians for altering vaginal pH to affect microscopic flora.

Many gynecologists believe that the healthy vagina cleanses itself and that the perineal area can be adequately cleaned with soap and water. Others seem to feel that douching, when done properly, promotes healthy vaginal tissues. The value of feminine deodorant sprays is also controversial. The efficacy of the sprays as deodorants is often questioned, and possible adverse effects, such as irritation of vaginal mucous membranes, have come to light since their appearance about 10 years ago.

In this chapter the word "hygiene" is not used in connection with these products because most of the products do not possess medicinal properties, especially the deodorant sprays. Their action and benefit are cosmetic. Furthermore, the few douche preparations that do have therapeutic properties should not be purchased for self-medication in the presence of disease; their use may delay the user from seeking medical attention. Nonprescription vaginal cleansing and deodorant products should always be used as cosmetics and toiletries unless a physician is supervising their use for therapeutic purposes.

Physiology of the vaginal tract

The important physiological considerations concerning the use of feminine cleansing and deodorant products include vaginal epithelial thickness and glycogen content, normal bacterial flora, vaginal pH, production of secretions and discharge, and production of objectionable odor. Vaginal surfaces are lined with squamous epithelium, and it is estrogens which are mainly responsible for the control of thickness of this lining. Epithelial cell height increases at menarche and decreases at menopause. Prior to menarche and after menopause the vaginal epithelium is apparently less resistant to infection. Glycogen content of vaginal epithelium is increased during the child-bearing years.

The health of the vagina depends on pH, normal bacterial flora, epithelial cellular height, and epithelial glycogen content. The normal vaginal bacterial flora include Doderlein's bacilli, diphtheroids, staphylococci, and anaerobic streptococci. Doderlein's bacilli (a strain of lactobacilli) metabolize epithelial glycogen to lactic acid. Vaginal pH is normally alkaline prior to menarche and following menopause but is normally acid during the child-bearing years as a result of this metabolic production of lactic acid by bacteria. Vaginal pH ranges from 3.0 to 6.1, but after about 10,000 observations, Karnaky[2] reported that pH is usually between 3.5 and 4.2.[3,4] The acidic vaginal pH and the presence of normal flora usually preclude the growth of pathogens, but a shift of the pH toward alkalinity may render the area more susceptible to infection.

Vaginal mucus originates in part from the endocervical mucus as well as from bacteria and desquamated epithelium of the vagina. This discharge is a natural cleansing mechanism, but in the absence of good hygiene, the mucus may accumulate on external genital surfaces. The vulvar/perineal area contains sebaceous, apocrine, and eccrine glands, each producing minimal secretions, as well as Bartholin's glands which secrete a very small amount of mucus during sexual stimulation. In addition, there is a clear, alkaline transudate in the vagina during sexual excitement. Vaginal discharge may increase noticeably during periods of emotional stress and ovulation.

The mucous, sebaceous, and apocrine secretions of the perineum and the vaginal discharge are subject to bacterial decomposition if left on the skin for long periods. This bacterial decomposition of normal secretions is the main cause of the production of objectionable odor. Malodor may also be associated with a forgotten tampon.

Vaginitis

Etiology and classifications

Besides cosmetic and deodorant considerations, the most common reasons for using douches and other feminine cleansing products are probably vulvar pruritus (and/or a burning sensation) and excessive vaginal discharge (leukorrhea). One of the most frequent causes of vulvar pruritus and leukorrhea is vaginitis. Vaginitis is an inflammation of vulvar and vaginal epithelium usually caused by disturbances of the normal flora or by pathogenic micro-organisms. In most instances, vaginitis causes more discomfort than danger to the patient.[5-7] A classification of vaginitis is given in Table 1, but most cases can be placed into one of four categories:

- *Trichomonas vaginalis* vaginitis
- *Candida albicans* (monilial) vaginitis
- Nonspecific vaginitis
- Atrophic vaginitis

The trichomonal and monilial types of vaginitis are the most common in women of child-bearing age. Prolonged use of tetracyclines, steroid therapy (including oral contraceptives), cancer, pregnancy, and diabetes are among the factors which may be predisposing to the overgrowth of monilial organisms (*C. albicans*).[8] Atrophic vaginitis occurs after menopause when vaginal epithelium thins. Proteus may be implicated in a significant number of

Table 1. Classification of Vaginitis

Type	Organism	Age group affected
Infectious		
Atrophic (senile)	Coliforms, staphylococci, streptococci	Postmenopausal (prepubertal, rarely)
Gonorrhea	*Neisseria gonorrhoeae*	Adult
Herpes II	Herpes II	All
Monilial	*Candida albicans*	Adult (especially if pregnant or diabetic)
Mycoplasma	Mycoplasma	All
Nonspecific	*Haemophilus vaginalis*,[a] coliforms, staphylococci, streptococci	All
Preadolescent (childhood vulvovaginitis)	Helminths, coliforms, staphylococci, streptococci	Prepubertal
Trichomonal	*Trichomonas vaginalis*	Adult (prepubertal, rarely)
Tuberculous	*Mycobacterium tuberculosis*	All
Noninfectious		
Allergic and chemical	—	All (when foreign chemicals are instilled vaginally)
Postirradiation	—	All (when irradiation is used for treatment of cervical carcinoma)
Traumatic	—	All

[a] *Haemophilus vaginitis* is frequently considered by itself because *H. vaginalis* is the most frequent pathogen in nonspecific bacterial vaginitis.

chronic cases of atrophic vaginitis. Although childhood vulvovaginitis is relatively uncommon, it usually has the same cause and manifestations as atrophic vaginitis. Monilial and trichomonal infections may occur simultaneously, and both organisms may be present in the normal, healthy vagina.[9, 10] *Trichomonas* and *Haemophilus* vaginitis are frequently transmitted by sexual contact.

Symptoms

The symptoms of vaginitis, leukorrhea and pruritus, may cause a woman to seek medical attention or to self-medicate. Offensive odor may be caused by discharge associated with trichomonal or *Haemophilus* organisms. The description of a purulent vaginal discharge should alert the pharmacist to the possibility of vaginitis and the need for a specific diagnosis and prescribed therapy. In postmenopausal women, a thin, watery discharge accompanied by pruritus indicates the possibility of atrophic vaginitis or malignancy. The pharmacist should determine if symptoms of vaginitis are present, how long they have persisted, and whether predisposing factors exist (prolonged use of tetracyclines or steroids, pregnancy, diabetes). The patient should also be asked if any previous attempts at self-treatment have been tried because symptoms may be an adverse reaction to an OTC product.

Depending on the specific diagnosis of vaginitis, antitrichomonal, antimonilial, or antibacterial therapy may be prescribed. In atrophic vaginitis, however, systemic or local estrogenic hormone therapy may be prescribed because estrogen stimulates vaginal epithelium, increasing its thickness and resistance to infection. Nonprescription feminine cleansing and deodorant products should be used in cases of vaginitis only when advised by a physician.

Pruritus and/or malodorous discharge may occur in conditions other than vaginitis, such as cystitis, urethritis, chemical irritation, venereal disease, or carcinoma of the cervix and endometrium. Regardless of the cause, these symptoms are an indication for diagnostic evaluation by a physician, especially if they are persistent, severe, or recurrent.

Vaginal douches

Douches may exert cleansing effects by lowering surface tension, mucolytic action, and proteolytic action, although standards for evaluating these effects have not been established.[11] Douche products are available as liquids, liquid concentrates to be diluted in water, powders to be dissolved in water, and powders to be instilled as powders. Common usage of the term "douche," therefore, is not limited to a stream of water. Douche products are also available in disposable or nondisposable form.

Ingredients

Recommended concentrations for many ingredients in feminine cleansing and deodorant products are listed in Table 2, but many manufacturers do not list concentrations.

Antimicrobial agents. Most antimicrobial agents in douche products are present in concentrations that provide preservative properties to the product per se not therapeutic activity. They include benzethonium and benzalkonium chlorides, parabens, hexachlorophene, and chlorothymol. Other compounds may be included for purported antiseptic or germicidal activity, such as boric acid, phenol, menthol, thymol, eucalyptol, cetylpyridinium chloride, oxyquinoline, and sodium perborate. However, the value of these ingredients as antimicrobials is questionable, depending in some cases on the concentration used. Because many manufacturers do not list concentrations of ingredients if the products are considered cosmetics, the assessment of efficacy is impossible. Boric acid (5 percent) under physician supervision is an effective antimicrobial for the treatment of monilial vaginitis, and povidone-iodine is an effective antimicrobial agent for adjunctive therapy in monilial and trichomonal vaginitis.[12, 13] The possibility of local irritation or sensitization exists with many antimicrobial agents found in douches, and if these effects are encountered, the patient should be instructed to discontinue use of the product and consult a physician.

Local anesthetics/antipruritics. Compounds such as phenol, menthol, and eucalyptol are included in douches for local anesthetic or antipruritic effects. Possible antipruritic effects are not substantiated. Eucalyptol, because of its fragrance, may also provide some deodorant effect by masking objectionable odor.

Counterirritants. Many douche products contain

substances such as menthol, thymol, and methyl salicylate for counterirritant effects, although their value has not been substantiated. Offensive odor may be masked by the fragrance of methyl salicylate.

Astringents. Astringent substances are included in some douches for reduction of local edema, inflammation, and exudation. They include ammonium and potassium alums, zinc oxide, and zinc sulfate. Micronized aluminum powder has also been used as an astringent douche.[3] The concentration of astringent is important because many astringents are irritants in moderate or high concentration.[14]

Proteolytics. At least one proteolytic agent, papain, is used in a douche product to remove excess vaginal discharge. Papain may elicit allergic reactions.

Surface active agents. Surface active substances such as sodium lauryl sulfate, nonoxynol 4 and dioctyl sodium sulfosuccinate are used to facilitate the spread of the douche over vaginal mucosa and the penetration of the mucosal folds and rugae.[2] Cetylpyridinium chloride also has surface active properties.

Substances affecting pH. Many vaginal douche products are buffered or contain substances that purposely render them either acidic or alkaline. For example, sodium perborate and sodium bicarbonate provide alkalinity; lactic acid and citric acid provide acidity. The significance of pH and buffering is discussed below.

Miscellaneous ingredients. Other ingredients occasionally found in douches are emollients, emulsifiers, keratolytics, and substances intended to raise the osmolarity of the preparation. Liquid vehicles are water, propylene glycol, alcohol, or combinations of these. Talc is used as a vehicle for douche powders intended to be instilled as powders (insufflations). Lactose may be added as a bacterial nutrient, but the reason for its inclusion is unclear. Aromatic agents (chlorothymol, eucalyptol, menthol, thymol, methyl salicylate) may be added for the general effect of producing a soothing and refreshing feeling.[11]

Types of syringes

Several types of syringes are available for administration of douches. The combination water bottle/syringe (fountain syringe) and the folding feminine syringe are held above the level of the hips while the douche liquid is instilled into the vagina via gravity. These syringes are supplied with the necessary tubing and tips for use with douches or with enemas. Patients should be advised of the difference between douche and enema tips. The main advantage to the combination (fountain) and folding feminine syringes is that fluids are administered with gentle gravity force only, thereby minimizing the chance of excessive fluid force upon instillation. Bulb-type feminine syringes are also available for administration of douche liquids via gentle squeezing of the bulb. The main advantage of bulb-type feminine syringes is ease of handling since the use of tubing and the holding of the syringe at an elevated level are avoided. Care must be exercised, however, to avoid excessive squeezing and excessive fluid force upon instillation of the douche.

Techniques of douching

To avoid the possible dangers of improper douching, several investigators have recommended procedures to ensure safe instillation:[8,15-17]

☐ Douches should never be administered with excess pressure. The force of gravity is sufficient if a bag, tube, and nozzle are used. The douche bag should not be more than 60 cm above the hips. If a syringe is used, minimum pressure should be applied.

☐ Most douches should be instilled while lying down, the knees drawn up, and the hips raised.

☐ Douching equipment should be thoroughly cleaned before and after use. Sterilization by boiling is also recommended. The use of disposable douche products eliminates the inconvenience of cleaning of equipment.

☐ Douches should not be used during pregnancy.

Recommendations concerning the frequency of douching vary widely. Long *et al.*[18] reported that 175 women douching daily had higher vaginal epithelial glycogen concentrations than 199 women douching less than daily, implying that the group douching more frequently experienced a beneficial effect. Water and a medicinal powder douche were used, but the ingredients and nature of the medicinal powder were not provided. Karnaky[2] stated that douching four to eight times daily is not harmful when using a "physiologic" douche.

Many studies recommend avoidance of routine douching altogether.[15,16,19] A common recommendation, however, is that a woman who insists on routine douching should not do so more than twice weekly unless otherwise advised by the pharmacist or physician. The potential for harm from frequent douching depends, in part, on formulation and technique of instillation, both of which may be incorrect. If properly prepared and properly instilled, a douche used twice a week should cause no harm, but it has not been proved that twice weekly or even less frequent douching is necessary at all.

An alternative self-bathing method for vaginal and perineal areas has been studied for benefits and possible adverse effects in more than 500 women, including 180 with symptoms or diagnosis of vaginitis.[20] The technique involves gentle washing with the fingers of the vulvar, perineal, and anal regions and the vagina, using only water and a mild soap. (See Chapter 27 for a discussion of antimicrobial soaps.) The technique was effective as a cleansing practice and was 94 percent effective in clearing the symptoms of vaginitis, the recurrence rate of which was slightly more than 5 percent.

Advisability of douching

Evaluation of the literature relative to the conflict on whether a woman should use a douche for routine vaginal cleansing is quite difficult; both sides are well represented. The current FDA position regarding safety and efficacy of vaginal douching is that there are no standards for evaluating or substantiating claims.[11]

Adverse effects of douches on vaginal pH, flora, and cytology have been cited as potential hazards of routine douching. However, the effects of acid, alkaline, and vinegar douches on vaginal pH and vaginal mucosal cytology are not significant.[4,21] An alkaline douche, however, is said to be more effective than an acid douche for removing vaginal discharge and relieving pruritus, and it is effective as adjunctive therapy in vaginitis.[21-23]

Reports by Karnaky[2,3] also support douching as a safe, effective cleansing mechanism that does not significantly alter vaginal pH if the douche preparation is unbuffered; Karnaky, however, advises acidic rather than alkaline douches because shifts toward alkalinity may inhibit normal flora and promote the growth of pathogens. Abruzzi[24] also reported that an acidic douche was harmless and was preferred, after studying the effects of douching in 250 women, of whom 78 were healthy and 172 had vaginitis or vaginal discharge. Of course, care should be

Table 2. Recommended Concentrations for Components of Feminine Cleansing and Deodorant Products[a]

Agent	Recommended concentration
Alum	0.5–5.0%[b]
Benzalkonium chloride	1:5,000 - 1:2,000 vaginally 0.02–0.2% externally
Benzethonium chloride	1:750[b]
Benzocaine	1.0–20%[b]
Boric acid[c]	1.0–4.0%[b]
Cetylpyridinium chloride	1:10,000 - 1:2,000 on mucous membranes 1:1,000 - 1:100 externally
Hexachlorophene	0.2%[d]
Menthol	0.1–2.0%[b]
Methylbenzethonium chloride	1:10,000 - 1:100[b]
Methyl salicylate	10–25%[b]
Oxyquinoline	1:1,000 vaginally or externally
Parabens (total)	0.05–0.3%[b]
Phenol	0.5–1.0%[b]
Phenylmercuric acetate	0.02% on mucous membranes 0.2% externally 0.002–0.125% as a preservative
Povidone-iodine[e]	10% (0.5–3.0% of available iodine)[b]
Resorcinol	2.0–20%[b]
Salicylic acid	2.0–20%[b]
Thymol	1.0%[b]
Zinc oxide	15–25%[b]
Zinc sulfate	0.25–4.0%[b]

[a] From "Remington's Pharmaceutical Sciences," 14th ed., A. Osol and J. E. Hoover, Eds., Mack Publishing, Easton, Pa., 1970.

[b] Recommendation does not specify difference in concentration between external skin and mucous membranes and should be viewed cautiously because mucous membranes may be more sensitive.

[c] From T. E. Swate and J. C. Weed, *Obstet. Gynecol.*, **43**, 893(1974).

[d] Present legal FDA maximum allowable concentration in OTC products. (From FDA Minutes of the OTC Panel on Contraceptives and Other Vaginal Drug Products.)

[e] From J. J. Ratzan, *Calif. Med.*, **110**, 24(1969).

taken that the douche is not excessively acidic, causing irritation or injury. In one study, douching caused no significant alterations in normal vaginal flora.[18] However, significant increases in vaginal epithelial glycogen content were observed in women who douched, and it was concluded in this study that douching was not only harmless but even beneficial to vaginal and cervical epithelium. Stock *et al.*[25] reported that a questionnaire regarding douching, administered to 1,600 women, revealed no evidence of harmful effects and no correlation between the incidence of vaginal infections and the practice of (or lack of) douching. No evidence was found in the literature that douche (or spray) ingredients may be absorbed systemically in significant quantities. Boric acid and phenylmercuric acetate may be absorbed but not in toxic amounts.[12 26]

If unbuffered douches do not significantly affect vaginal pH or normal flora, it seems that choosing between an acidic or alkaline douche is not important. It is reasonable to assume, however, that if a douche is used in the absence of disease or symptoms, it should approximate vaginal pH as nearly as possible. An alkaline douche may provide more efficient cleansing and relief of symptoms in women whose vaginal discharge is excessive, is retained on perineal surfaces, and causes irritation.

A significant number of case reports described adverse effects, suggesting that douching may be unwise without specific indication. Hirst[17] described five cases in which salpingitis, endometritis, or pelvic inflammatory disease was associated with douching. Pressure of instillation of the douche fluid was implicated in each case. Other conditions linked to douching are infection, hemorrhage, trauma, embolism, and chemical peritonitis.[15 16 20 27]

Perhaps the most frequent adverse effects of douches are direct, primary mucosal/dermal irritation or allergic contact sensitivity from specific ingredients. No well-controlled clinical studies of these effects on vaginal mucosa after douching could be found, but many ingredients of douche preparations have been implicated in these effects on the dermis. Dermal irritants or sensitizers may similarly affect the vaginal epithelium. Compounds incorporated into douche products which cause direct chemical effects, especially allergic contact sensitivity, include benzocaine, parabens, propylene glycol monostearate, triethanolamine, phenol, chlorhexidine, chloroxylenol, and benzalkonium and benzethonium chlorides.[28-33]

Potential hazards must be weighed against the questionable value of routine douching in the absence of symptoms. Hirst[17] summarized an excellent position regarding the advisability of douching by stating that, in spite of reported adverse effects, we must "recognize that a douche properly prepared and administered is harmless." This position is still applicable but only to properly prepared and properly administered douches.

The available douche products should not be considered contraceptive agents. Douches of normal volume, properly instilled, are ineffective in removing seminal fluid.[19] Precoital douches are also ineffective as contraceptives.[17] The use of douches postcoitus is preferred by some women, but the benefits are probably psychological or placebo because the superiority of douching over cleansing with soap and water has not been conclusively demonstrated. Douches should be used no sooner than 6 to 8 hours after the use of a spermicide because spermicidal agents may be removed in the douching process.

Feminine deodorant sprays

Feminine deodorant sprays are aerosol products intended for use on the external genital area to reduce or mask objectionable odor. They are available as spray mists and spray powders. A typical formula includes an antimicrobial agent, an emollient carrier, perfume, and a propellant. Talc is added to spray powders. The FDA considers these products cosmetics and prohibits references to "hygiene" by manufacturers.[34] The sprays do not possess therapeutic or medicinal properties. They may be used as deodorants or simply for placebo or psychological benefits as toiletries.

Ingredients

Some concentrations of feminine deodorant spray ingredients may be for external skin and not necessarily for vaginal mucosa.

Perfumes. Fragrances, or perfumes, are the main ingredients of feminine deodorant sprays. They are responsible for deodorant activity. Fragrances should be selected with care because some may be irritating to mucous membranes.[35] Carsch[1] has characterized the fragrances, including comments as to whether the fragrances are mild or strong, short or long lasting, sweet, medicinal, floral, etc. Some products contain encapsulated perfumes which are slowly released upon contact with moisture.

Antimicrobials. Antimicrobial compounds in these sprays include benzethonium and benzalkonium chlorides, hexachlorophene, and chloroxylenol. These and similar compounds are preservative rather than therapeutic in action. Although a deodorant action can be achieved by inhibiting or eradicating vulvo/perineal bacteria, the available sprays do not deodorize in this manner. They do not alter normal vulvo/vaginal flora if properly used but may, if used improperly.[36] Holding the spray too close to the body may result in an excessively high surface concentration of the antimicrobial agent or the entrance of the agent into the vagina where concentration also may be excessive.

Emollients. A number of emollient substances are included in these formulations as vehicles and for their soothing effect on the skin. The most commonly used are fatty esters such as isopropyl myristate, polyoxyethylene derivatives of fatty esters, and fatty alcohols. Unfortunately, some of these substances may also be sensitizers.[29, 31, 35]

Propellants. The fluorinated hydrocarbon propellants used in feminine deodorant sprays may also be responsible for some adverse reactions. If the spray is held too close to the body and the propellant reaches the skin, the chilling effect upon evaporation may cause irritation and edema.[35, 37, 38] With proper application, propellants are not likely to be irritants.

Advisability of sprays

As with douche products, the advisability and benefits of using feminine deodorant sprays are controversial. Their efficacy even as deodorants has been questioned, and adverse effects have been reported.[39] When used as directed, however, manufacturers report that extensive testing fails to demonstrate adverse effects.

Kass *et al.*[40] reported evaluations of a feminine deodorant spray in 1,400 women after more than 200,000 test applications by direct application and patch testing. Evaluation of the study is difficult because many of the details were not provided. The authors felt their study supported the position that the sprays were nonirritating and nonsensitizing. It was also reported that in one group of 300 women, 8 percent of the control group experienced erythema from soap and water, but only 3 percent of those using the spray experienced this effect. The authors offered other possible explanations for consumer complaints of vulvar irritation after the use of these sprays:

- ☐ Close-fitting and/or nonabsorbent undergarments may cause vulvar irritation even if no spray has been applied.
- ☐ The symptoms may appear if sprays are used immediately after intercourse.
- ☐ The sprays may be held too closely to the body when applied.

In another study, only one case of erythema and one of irritation were reported, and it was concluded that the preparation was suitable for use.[41] Other authors also have attested to the safety of feminine deodorant sprays.[37, 42]

Despite reports that these aerosol products are not hazardous when evaluated in controlled studies and when they are properly used, there is evidence that hazards exist. Physicians in private practice have reported vulvar irritation in some of their female patients.[43-45] Feminine deodorant sprays were strongly suspected as the cause. There are many reports received by FDA of adverse local reactions, all locally severe and all attributed to the use of these products.[46] In most of these cases, systemic steroid treatment was required even when the sprays were discontinued. The specific ingredients responsible for adverse effects, however, were not identified. Fisher[35] reported four positive patch-test reactions to specific ingredients after testing 30 women and 2 men with the individual ingredients in 12 different sprays. The ingredients eliciting positive responses were benzethonium chloride, chlorhexidine, isopropyl myristate, and perfume. Ingredients in douches which cause either direct primary irritation or allergic contact sensitization are also frequently found in feminine deodorant sprays. Women who use sprays immediately prior to sexual intercourse may also exhibit local reactions.[35]

Most of the evidence criticizing the use of feminine deodorant sprays is from case reports or complaints received by manufacturers, physicians, and FDA; most of the evidence in defense of these products is cited by the authors as the findings of controlled studies. Perhaps this is because in controlled studies, subjects are given instructions on proper application. The use of sprays throughout the population is uncontrolled, especially in terms of assessing the incidence of improper application. It seems that feminine deodorant sprays are harmless to most users, but reports of adverse effects are too frequent to be ignored and there are significant potential hazards which must be considered. Furthermore, the superiority of these sprays over soap and water has been questioned.[47, 48] In the absence of conclusive demonstrations of prominent adverse effects, they continue to be available.

Proper application of sprays

Most manufacturers recommend that sprays be held at least 8 inches from the body when applying. By following this, premarketing evaluations of sprays consistently demonstrate safety. The most frequent adverse effect resulting from applying a spray held too closely is irritation as a result of:

- ☐ Evaporation and "chilling" from propellants inappropriately reaching the skin,
- ☐ Excessive concentrations of ingredients on cutaneous surfaces, or
- ☐ Accidental penetration of ingredients into the vagina from the force of the spray (ingredients are intended only for external use).

The relationship between frequency of use and the incidence of adverse effects has not been described well in the literature. It is reasonable to assume, however, that frequent application, perhaps several times a day, elicits more frequent local reactions than less frequent use. If women are fully informed of the possibility and nature of side effects, they can, with the help of the pharmacist, determine a desirable frequency of application for themselves.

Miscellaneous products

Although their uses and ingredients are similar to the douche or spray formulations, some OTC vaginal products are available in different dosage forms. They include suppositories, premoistened towelettes, and a local anesthetic cream.

The antimicrobial agents used in vaginal antiseptic suppositories are chloramine and phenylmercuric acetate, each contained in a greaseless, water-dispersible suppository base. Both compounds are effective antimicrobial agents *in vitro,* but subjective appraisal of their clinical efficacy is impossible because the concentration of the agents in the vagina following dispersion is unknown.[49 50] Both chloramine and phenylmercuric acetate can produce local irritation in sufficient concentration or in sensitive individuals. Because these suppositories are used for purposes similar to those for douches, the same considerations concerning benefits and risks apply.

Premoistened towelettes are used for their deodorant, cleansing, and/or cosmetic properties. Except for the propellants in sprays, ingredients of these towelettes are the same as those of spray products. Women who are sensitive to aerosol propellants might be informed of the towelette formulations. Direct irritation or sensitization from other towelette ingredients may occur.

A vaginal cream (Vagisil) for local anesthetic/antipruritic effect contains benzocaine as the local anesthetic and resorcinol for antimicrobial effects. Concentrations of benzocaine and resorcinol in this cream are not provided so efficacy cannot readily be determined. Both ingredients can cause local irritation or sensitization.[14 28 29] The intended purpose and use of this product present another significant hazard—the masking of symptoms of vaginitis. In the presence of symptoms possibly indicating vaginitis, the pharmacist should not recommend this or similar local anesthetic vaginal products without concurrent recommendation by the woman's physician.

Guidelines for product selection

In the absence of physician supervision, products should be selected only for cosmetic use. The pharmacist should determine persistence, recurrence, and severity of any symptoms or ascertain signs of infection or disease before attempting to recommend a product. If infection or disease is possible, the patient should be referred to a physician. Patient history or medication profiles may reveal predisposing factors for vaginitis such as pregnancy, diabetes, and chronic use of steroids (including oral contraceptives) or antibiotics (especially tetracyclines). If infection or other disease is suspected, a specific diagnosis and prescription products are nearly always indicated.

When satisfied that an OTC product may be safely used, the pharmacist should recommend that:

☐ Douches used routinely in the absence of symptoms should probably be acidic or as nearly physiologic as possible.

☐ If a douche is used for removal of excessive discharge, an alkaline douche may be more effective.

☐ Douches and sprays should be avoided before coitus.

☐ Douches are not contraceptive and should be used after coitus only for cleansing.

☐ Proper techniques of application should be followed.

☐ If irritation occurs, the product should be discontinued.

☐ Deodorant sprays may be indicated when frequent bathing is not possible or in the presence of menstrual odor.

☐ Regardless of the reasons for seeking a vaginal product, thorough cleansing with soap and water of the vulvar, perineal, and anal regions may be equally or more effective.

Summary

The benefits and hazards of vaginal cleansing and deodorant products are controversial. It is not universally accepted that these products have an advantage over cleansing with soap and water. Benefits may be largely placebo or psychological. The products may be misused in terms of frequency of use, preparation, and technique of application—perhaps the greatest problems are with the user, not the product. They may also cause direct contact irritation or allergic sensitization. The incidence of adverse effects may be small, but according to many gynecologists, potential benefits may be even less.

Most manufacturers state that products are extensively evaluated before marketing, and that in controlled studies the products have proved to be safe and effective. These claims seem to be justified because the studies were controlled (especially proper preparation and proper application). There is no guarantee that women in the general population prepare and apply these vaginal products properly, and this is one important reason for the occurrence of adverse effects. With reports of questionable benefits and potential hazards, the available literature is not convincing that vaginal cleansing and deodorant products are advisable for routine use. These products should be used only upon the advice of a pharmacist or physician, and their use without specific indication is unjustified. Women who insist on routine use of these products as part of their habits of personal cleanliness, however, should be fully informed of product expectations and limitations.

References

1. G. Carsch, *Soap Chem. Spec.*, **47,** 38(1971).
2. K. J. Karnaky, *Am. J. Surg.*, **101,** 456(1961).
3. K. J. Karnaky, *Am. J. Obstet. Gynecol.*, **115,** 283(1973).
4. R. Glynn, *Obstet. Gynecol.*, **20,** 369(1962).
5. E. A. Banner, *Med. Clin. North Am.*, **58,** 759(1974).
6. J. C. Hartgill, *Practitioner,* **202,** 363(1969).
7. G. J. Dennerstein, *Drugs,* **4,** 419(1972).
8. F. Sadik, *J. Am. Pharm. Assoc.*, **NS12,** 565(1972).
9. Tran-Dinh-De, Nguyen-Van-Tu, *Am. J. Obstet. Gynecol.*, **87,** 92(1965).
10. L. A. Gray and M. L. Barnes, *Am. J. Obstet. Gynecol.*, **92,** 125(1963).
11. FDA, Summary Minutes of the OTC Panel on Contraceptives and Other Vaginal Drug Products, Rockville, Md., September 20 and 21, 1974.
12. T. E. Swate and J. C. Weed, *Obstet. Gynecol.*, **43,** 893(1974).
13. J. J. Ratzan, *Calif. Med.*, **110,** 24(1969).
14. "Remington's Pharmaceutical Sciences," 14th ed., A. Osol and J. E. Hoover, Eds., Mack Publishing, Easton, Pa., 1970.
15. J. Barnes, *Practitioner,* **184,** 668(1960).
16. J. F. Byers, *Am. Fam. Physician,* **10,** 135(1974).
17. D. V. Hirst, *Am. J. Obstet. Gynecol.*, **64,** 179(1952).
18. J. H. Long *et al.*, *West. J. Surg. Obstet. Gynecol.*, **71,** 122(1963).
19. H. A. Kaminetzky, *J. Am. Med. Assoc.*, **191,** 154(1965).
20. L. McGowan, *Am. J. Obstet. Gynecol.*, **93,** 506(1965).
21. R. Glynn, *Obstet. Gynecol.*, **22,** 640(1963).
22. M. H. Gotlib and D. N. Adler, *Med. Times,* **96,** 902(1968).
23. R. S. Cohen *et al.*, *Curr. Ther. Res.*, **15,** 839(1973).
24. W. A. Abruzzi, *J. Am. Med. Women's Assoc.*, **21,** 406(1966).
25. R. J. Stock *et al.*, *Obstet. Gynecol.*, **42,** 141(1973).
26. FDA, Summary Minutes of the OTC Panel on Contraceptives and Other Vaginal Drug Products, Rockville, Md., February 7 and 8, 1975.
27. G. F. Egenolf and R. McNaughton, *Obstet. Gynecol.*, **7,** 23(1956).
28. F. H. Downer and C. J. Stevenson, *Adv. Drug React. Bull.*, **42,** 136(1973).
29. C. D. Calnan, *Proc. R. Soc. Med.*, **55,** 39(1962).
30. *Med. Lett. Drugs Ther.*, **10,** 27(1968).
31. A. A. Fisher *et al.*, *Arch. Dermatol.*, **104,** 287(1971).
32. A. A. Fisher and M. A. Stillman, *Arch. Dermatol.*, **106,** 169(1972).
33. E. Shmunes and E. J. Levy, *Arch. Dermatol.* **106,** 169(1972).
34. *Fed. Regist.*, **40,** 8926(1975).
35. A. A. Fisher, *Arch. Dermatol.*, **108,** 801(1973).
36. J. Meyer-Rohn and V. Kassebart, *Kosmetologie,* **4,** 159(1971).

37. J. A. Cella, *Am. Cosmet. Perfum.*, **86(10)**, 84(1971).
38. R. W. Pfirrman and P. Geistlich, Feminine Hygiene Spray Deodorant Compositions, U.S. Patent No. 3,574,821 (1971).
39. G. McBride, *J. Am. Med. Assoc.*, **219**, 449(1972).
40. G. S. Kass *et al.*, Feminine Hygiene Deodorant Sprays, Presented at XIV International Congress of Dermatology, Venice, Italy, May 22, 1972.
41. A. Kantner, *Am. Cosmet. Perfum.*, **87(2)**, 31(1972).
42. Y. M. Kapadia, Warner Lambert Research Institute, Personal Communication, May 15, 1975.
43. B. A. Davis, *Obstet. Gynecol.*, **36**, 812(1970).
44. B. M. Kaye, *J. Am. Med. Assoc.*, **212**, 2121(1970).
45. B. A. Davis, *Obstet. Gynecol.*, **37**, 949(1971).
46. J. M. Gowdy, *N. Engl. J. Med.*, **287**, 203(1972).
47. *Med. Lett. Drugs Ther.*, **12**, 88(1970).
48. M. Morrison, *FDA Consumer*, **7**, 16(1973).
49. A. E. Elkhouly and R. T. Yousef, *J. Pharm. Sci.*, **63**, 681(1974).
50. "National Formulary," 10th ed., American Pharmaceutical Association, Washington, D. C., and Lippincott, Philadelphia, Pa. 1955.

Products 18 FEMININE CLEANSING AND DEODORANT

Product (manufacturer)	Antimicrobial	Local anesthetic/ antipruritic/counterirritant	Other
Betadine Douche (Purdue Frederick)	povidone-iodine	—	—
Bo-Car-Al (Calgon)	boric acid	phenol menthol methyl salicylate eucalyptol thymol	potassium aluminum sulfate
Demure (Vick)	benzethonium chloride	—	—
Dismiss Disposable Douche (Richardson-Merrell)	—	—	ceteareth-27 cetearyl octoate sodium chloride sodium citrate citric acid
Femidine Douche (A.V.P.)	povidone-iodine	—	—
Jeneen (Norwich)	—	—	lactic acid sodium lactate propylene glycol
Lysette (Lehn & Fink)	—	—	triethanolamine dodecylbenzene sulfonate alcohol, 31%
Massengill Disposable Douche (Beecham Products)	cetylpyridinium chloride	—	alcohol lactic acid octoxynol fragrance
Massengill Douche Powder (Beecham Products)	boric acid	—	ammonium aluminum sulfate berberine fragrance
Massengill Liquid (Beecham Products)	—	—	alcohol lactic acid sodium lactate octoxynol aromatics
Meta-Cine (Chattem)	chlorothymol, 0.1%	methyl salicylate, 0.5% eucalyptol, 0.25% menthol, 0.25%	lactose, 840 mg/g citric acid, 135 mg/g papain, 10 mg/g eucalyptus oil, 0.25%
PMC Douche Powder (Thomas & Thompson)	boric acid, 82%	thymol, 0.3% phenol, 0.2% menthol	ammonium aluminum sulfate, 16% eucalyptus oil peppermint oil
Stomaseptine (Cooper)	—	menthol, eucalyptol, thymol } 2%	sodium perborate, 18% sodium chloride, 28% sodium borate, 25% sodium bicarbonate, 25%
Trichotine (Reed & Carnrick)	—	—	sodium perborate sodium borate aromatics sodium lauryl sulfate alcohol, 8%
V.A. (Norcliff-Thayer)	boric acid 8-hydroxyquinoline citrate	—	potassium aluminum sulfate zinc sulfate
Zonite (Norcliff-Thayer)	benzalkonium chloride	menthol thymol	propylene glycol buffer

Otic Products

Keith O. Miller

Questions to ask the patient

Do you feel pain? Is it constant or is it increased by chewing?

Do you have loss of hearing or ringing in the ears?

Do you have a cold or the flu?

Do you have a fever or malaise?

Do you have a discharge from the ear?

How long have these symptoms been present?

Have you been swimming within the past several days?

Do you have diabetes or other chronic diseases?

If the patient is a child, what is the age of the patient?

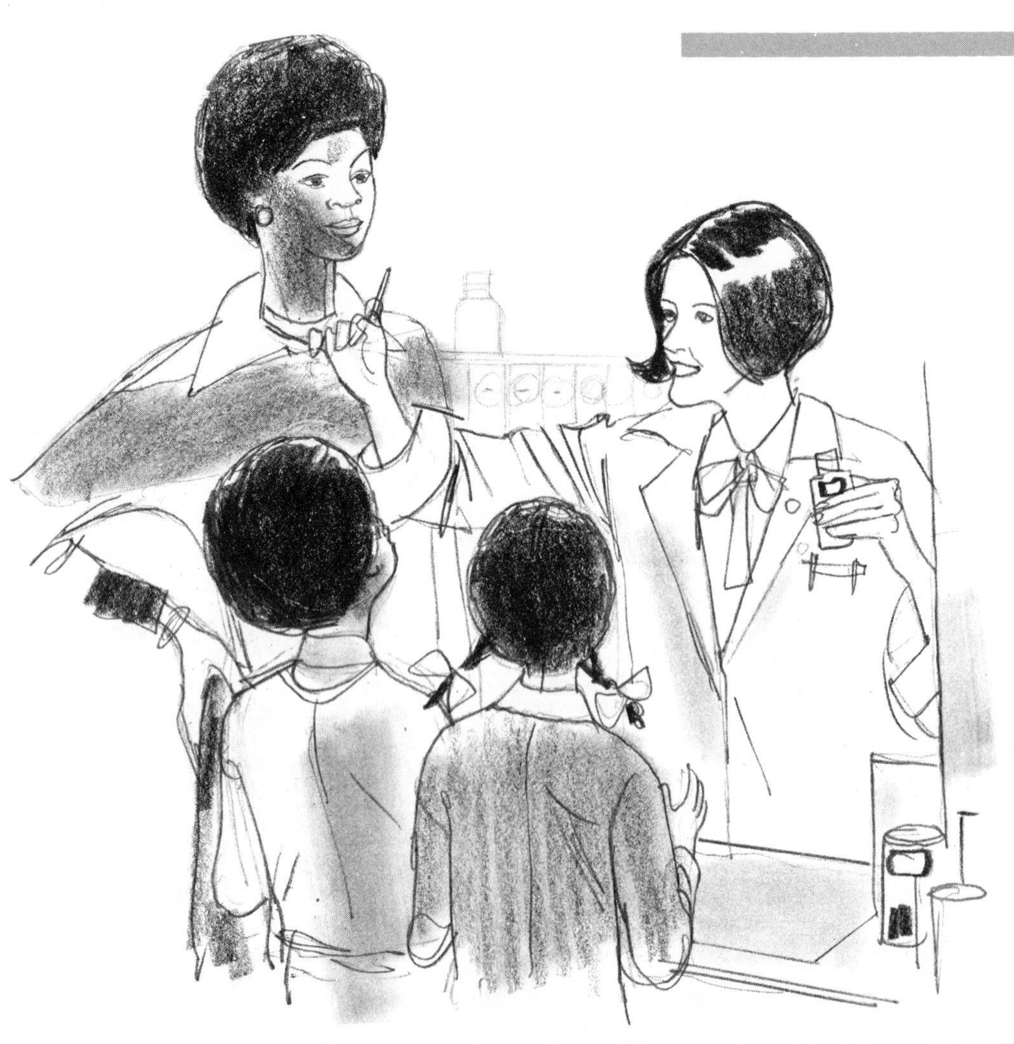

CHAPTER 19

Ear disorders are very common and, in most cases, cause discomfort. Patients usually have complaints or symptoms such as an "earache," "impacted ear," "running ear," "cold in the ear," or a combination of these. Attempts to advise patients with ear disorders of this nature to self-treat without further information regarding the symptoms are unwise. It is vitally important to obtain a clear picture of the symptoms of ear disorders and their corresponding pathophysiology in order to understand the recommended plans of treatment.

Ear disorders can be caused by a disease process of the auricle, external auditory meatus (external ear canal), or middle ear or by a disease process in another area of the head or neck region. A traumatic or pathologic condition of the tongue, mandibles, oropharynx, tonsils, or paranasal sinuses may cause referred pain to the ear and may appear to the patient as an "earache."

Home remedies and nonprescription drugs are usually restricted to conditions related only to the external ear. Self-medication should be reserved for minor conditions. It can also be used effectively for prophylaxis to aid the normal body defenses and to improve the integrity of the skin lining of the auricle and external auditory canal.

Anatomy and physiology of the ear

The external ear is composed of the auricle (pinna) and the external auditory meatus (ear canal) (Figs. 1 and 2). The auricle is the external appendage consisting of cartilage (elastic type) covered by a thin layer of normal skin, except for the lobule, which is mainly fatty tissue. A thin layer of tissue called the perichondrium covers both the cartilaginous auricle and cartilaginous portion of the external auditory canal.[1] The periostium covers the bony portion of the external auditory canal.

The external auditory meatus is tubelike and forms a channel for sound waves to pass to the tympanic membrane (drum head); it also protects the membrane from injury. The external auditory canal of adults is about 24 mm long and has a volume of about 0.85 ml (17 drops).[2] The outer half of the external auditory canal is cartilaginous and the inner half is bony tissue. At about 7 mm from the tympanic membrane, the channel narrows; this area is called the isthmus.[3] At the isthmus, the meatus bends posteriorly, and it is often necessary to straighten it by upward traction on the auricle to permit direct visual examination of the tympanic membrane.

The skin of the auricle is continuous and lines the entire auditory meatus and the outer covering of the tympanic membrane.[4] The skin of the cartilaginous part of the canal contains hair follicles, sebaceous glands which either open to the surface of the skin or into the lumen of the hair follicles, and ceruminous glands.[2] There are between 1,000 and 2,000 ceruminous glands in the average ear, less in older people.[2] Neither hair follicles nor sebaceous or ceruminous glands are found in the inner half of the external auditory canal.

The secretory product of the ceruminous glands is colorless, watery fluid (cerumen). Cerumen is derived from the watery secretions of the ceruminous glands and the oily secretions of the sebaceous glands.[2] Its composition is a mixture of polypeptides, lipids, fatty acids, amino acids, and electrolytes.[2,5] Cerumen looks brown because it mixes with desquamated epithelial cells and dust particles. It lubricates the skin and entraps foreign material entering the external auditory canal, providing a protective barrier.[3] Under normal conditions, the cerumen forms small, round droplets and dries into a semisolid. It is then expelled unnoticed by a process called epithelial migration, which is the movement of epithelial cells across the surface of the tympanic membrane and across the epithelial lining of the external auditory meatus to the outside. The normal pH of the healthy external auditory meatus is between 5.0 and 7.2.[2]

The tympanic membrane is pearly-gray, egg shaped, semitransparent and is about 0.1 mm thick and 8 to 9 mm wide (the narrow portion is at the bottom).[2] The outer layer of its epithelium is continuous with the epidermis of the external auditory canal; the middle layer is tough, fibrous tissue; and the innermost layer is a mucous membrane continuous with the lining of the tympanic cavity.[6] In adults the membrane forms about a 45° angle with the floor of the external meatus, and it is almost horizontal in infants.[2] Anatomically, the tympanic membrane is considered with the external auditory canal because it is attached to the medial terminal end of the canal. Functionally, it is considered with the middle ear (tympanic cavity).[3]

Common problems of the ear

Auricle

Trauma. Lacerations, including scrapes and cuts, involving only the skin of the auricle usually heal spontaneously. Deep wounds that may involve injury to the cartilage should be inspected by a physician. Injury to the auricle that does not perforate the subperichondrium may cause a hematoma (bruise). A bruise is caused by subcutaneous bleeding.

Symptoms of trauma include red-blue swelling which may obliterate the normal contours of the auricle, local pruritus, and pain upon touching. A flatulent hematoma requires aspiration or incision by a physician. If not aspirated, hematomas frequently result in perichondritis or cauliflower ear. A wound that does not heal normally should be checked by a physician.

Boils. Boils (furuncles) are usually localized infections of the hair follicles predisposed by irritation, pressure, friction, and scratching. Other factors suspected for recurrent lesions are diets rich in sugars and fats and states of lowered resistance such as anemia, alcoholism, diabetes mellitus, malnutrition, poor bathing habits, and poor body hygiene.

Boils usually involve the anterior part of the external auditory meatus. They usually begin as a red papule and may progress into a round or conical, superficial pustule with a core of pus and erythema around the base. The lesion gradually enlarges, becomes firm, then softens and opens spontaneously (after a few days to as long as 2 weeks) to discharge the purulent contents. Because the skin is tightly attached, minimal swelling may cause severe pain.

Boils usually are self-limiting; however, they may be severe, autoinoculable, and multiple. Deeper lesions may lead to perichondritis. The pus-producing species found in boils is usually *Staphylococcus*.

Usually, small boils can be treated by good hygiene and topical compresses, and/or antibiotic ointment. Hot compresses of saline solution may be applied to the auricle and the side of the face. Antibiotic ointments do not help heal boils, but they do prevent spreading. Cases of boils which do not respond rapidly to antibiotic ointment and/or to topical dressings should be referred to a physician. Recurring conditions should also be referred to rule out predisposing causes.

Perichondritis. Perichondritis is an infection involving the perichondrium, usually following a poorly treated or untreated burn, injury, hematoma, or local infection.

The onset of perichondritis is characterized by a sensation of heat and stiffness of the auricle. Pain is pronounced. As the condition progresses, an exudate forms, and the auricle becomes dark red, diffuse, and swollen. The entire auricle becomes shiny and red with uniform thickening caused by edema and inflammation.[1] The lesions usually are confined to the cartilaginous tissue of the auricle and external canal. Constitutional disturbances may include generalized fever and malaise.

Perichondritis frequently results in severe deformity of the auricle, and atresia (a pathological closure) of the external auditory canal may occur. A patient suspected of having symptoms of perichondritis should be seen by a physician.

Dermatitis of the ear. An inflammatory condition can result from an abrasion of the auricle, and if left untreated, may develop into an infection of these skin layers. Inflammatory conditions such as seborrhea, psoriasis, contact dermatitis (e.g., poison-ivy and poison-oak) also may affect the skin of the auricle and the external ear canal. Often, dermatitis of the ear is associated with seborrhea of the scalp. Contact dermatitis also may be caused by an allergic response to jewelry, cosmetics, detergents, or topical application of drugs. The lesions may spread to the auditory canal, neck, and facial areas, and from one person to another by contact.

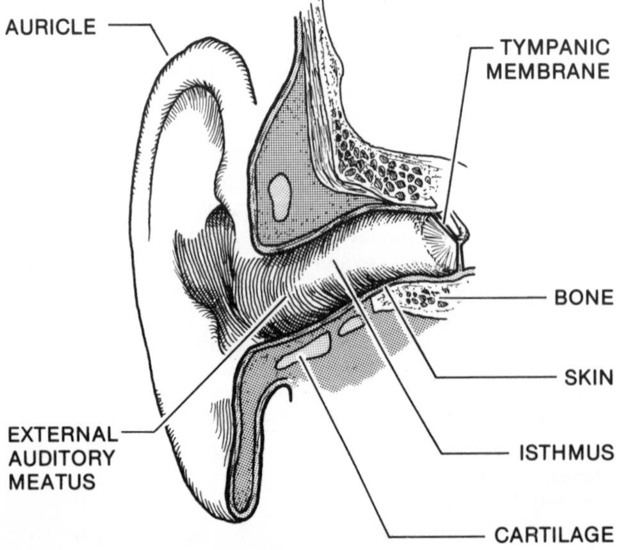

Figure 1. Anatomy of the auricle.

The symptoms of dermatitis of the ear usually include severe itching and local redness followed by vesication, weeping, and erythema. The lesions form scales and yellow crusts on the skin.[6] They may spread to adjacent unaffected areas, and excessive scratching may cause them to become infected. Topical drugs should be used cautiously with dermatitis due to their potential allergenicity. Seborrheic dermatitis of the ear is usually associated with dandruff, and treatment with dandruff control shampoos is recommended. Cases which are difficult to control and generalized dermatitis around the ear should be referred to a physician.

External auditory canal

Boils. Boils of the external auditory canal are pathologically similar to those found on the auricle. Symptoms include pain of the infected site which is usually exacerbated by mastication. The meatal opening may be partly occluded by swelling; however, hearing is impaired only if the opening is completely occluded. Edema and pain over the mastoid bone directly behind the auricle may occur. Traction on the auricle or the tragus is very painful. Patients with boils in the external auditory canal should be referred to the physician because unresolved conditions may lead to a generalized infection of the entire external auditory canal.

Otomycosis. Otomycosis is external fungal infection of the ear. It is more common in warmer, tropical climates than in mild, temperate ones. *Aspergillus* sp. and *Candida* sp. are the most common causative agents.[4, 7] Antibiotic treatment of a bacterial ear infection, with resultant suppression of normal bacterial flora, may predispose an individual to a mycotic external ear infection.[7]

A superficial mycotic infection of the external auditory meatus is characterized by pruritus with a feeling of fullness and pressure in the ear and itchiness. Pain is usually present and increases severely with mastication and traction on the pinna and the tragus. The fungus forms on a mass of epithelial debris, exudate, and cerumen and, in the acute stage, may clog the external auditory meatus. Hearing impairment may occur. Depending on the nature of the fungus, the color of the mass may vary. *Apergillus* sp. infections usually appear dark gray, dark brown, or black in color, and *Candida* sp. infections usually appear creamy colored to gray. The skin lining the external auditory canal and the tympanic membrane becomes beefy red, scaly, and may be eroded or ulcerated.[2] A scant, colorless discharge is common. Otomycosis is particularly serious in diabetic patients because of the microangiopathy and cutaneous manifestations common to diabetes mellitus.[4] Mycotic infections of the ear must be treated by a physician.

Keratosis obturans. This condition is rare, and its etiology is unclear.[4] Wax accumulates in the deeper parts of the external auditory canal and, with adjacent epithelial cells that contain cholesterol, forms a mass and exerts pressure on the surrounding tissue. The mass is a shiny, white, pluglike occlusion of the external auditory canal. It may cause a ring of pressure and erosion of the epithelial tissues surrounding it, forming a potential entrance for organisms to initiate a bacterial infection.[1] The infection may form abscesses in the subcutaneous tissue and mastoid bone tissue.

Pain in the ear and decreased hearing are common symptoms. A discharge and tinnitus may also occur. Mechanical removal of the obstruction is necessary and is often difficult. The removal should be reserved for a physician; patients should not attempt to remove the obstruction themselves.

Foreign objects in the ear. Young children invariably use the ear canal for inserting precious "gems" such as beans, peas, marbles, pebbles, or beads. If the objects become lodged in the ear canal, they may cause significant hearing loss. Vegetable seeds, such as dried beans or dried peas, lodged in the external auditory meatus swell when moistened during bathing or swimming and become wedged in the bony portion of the canal, causing severe pain. Furthermore, an obstruction of the external auditory meatus, if not removed promptly, may provide a potential culture medium for organisms, resulting in acute bacterial external otitis.

Foreign objects lodged in the ear canal may not cause symptoms and may be found only during a routine physical examination. Usually, a hearing deficit is observed with pressure in the ear on mastication. Pain may be present. Exudate may form because of secondary bacterial infection. Insects may enter the meatus and cause distress by beating their wings and crawling. Mechanical removal should be reserved for a physician because unskilled attempts at removal often result in damage to the skin surrounding the external auditory meatus.

Impacted cerumen. The accumulation of cerumen in the external auditory meatus may be caused by overactive ceruminous glands, an abnormally shaped external auditory meatus, or abnormal cerumen secreted by the ceruminous glands. Overactive ceruminous glands cause cerumen to accumulate in the external auditory canal. A tortuous or small canal or abnormal narrowing of the canal may not permit normal migration of the cerumen to the outside, causing the cerumen to accumulate. Abnormal cerumen is drier or softer than normal cerumen and may interfere with the normal epithelial migration. It is often packed deeper into the external auditory meatus by repeated attempts to remove it, which is the most common cause of impacted cerumen. There usually is no cerumen in the inner half of the external auditory canal unless pushed there.

In the elderly, cerumen often is admixed with long hairs in the external auditory canal, preventing normal expulsion and forming a matted obstruction.

External otitis. External otitis (an infection of the skin lining the external auditory canal) is one of the most common diseases of the ear. It is very painful and annoying. The external auditory canal is considered a blind canal lined with skin. It is a cul-de-sac that is dark, warm, and well suited for the collection of moisture. Prolonged exposure to moisture tends to disrupt the continuity of the epithelial cells, causing maceration and fissuring of the skin and providing an area of fertility for the growth of bacteria. Additionally, this prolonged exposure to moisture tends to raise the normal pH of the skin, improving the growth media for bacteria. Factors contributing to susceptibility to external otitis include race, heredity, age, sex, climate, diet, and occupational background.[7] The most common causative organisms of external otitis include *Pseudomonas* sp., *Staphylococcus* sp., *Bacillus* sp., and *Proteus* sp.

There is very little subcutaneous tissue between the skin which is tightly bound to the perichondrium on the cartilaginous portion and the periostium on the bony portion of the external auditory canal. Consequently, there is a disparity between the size of the visible swelling and the amount of pain associated with the condition. The lack of space available for expansion increases the tension on the skin, and inflammation causing edema provokes severe pain in the inflamed skin which is out of proportion to visible swelling. As the inflammation increases, the pain may be significantly increased during mastication. Symptoms often develop following attempts to clean the ear (with cotton swabs, hair pins, match sticks, pencils, fingers, or other objects) of foreign debris or to scratch the ear to relieve itching. The instruments may traumatize and damage the horny skin layer, forming an opening for the invasion of organisms.

A normal, healthy external auditory canal is impervious to the invasion of pathological organisms. Generally, individuals must be susceptible to bacterial infections and the integrity of the skin must be interrupted before an organism can produce an infected lesion.

Another type of trauma-induced external otitis is called "swimmer's ear," or desquamative external otitis.[7] This condition is caused by excessive moisture in the external auditory meatus. After bathing or swimming, patients frequently attempt to clear the ear canal of water with instruments which cause abrasions or lacerations of the skin lining. Also, cerumen, which absorbs water, accumulates in the external auditory meatus, causing the cerumen to expand (increasing its bulk) and entrap water, providing a basis for infection.[3] Within a few hours to one day following exposure to excess water, symptoms occur. They are itching, pain, and possible draining from the ear with partial occlusion. In many cases this condition is related to climatic conditions where the relative humidity and temperature are high and where dust and sand storms occur.[3]

A bacterial infection of the external auditory canal leads to inflammation and epidermal destruction of the skin lining the tympanic membrane. The infection may progress through the fibrous layer of the tympanic membrane and cause perforation and spreading of the infection into the middle ear, resulting in intense pain and discomfort. External otitis, like otomycosis, is particularly difficult to control in diabetics.[4, 8]

Symptoms of external otitis are related to the severity of the pathological conditions. There usually is mild or moderate pain that becomes pronounced by applying trac-

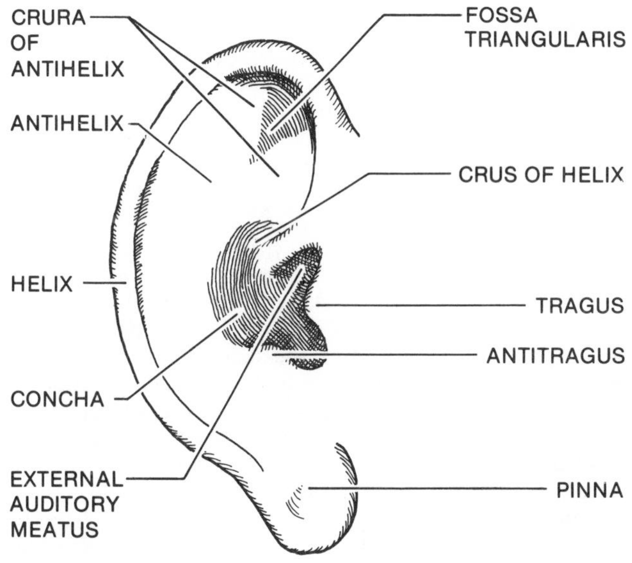

Figure 2. Anatomy of the external ear.

tion to the auricle or applying pressure on the tragus. There may be a discharge. Hearing loss may occur if the ear canal has been obstructed by swelling and edema or by debris.

Chronic external otitis is usually caused by the chronicity of predisposing factors. The most common symptom is itching, which prompts patients to attempt to "scratch the ear canal" to reduce or relieve the itch. This scratching causes the skin to become obliterated or broken.

In allergic external otitis and dermatitis of the external auditory canal caused by seborrhea, a common symptom is itching, burning, or stinging of the lesions. Often, the complaints seem excessive compared to the visible signs.

Chronic cases and the more severe cases with symptoms of severe pain, lymphadenopathy, discharge, possible hearing deficit, and fever should be referred to a physician.[3] Tender nodes may be felt anteriorly to the tragus, behind the ear, or in the upper neck just below the pinna. Minor cases can often be adequately treated with OTC products. Often, chronic and allergic external otitis can be treated prophylactically with OTC products, especially for "swimmer's ear" otitis.

Middle Ear

Disorders involving the middle ear should not be treated with nonprescription otic products, but a brief overview of the common conditions involving the middle ear will aid the pharmacist in the evaluation of symptoms. Some symptoms of middle ear disorders are the same as those of external ear disorders; others are not. All bacterial infections of the middle ear should be evaluated and treated by a physician. The usual treatment is systemic antibiotics.

Otitis media (serous and purulent). Otitis media is an inflammatory condition of the middle ear that most often occurs during childhood. Conditions which interfere with the eustachian tube function, i.e., upper respiratory tract infection, allergy, adenoid lymphadenopathy, cleft palate, etc., predispose individuals to otitis media. With eustachian tube dysfunction, the oxygen in the middle ear cleft is absorbed, leaving a relative negative pressure or vacuum, resulting in a transudation of fluid into the middle ear cleft. If the serous fluid in the middle ear cavity remains sterile, the condition is referred to as serous otitis media; if it becomes infected, it is called purulent otitis media.

Children often experience repeated eustachian tube obstruction episodes which are caused by masses of adenoids that become edematous and block the eustachian tube openings. Usually, an adenoidectomy prevents future episodes. In adults, recurrent otitis media may be caused by a nasopharyngeal tumor.

The most common symptoms in the acute phase of purulent otitis media are pain, hearing loss, and constitutional disturbances such as fever [often as high as 104° F (40° C)] and malaise.[9] The severity of these symptoms is increased as the condition worsens. Pain arises from the pressure of the fluids in the middle ear causing an outward tension on the tympanic membrane, which is innervated with sensory nerves. The rapid production of fluid and tension in a short period is responsible for the acute pain, described as sharp, knifelike, and steady. It is usually not increased with mastication or when traction is applied to the auricle or tragus. Excessive nose blowing may force additional purulent mucus into the eustachian tube, perpetuating the condition. If patients are not properly treated, the pressure may increase to the point where the tympanic membrane ruptures, resulting in a mucopurulent discharge. This discharge may cause secondary bacterial external otitis infection. The appearance of a discharge usually is accompanied by a lessening of pain due to the decreased tension on the tympanic membrane. The initial discharge may be bloodstained, followed by a foul-smelling, purulent, serous fluid. The tympanic membrane usually loses its pearlish-gray luster and appears yellow to orange-pink, another important factor in diagnosing.

The symptoms of serous otitis media include a sensation of fullness in the ear with accompanying loss of hearing. The condition worsens as the fluid accumulates and fills the middle ear cleft. The feeling of fullness is associated with voice resonance, a stopped-up feeling in the ears, a hollow sound, or a popping or cracking noise in the ears, especially during swallowing or yawning. These symptoms usually are not present in external otitis.

Potential complications

Conductive hearing loss. Conductive hearing loss (mechanical deafness) is a deficiency in the conduction of sound waves from the air through the tympanic membrane and ossicles to the nerve fibers in the inner ear. It may occur with external otitis, otomycosis, a foreign body in the external auditory meatus, impacted cerumen, a perforated tympanic membrane, acute serous otitis media, mastoiditis (an inflammation of the mastoid bone-cleft surrounding the middle ear), and otosclerosis.

Neural hearing loss. Neural hearing loss is usually accompanied by tinnitus and a sensation of disequilibrium. It may be caused by a viral or bacterial infection or a vascular or metabolic condition. Patients with neural hearing loss should be under the care of a physician. The above characteristics are very important for differential diagnosis.

Chronic otitis media (serous and purulent). In chronic, serous otitis media the fluid in the middle ear may be thin and serous or thick and viscous ("glue ear").[4] Chronic, serous otitis media occurs most often in small children. It may be caused by inadequate treatment of previous episodes of acute otitis media or by recurrent upper respiratory tract bacterial or viral infections associated with eustachian tube dysfunction.

The most common symptom is impaired hearing, but the onset is often insidious, and the child may have no acute symptoms. Frequently, parents accuse the child of being inattentive and disobedient. Pain is usually absent. The tympanic membrane appears yellow or orange, is lusterless, and its mobility is lost.[4] It is not perforated but often appears to be retracted.

Chronic purulent otitis media is usually secondary to a persistent tympanic membrane perforation. With exacerbation the patient may exhibit the symptoms of acute purulent otitis media as well as mucopurulent discharge.

Perforation of the tympanic membrane. The most common causes of traumatic perforation of the tympanic membrane are water sports, such as diving or water skiing.[6] Any corrosive agent introduced into the ear canal has the potential for producing tympanic membrane perforation. Other causes of perforation include blows to the head with a cupped hand, foreign objects entering the ear canal with excessive force, and forceful irrigation of the ear canal. At the moment of the injury, pain is severe, but it decreases rapidly. Hearing acuity will usually diminish. An untreated injury may lead to an infection of the middle ear (otitis media). Other complications may include tinnitus, nausea, and vertigo.

Treatment of otic disorders

Normally, the skin lining the external auditory meatus provides adequate protection against bacterial or fungal infection; cerumen provides a lubricant to the skin to maintain its integrity. The hairs help stop dust and debris from entering the meatus. Cerumen provides a continuing, self-cleaning process which removes particulate matter and debris from the external auditory meatus. An infection of the auricle or external auditory meatus is an infection of the skin and should be treated as such.

More serious conditions of the ear should be treated by a physician. Impacted cerumen or other debris lodged in the external auditory meatus should only be removed by a physician. Surgical intervention may be necessary for deep cuts, bruises, or abrasions. Severe infections often require systemic and local antibiotics. External otitis that is not treated properly is likely to spread to the mastoid bone or to the middle ear cavity, causing severe patient disability. Permanent hearing loss may occur.

Ingredients in OTC products

Nonprescription products used for palliative treatment of ear disorders of the auricle should include those used for the treatment of all topical skin disorders (see Chapter 27). Antibiotic ointments, such as neomycin and bacitracin ointments, alone or in combination with polymyxin B sulfate, are adequate for treating minor lesions of the auricle. Antibiotics cannot penetrate into abscesses because of the intrinsic nature of abscesses to wall themselves off. Antibiotic ointments can prevent the spread of autoinoculation when applied to surrounding tissue. They also help keep the surrounding skin soft and moist.

Ichthammol. Ichthammol is a weak antiseptic and irritant with demulcent and emollient properties. Its primary contribution is as an emollient, not as an antiseptic. Ichthammol ointment (NF), 10 percent, is used for treating local inflammation associated with minor boils or a wound which has become walled off.[10 11] Ichthammol (10 percent) in glycerin has been used as ear drops for treating minor inflammatory conditions of the external ear.

Aluminum acetate (Burow's) solution. External otitis or local itching of the external ear caused by external ear dermatitis can be treated with an astringent such as 1:20 or 1:40 aluminum acetate solution.[3 10 12] It is available in tablets or packets. One tablet or packet dissolved in 1 pint of water yields a concentration of 1:40. Aluminum acetate solution is widely used for conditions involving the external ear. Its principal value is its acidity, which restores the normal antibacterial pH of the ear canal. Astringents are applied locally as protein precipitants.[11] They cause the affected area to become drier by reducing the secretory function of the glands in the skin. Contraction and wrinkling of the affected tissue can be seen; astringents also toughen the skin to prevent reinfection.

A wet compress of aluminum acetate solution can be used with a gauze dressing on the auricle.[3] Drops can be instilled into the external auditory meatus. The usual dose is four or six drops every 4 to 6 hours until symptoms of itching or burning subside. Aluminum acetate solution drops can also be used prophylactically against swimmer's ear. They help clean and dry the ear canal after swimming or bathing. Aluminum acetate solution can be used by children and adults. It is nonsensitizing and well-tolerated when used property. Adverse reactions to aluminum acetate solution are rare.

Acetic acid solution. Weak acetic acid solutions are used to treat mild forms of external otitis. A concentration of 2 or 2.5 percent can easily be made in the pharmacy from glacial acetic acid or from white distilled household vinegar, which is usually 5 percent acetic acid. A 50-50 mixture of distilled household vinegar with either water, propylene glycol, glycerin, or rubbing alcohol (either 70 percent isopropyl alcohol or 70 percent ethanol) can be used.[13] (Patients should be cautioned that the denaturants in commercial denatured alcohol may cause sensitization.) The mixture is convenient to make and inexpensive. The acetic acid increases the acidity of the normal skin of the external auditory canal. This creates an undesirable environment for the growth of bacteria, especially *Pseudomonas*.[10] Rubbing alcohol is a local anti-infective and provides a local drying effect for prophylaxis against swimmer's ear.[6 14 15]

Propylene glycol. Propylene glycol is a solvent that has preservative properties and is a useful humectant. It is used in many otic preparations (prescription-only and OTC). Propylene glycol is a clear, colorless, nonirritating, viscous liquid. Its viscosity provides increased contact time to the tissues of the external auditory meatus. The addition of acetic acid to propylene glycol increases the acidity of the solution, enhancing its anti-infective properties.[6 16]

Glycerin. Glycerin can be used as a solvent, a vehicle, an emollient, and a humectant. It acts as a humectant because of its hygroscopicity and its viscosity. Glycerin is widely used as a solvent and a vehicle in many otic preparations (prescription-only and OTC). It is safe and nonsensitizing when applied to open wounds or abraded skin.

Olive oil (sweet oil). Olive oil is a fixed oil containing mixed glycerols of oleic acid (about 83 percent).[17] It is used as an emollient and topical lubricant. Often, olive oil is instilled into the ear canal to alleviate itchiness and burning and can be used for softening earwax.[10]

Thymol. Thymol, a phenol obtained from thyme oil, has a more agreeable odor than phenol. It has antibacterial and antifungal properties in concentrations of 1 percent.[11] In the presence of large amounts of proteins, its antibacterial activity is greatly reduced. It has traditionally been used in topical preparations partly because of its deodorant properties. Its clinical effectiveness for ear disorders has not been substantiated.

Menthol. Menthol is included in some earwax softeners. It is an antipruritic and counterirritant. Menthol provides a local feeling of coolness when applied to the tissues. Its clinical effectiveness in treating ear disorders has not been substantiated.

Camphor. Camphor is used in eardrop preparations and earwax softeners. It is a weak antiseptic and a mild anesthetic. It is intended to suppress itching, but its effectiveness has not been substantiated.

Chloroform. Chloroform is an irritant and preservative. It is used in some eardrop preparations. Chloroform is volatile and usually evaporates following exposure to the air. Its effectiveness for treating ear disorders has not been substantiated.

Boric acid. Boric acid is an ingredient in several ear preparations. It is a weak, local anti-infective and is nonirritating to intact skin in a dilute solution of 1 to

5 percent. Boric acid in low concentration with isopropyl alcohol enhances the acidity of the alcohol. Acetic acid and boric acid increase the acidity of dosage forms, increasing the normal acidic nature of the skin.[10] Because of its toxicity, boric acid should be used with caution, particularly with children and on open wounds, where the potential for systemic absorption is high.

Phenol–glycerin. Phenol–glycerin was once recommended for the treatment of pain caused by ear disorders.[18] Presently, its use is not recommended because of its inherent dangers of necrosis and perforation of the tympanic membrane.[19]

Benzocaine (ethyl aminobenzoate). Benzocaine is a local anesthetic that is commonly used for skin ulcers, wounds, mucous membranes, hemorrhoids, and skin irritations, including sunburn and insect bites. Benzocaine is poorly soluble in water. It is very slowly absorbed and relatively nontoxic. The localized anesthesia produced is not complete but is long acting due to its poor solubility and slow absorption.

Benzocaine has been used as a local anesthetic to treat pain associated with external otitis and other disorders of the auricle and/or ear canal. The usefulness of benzocaine or other local anesthetics for local analgesia in the ear canal is not clear. Its application to weeping wounds or fulminating infections is usually not effective because of the drainage of body fluids away from the wound. A therapeutic concentration cannot be achieved at the site of pain. Furthermore, the relief of the symptomatic pain may disguise the symptoms of an infection that in fact may be worsening.

Carbamide peroxide (urea hydrogen peroxide). The antibacterial properties of carbamide peroxide are due to its release of nascent oxygen. Its main value is to clean wounds. The effervescence caused by the release of oxygen mechanically removes debris from inaccessible regions. In otic preparations, the effervescence disorganizes wax accumulations. Carbamide (urea) helps debride the tissue. These actions soften the residue in the ear, and the liquefied cerumen can then be removed by warm water irrigation.

Other cerumen-softening products. Other products used to soften earwax include light mineral oil, a mixture of warm water and 3 percent hydrogen peroxide (in a ratio of 1:1), or a 3 percent hypertonic sodium chloride solution.[10] Cerumen-softening agents only soften the hardened, impacted cerumen. They do not and should never be expected to both soften and remove cerumen. If the tympanic membrane is perforated or if it is not known whether or not the tympanic membrane is intact, these cerumen-softening drug products should be used only under the direct supervision of a physician.

More than 90 percent of all cases of external otitis can properly be treated with aluminum acetate solution or acetic acid (2 percent) in either 70-percent alcohol or propylene glycol, four to six drops every 4 to 6 hours. This is the preferred treatment except in diabetics and in unusually severe cases of external otitis. In severe cases these solutions are often used to irrigate the debris from the ear canal to improve the effectiveness of topical antibacterial otic drops. Patients with a known tympanic membrane perforation should not use otic preparations without the consent of their physician. All nonprescription otic preparations may be contraindicated because of local irritation and hypersensitivity caused by the ingredients. Patients should be advised that if a rash, local redness, or noticeable adverse symptom occurs, the medication should be discontinued.

Guidelines for product selection

Patient considerations

The pharmacist's evaluation of the patient's present health status must be based on information on the medical and drug history, including present symptoms. This information should include the presence of chronic diseases that may impair healing, e.g., diabetes mellitus (is the patient taking insulin or oral hypoglycemics?), or that may influence the patient's response to self-medication, e.g., dandruff. Other considerations include deformities or scarring of the ear. An earache due to otitis media, secondary to an upper respiratory tract infection, should be ruled out before considering initiating treatment of an external ear disorder. A history of pressure in or referred pain to the ear may be caused by a tumor in the area around the ear. Recent injury or trauma in the head or neck regions also may cause referred pain to the ear. Adults with recurrent otitis media may respond very poorly to treatment.

Management of ear disorders may often be difficult due to underlying diseases or to predisposing factors. The skin of patients with diabetes mellitus is more prone to infection (bacterial and fungal), especially when the diabetes is uncontrolled, and infections clear up more slowly and recur more frequently. The increased predisposition to infection is related to circulatory impairments of the skin, increase in glucose concentrations, and abnormalities in immunologic responses. Ear disorders, especially external otitis, are difficult to treat in diabetic patients. Rigid control of diabetes cannot be overemphasized for favorable outcome of treatment.

The pharmacist should ask specific questions regarding the patient's medical history, e.g., has the patient experienced similar symptoms previously? If so, when and how were they treated? The pharmacist should ask the patient to describe the symptoms. The patient's history should reveal underlying disease states and predisposing factors, including allergies, which may influence the response to self-medication.

The pharmacist should first consider whether the patient can be treated appropriately with nonprescription drugs. Nonprescription drug products can often be relied upon to provide the appropriate therapeutic response only if the pharmacist becomes well acquainted with the symptomatology of the patient and the pathophysiology of the illness and if the pharmacist instructs the patient in the use of the medication. Medical treatment by a physician may be indicated. This depends on the severity of illness.

Patient consultation

Many physicians feel that cleansing procedures and the use of self-medication in treating ear disorders should be delegated neither to the patient nor to anyone who does not have sufficient information and know-how pertaining to the treatment of the condition. Patients must be evaluated for their ability to understand the hazards of inappropriate use of self-medication. The pharmacist can usually make these value judgments.

The use of nonprescription drugs for the ear should be supervised as other drug products dispensed by the pharmacist. The proper use of medicine droppers for administering ear drops into the ear and ear syringes for irrigating the ear should be fully understood by the patient. Ear drops should be warmed to body temperature.

This can be accomplished by holding the medication container in the palm of the hand or in a vessel of warm water for a few moments prior to administration.

A cotton plug can be gently inserted to help maintain the medication in the ear canal. Cotton wicks, however, usually require insertion with instrumentation and should only be used by trained personnel. Pulling the auricle back may facilitate the medication to reach a greater depth in the ear canal. Patients must also be advised that if the symptoms persist or increase in severity within a few days following the initiation of self-medication, a physician should be consulted. Symptoms usually begin to subside within 1 or 2 days if self-medication is useful. If symptoms persist or if an adverse reaction to the medication occurs, the patient should be referred to a physician.

Other self-therapy procedures

During recovery of an ear disorder, general measures are advisable to assist the natural healing process and to prevent reinfection.[20]

The external auditory canal must not be exposed to water. A bathing cap should be worn while taking a shower, and swimming should be avoided during and immediately following an infection. Patients prone to recurrence should swim only after consulting a physician. If water enters the external auditory canal, the head should be tilted for the water to drain out by gravity. If the water does not drain out, an appropriate nonprescription otic preparation can be used to aid in drying the external auditory canal. To clean the auricle, a soft cotton cloth should be wrung out in soapy water and wiped over the auricle, followed by wiping the auricle again with a damp soft cloth rinsed in clear water, then drying with a clean towel.

Objects such as hair pins, pencils, match sticks, cotton swabs, or other sharp instruments should never touch the external auditory canal. Objects larger than a finger draped with a clean washcloth should never enter the external auditory canal. Good personal hygiene should be maintained. This includes maintaining clean facial and neck areas. Dandruff and dirty hair can be controlled with appropriate shampoos and bathing. A skin infection must not be neglected because transfer of infection to uninfected areas is very easy.

References

1. I. Hall and B. Colman, "Diseases of the Nose, Throat and Ear," 10th ed., Williams and Wilkins, Baltimore, Md., 1973, pp. 278, 315, 324.
2. I. Friedmann, "Pathology of the Ear," Blackwell Scientific Publications, London, England, 1974, pp. 10, 14, 15, 27.
3. D. DeWeese and W. Saunders, "Textbook of Otolaryngology," 4th ed., Mosby, St. Louis, Mo., 1973, pp. 235, 245, 272-274, 327, 328, 336, 337, 346.
4. M. A. Paparella and D. A. Shumrick, "Otolaryngology," vol. 2, Saunders, Philadelphia, Pa., 1973, pp. 24, 26, 29, 30, 37, 85, 103.
5. S. Riegelman and D. L. Sorby, in "Dispensing of Medication," 7th ed., E. W. Martin, Ed., Mack Publishing, Easton, Pa., 1971, p. 908.
6. "Diseases of the Nose, Throat and Ear," 11th ed., J. J. Ballenger *et al.*, Eds., Lea and Febiger, Philadelphia, Pa., 1969, pp. 505, 604, 609, 610, 612.
7. S. R. Mawson, "Diseases of the Ear," 3d ed., Williams and Wilkins, Baltimore, Md., 1974, pp. 218, 236, 237, 245, 251.
8. A. Cohn, *Arch. Otolaryngol.*, **99**, 138(1974).
9. D. Elliott *et al.*, *Patient Care*, **5**, 21(1971).
10. "AMA Drug Evaluations," 2d ed., Publishing Sciences Group, Acton, Mass., 1973, pp. 388, 664, 732-734.
11. E. A. Swinyard and S. C. Harvey, in "Remington's Pharmaceutical Sciences," 14th ed., Mack Publishing, Easton, Pa., 1970, pp. 768, 775, 1191.
12. "Drugs of Choice 1974-1975," W. Modell, Ed., Mosby, St. Louis, Mo., 1974, p. 603.
13. Personal Communications.
14. D. Wright and F. Alexander, *Arch. Otolaryngol.*, **99**, 16, 18(1974).
15. D. Wright and M. Dinen, *Arch. Otolaryngol.*, **95**, 245(1972).
16. Burroughs Wellcome Co., "Medical notes of external otitis," 1972.
17. "The United States Dispensatory," 27th ed., A. Osol and R. Pratt, Eds., Lippincott, Philadelphia, Pa., 1973, pp. 199, 804.
18. M. S. Ersner, in "Diseases of the Nose, Throat and Ear," 1st ed., C. Jackson and C. L. Jackson, Eds., Saunders, Philadelphia, Pa., 1945, p. 266.
19. L. R. Boies, "Fundamentals of Otolaryngology" Saunders, Philadelphia, Pa., 1950, pp. 66-67.
20. R. D. Stride, *J. Laryngol. Otol.*, **73**, 48(1959).

Products 19 OTIC

Product (manufacturer)	Ingredients
Aquaear (Miller and Morton)	boric acid, 2.5%; isopropyl alcohol
Aqua-Otic-B (Ortega)	aluminum acetate; boric acid, 1%; acetic acid, 1%; benzocaine, 1%; propylene glycol
Aurinol (National)	acetic acid, 2%; chloroxylenol, 0.12%; benzalkonium chloride, 0.09%; propylene glycol; glycerin
Auro-Dri (Commerce)	boric acid, 2:75%; isopropyl alcohol
Auro Ear Drops (Commerce)	camphor, thymol, propylene glycol
Columbia Ear Drops (Columbia Medical)	carbamide, propylene glycol, glycerin, chlorobutanol
Debrox Drops (International)	carbamide peroxide, 6.5%; anhydrous glycerol
Ear-Dry (First Texas)	boric acid, 2.75%; isopropyl alcohol
E.R.O. (First Texas)	glycerin, 95%; propylene glycol, 5%
Kerid Ear Drops (Blair)	glycerin, 30%; urea, 0.1%; propylene glycol
Oil for Ear Use (DeWitt)	cajeput oil, 1.6%; white thyme oil, 1.6%; camphor, 0.5%; menthol, 0.3%
Stall Otic Drops (Cenci)	salicylic acid, 0.5%; thymol, 0.5%; isopropyl alcohol, 70%

Ophthalmic Products

Paul W. Lofholm

Questions to ask the patient

Is your vision blurred? Is your eye painful as opposed to itching or stinging?

What are the symptoms of the eye condition—redness, swelling, discharge (purulent or watery), itching, and dryness?

Do you have an anatomical dysfunction of the eye?

Are you under the care of a physician for any conditions (e.g., glaucoma or diabetes)?

Do you wear contact lenses?

Do you have any allergies?

Have your eyes recently been exposed to irritants such as smog, chemicals, or sunglare?

Do you use eye cosmetics?

Have you used an OTC ophthalmic product recently? Which one(s)? For what symptom?

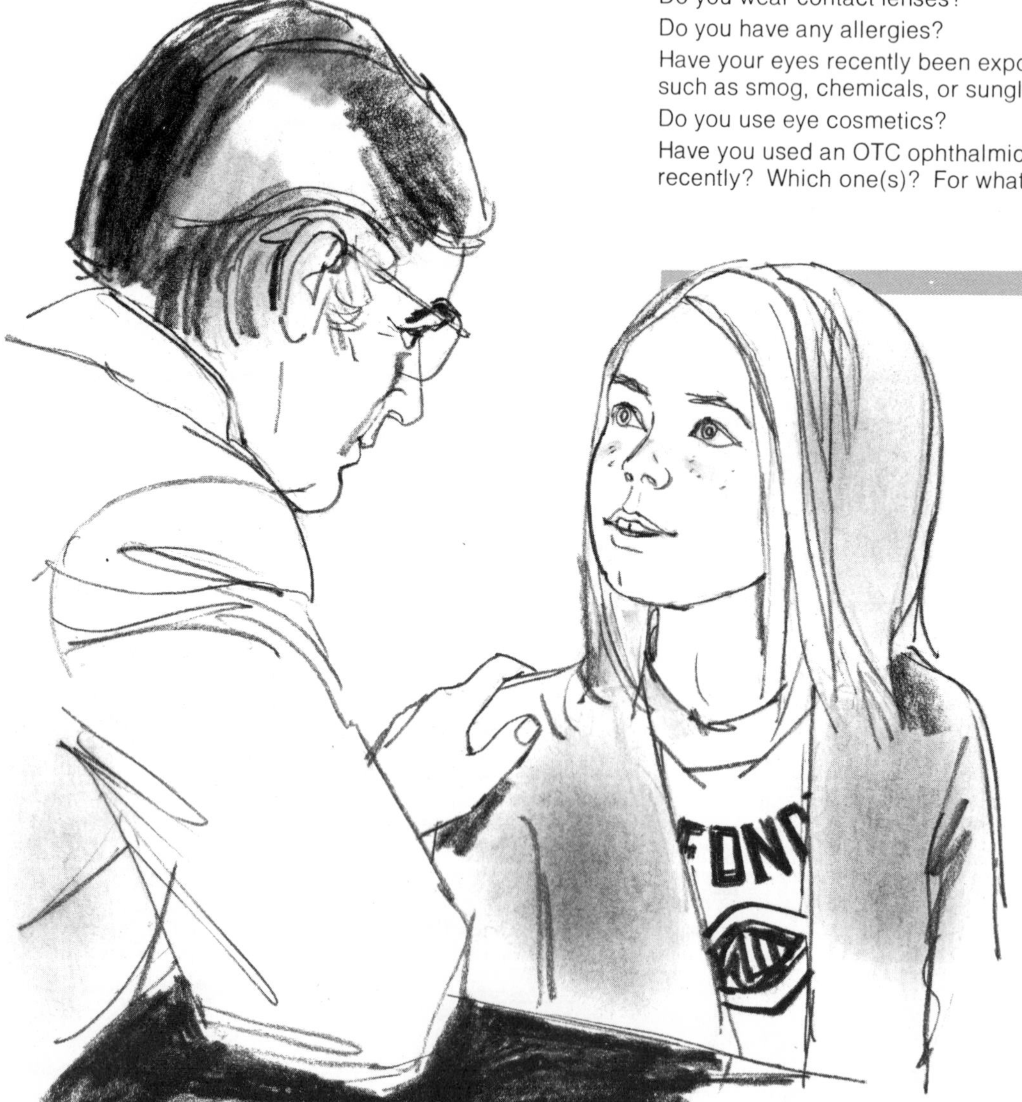

CHAPTER 20

Persons experiencing ocular discomfort usually seek initial relief by self-treatment and often ask the advice of a pharmacist. Therefore, to assist such patients, pharmacists must be familiar with the anatomy and physiology of the eye and the various conditions that can affect it. Pharmacists and patients must recognize that some ocular disorders that initially appear minor may be manifestations of serious underlying problems that require treatment by a physician, preferably an ophthalmologist.

Generally, an OTC ophthalmic product is safe only for the relief of symptoms such as stinging, itching, tearing, "tired eyes" or "eye strain," and/or other minor (painless) ocular discomforts. Patients who experience ocular pain and/or blurring of vision should be discouraged from self-treatment and directed to consult an ophthalmologist promptly.

Anatomy and physiology of the eye

The eyeball (or globe) (Fig. 1) is covered by three layers of tissue: the sclera, the choroid, and the retina. The sclera (white of the eye) is the tough, fibrous connective tissue surrounding the globe and covers the posterior portion of the eyeball. It is continuous with the cornea, which is transparent and covers the anterior portion of the globe. The choroid is the middle layer which anteriorly becomes the ciliary tissue which, in turn, is nearly continuous with the iris. These latter tissues contain most of the blood vessels and the pigment cells found in the eye. The retina, the innermost layer, is composed primarily of nervous tissue.

The eyeball consists of the interior compartment, which contains gellike vitreous humor, and the forward compartment, which contains the aqueous humor; the compartments are separated by the lens. The aqueous humor compartment has two chambers: the posterior chamber is situated between the lens and the iris, and the anterior chamber is located between the iris and the cornea. Aqueous humor is produced constantly by the ciliary body in the posterior chamber and drains out into the anterior chamber at the chamber angle into the canal of Schlemm. The cornea, the lens, and the humor compartments are avascular, and all exchanges of substances in these areas take place primarily by diffusion.

Although the eyes constantly are exposed to airborne pathogens, they are not continually infected because the tears lubricate, hydrate, and remove debris from the ocular surfaces. In addition, the tears contain lysozyme, an enzyme that catalyzes the hydrolysis of 1,4-glycosidic bonds characteristic of the polysaccharide coat of many airborne bacteria.[1]

Tears are a mixture of secretions produced by the lacrimal and sebaceous glands of the eye and contain mucus, water, and oil.[2] The tear layer next to the eye contains mucus, which allows the water phase to spread over the eye by altering the surface chemistry of the lipid layer of the cornea. The oily component of tears may stabilize the aqueous phase of the tears. The tears are 0.7-percent protein (e.g., albumin, mucin, and globulins, mainly IgA) and are slightly alkaline. They flow over the corneal surface and are collected in the conjunctival cul-de-sac, which is drained by the puncta located on the inside of the upper and lower lids.

The eyelids contain sebaceous glands, sweat glands, hair follicles, and muscles to operate the blink reflex. They also contain the openings of the nasolacrimal system which drains the tears from the eyes into the nose through the nasolacrimal duct. The oily secretions of the sebaceous glands help lubricate and prevent maceration of the lids by the aqueous tears.

Etiology of ocular inflammation/discomfort

Ocular inflammation and discomfort result from various conditions including anatomical anomalies such as incomplete closure of the eyelids, abnormal physiological states such as inadequate tearing, and ocular irritants. Irritants often implicated in cases of ocular inflammation include bacterial, viral, fungal, or parasitic infections; exposure to excessive U.V. radiation from snow- or sunglare or from a therapeutic lamp; drying winds; or volatile chemical components of smog. Ocular irritation also may result from generalized allergic reactions or a response to the application of a nonphysiologic or nonophthalmologic preparation to the eye. A guide to the differential diagnosis of ocular inflammation is provided in Table 1.

The reddened eye is a common sign of conjunctivitis, a condition that may involve one or both eyes. Ocular redness is also a sign of iritis, acute glaucoma, or eye trauma. Conjunctivitis may be distinguished from the latter conditions by the general absence of pain and/or visual disturbances.

External ocular conditions

Conjunctivitis. Conjunctivitis is a common external eye problem involving inflammation of the mucous membrane covering the anterior surface of the eyeball and the lining of the eyelids (conjunctiva).

The symptoms of conjunctivitis are a diffusely reddened eye with a purulent or serous discharge accompanied by itching, smarting, stinging, or a scratching, "foreign body" sensation. They cause considerable discomfort, but the complaints usually are out of proportion to the degree of irritation.

Conjunctivitis may be bacterial, fungal, parasitic, viral, allergic, or chemical in origin, thus making diagnosis difficult (Table 2). If the patient has not experienced pain or blurred vision, the reddened eye usually indicates a type of conjunctivitis. Bacterial conjunctivitis is usually self-limiting, and vision will not likely be impaired. If the patient awakens with the eyelids stuck together by dried exudate or if there is discharge or signs of swelling of the preauricular lymph node, the etiology of the conjunctivitis is probably bacterial. In such cases, OTC ophthalmic products have only limited efficacy.[3] Recovery from bacterial conjunctivitis can be hastened more readily by the use of an appropriate prescription drug, i.e., a sulfonamide or antibiotic-containing ophthalmic product. Without treatment, most bacteria-induced conjunctivitis lasts 10 to 14 days, although *Staphylococcus* and *Moraxella* infections may become chronic. A purulent discharge characterizes the more common forms of bacterial conjunctivitis (staphylococcal or diplococcal). In contrast to bacterial conjunctivitis, corneal infections can rapidly obliterate vision. Therefore, an accurate diagnosis is important.

Pinkeye, a bacterial infection caused by *Haemophilus aegyptius* in warm climates, and *Pneumococci* in temperate climates, is characterized by diffuse redness of the eye, photophobia, and pain and is moderately contagious.

Fungal and parasitic conjunctivitis are much less common than other types. Trachoma and inclusion conjunctivitis (TRIC) are chronic diseases of the eye caused by closely related micro-organisms. The clinical manifestations of the infections range from mild and self-limited to severe and blinding eye disease. Bacterial superinfection undoubtedly contributes to the severity of this eye disease. TRIC infection is rare in most parts of the U.S. Although this infection is endemic to some parts of the Southwest, it rarely leads to visual impairment because bacterial superinfection does not occur.

Viral conjunctivitis may resemble chemically induced conjunctivitis, i.e., red, perhaps swollen, watery, itching eyes and swollen preauricular lymph nodes. Unlike chemical irritations, however, viral conjunctivitis is often accompanied by systemic symptoms. Careful questioning of the patient by the pharmacist may suggest that the patient also has the flu. The reddened eyes in such cases suggest viral conjunctivitis, which is not amenable to specific drug therapy.

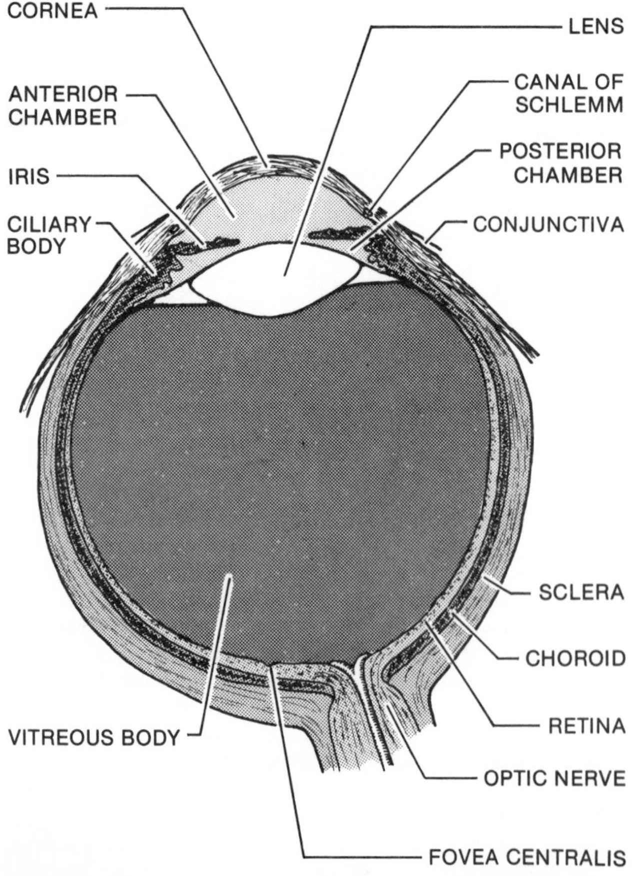

Figure 1. Horizontal cross section showing the anatomy of the eyeball.

Allergic conjunctivitis usually occurs on warm, windy days in the spring and during hay fever season. The discomfort is associated with a typical allergic response—swollen, congested, stinging, watery, and itching eyes. The irritation is bilateral as opposed to the reddened eye caused by a foreign body in the eye.

Chemical conjunctivitis, caused by airborne irritants such as smoke, smog, or garden sprays, also involves both eyes, an important observation for the pharmacist determining the nature of the patient's discomfort.

The majority of OTC ophthalmic products are promoted for the relief of allergic or chemical conjunctivitis. If an irritant has not been directly sprayed or instilled into the eye and if the cornea is not abraded, OTC decongestants are useful in relieving the discomfort. Ophthalmologists often use steroids to treat allergic conjunctivitis. Pharmacists must be aware of the chronic use of steroids as evidenced by repeated requests for prescription renewals because the long-term use of steroids may lead to the development of glaucoma or cataracts.

Disorders of the eyelids. These conditions include blepharitis and sties.

Blepharitis. Blepharitis is the most common disease of the eyelids, and its symptoms include a feeling of sand in the eyes, red-rimmed lid margins, burning, and itching. Flaking or scaling of the skin surrounding the lid may occur. The flaking may be bacterial (staphylococcal), seborrheic, parasitic (lice infestation), or allergic (cosmetic) in origin.

Sties. Abscesses involving the hair follicles or sebaceous and sweat glands of the eyelids are called sties. The causative organism most often involved is a *Staphylococcus.* The area surrounding a sty is red, swollen, tender, and painful, depending on the extent to which the skin is stretched. Although sties usually are self-limiting, they may spread to involve large areas of the eyelid. Sties do not endanger vision but those persisting for more than 48 hours should be drained surgically by a physician. Pain is reduced when the swelling is relieved.

Foreign body. Foreign bodies in the eye are a common cause of ocular discomfort. Symptoms vary from little or no discomfort to severe pain. The patient usually has a sensation of a foreign body in the upper eyelid, and the presence of a foreign body may be associated with tearing, photophobia, and redness of the affected eye. Unless the foreign object can be removed by irrigating the eye with sterile saline, the patient should be referred to an ophthalmologist. When objects embedded in the eye are removed, antibiotic therapy may also be necessary to prevent secondary bacterial infection.

Internal ocular conditions

Glaucoma. Glaucoma is characterized by an abnormal increase in intraocular pressure and may be classified as primary or secondary. Primary adult glaucoma is differentiated as either open-angle (wide-angle) or angle-closure (narrow-angle) glaucoma.

Open-angle glaucoma results from a resistance to the outflow (drainage) of aqueous humor from the anterior chamber of the eye in individuals with apparently normal chamber angles. The resistance may result from hemorrhage, inflammation, or swelling and congestion of the ciliary body and occurs in the meshwork of the chamber angle, the canal of Schlemm, the aqueous veins, or the ciliary veins.

In persons with angle-closure glaucoma (narrow chamber angles), any sudden dilation of the pupil, e.g., from mydriatics, swelling of the iris, or swelling of the lens, may produce a sudden and complete obstruction to the outflow of the aqueous humor. This obstruction results in a rapid increase in the intraocular pressure accompanied by pain and varying degrees of visual impairment.

Acute glaucoma. Acute glaucoma is associated with the inflammation of the eye in which the iris appears congested and discolored. Severe eye pain with violent headaches and a rapid failure in eyesight occur. The headaches may be accompanied by nausea and vomiting. Recurrent attacks of acute glaucoma lead to progressive loss of vision.

Uveitis. The uvea is the vascular coat of the eye which nourishes the eyeball and is composed of the iris, the ciliary body, and the choroid. The latter three are so close anatomically that, when one becomes diseased, the others usually are affected.

Inflammatory lesions of the uvea result from various exogenous and endogenous causes including infection and trauma, anatomic abnormalities (e.g., cataracts), and systemic inflammatory disease. Thus, depending on its specific etiology, uveitis may involve the anterior uvea or the posterior uvea or may diffusely involve the entire uveal tract.

Other ocular conditions

Keratoconjunctivitis sicca. Keratoconjunctivitis sicca is relatively uncommon, occurring primarily in postmenopausal women with rheumatoid arthritis. The symptoms are reddening and drying of the eyes. This condition is evaluated by performing the Schirmer test, which measures the tear flow in the conjunctival sac for 5 minutes, and by staining the eye with 1 percent rose bengal and examining the eye with a slit lamp to detect epithelial abnormalities.

Dry eye in the elderly. Although some ocular diseases are caused by insufficient lacrimal fluid, increasing age also gives rise to dry eyes. Although the eyes of elderly patients may be sufficiently moist upon awakening, they may become drier during the day. During sleep, the tears are not readily lost to the environment because the lids are closed. However, during the waking hours, there are insufficient tears to adequately hydrate the outer layer of the cornea, and the patient experiences a dry eye sensation. Tear substitutes are appropriate for these patients.[4]

Cosmetic-induced conditions. The use of eye cosmetics may lead to allergic reactions and bacterial infections of the eye because cosmetic products contain allergic constituents and frequently become contaminated while in use. Of 428 products sampled at a student health center, 12 percent were contaminated with fungi and 43 percent with bacteria, mostly gram-positive micrococci.[5] The conclusions drawn from the studies were that all the tested products supported microbial growth and that the occurrence of contamination was associated with the

Table 1. Differential Diagnosis of Common Causes of Inflamed Eye[a]

Parameter	Acute Conjunctivitis	Acute Iritis[b,c]	Acute Glaucoma[b,d]	Corneal Trauma or Infection[b]
Incidence	Extremely common	Common	Uncommon	Common
Discharge	Moderate to copious	None	None	Watery or purulent
Vision	Normal	Slightly blurred	Markedly blurred	Usually blurred
Pain	None	Moderate	Severe	Moderate to severe
Conjunctival redness	Diffuse	Mainly circumcorneal	Diffuse	Diffuse
Cornea	Clear	Usually clear	Steamy	May be abraded, lacerated, ulcerated, or show foreign body
Pupil size	Normal	Small	Moderately dilated	Normal
Pupillary light response	Normal	Poor	Poor	Normal
Intraocular pressure	Normal	Normal	Elevated	Normal
Conjunctival smear	Causative organisms	No organisms	No organisms	Organisms found only in corneal ulcer

[a] D. Vaughan *et al.*, "General Ophthalmology," 4th ed., Lange Medical Publications, Los Altos, Calif., 1965.
[b] A pharmacist should refer all patients with iritis, acute glaucoma, or corneal injury to a physician.
[c] Acute anterior uveitis.
[d] Angle closure glaucoma.

length and frequency of use, the personal habits of the user, the formulation of the product, and the presence or absence of preservatives (parabens). Because cosmetics are a source of ocular infection, patients should be advised to avoid the application of eye makeup for at least 1 week prior to ocular surgery. Mascara should not be used to hide blepharitis because it may aggravate and prolong the condition.

Two other studies supply additional evidence supporting cosmetics as causes of ocular problems. In one report, 75 female high school students developed trachoma after using one student's eye makeup.[6] The other study involved conjunctival pigmentation in subjects who had applied pencil eyeliner to the conjunctival side of their eyelashes.[7] Women with signs and symptoms of blepharitis or conjunctivitis should be interviewed carefully by the pharmacist to ascertain if eye cosmetics are used routinely.

Treatment

General guidelines

Except for a dry eye condition, autotherapy should not be used for more than 48 hours before consulting a physician. If symptoms of internal eye disease are present, e.g., pain or blurring of vision, medical help should be obtained immediately.

Eye washes aid in the removal of foreign particles from the eye. In an emergency, when sterile eyewashes are not immediately available in large amounts or especially when chemicals come in contact with the eye, the eye should be irrigated with large amounts of tapwater. Although only slight corneal edema similar to the effects of swimming underwater with one's eyes open may occur, it is important to immediately wash away the noxious agent to prevent further damage. If acids or bases are accidentally splashed into the eyes, water in large amounts is the preferred emergency treatment. Neutralization should not be considered in these cases because the heat that would be generated could damage delicate tissue.

Many external ocular conditions are self-limiting. The symptoms of allergic conjunctivitis can be relieved and the spreading of sties can be reduced by OTC medication. Sties should be drained surgically and/or treated with antibiotics if they have not resolved within 48 hours. If left untreated, nonallergic conjunctivitis is self-limiting in 2 weeks. A physician may advise specific prescription-only therapy, including antibiotic, anti-infective, or anti-inflammatory agents.

Dry eyes can be lubricated with artificial tears, and this condition is usually treated with OTC products by a physician. Surgery is sometimes indicated for this condition to provide ancillary tubes to carry tears directly to the eye.

Whatever the cause of blepharitis, the treatment objective is to remove the source of the irritation and inflammation. Any scaling should be removed daily with warm compresses, and the area should be kept clean. The patient should avoid the use of allergenic substances such as cosmetics. If the etiology of a chronic condition is bacterial, infection of the other members of the household can be avoided by isolation of the patient's towels and decontamination of the eyecups and droppers used in treatment.

Patients with ocular infections should be referred to a physician for appropriate treatment. In some cases, a bland ointment reduces the irritation by protecting the skin from topical irritants. Warm compresses and an antibacterial ointment can be applied; however, an ointment for sties such as cod liver oil, boric acid, zinc sulfate, mer-

Table 2. Differential Diagnosis of Conjunctivitis[a]

Parameter	Viral	Bacterial: *Purulent*	Bacterial: *Nonpurulent*	Fungal and Parasitic	Allergic
Discharge	Minimal	Copious	Minimal	Minimal	Minimal
Tearing	Copious	Moderate	Moderate	Minimal	Moderate
Itching	Minimal	Minimal	None	None	Marked
Infection	Generalized	Generalized	Localized	Localized	Generalized
Localized conjunctival lesions	None	None	Frequent	Frequent	None
Preauricular node	Common	Uncommon	Common	Common	None
Stained smear	Monocytes	Bacteria P.M.N.'s	Bacteria P.M.N.'s	Usually negative	Eosinophils
Associated sore throat and fever	Occasionally	Seldom	None[b]	None	None

[a]D. Vaughan *et al.*, "General Ophthalmology," 4th ed., Lange Medical Publications, Los Altos, Calif., 1965.

[b]Diphtheritic conjunctivitis occurs only as a complication of diphtheria, and so the other manifestations of the disease are present also. It may be purulent.

curic oxide, or yellow mercuric oxide should not be used.

All ophthalmic products should have an expiration date of several months from the date of opening. The hazard of introducing drug crystals in the eye is a problem associated with all ophthalmic solutions if the drug crystallizes on the lip of the bottle or the dropper tip. However, the probability of contamination is more serious. All ophthalmic solutions that are cloudy, discolored, more than 3 months old, or that contain foreign particles should be discarded.

The pharmacist can recommend several products for self-medication of ocular conditions: artificial tears, eyewashes, antiseptic drops or ointments, and decongestants. Application of these products should be limited to conditions where vision is not likely to be impaired, i.e., where ocular damage is not likely to result if medical advice is not sought and the product intended for use is safe for the particular patient. The responsibility of the pharmacist in advising patients is to determine whether the patient has a condition requiring medical attention.

Drugs used in ocular therapy

Decongestant ophthalmic solutions. Ocular congestion is caused by the dilation of capillaries of the conjunctiva or sclera and the transudation of fluid into the surrounding tissue. The tissue swells, producing local irritation characterized by itching and possibly pain. The lacrimal glands are stimulated and tearing occurs. The ophthalmic decongestants useful in relieving ocular congestion include vasoconstrictors and hypertonic solutions of sodium chloride.

If an ophthalmic decongestant is used when there is disease of the interior of the globe, no relief can be expected, and complications from the lack of primary treatment may occur. Furthermore, bacterial or other infections may be masked by the use of symptomatic treatment. Therefore, if an ocular condition persists, the patient should be instructed to consult a physician.

Products marketed as "eye whiteners" or decongestants are less effective than the newer solutions. Zinc salts have no decongestant action and are not effective as promoted. They are mild vasodilators in the concentrations used, but the only indication in ophthalmology for zinc sulfate is for a rare form of conjunctivitis caused by the gram-negative diplobacillus, *Moraxella lacunata.* This chronic conjunctivitis also responds to sulfonamides.

Vasoconstrictors. The OTC vasoconstrictors lessen the discomfort of certain types of conjunctivitis. If the conjunctivitis is caused by hay fever, oral antihistamines also may be considered, and physical measures such as moist heat or cold can be used. Reddened eyes are usually rapidly whitened by vasoconstrictors, which limit the local vascular response by constricting the blood vessels. The vasoconstrictors not only affect the vascular receptors but also stimulate other receptors such as the nerves that control pupillary size. To minimize pupillary dilation, which can adversely affect some patients, most ocular decongestants contain low concentrations of vasoconstrictors.

Ophthalmic products containing vasoconstrictors carry a warning that they should not be used in patients with glaucoma. If the patient has narrow-angle glaucoma, mydriasis secondary to the instillation of vasoconstrictors probably will precipitate a glaucomatous attack.[8] However, vasoconstrictors are not contraindicated for all glaucoma patients, only those with narrow-angle glaucoma. Anticholinergic drugs, e.g., belladonna, scopolamine, and antihistamines (OTC or prescription), also carry warnings against their use in patients with glaucoma because these drugs may cause mydriasis. Again, this effect is significant only in patients with narrow-angle glaucoma.[8] Patients often do not know what type of glaucoma they have. Therefore, the pharmacist should consult the patient's ophthalmologist and record the particular type of glaucoma on the medication record.

The use of epinephrine (the classic vasoconstrictor) as an ophthalmic decongestant is limited by the drug's instability in solution, by its irritating properties, by its relatively short duration of action, and by the production of rebound congestion. However, epinephrine has a long duration of action when used to lower intraocular pressure and is used by ophthalmologists in treating open-angle glaucoma.

OTC decongestant preparations contain other sympathomimetics, including ephedrine, naphazoline, phenylephrine, and tetrahydrozoline. In general, these sympathomimetic drugs are effective vasoconstrictors and do not produce mydriasis or systemic effects if absorbed or accidentally ingested.[9] Products containing these agents should be stable, nonirritating, and sterile and should not mask infection.

Ephedrine is similar to epinephrine in that it is short acting and produces rebound congestion. However, it is more stable than epinephrine.

Phenylephrine is the most commonly used vasoconstrictor in OTC ophthalmic products.[10] Its relative instability accounts for its variable effectiveness. In solution, it usually is effective initially, but with continued use, oxidation may significantly reduce the product's activity even though the product may not become discolored.[11] Furthermore, phenylephrine products in polyethylene containers may be less stable than those packaged in glass.[12] The oxygen diffuses through the polyethylene and hastens oxidation of the amine unless an oxygen-resistant coating is put over the plastic bottle. Patients who are allergic to epinephrine may show cross-sensitivity to phenylephrine.[6]

The imidazoline derivatives, naphazoline and tetrahydrozoline, are more stable and have a longer duration of action than epinephrine.[13] They are buffered to pH 6.2.[14] Naphazoline is used in prescription ophthalmic solutions at a 0.1-percent concentration and in OTC nasal solutions at 0.05 percent. In OTC ophthalmic products, it is used at a 0.012-percent concentration with camphor. Tetrahydrozoline is used as a nasal solution (0.1-percent concentration for adults and 0.05-percent for children) and as an OTC ophthalmic at 0.05-percent concentration, without camphor. Because camphor is irritating, useless, and perhaps harmful, and because the concentration of naphazoline in OTC ophthalmic products is significantly lower than that of tetrahydrozoline, the use of naphazoline as formulated is unwarranted.

Untoward effects occurring after using imidazoline derivatives have been reported, particularly CNS stimulation after accidental ingestion by children.[15] Although rebound congestion was reported after intranasal use of naphazoline, it has not been reported after ophthalmic use.

Hypertonic solutions. When applied to the eye, hypertonic solutions act as decongestants because of their osmotic effect on edematous tissue. Sodium chloride solutions (2 to 5 percent) are used for this purpose. Products that are only slightly hypertonic can be used for patients whose eyes become edematous after swimming.

Antibacterials. There is little rationale for inclusion of antibacterial ingredients (boric acid solution and mercuric oxide) in ophthalmic products.

Boric acid solutions. Boric acid solution (NF XII)

is commonly used as an eyewash. Although classified as an antibacterial, it is a traditional ophthalmic irrigating solution and cannot be recommended to act in a way other than its physical washing ability.[16] Boric acid is distributed as a saturated solution to reduce contamination. The isotonic concentration is prepared by diluting the saturated solution with an equal amount of water and boiling it in a clean, covered container or by adding a teaspoon of boric acid powder to a pint of water and boiling it. If the solution is not used within 1 day of preparation, it must be discarded.[17] This recommendation reflects the lack of antibacterial effects of these solutions. The patient should not rely on these solutions to treat an ocular injury or infection. The disadvantages of boric acid solution can be lessened if a preservative is added and if the packaging is modified to reduce contamination. Unused portions should be discarded once the bottle is opened.

The significant risk of toxicity associated with absorption of boric acid through broken skin, or through inadvertent oral ingestion, has prompted some medical authorities to discourage the use or distribution of boric acid for any medical purposes.

Mercuric oxide. Mercuric oxide ointments are useless because of the insolubility of the mercury salt. The antibacterial activity in mercury preparations is a function of the amount of free mercuric ion. The concentration of mercuric ion in mercuric oxide (associated with the amount of mercury in solution) is insufficient to prevent the growth of *Staphylococcus.*

In 1933, Hosford and McKenney[18] stated, "We doubt the wisdom of ever prescribing it [yellow mercuric oxide ophthalmic ointment] for home use," and suggested that mercuric oxide was useful only for its abrasive properties. However, they note that this product might have been effective in the past. Mercuric oxide is made from mercuric chloride and sodium hydroxide. If the resultant precipitate was not thoroughly washed free of mercuric chloride, there might have been enough free mercuric ion left over to exert an antibacterial effect. More recently, however, mercuric oxide must be free from contamination as specified in the National Formulary. With this purification, the active ingredient of this preparation, the soluble mercuric salt, is removed. It is recommended that mercurials not be used at all, but if they are, a soluble form of mercury (e.g., thimerosal) is recommended. When in solution, mercurials are only bacteriostatic and are not only slow acting but also are allergenic.

Artificial tears. Several viscous, surface-active solutions are marketed as tear replacement fluids for a dry eye condition. An ophthalmic ointment (ocular lubricant) also is available for this condition. Components of these formulations include polyvinyl alcohol, methyl- and substituted hydroxyethylcelluloses, polyethylene glycols, povidone, propylene glycol, glycerin, and dextrans.[19] These polymers are used because of their clarity and pharmaceutical compatibilities.

There are no apparent differences among artificial tear products. In general, products containing viscosity agents are retained about twice as long as a saline solution (several minutes). The retention time depends on the viscosity and the drainage rate, not on the concentration of the polymer.[20] Methylcellulose solutions as formulated are more viscous than polyvinyl alcohol solutions and, thus, tend to form crusts on the eyelids which may be annoying to some patients. However, the methylcellulose solutions are retained longer than the polyvinyl alcohol solutions. Products containing polyethylene glycol polymers are claimed to have mucomimetic properties. In the presence of these glycols, gelatin, or bovine mucin, the surface of the cornea is easier to wet.

Other components of ophthalmic formulations. Ophthalmic products generally are formulated to be self-sterilizing, isotonic, buffered for stability, and viscous. The typical preservatives are chlorobutanol, benzalkonium chloride, and thimerosal.[21] Chlorobutanol (0.5 percent) is an effective antibacterial agent, but it may decompose in the presence of heat or alkalinity or when stored in polyethylene containers.[22] Benzalkonium chloride (0.01 percent) is also an effective antibacterial agent, especially when edetic acid is added. However, when concentrations higher than 0.013 percent were experimentally applied to rabbit eyes, corneal damage was reported.[23] Thimerosal is also used, but this preservative is slow acting, is a possible contact allergen, and is incompatible with edetic acid.[24,25]

Edetic acid is included in the formulations because it enhances the preservative activity of benzalkonium chloride. Ophthalmic products containing edetic acid may cause allergic manifestations.[26,27] In one study, edetic acid in ophthalmic products was established as the primary sensitizer, causing acute allergic conjunctivitis and periorbital dermatitis.[28] However, the investigators commented that "in view of the compound's widespread use and absence of previously reported reactions, we feel it must be a weak sensitizing compound."

Specific ingredients in a product may be incompatible with other products used concurrently. For example, contact lens cleaning products often are slightly alkaline to improve their efficacy in removing proteinaceous substances. Patients should not simultaneously use alkaline products containing borates and products containing polyvinyl alcohol because gel systems may form, resulting in gummy deposits.[29,30]

Tears are produced by reflex when there is corneal or conjunctival irritation. Nonphysiologic drug formulations also produce such irritation, and tearing may occur when these solutions are instilled.

Considerations in product selection

Patient considerations

The following general guidelines will aid the pharmacist in selecting the most suitable OTC ophthalmic product for the patient.

- ☐ OTC ocular medications should not be recommended to patients who have demonstrated an allergy to any of the active ingredients or preservatives.
- ☐ Patients with narrow-angle glaucoma should not receive sympathomimetics.
- ☐ Topical anesthetics should never be instilled into the eye because the anesthetic agent seriously compromises the body's defense mechanisms.
- ☐ Pain should be treated with oral analgesics.

Patients who have had an eye condition for more than several days may not have a self-limiting condition and should consult a physician. Ocular pain or blurring of vision are contraindications to self-medication. Cosmetics should be considered as the possible cause for a reddened eye. If soft contact lenses or Ocuserts are worn, OTC medications should not be used unless they are specifically formulated for soft lenses.

Using the product

The pharmacist should instruct the patient on the proper use of ophthalmic products. Before instillation, the hands should be washed and the product should be inspected for expiration date, contamination, discoloration, and other abnormalities. The dropper tip should not touch the eye or eyelid and should be replaced on the bottle immediately after use. Ointments should be applied in a thin line to the inside of the lower lid. The eyelids should then be closed and the eye gently massaged. Transient blurring or stinging may occur. If the patient is a child, the hand holding the product should be rested on the child's cheek so that if the child makes an abrupt move, the tip will not enter the eye. A nose bridge guiding device is available to help patients guide the bottle into the proper position for self-administration. Several companies market a sprayer top with pump (no propellant) so that the ophthalmic medication may be sprayed into the eye. All of these devices should be considered when a patient is seeking an OTC ophthalmic product.

Summary

Knowledge of ocular diseases and the indications for OTC drugs is important to the pharmacist. Patients depend on the pharmacist for advice on the safe and effective use of drugs. Because the pharmacist may be the first health care practitioner consulted by the patient with ocular discomfort, good judgment is essential.

References

1. P. Handler *et al.*, "Principles of Biochemistry," 2d ed., McGraw-Hill, New York, N.Y., 1959, p. 723.
2. M. A. Lemp *et al.*, *Arch. Ophthalmol.*, **83,** 89(1970).
3. D. Vaughan *et al.*, "General Ophthalmology," 4th ed., Lange Medical Publications, Los Altos, Calif., 1965, p. 69.
4. F. K. Goodner, "Ocular Pharmacology and Therapy," Davis, Philadelphia, Pa., 1963, p. 114.
5. A. Wilson *et al.*, *Am. J. Ophthalmol.*, **79,** 596(1975).
6. S. Aronson and E. Yamamoto, *Invest. Ophthalmol.*, **5,** 75(1966).
7. B. D. Zuckerman, *Am. J. Ophthalmol.*, **62,** 672(1966).
8. W. H. Havener, "Ocular Pharmacology," 3d ed., Mosby, St. Louis, Mo., 1974, p. 236.
9. H. C. Menger, *J. Am. Med. Assoc.*, **170,** 178(1959).
10. R. N. Shaffer and D. I. Weiss, *Arch. Ophthalmol.*, **68,** 727(1962).
11. G. B. West and T. D. Whittet, *J. Pharm. Pharmacol.*, **12,** 113T(1960).
12. H. Beal *et al.*, *J. Pharm. Sci.*, **56,** 1310(1967).
13. E. Smissman, in "Textbook of Organic, Medicinal and Pharmaceutical Chemistry," 4th ed., C. O. Wilson *et al.*, Eds., Lippincott, Philadelphia, Pa., 1962, p. 405.
14. A. J. Spiegel and C. F. Gerber, *J. Am. Pharm. Assoc. Pract. Ed.*, **20,** 404(1959).
15. R. Mindlin, *N. Engl. J. Med.*, **275,** 112(1966).
16. D. E. Francke, in "American Hospital Formulary Service," American Society of Hospital Pharmacists," Washington, D. C., 1967, 54:04. 12.
17. "National Formulary," 12th ed., American Pharmaceutical Association, Washington, D. C., 1965, p. 59.
18. G. Hosford and J. P. McKenney, *J. Am. Med. Assoc.*, **100,** 17(1933).
19. W. H. Havener, "Ocular Pharmacology," 3d ed., Mosby, St. Louis, Mo., 1974, p. 494.
20. T. F. Patton and J. R. Robinson, *J. Pharm. Sci.*, **64,** 1312(1975).
21. W. H. Havener, "Ocular Pharmacology," 3d ed., Mosby, St. Louis, Mo., 1974, p. 415.
22. W. T. Friesen and E. M. Plein, *Am. J. Hosp. Pharm.*, **28,** 507(1971).
23. M. A. Lemp, *Ann. Ophthalmol.*, **5,** 22(1973).
24. M. R. W. Brown, *J. Pharm. Sci.*, **57,** 389(1968).
25. P. P. Hoof, *Manufacturing Chemist*, **24,** 444(1953).
26. T. T. Provost and O. F. Jillson, *Arch. Dermatol.*, **96,** 231(1967).
27. E. Epstein and H. I. Maibach, *Arch. Dermatol.*, **98,** 476(1968).
28. J. Z. Raymond and P. R. Gross, *Arch. Dermatol.*, **100,** 436(1969).
29. Product Insert on Lensine, the Murine Company.
30. R. K. Schultz and R. Myers, *Macromolecules,* **2,** 281(1969).

General references

D. Vaughan *et al.*, "General Ophthalmology," 6th ed., Lange Medical Publications, Los Altos, Calif., 1971.

W. H. Havener, "Ocular Pharmacology," 3d ed., Mosby, St. Louis, Mo., 1974.

S. Riegelman and D. Sorby, in "Husa's Pharmaceutical Dispensing," 6th ed., Mack Publishing, Easton, Pa., 1966.

Archives of Ophthalmology, annual reviews on structures of the eye and a review of ophthalmic pharmacology and toxicology.

Products 20 OPHTHALMIC DECONGESTANT

roduct (manufacturer)	Viscosity agent	Vasoconstrictor	Preservative	Buffer	Other
lerest (Pharmacraft)	—	naphazoline hydrochloride, 0.012%	thimerosal, 0.005%	boric acid sodium carbonate	potassium chloride camphor zinc sulfate
lear Eyes (Abbott)	methylcellulose	naphazoline hydrochloride, 0.012%	edetate disodium, 0.1% benzalkonium chloride, 0.01%	boric acid sodium borate	—
ollyrium Drops (Wyeth)	—	ephedrine, 0.1%	thimerosal, 0.002%	boric acid sodium borate	antipyrine, 0.4% sodium salicylate, 0.056%
egest 2 (Barnes-Hind)	hydroxyethylcellulose	naphazoline hydrochloride, 0.012%	edetate disodium, 0.02% benzalkonium chloride, 0.0067%	sodium citrate	antipyrine, 0.1%
ye Cool (Milroy)	—	phenylephrine hydrochloride, 0.08%	edetate disodium, 0.05% thimerosal, 0.002%	sodium borate boric acid	menthol eucalyptus oil sodium chloride sodium bisulfite

Products 20 OPHTHALMIC DECONGESTANT

Product (manufacturer)	Viscosity agent	Vasoconstrictor	Preservative	Buffer	Other
20/20 Eye Drops (S.S.S.)	—	naphazoline hydrochloride, 0.012%	thimerosal, 0.005%	boric acid sodium carbonate	potassium chloride zinc sulfate
Isopto-Frin (Alcon)	hydroxypropyl methylcellulose, 0.5%	phenylephrine hydrochloride, 0.12%	benzethonium chloride	sodium citrate sodium phosphate sodium biphosphate	—
Naphcon (Alcon)	—	naphazoline hydrochloride, 0.012%	benzalkonium chloride, 0.01%	—	—
Ocusol Drops (Norwich)	methylcellulose	phenylephrine hydrochloride	benzalkonium chloride	boric acid sodium borate	sodium chloride
Phenylzin (Smith, Miller & Patch)	hydroxypropyl methylcellulose, 0.1%	phenylephrine hydrochloride, 0.12%	benzalkonium chloride, 0.01% edetate disodium, 0.01%	boric acid, 1.1% sodium carbonate, 0.02%	zinc sulfate, 0.25% sodium bisulfite, 0.01% potassium chloride
Prefrin (Allergan)	polyvinyl alcohol, 1.4%	phenylephrine hydrochloride, 0.12%	benzalkonium chloride, 0.004%	sodium phosphate sodium biphosphate	antipyrine, 0.1%
Prefrin Z (Allergan)	polyvinyl alcohol, 1.4%	phenylephrine hydrochloride, 0.12%	thimerosal, 0.005%	sodium hydroxide sodium citrate	zinc sulfate, 0.25% sodium chloride sodium bisulfite
Tear-efrin (Smith, Miller & Patch)	hydroxypropyl methylcellulose, 0.5%	phenylephrine hydrochloride, 0.1%	benzalkonium chloride, 0.01% edetate disodium, 0.01%	—	sodium bisulfite, 0.05% sodium chloride
Visine (Leeming)	—	tetrahydrozoline, 0.05%	edetate disodium, 0.1% benzalkonium chloride, 0.01%	boric acid sodium borate	sodium chloride
Zincfrin (Alcon)	—	phenylephrine hydrochloride, 0.12%	benzalkonium chloride, 0.01%	barbital barbital sodium	zinc sulfate, 0.25%

Products 20 ARTIFICIAL TEARS

Product (manufacturer)	Viscosity agent	Preservative	Other
aqua-Flow (Flow)	polyvinyl alcohol, 1.4% hydroxyethylcellulose	edetic acid, 0.025% benzalkonium chloride, 0.005%	—
Bro-lac (Riker)	hydroxypropyl methylcellulose	benzalkonium chloride, 0.02%	glycerin, sodium borate, boric acid
Contique Artificial Tears (Alcon)	polyvinyl alcohol, 2%	benzalkonium chloride, 0.01% edetate disodium	sodium chloride, potassium chloride, calcium chloride, magnesium chloride, sodium acetate, sodium citrate, sodium hydroxide
Goniosol Ophthalmic Solution (Smith, Miller & Patch)	hydroxypropyl methylcellulose, 2.5%	edetate disodium, 0.01% benzalkonium chloride, 0.01%	boric acid, 1.1%; sodium carbonate; potassium chloride
Isopto Alkaline (Alcon)	hydroxypropyl methylcellulose	benzalkonium chloride, 0.01%	—
Isopto Plain (Alcon)	hydroxypropyl methylcellulose, 0.5%	benzalkonium chloride, 0.01%	—
Isopto Tears (Alcon)	hydroxypropyl methylcellulose, 0.5%	benzalkonium chloride, 0.01%	—

Products 20 ARTIFICIAL TEARS

Product (manufacturer)	Viscosity agent	Preservative	Other
Lacril (Allergan)	hydroxypropyl methylcellulose gelatin	chlorobutanol, 0.5%	potassium chloride, sodium chloride, calcium chloride, magnesium chloride, sodium acetate, sodium citrate, sodium borate, acetic acid, polysorbate 80, dextrose
Liquifilm Forte (Allergan)	polyvinyl alcohol, 3.0%	chlorobutanol, 0.5%	dextrose
Liquifilm Tears (Allergan)	polyvinyl alcohol, 1.4%	chlorobutanol, 0.5%	sodium chloride
Lyteers (Barnes-Hind)	hydroxypropyl methylcellulose, 0.2%	edetic acid, 0.05% benzalkonium chloride, 0.01%	sodium chloride, potassium chloride
Tearisol (Smith, Miller & Patch)	hydroxypropyl methylcellulose, 0.50%	benzalkonium chloride, 0.01% edetate disodium, 0.01%	boric acid, sodium carbonate, potassium chloride
Tears Naturale (Alcon)	water-soluble polymeric system	benzalkonium chloride, 0.01% edetate disodium, 0.05%	—
Ultra Tears (Alcon)	hydroxypropyl methylcellulose, 1%	benzalkonium chloride, 0.01%	—

Products 20 EYEWASH

Product (manufacturer)	Buffer	Preservative	Other
Blinx (Barnes-Hind)	boric acid, sodium borate	phenylmercuric acetate, 0.004%	—
Collyrium (Wyeth)	boric acid, sodium borate	thimerosal, 0.002%	antipyrine, 0.4%; sodium salicylate, 0.056%
Dacriose (Smith, Miller & Patch)	boric acid, sodium carbonate	benzalkonium chloride, 0.01%; edetate disodium, 0.01%	potassium chloride
Enuclene (Alcon)	—	benzalkonium chloride, 0.02%	tyloxapol, 0.25%
Eye-Stream (Alcon)	—	benzalkonium chloride, 0.013%	sodium chloride, potassium chloride, calcium chloride, magnesium chloride, sodium citrate, sodium acetate
auro Eye Wash (Otis Clapp)	boric acid, sodium borate	—	sodium chloride
M/Rinse (Milroy)	sodium borate, boric acid	edetate disodium, 0.1%; thimerosal, 0.004%	sodium chloride, potassium chloride
Murine (Abbott)	boric acid, potassium bicarbonate, potassium carbonate	benzalkonium chloride, 0.004%; thimerosal, 0.001%	hydrastine, berberine, glycerin
Ocusol Eye Lotion (Norwich)	boric acid, sodium borate	edetate disodium, 0.05%; benzalkonium chloride, 0.01%	phenylephrine hydrochloride, sodium chloride
Op-thal-zin (Alcon)	—	benzalkonium chloride, 0.01%	zinc sulfate, 0.25%
risol Eye Wash (Buffington)	boric acid, sodium borate	—	sodium chloride

Contact Lens Products

Peter P. Lamy
Ralph F. Shangraw

Questions to ask the patient

What types of problems are you having with your lenses? Are they related to eye irritation or changes in vision?

What type lenses do you wear?

How long have you been wearing lenses?

What drugs are you currently using?

Have you become pregnant or begun using oral contraceptives since you were fitted for lenses?

Which products do you use for cleaning, sterilizing, and wetting your lenses?

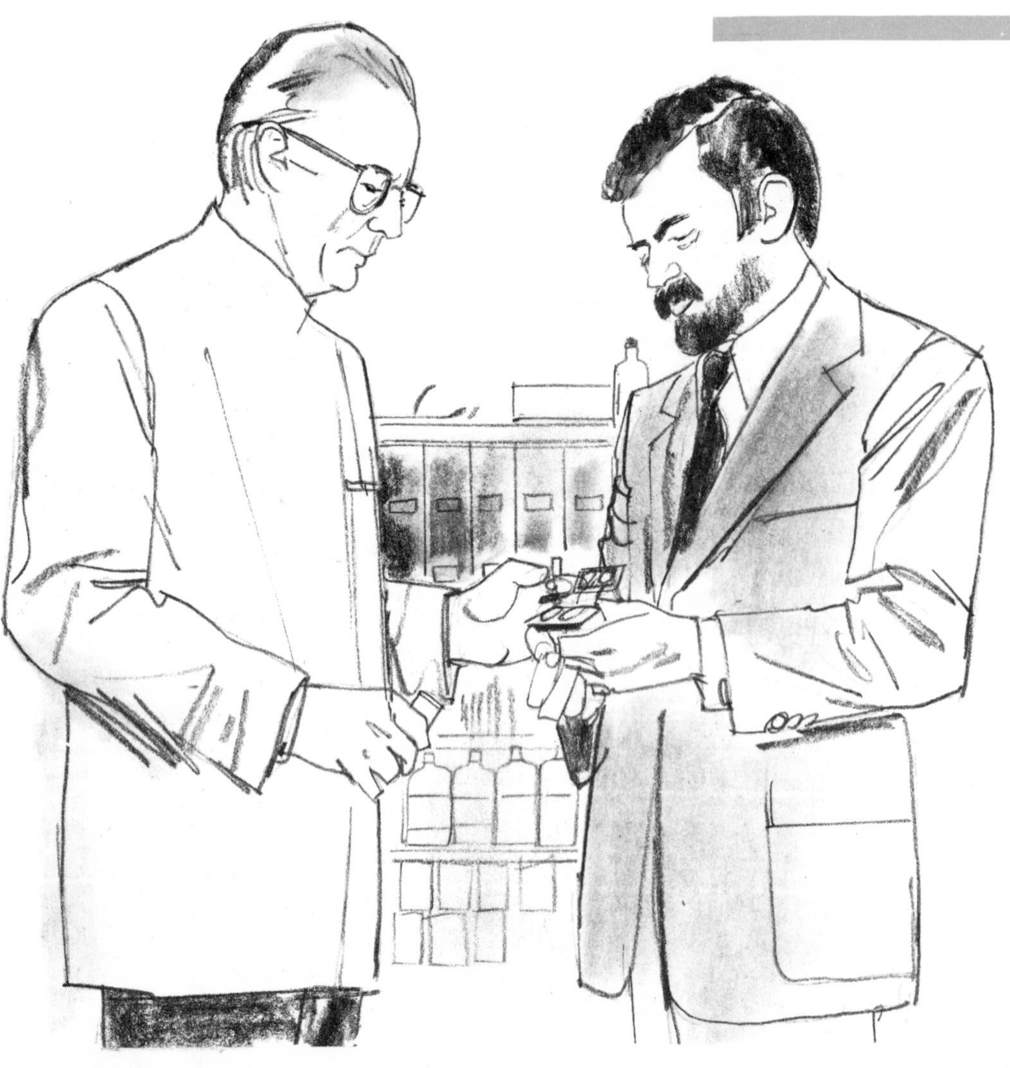

CHAPTER 21

About 90 million Americans must use corrective lenses, and of these, almost 10 percent use contact lenses. (The term "contact lens" is somewhat of a misnomer—a properly fitted lens is never in contact with the cornea but floats freely on the precorneal fluid and mucous secretions.) Most frequently, contact lenses are used by young, middle-class women. Although contact lenses are often used for therapeutic reasons, e.g., for corneal scarring, the majority of contact lens wearers use them for cosmetic reasons, i.e., for correction of vision of the otherwise healthy eye. (See Chapter 20 for a discussion of the anatomy and physiology of the eye.) Psychological reasons based on improvement of the wearer's appearance are often cited for the rapid acceptance of the lenses by the public.

In 1968, the FDA announced that all contact lenses would be classified as drugs but that hard contact lenses, due to a history of safe use, would automatically be accepted, as would their solutions. In contrast, each soft lens system would have to be approved, i.e., the specific lens together with the solutions specifically designed for that lens. Soft contact lenses (Table 1) would have to follow the procedures set forth for new drugs. [Aosoft (American Optical) lens has been approved for distribution in the U.S. as of Fall, 1976.]

The FDA's Bureau of Devices and Diagnostics (BuDD) Ophthalmic Advisory Panel has requested that the FDA Commissioner consider poly(methyl methacrylate) (PMMA) lenses "hard" lenses and all others "soft" lenses. This is of considerable interest because there are soft lenses in various stages of development, not based on 2-hydroxymethyl methacrylate (HEMA) but on other substances, that would then be required to undergo scientific review.

Composition and properties of hard and soft lenses

The polymerized products of esters of acrylic acid and those of methacrylic acid are the resins used in the production of hard contact lenses.[1] Poly(methyl methacrylate) (Lucite or Plexiglas) is the plastic most often used. It contains relatively few hydrophilic groups and many closely packed methyl groups which give the plastic its hydrophobic properties.[2] The plastic allows light transmission of 90 to 92 percent, and lenses made of this plastic absorb about 1 percent of water after prolonged immersion.[3] The index of refraction of PMMA is 1.49.

All of the common hydrophilic lenses (soft lenses) are made of 2-hydroxymethyl methacrylate (HEMA) which has been cross-linked to varying degrees.[4] Cross-linkages produce distinct chemical entities, and each iens, therefore, has well-defined physical and chemical properties. These differences have been described as "significant" for cosmetic use and "crucial" for therapeutic use.[5]

Water content of soft lenses varies widely and is inversely proportional to the degree of cross-linking. HEMA absorbs about 47 percent water by weight, if the water is pure, and about 30 percent when immersed in normal saline solution.[6] The refractive index changes from 1.53 in the dry state to 1.43 when material is fully hydrated in normal saline.[7]

When it is hydrated, a HEMA lens expands about 18 percent in all directions.[8] Oxygen exchange, although probably better than with PMMA, is still insufficient to support the cornea without additional oxygen provided by tears.[8] Generally, HEMA lenses are larger than the cornea and are untinted. They are comfortable only when they are as large or larger than the corneal diameter, have very thin edges, and have limited movement, all of which produce minimum contact between the lens and eyelids.[6] Hard contact lenses could be manufactured to meet these specifications, but, because they are inflexible, normal tear exchange would not occur; soft lenses flex with each blink.[6]

In contrast to hard lenses, soft lenses can absorb drugs and preservatives from ophthalmic solutions.[9, 10] This can cause altered therapeutic effects and possible irritation. Some drugs may cause discoloration of soft lenses because of oxidative breakdown of the plastic or binding onto it.[11] All manufacturers of HEMA lenses indicate that "no ophthalmic solution or medicament, including conventional contact lenses solutions, can be used by the lens wearer prior to or while the lens is in place in the eye."

A less common soft lens is made of a cross-linked dimethyl polysiloxane, hydrocarbon-substituted rubber (silicone). The rubber is extremely hydrophobic, and lenses made of this material absorb only 0.5 percent water by weight—less than the conventional hard lenses. This material is chemically and physiologically inert, flexible, and rubbery, but it has a certain innate rigidity. It is pliable in the dry state, and fingernails can penetrate it. The lens is less flexible than the hydrogel lens.

The silicone lens is not permeable to liquids, has a refractive index of 1.439, and permits light transmission of 86 percent in the dry state and 91 percent when it is wet.[12-15]

Contact lenses or eyeglasses

Contact lenses have gained wide patient acceptance, mainly because of their cosmetic and improved vision qualities. A few patients (high hypermetropes and high myopes) have much better vision with contact lenses than with eyeglasses, and contact lenses are essential for patients with a conical cornea or corneal scarring. The effects of corneal scars (except for loss of light transmission) can often be corrected much better with contact lenses.[16] Binocular vision without contact lenses cannot be achieved in cases of unilateral aphakia (cataract extraction) and anisometropia (markedly different refractive errors in each eye). Some myopic contact lens wearers perceive improved vision, because the lens produces a slight magnification of the retinal image and a slight increase in light transmission. Also, lenses do not produce the obstruction frequently encountered by the frame of eyeglasses.[17-19]

These factors may not actually improve visual acuity, but patients have mistaken increased sensitivity to light with increased visual acuity.[20] Visual acuity is, in fact, noticeably lower for many lens wearers.[21] There is a considerable difference in the retinal image—the lens wearer views all objects through the optical center of the lens; the eyeglass wearer observes aberrations when viewing objects through the periphery of the glasses.[21] Contact lens wearers must have their eyes and lenses examined more frequently than eyeglass users, thus the long-term cost of lenses is usually much higher than that of eyeglasses.[21]

In general, there does not seem to be an appreciable difference between the effectiveness of eyeglasses and lenses. In a study of 3,458 eyes (myopic, hyperopic, and aphakic), 3,167 eyes (91.6 percent) achieved a visual acuity of 20/25 or better with eyeglasses, and 2,881 eyes (83.3 percent) achieved a visual acuity of 20/25 or better with contact lenses.[22]

Comparison of hard and soft lenses

Most patients seem to adjust well to the wearing of contact lenses. In a study of hard lenses in 200 patients, only 22 percent failed partly or completely to adjust.[23] In another group fitted with soft contact lenses for errors of refraction, 57 percent were counted as successful.[22] Published success rates vary probably because there are no standards to which "success" can be compared. Subjective criteria such as wearing time, comfort, and vision should be considered as well as objective criteria such as ocular tissue changes and patient appearance. Using these standards, another study found 73 percent of 122 patients to be successful in adapting to lens wear.[24]

PROBLEMS IN ADAPTING TO HARD LENSES

☐ A slight burning sensation caused by the lack of oxygen.

☐ Difficulty in looking up which disappears when eyelids learn to tolerate the "foreign body" in the eye.

☐ Blurring of vision upon removal of the lenses.

☐ Photophobia, which can be expected in the early stages of wear. This problem can be diminished by good sunglasses.

☐ Reflections (more noticeable at night).

☐ Redness of the eyes. This is caused by the normal response of the eye to the "foreign body."

☐ Fogging of the lenses until the fluid exchange rate is adjusted.

☐ Excessive tearing.

☐ Tendency for lens to slip off center or fall out because of excessive tearing.

☐ Excessive blinking. This is normal because the body tries to provide a better flow of fluids.

☐ Difficulty in focusing on nearby objects.

☐ Itching.

☐ Excessive tiredness at the end of the wearing period.

These symptoms usually disappear in time if the wearing schedule is followed conscientiously.

The community pharmacist may be confronted by a patient experiencing a typical overwear syndrome (due to hard lenses). This can be an extremely painful condition caused by irritation of the cornea which the patient usually does not notice until the lenses are removed. In most instances, the cornea regenerates within 24 hours. First aid treatment might consist of eye patches (for both eyes) cold compresses, and lubricant drops. The patient should guard against infection; a physician will often prescribe Neosporin drops.

Many people prefer the comfort of soft lenses to the superior vision offered by hard lenses.[25] The literature agrees that soft lenses are more comfortable and are more easily tolerated, that good visual acuity cannot be achieved by all soft lens wearers, and that overall visual acuity with soft lenses is not as good as that achieved with hard lenses.[21] Soft lenses conform to the cornea and, therefore, tend not to correct corneal astigmatism. Vision with soft lenses may fluctuate as the state of hydration of the lens fluctuates.[21] On the other hand, people tend to lose hard lenses more frequently than soft lenses.[26] Soft lenses are particularly good for occasional wear and sports (except swimming) and do not require the disciplined daily schedule of hard lenses. Soft lenses are less easily dislodged, and dust particles do not get caught easily under the lens.

The relative permeability of hard and soft lens material to gases has been extensively investigated because oxygen depletion may cause corneal lesions.[27,28] It appears that the soft lens causes less injury than the hard lens, but the soft lens may inhibit tear flow more.[29] There may be more depletion of glucose under hard contact lenses, but there is no difference in the metabolites of pyruvate, lactate, the lactate/pyruvate quotient, or in concentrations of adenosine triphosphate, adenosine diphosphate, adenosine monophosphate, and glucose 6-phosphate.[29,30] An increase in corneal thickness can be observed with all lens wear, but more so with hard lenses than with soft ones. The increase may be caused by an osmolarity effect, a decrease in glycogen content of the cornea, or a significant decrease of transcorneal potential.[31] In some cases (13 of 445 eyes), vascularization was reported with soft lens wear.[32] Increased vascularization of the cornea, which normally is vascularized, occurs in pathologic conditions and where 24-hour lens wear is required. It is probably related to hypoxia and rarely causes a significant decrease of visual acuity.

The soft lenses are apparently considerably more comfortable for the average wearer than the hard lenses. They do not diminish corneal sensitivity.[33] Flare, glare, and photophobia are practically nonexistent, although people with large pupils may complain about flares, particularly at dusk or at night.[34] The soft lens wearer may freely alternate between lenses and eyeglasses, and there seems to be no need for an adaptation period and no overwearing syndrome in most users. The "contact lens look," i.e., holding the chin up, blinking frequently, restraining from quick eye movement, or avoiding looking up to the ceiling, is not seen with soft lenses.[35] Soft lens users seem to complain less about atmospheric pollutants than hard lens wearers.[36]

Soft lenses can be considerably more expensive than the hard ones. They may have to have a power change within 2 months of the original fitting.[33] Although an average use of 2 years is usually mentioned in the literature, references to a lifespan of 1 year are encountered.[37]

Soft lenses may be uncomfortable if debris is caught between the lens and the eye, if they are too loose, or if they are hydrated with improper solutions.[35] Variable vision, which is caused by poor centering, and poor return of the lens after blinking may occur.[33] In some cases there may be "start-up" problems, i.e., vision is "watery." This will usually disappear but may take as long as 2 months. Soft lenses cannot be marked "left" and "right," and a soft lens wearer who loses correct identification of the lenses may have to return to an optometrist or ophthalmologist for identification.

Sampson[38] has summed up the differences between hard and soft lenses by observing that soft contact lenses have proved to be safe and effective, although hard corneal lenses are the modality of choice for the majority of candidates for contact lens wear. Whether a hard or soft lens is chosen, lens-induced corneal edema is one of the most serious obstacles to successful lens wear. The edema is caused by localized hypoxia, and its symptoms are photophobia, dryness, burning, and tearing.[39] In hot and stuffy areas, congestion and watering of the nose and reflex vasodilation in the rosacea areas of the face in susceptible individuals have been observed.[40] Corneal edema increases with length of wear but disappears rapidly upon removal of the lens.

Use of contact lenses

Indications

Contact lenses can be used in all cases of myopia and astigmatism, aphakia, anisometropia, certain eye diseases, and to control keratoconus.[41] In aphakia (absence of the crystalline lens), eyeglasses with very thick convex lenses usually had to be used. They produced disturbing aberrations and magnification. Contact lenses minimize these aberrations and reduce the size of the image to nearly that of the retinal image of the normal eye.

Contraindications

Corneal contact lenses are contraindicated in active intraocular or corneal pathologic conditions but can be used in cases of open-angle glaucoma.[41] They are contraindicated in older people because of lacrimal insufficiency or where arthritis may restrict the movement and dexterity needed to insert the lenses. They are also contraindicated in blepharitis, and many people with hay fever cannot wear them. Contact lenses are contraindicated in people who have a tear deficiency, excessive tear production, an obstructed nasolacrimal duct, chronic allergies, anatomic or physiologic abnormalities, and various clinical conditions, such as herpes simplex.[42]

Dry spots on the cornea, often found in postmenopausal women, prevent the successful use of lenses.[43] They may be caused by the absence of precorneal film and are often identified with lacrimal insufficiency or as the result of subclinical hypothyroidism. The corneal topography may be altered by pregnancy or by oral contraceptives.[42 43] Microedema caused by hormonal therapy and premenstrual edema are also contraindications to the use of contact lenses.

Cautions

Contact lenses should be used with caution in patients with epilepsy, diabetes mellitus, high blood pressure, heart disease, or severe arthritis. Restricted use of lenses may be necessary when a person's occupation is connected with chemical vapors or dust.

Many systemic medications, e.g., diuretics, affect the eyes and can, therefore, influence successful lens wear.[44] Orally administered antihistamines and decongestants can exert a drying effect on the tears and the cornea, interfering with lens wear.[45]

During the adaptive period to contact lenses, the eyelids may become hyperemic which can lead to blepharitis, especially in the upper lid.[39] Short pseudoblinks often found with new wear of hard lenses, can cause irritation of the conjunctiva of the upper eyelid. A poor blinker or nonblinker may be helped by a fenestrated lens (UF-9) or an otherwise adapted one.[46] Chin elevation and squinting may result from irritating lenses.[39]

Many cosmetics have an oily base which, if deposited on the lens, may cause blurred vision and irritation. They must be chosen with care, and only those that have an aqueous base should be used. Powders can also be irritating if small particles become lodged under the lens. Mascara should be applied only to the very tips of the lashes. Hair sprays, in particular, must be used with caution. They can be very irritating if some of the spray particles are trapped in the tear layer beneath the lens, and some sprays can actually damage the lens. Nail polish, hand creams, and perfumes should be applied only after the lens has been inserted. Men frequently contaminate their lenses with hair preparations, and special care must be taken to clean hands after using these products.

Table 1. Soft Contact Lenses

Aquaflex[ab] (Union Corp.)
Contaflex (Canadian Contact Lens)
Dominion (Dominion Soft Lens)
Gelflex (Calcon)
Hydracon (Kontur Kontact)
Hydralens (Ophthalmos)
HydroCurve[a] (Soft Lenses, Inc.)
Hydro Marc (Frontier)
Jel Soft (Invisible)
Lacrophilic (N&N)
Opti Contact (Opti-Con)
Perma-Lens (Cooper Laboratories, Inc.)
Soflens[a] (Bausch & Lomb)
Softcon[a] (Warner-Lambert)
Urosoft (Urocon)
Verazel (Veracon)

[a]Approved by FDA for distribution in the U.S.

[b]An NDA was approved in June 1976 for the Aquaflex tetrafilcon A soft lens (UCO Optics, a subsidiary of Union Corp.). The lens contains 42.5% water when fully hydrated and consists of a network of terpolymer chains linked by divinylbenzene crosslinks.

Removal of lenses in comatose patients

When blinking reflexes are absent, as in the comatose patient, a contact lens will not move enough to keep tears circulating between it and the cornea. There may be permanent corneal damage if a lens is left in place. It is probably safest to remove the lens by irrigation as described below.

> ". . . With the patient supine, turn the head toward the side to be irrigated and separate the lids. Irrigate gently with sterile saline solution from the nasal side, and the lens will simply float out of the eye.
>
> "If irrigation is unsuccessful, try to remove the contact lenses by the rubber suction-cup method. Wet a small contact lens suction cup with sterile saline solution and place it gently on the center of the contact lens. Pressure on the cup is then slowly released and suction will form so that the lens can be lifted from the eye. Great care must be exercised in applying the suction cup to the contact lens; rough handling can result in permanent scarring of the cornea.
>
> "When the above methods fail or in an extreme emergency, the contact lenses can be moved temporarily onto the sclera. Gently, push the lower lid against the bottom edge of the contact lens. This will slide the lens off the cornea onto the bulbar conjunctiva where it can rest safely until an ophthalmologist can remove it. Make a note on the chart that the contact lens is still in the eye, and to have it removed as soon as possible."[47]

Hard lens solutions

The use of hard contact lenses necessitates the concurrent use of special solutions, formulated to help the user in achieving maximum compliance, comfort, and safety. In selecting or recommending a procedure for lens care, the individual's personality, temperament, physical capabilities, and characteristics should be taken into account. If a specific regimen is not suitable, it will probably be disregarded or followed poorly, with possibly detrimental effects.[48]

Chemical composition, sterility, tonicity, stability, and, of course, effectiveness must all be considered when formulating a hard contact lens solution. The solution should have cleaning and antiseptic action and should be self-preserving. It must be actively bactericidal because viable organisms may not only cause decomposition of the solution but also may adversely affect the eye.

Standards for evaluation of preservatives in these solutions are necessary, but none have been developed that are universally acceptable. Several of 34 commercially available solutions failed to suppress microbial growth even after 24-hour contact.[49]

A number of ingredients are required for buffering, adjusting tonicity, wetting, and cushioning. When the solution vehicle evaporates, a crystalline or granular residue may form, interfering with wearing comfort. An inadequately formulated solution can cause burning, stinging, excessive tearing, and possibly more serious side effects. It can exert an adverse effect on the lacrimal fluid and the eye and can cause damage to the contact lens.

Contact lens solutions are not considered drug products and their formulations are not, therefore, governed by the formulation and manufacturing restrictions placed on therapeutic ophthalmic solutions. However, in contrast to ophthalmic solutions, they are used over a long period, and their cumulative effect might be more severe. Contact lens solutions are used without medical supervision by inexperienced people; therefore, all ingredients, including preservatives, must have a high margin of safety.

Wetting solutions

Because hard contact lenses are hydrophobic, the lenses resist wetting by the lacrimal fluids, producing a foreign body sensation upon insertion. Tears contain protein compounds which are conjugated with highly hydrated polysaccharides. They have a wetting effect on the lens, but it might take as long as 15 minutes after insertion, possibly causing severe discomfort.[2] For maximum wetting of hard lenses, a solution should have a surface tension of less than 39 dyn/cm^2. Normal tear fluid has a surface tension of about 46 dyn/cm^2, which accounts for the slow wetting.

A wetting solution is "an agent which coats the contact lens uniformly with a film which is intended to minimize the friction of the contact lens against the palpebral conjunctiva and cornea." [50] It should be partly retained on the lens surface after "rinsing under a stream of slowly flowing cold water for approximately five seconds." [51] The ideal wetting solution should spread over the entire surface of the lens.[52] It should form a film that does not wash away easily; be nonirritating and nonsensitizing; not leave a residue on the lens after drying; have a cleansing and antiseptic action; be self-sterilizing; and have the proper degree of viscosity for efficient lubrication.[3]

Another function of a wetting solution is to provide a viscous coating for the contact lens which prevents direct contact with fingers during insertion. This, in turn, prevents transfer of oily deposits on the lens. Wetting solutions are directly applied to the cornea and should act as a substitute for tears. They should, therefore, have a viscosity approximating that of tears so that the normal emollient action of the precorneal film is not reduced.

The wetting solution must act as a cushion between the cornea and the lens. The precorneal film has a regulated viscosity and wetting properties which must be obtained for optical clarity. The cushion also acts as a shock absorber to prevent the lens from making sudden movements when the eyes are turned.

Because of the need for this cushioning effect, wetting solutions usually contain methylcellulose, hydroxypropyl methylcellulose, or polyvinyl alcohol (PVA) to increase the viscosity of the solution. Too high a concentration of viscosity-building agents can cause crusting on eyelids and storage cases and transient blurring of vision; too low a concentration will cause discomfort. Studies have been conducted to determine the optimum level.[53] Solutions of varying viscosity (9 to 26 cP) were instilled in the sub-

Table 2. Comparison of Some Contact Lens Cases

	Volume fluid ml (two lenses)	Cleaning accessibility	Compartment letter coding	Compartment color coding	Leakproofness	Patient identification	Lens cleaning provision	Lens rinsing provision	Complete lens submersion	Lens protection	Mirror	Absence of metal components	Lens placement and retrieval	Boilability	Screw, snap or sliding closure	Light background color	Living hinge	Plastic optimal hardness
Kelley-Hueber Mailer	(1.8)	yes	yes	no	no	no	no	no	no	no	no	yes	yes	no	yes	yes	no	yes
Multi-Pack	(0.8)	yes	yes	yes	no	yes	no	no	no	no	yes	yes	yes	no	yes	yes	no	yes
W/J B-Lens Mailer	(2.8)	yes	yes	no	no	no	no	no	no	no	no	yes	yes	no	yes	yes	no	yes
Slim Jim	(0.8)	yes	yes	yes	no	yes	no	no	no	no	no	yes	yes	no	yes	yes	no	yes
Hydra-Kit	(5.0)	no	yes	yes	no	no	no	no	yes	no	no	no	yes	no	yes	yes	no	yes
Aquacell Mates	(6.5)	no	yes	yes	no	yes	no	yes	yes	no	no	yes	no	no	yes	yes	no	yes
Antisept Jeweled	(1.2)	no	yes	no	yes	no	no	no	no	no	no	yes	no	no	yes	no	no	yes
Guardian	(6.0)	yes	yes	no	yes	yes	no	no	yes	no	no	yes	no	no	yes	yes	no	yes
Ideal	(5.6)	no	yes	no	yes	yes	no	no	yes	no	no	yes	no	no	yes	yes	no	yes
Multimaster	(7.7)	no	yes	no	yes	no	no	no	yes	no	no	yes	no	no	yes	yes	no	yes
Comfort Case	(6.0)	no	no	yes	yes	no	no	no	yes	no	no	yes	no	no	yes	yes	no	yes
Sentinal	(7.4)	yes	yes	yes	yes	yes	no	no	yes	no	yes	yes	no	no	yes	yes	no	yes
Clean-N-Stow	(8.0)	no	yes	yes	yes	no	no	yes	yes	yes	no	yes	yes	yes	no	yes	no	yes
Clean-N-Soakit	(4.7)	no	yes	yes	yes	no	no	yes	no	yes	no	yes	yes	yes	no	yes	no	yes
Porta-FLOW	(4.0)	yes	yes	yes	yes	yes	yes	yes	yes	yes	yes	yes	yes	yes	yes	yes	yes	yes
Una-Pac	(6.5)	no	yes	yes	yes	no	no	yes	no	yes	no	no	no	yes	no	yes	no	yes
Hydra-Mat	(30)	no	yes	no	yes	no	yes	yes	yes	yes	no	yes	no	no	no	yes	no	yes
Tote and Soak	(8.0)	no	no	yes	yes	no	no	yes	no	yes	no	yes	yes	yes	yes	yes	yes	yes
Lensine	(1.8)	yes	yes	no	no	no	no	no	no	no	no	yes	no	yes	yes	yes	no	yes
Dispos-A-Kit	(7.0)	no	yes	no	no	no	no	no	no	no	no	yes	yes	no	yes	yes	no	yes

Adapted from J.Z. Krezanoski and J.B. Lowry, *Contact Lens Soc. Am. J.*, **7 (3)**, 13 (1973).

jects' eyes and patients were evaluated subjectively. Complaints were lack of comfort (with low viscosity solutions) and transient, blurry vision (with high viscosity solutions). On the basis of this simple test, the optimal viscosity range was found at 15 to 20 cP. The viscosity of most products is not listed on the label and can vary to some extent from batch to batch because of the variability in the polymers.

Sodium chloride is used to make wetting solutions isotonic. Some solutions are made mildly hypertonic (1.1 percent sodium chloride) because the tonicity of tears approximates an equivalent of 1 percent sodium chloride. Although a mildly hypertonic solution is said to be better tolerated and reduce superficial edema and swelling, these conclusions are questionable.[54]

Wetting solutions contain a buffer system to adjust the pH and keep it at a predetermined level. It is best to adjust the pH to that of the lacrimal fluid ($\sim$ 7.2) as this would cause the least discomfort. However, Gould and Inglima [55] investigated 14 wetting solutions and found two below pH 4.0, eight between pH 4.0 and 5.0, two between 6.0 and 7.0, and two above pH 7.0. Solutions that are adjusted to a pH which is significantly below the physiological pH of tears should have a minimal buffer capacity so that the natural fluids of the eye can quickly adjust them to correct physiologic pH. When adjusting pH, other factors such as the stability of the preparation must also be considered. Partly acetylated PVA, for example, necessitates formulation of solutions at an acidic pH to prevent hydrolysis of the polymer.

All contact lens solutions are exposed to a high degree of contamination, and special care must be exercised in selecting a preservative. Also, continual application of bactericidal agents to the eye may be irritating. Wetting solutions, once they have been applied, have no germicidal activity, because the contact time is too short.[56]

The acceptable preservatives used in contact lens solutions are limited, and they vary in their bactericidal action and sensitizing potential. Agents include a quaternary ammonium compound (benzalkonium chloride), chlorobutanol, and organic mercurials. Benzalkonium chloride was first proposed in 1947 as a preservative for ophthalmic solutions.[57] For it to be effective, particularly against *Pseudomonas aeruginosa*, a sufficiently strong solution must be used. However, too strong a solution may produce liquefaction of intercellular cement, desquamation of the epithelium, and edema. Conjunctival and corneal lesions have been found when benzalkonium chloride was used in a strength of 0.1 percent.[58] Because the effect is cumulative, a single application may be well tolerated, but the second or third may produce irritation. Solutions of 0.02 percent apparently are tolerated, even when they are used three or four times a day.[48] The bactericidal activity of benzalkonium chloride is reduced by soaps, metallic ions, and rubber.

Chlorobutanol is a volatile, relatively insoluble, slow-acting bactericide that does not seem to have an advantage over benzalkonium chloride. It usually is used at a concentration of 0.5 percent, although concentrations of as low as 0.15 percent have been used. It is effective only after it permeates into the bacterial cell. Chlorobutanol is unstable in alkaline medium and is seldom used in contact lens solutions, unless the pH is 6 or lower.

The two most commonly used organic mercurial compounds are thimerosal and phenylmercuric nitrate. They have a slow rate of kill, and they act through the sustained release of the mercurial ion which penetrates into the bacterial cell and combines with various respiratory enzymes to inhibit metabolism.[59] Thimerosal is a basic salt and must be used in neutral or slightly alkaline solutions. Phenylmercuric nitrate is an organic mercurial which is used in dilute concentrations. It differs from other organic mercurials in that it is not precipitated in an acid pH.

Many wetting solutions contain a small concentration of edetate disodium which, when combined with benzalkonium chloride, chlorobutanol, or thimerosal, enhances the bactericidal properties of these agents when tested against *P. aeruginosa.* It apparently disrupts the integrity of a lipid or lipid-protein complex in the cell wall, increasing the permeability of the obstructing layer of the cell wall to the bactericidal agent.[60]

Soaking solutions

A soaking solution should provide for hydration of the lenses which facilitates wetting; for removal of adsorbed organic substances which, if allowed to remain, inhibit wetting of the lens; and for antisepsis.[7]

PMMA contact lenses become hydrated when they are in contact with aqueous solutions and are dehydrated when exposed to dry air.[61] Hydration produces a lens of longer radius, i.e., a flatter lens. Because lenses become hydrated when they are worn, they should be kept hydrated when not worn, in order to maintain constant dimensional stability. The average amount of precorneal fluid absorbed by dry lenses is about 30 percent more than that absorbed by those stored in a soaking solution.[62]

Bacterial contamination and the relative effect of a wet or dry storage regimen on lens wettability have been studied extensively. [55,63,64] Insertion of the contact lens in a dry state may cause discomfort for several minutes to an hour; wet storage can increase comfort. Soaking solutions gently remove adsorbed material which has accumulated on the lens during wearing. This prevents the accumulation from drying onto the surface and into the pores of the lens which can cause surface chemical change and "fogging."

The original argument against wet storage was that soaking solutions could possibly be the source of *Pseudomonas* infections.[63,65,66] It is now known that infections may have been caused by failure of the patient to renew the soaking solution or by adding new solution to the old one. It also has been shown that the original storage containers made of soft, colored plastic or those with rubber inserts can release highly irritating products which reduce the bactericidal activity of the solution and alter its pH.[55] To overcome this, it is recommended that containers not include sponge rubber pads and that they be filled with soaking solution for 15 minutes, which is then discarded, new solution added to the container, and the lenses stored. Lenses stored in soaking solutions are less subject to bacterial contamination and cause less discomfort than lenses stored in a dry state.[2]

To sterilize lenses, soaking solutions often contain both benzalkonium chloride and chlorobutanol. This combination has a synergistic effect.[67] Increasing the concentration of benzalkonium chloride in soaking solutions does not seem to increase effectiveness.[68,69] Other antimicrobial agents included in soaking solutions are polymyxin B sulfate, organic mercurials, benzoic acid esters, and certain phenols and substituted alcohols.[56]

Cleaning solutions

Lenses must be clean for maximum hydration. They absorb water from the lacrimal fluid, trapping mucus and salts on the surface which attach firmly to the lens surface forming a thin film; oily residue may also be left on the lens surface during insertion. These contaminants are a barrier to the wetting action of tears, can impair vision, and can cause irritation and infections. Cleaning solutions contain nonionic surfactants which reduce surface tension, emulsify lipids, and solubilize other debris. Lipids and proteins, which are often found on contact lenses, are soluble in alkaline media, but strongly alkaline solutions can chemically decompose the plastic.

All-purpose solutions

These solutions, also called multi-purpose or convenience solutions, are designed as a compromise between patient convenience and optimal lens care. Many formulation problems are encountered, and some of the necessary functions, e.g., wetting, may not be as effectively achieved as with an individual solution. However, it is felt that compliance can often be improved with use of multi-purpose solutions. There are other solutions which can be used on an intraocular basis (for wetting and cushioning) and some used on an extraocular basis (for hydration, disinfection, and cleaning).[70-72]

Artificial tears

Artificial tears are solutions that provide an emollient and lubricating effect in cases of lacrimal insufficiency. They can also be used to relieve ocular irritation. These solutions are not recommended for use while the lenses are in place. They usually contain tonicity agents, such as sodium chloride; viscosity-increasing agents, such as methylcellulose; and a bactericidal agent, such as benzalkonium chloride. The pH of these solutions is usually adjusted to simulate the physiologic pH of tears.

Ocular decongestants

Prolonged wearing of contact lenses, especially in the adaptation stage, can cause conjunctivitis. Many ocular decongestant products are available, most of which contain phenylephrine hydrochloride at about a 0.1-percent concentration. There is no clinical evidence that one product is better than another. These solutions are applied after the lenses have been removed to hasten the regression of the inflammation by reducing the size of the engorged small vessels. They are not to be used with the lens in place.

Miscellaneous

Many specialized solutions have been marketed for use with hard contact lenses. It is questionable whether they offer a significant advantage over the products already discussed. In many cases, it seems that they are attempts at increasing product lines and sales volume.

In-the-eye cleaning solutions. These solutions supposedly clean lenses while they are being worn. They contain surfactants to remove deposits (mucus and dirt) from the lens surface by surface activity and lid-wiping action.

Preinsertion solutions. These solutions are a kind of artificial tears which have a high relative viscosity to enhance cushioning and reduce irritation during the "breaking-in" period. Their viscosity can cause problems with visual acuity immediately after insertion.

Conditioners. Conditioners are recommended in cases where tears do not supply sufficient wetting action or cushioning effect. They are also used to clear the eye of potential debris-forming substances prior to lens insertion. They can be applied to the eye as frequently as three or four times a day while the lens is being worn.[73]

Guidelines for product selection

Based on current information, it is very difficult to recommend objectively a particular contact lens solution as the preferred product. A person's temperament, personality, physical characteristics, and capabilities must be taken into account. If a specific regimen is not suitable, it will probably be disregarded or followed poorly.

Ocular discomfort may be caused by lens-induced corneal edema, and removal of the lens makes the symptoms disappear. It can also be caused by a person's inability or lack of determination to follow a particular regimen. In these cases, multi-purpose or all-purpose solutions may be helpful. A specific product which has too high a content of total solids may cause ocular discomfort. Changing to a mildly hypertonic solution or a solution with a different viscosity-increasing agent may help.

Contact lens wearers may encounter problems when placed on a therapy involving antihistamines, oral decongestants, or diuretics, all of which decrease lacrimal fluid volume. Patients whose tears do not produce enough wetting action or who do not achieve enough cushioning with a wetting solution may be helped by a conditioner which can be instilled while the lens is worn. Ocular irritation is sometimes relieved by use of artificial tears.

It is not good practice to mix solutions from different manufacturers without checking contents. This could lead to concurrent use of solutions with anionic and cationic agents which might inactivate one or both agents and possibly cause precipitation.

Contact lens remover

The DMV Contact Lens Remover is sometimes recommended to elderly patients to help in removal of lenses. The pharmacist must be aware that good patient instructions are needed. The contact lens remover uses a suction cup, and if the patient places the cup on cornea instead of lens, corneal damage may result.

Contact lens cases

Several devices are available for mailing, soaking and cleaning, and storing hard contact lenses. Standards for these have been recommended, and their effectiveness can be judged by the categories in Table 2.[74]

Soft lens solutions

Conventional contact lens solutions cannot be used with soft lenses because all chemicals, especially benzalkonium chloride, seem to bind to the soft lens material.[75] Originally, the problem of lens sterility was anticipated, based on the premise that bacteria and fungi would penetrate into the lens matrix. It was found, however, that the problem was not the penetration, but the enzymatic degradation of the lens material by bacteria and fungi.[76] Another problem was not anticipated and has not been solved satisfactorily—deposits of protein, particularly mucoproteins, meibomian oils, fungus remnants, and occasional calciferous deposits, have been found on soft lenses. Thus, separate cleaning and sterilization cycles had to be developed for the care of soft lenses.

Cleaning cycle: general

Dirty lenses still are the major complaint of soft contact lens wearers. Literature is available on cleaners and cleaning procedures of soft lenses, including concern for the basic solution used in cleaning and rinsing of the lenses.[77-83]

If lenses are adequately cleaned before boiling, the sterilization cycle can be fully effective, and cumulative deposits on the lens can be prevented. Rubbing and rinsing with normal saline solution is still the recommended procedure. If the solution is freshly prepared according to instructions, there should be no problems. A saline solution with a preservative prevents microbial growth in the solution while it is not in use. The mineral and iron content of the water used to prepare the solution may cause discoloration of the lenses.

More effective cleaners have been proposed. They include surfactants, oxidative systems, and enzymes. Surfactants alone may remove deposits which are amenable to a reduction of interfacial tension; however, they would not remove proteins. Surfactant residue could probably produce a permanent coating of the lens, if the lens is subjected to repeated heat treatment for purposes of sterilization.[83]

Oxidative systems, mainly hydrogen peroxide, can remove lens deposits, but if they are not specially formulated, the basic polymer chain could be affected by the solution. Although a cleaning action has been ascribed to hydrogen peroxide, it is not clear whether this solution has a better cleaning action than either water or isotonic sodium chloride solution. In some instances, as a matter of fact, the hydrogen peroxide solution may enhance the rate of protein deposition on the lens because it denatures proteins due to its oxidative reactivity.

Enzymatic agents have also been proposed. They remove proteins from the lens and are not damaging to the lens. Although enzymatic cleaners have been available outside the U.S. for some time, it has been thought that they might be sensitizing to the eye. However, the FDA has approved for use in the U.S. one cleaner based on the enzymatic principle.

Several prophylactic cleaners are in various stages of development and testing. A typical solution contains nonionic surfactants, edetate sodium, and, in some cases, cellulose derivatives.

Sterilization cycle: general

Soft lenses are kept hydrated for patient comfort, but hydration, theoretically, increases the chances for microbial contamination.[84] Although research shows that *Escherichia coli* and *P. aeruginosa* cannot enter the hydrogel, the FDA demands "sterilization" of the lens.[36]

It has been suggested that the term "sterilization" is not really appropriate to use; the lens must be rendered free from (potential) pathogens, a process more accurately called "disinfecting" or, by one manufacturer of a soft lens, "asepticizing." [76]

So far, the FDA has approved only boiling as the process for sterilizing all approved soft lenses.[85] The manufacturer of one lens has asked for approval of the use of hydrogen peroxide solution as a sterilizing solution.

Boiling of lenses destroys pathogens satisfactorily but fails to kill spores. Although the effectiveness of boiling itself is not questioned, a number of factors can influence its effectiveness—the boiling cycle is tedious and inconvenient, it decreases the lifespan of the lens, or it may not last long enough to sterilize.[86]

Another disadvantage of sterilization is the cumbersome containers, which may be convenient for home use but are unacceptable for travel. Distilled water may leave a residue, but it can be wiped away with a paper towel.[33] It is possible that lenses that are not completely clean are covered with proteins which could be denatured by the boiling process. This material would then have a tendency to accumulate on the lens, shortening the effective life of the lens. Some cold sterilizing solutions are in various stages of development and trial. A suggested approach involves the use of an iodophore concentrate (0.1 percent iodine) followed by treatment with a thiosulfate neutralizing solution. Iodine causes rapid kill and has a broad spectrum of antimicrobial activity. An advantage of this system is its color reaction. As long as a distinctive blue color persists, the disinfecting process is still going on; when solution and lenses are clear, lenses can be inserted and worn safely.[86, 87] Several other solutions which contain chlorhexidine gluconate, thimerosal, and edetate sodium also are being investigated.[88]

Care of the Softcon lens

The Softcon vifilcon A lens was formerly called the Griffin or Bionite Naturalens. It is approved only for therapeutic use. The lens wearer must be completely familiar with the correct lens care procedures. This lens has been described as "dynamic," i.e., it changes its profile with drying and pH fluctuations. The wearer must learn how to respond to these lens changes, which are also encountered with the other soft lenses.[89]

Cleaning. The lens is cleaned by gently rubbing both sides between the fingers, using Lensrins solution. This is a normal saline solution, buffered to pH 7.0 to 7.1, which contains thimerosal and edetate disodium. It is used to prevent changes in the lens caused by an acid pH. Other solutions have been investigated for use with this lens. They contain chlorhexidine gluconate, edetic acid, and thimerosal.[90]

Sterilization. Any lens should be disinfected before being reapplied to the eye. Boiling is the only approved method for this process. The lens should be immersed in Lensrins solution and boiled for at least 15 minutes in either a boiling water bath or an office sterilizer.

It has been suggested that a peroxide cycle can be used to sterilize the lens.[91] It would seem that more research is needed in the area of peroxide use. Although the minimum inhibitory concentration (MIC) of hydrogen peroxide is extremely low, the kill rate varies directly with the concentration. Because hydrogen peroxide is unstable, it is usually formulated at an acid pH, which is undesirable for comfort and lens stability.[84]

Thus, in the originally proposed peroxide cycle, the lens was first soaked in peroxide, which was then discarded. A solution of sodium bicarbonate was then added which interacts with the peroxide, forming water and oxygen, thus neutralizing the acidic pH.

Lensept, a hydrogen peroxide solution which obviates the use of sodium bicarbonate is now available. A 10-minute soaking is suggested, followed by two rinsings and storage in Lensrins. The lens should be rinsed again before insertion into the eye.[35] It should never be stored in plain water. The case in which the lens is boiled and/or stored should be tightly sealed.

Therapeutic use. The Softcon lens is a corneal bandage lens which covers the cornea and the adjacent sclera. It has been in use as a therapeutic bandage, designed to aid corneal healing, to relieve pain, to reduce corneal edema and, in selected cases, to improve vision. Supplemental requests for its use in other corneal pathologies have been submitted. The Softcon lens is often used with a 5-percent saline (hypertonic) solution which does not contain preservatives or methylcellulose. This solution is usually used three to five times a day.[92]

Care of the Soflens lens

The Soflens polymacon lens was developed for the correction of refractive errors. It is also used in the treatment of dry eye and corneal edema.[10] It is smaller and thinner than the other soft lenses and, therefore, might be somewhat less effective in promoting the healing of indolent corneal ulcers. The most frequent disadvantage is erratic, often poor visual acuity, far and near. Lens durability, especially with regard to torn edges, is not good.[7]

The lenses are packaged sterilely in normal saline solution in glass vials. A Patient Care Kit (aseptor-patient unit) is supplied which contains a carrying case, 200 salt tablets, a small plastic squeeze bottle in which normal saline solution is mixed and stored, an instruction booklet, and an asepticizer.

Cleaning. In the past, normal saline solution was the only cleaning agent used. It is applied to the lens, and the lens is rubbed between the fingers. The lens is then rinsed under running water and returned to normal saline solution for storage (note: normal saline solution used in the care of this lens should not contain thimerosal). If tapwater or an improper number of salt tablets is used, an imbalanced storage solution results, causing changes in lens dimensions and light transmission.[93]

Now, the Soflens Enzymatic Contact Lens Cleaner has been approved for use in the U.S. The cleaner most likely contains a specially purified enzyme (papain) designed to remove proteinaceous lens deposits. It is purified to prevent eye irritation. Also under development is a "new sterilizing system," a solution claimed to have broad-spectrum germicidal and fungicidal action. Designed as a soaking solution, it contains a quaternary ammonium compound and a surfactant to cleanse the lenses of oil and mucus. A "special detoxifying agent," not identified in the literature, appears to be the major ingredient.

Sterilization. The lenses should be sterilized daily by boiling them in the asepticizer for 15 minutes, until all of the solution is boiled away. They should be stored in isotonic normal saline solution. Hypotonic solutions or plain water make lenses tacky and sticky and cause discomfort until tonicity is achieved by tears. Hypertonic solutions cause stinging, lacrimation, and hyperemia.[85]

Use. Before insertion of the lens, sufficient normal saline is again applied to the lens to wet it well, the lens is rubbed between the thumb and forefinger, and it is flushed with normal saline solution. If it is difficult to remove the lens from the eye, a "pinching" procedure is recommended because the lens firmly adheres to the eye, and air must be allowed to come between the lens and eye before the lens can be removed.

Care of the Hydrocurve lens

The Hydrocurve hefilcon A lenses are approved for the correction of visual acuity in people with nondiseased eyes. As with all soft lenses, these lenses must be cleaned and boiled every day.

Cleaning. Softmate is the suggested cleaning solution. It contains a nonionic surfactant, hydroxyethylcellulose in isotonic sodium chloride solution, thimerosal, and edetate sodium. The solution is formulated at an alkaline pH which is claimed to facilitate the removal of proteins, meibomian oils, and cholesterol lipids.

Pliagel can also be used. It is a sterile isotonic cleanser that contains a surfactant, sorbic acid as a preservative, and edetate trisodium.

Sterilization. The lens should be boiled for 15 minutes. Boiling and subsequent storage are recommended in Boil-n-Soak, a preserved isotonic solution. A particular unit is recommended, but the process can be accomplished by boiling the lenses in their carrying case in a pan of water.

CAUTIONS FOR THE CARE OF SOFT LENSES

☐ A solution designed for use with hard lenses should not be used on soft lenses.

☐ The system approved by the FDA for the care of particular lenses should be used.

☐ No ophthalmic solutions or medicants, including conventional contact lens solutions, can be used by soft lens wearers prior to or while lens is in place on the eye.

☐ The prescribed regimen should be followed exactly.

Problems arise when the lens is not cleaned carefully before sterilization. This can lead to ocular irritation and clouded lenses.

References

1. "Modern Plastics Encyclopedia," vol. 1, Breskin, New York, N.Y., 1947, p. 129.
2. O. H. Dabezies, in "Corneal and Scleral Contact Lenses," L. J. Girard, Ed., Mosby, St. Louis, Mo., 1967, pp. 347-361.
3. H. W. Hind and I. J. Szekely, *Contacto,* **3**, 66(1959).
4. R. E. Phares, in "Soft Contact Lens," A. R. Gasset and H. E. Kaufman, Eds., Mosby, St. Louis, Mo., 1972, pp. 233-239.
5. H. E. Kaufman *et al.*, in "Soft Contact Lens," A. R. Gasset and H. E. Kaufman, Eds., Mosby, St. Louis, Mo., 1972, pp. 175-183.
6. "Contact Lens Practice," R. B. Mandell, Ed., Charles C Thomas, Springfield, Ill., 1974, pp. 437-454.
7. N. J. Bailey, in "Soft Contact Lens," A. R. Gasset and H. E. Kaufman, Eds., Mosby, St. Louis, Mo., 1972, pp. 61-71.
8. F. B. Hoefle, *Trans. Am. Acad. Ophthalmol. Otol.*, **78**, OP-386-390(1974).
9. H. E. Kaufman *et al.*, in "Symposium on Contact Lenses," Mosby, St. Louis, Mo., 1973, pp. 174-180.
10. H. M. Leibowitz, in "Soft Contact Lens," A. R. Gasset and H. E. Kaufman, Eds., Mosby, St. Louis, Mo., 1972, pp. 199-209.
11. J. Sugar, *Arch. Ophthalmol.*, **91**, 11(1974).
12. W. E. Long, in "Symposium on the Flexible Lens," J. L. Bitonte and R. H. Keates, Eds., Mosby, St. Louis, Mo., 1972, pp. 73-79.
13. "Contact Lens Practice," R. B. Mandell, Ed., Charles C Thomas, Springfield, Ill., 1974, pp. 519-522.
14. A. B. Rizzuit, *Ann. Ophthalmol.*, **6**, 596(1974).
15. C. J. Black, in "Soft Contact Lens," A. R. Gasset and H. E. Kaufman, Eds., Mosby, St. Louis, Mo., 1972, pp. 126-138.
16. C. Thranberend, *Klin. Monatsbl. Augenheilkd.*, **164**, 509(1974).
17. F. Dickenson, *Contacto*, **11(2)**, 12(1967).
18. C. H. May, *Contacto*, **4(2)**, 51(1960).
19. T. F. Gumpelmayer, *Am. J. Optom.*, **47**, 879(1970).
20. M. Millodot, *Arch. Ophthalmol.*, **82**, 461(1969).
21. M. G. Harris, in "Contact Lens Practice," R. B. Mandell, Ed., Charles C Thomas, Springfield, Ill., 1974, pp. 83-116.
22. J. A. Baldone, *Trans. Am. Acad. Ophthalmol. Otol.*, **78**, OP-406(1974).
23. F. B. Sannin, in "Corneal and Scleral Contact Lenses," L. J. Girard, Ed., Mosby, St. Louis, Mo., 1967, pp. 170-173.
24. M. D. Sarver and M. G. Harris, *Am. J. Optom.*, **48**, 382(1971).
25. R. L. Sutherland and W. N. Van Leeuwen, *Can. Med. Assoc. J.*, **107**, 49(1972).
26. *Optom. Weekly*, **63(45)**, 25(1972).
27. I. Fatt and R. St. Helen, *Am. J. Optom.*, **48**, 545(1971).

28. D. R. Morrison and H. F. Edelhauser, *Invest. Ophthalmol.*, **11**, 58(1972).
29. L. Krejci and H. Krejcova, *Br. J. Ophthalmol.*, **57**, 675(1973).
30. R. L. Farris *et al.*, *Arch. Ophthalmol.*, **85**, 651(1971).
31. S. G. El Hage *et al.*, *Am. J. Optom. Physiol. Optics*, **51(1)**, 24(1974).
32. C. H. Dohlman, *Trans. Am. Acad. Ophthalmol. Otol.*, **78**, OP-399(1974).
33. C. J. Black, in "Symposium on the Flexible Lens," J. L. Bitonte and R. H. Keates, Eds., Mosby, St. Louis, Mo., 1972, pp. 30-32.
34. H. I. Moss, in "Soft Contact Lens," A. R. Gasset and H. E. Kaufman, Eds., Mosby, St., Louis, Mo., 1972, pp. 83-86.
35. A. A. Isen, in "Symposium on the Flexible Lens," J. L. Bitonte and R. H. Keates, Eds., Mosby, St. Louis, Mo., 1972, pp. 35-51.
36. R. H. Keates, in "Symposium on the Flexible Lens," J. L. Bitonte and R. H. Keates, Eds., Mosby, St. Louis, Mo., 1972, pp. 222-234.
37. *Br. Med. J.*, **3**, 254(1972).
38. W. G. Sampson, *Trans. Am. Acad. Ophthalmol. Otol.*, **78**, OP-423(1974).
39. C. J. Black, in "Symposium on Contact Lenses," Mosby, St. Louis, Mo., 1973, pp. 1-12.
40. I. A. Mackie, in "Symposium on Contact Lenses," Mosby, St. Louis, Mo., 1973, pp. 65-81.
41. L. J. Girard, in "Corneal Contact Lenses," L. J. Girard, Ed., Mosby, St. Louis, Mo., 1972, pp. 107-120.
42. L. J. Girard, in "Corneal and Scleral Contact Lenses," L. J. Girard, Ed., Mosby, St. Louis, Mo., 1967, pp. 40-48.
43. "Corneal and Scleral Contact Lenses," L. J. Girard, Ed., Mosby, St. Louis, Mo., 1967, pp. 1-17.
44. H. M. Rosenwasser, *Opt. J. Rev. Optom.*, **100(22)**, 41(1963).
45. O. W. Cole, *Contacto*, **15(2)**, 5(1971).
46. G. P. Halberg, in "Symposium on Contact Lenses," Mosby, St. Louis, Mo., 1973, pp. 42-52.
47. R. F. Meyer and J. W. Henderson, *Clin. Med.*, **82(2)**, 26(1975).
48. *Contacto*, **15(3)**, 20(1971).
49. D. A. Norton *et al.*, *J. Pharm. Pharmacol.*, **26**, 841(1974).
50. H. L. Gould, *Eye Ear Nose Throat Mon.*, **41**, 359(1962).
51. *Contacto*, **3**, 262(1959).
52. I. J. Szekely, *South. Pharm. J.*, **52**, 17(1960).
53. B. F. Rankin, *Optom. Weekly*, (May 25, 1961).
54. J. Z. Krezanoski, *J. Am. Pharm. Assoc.*, **NS10**, 13(1970).
55. H. L. Gould and R. Inglima, *Eye Ear Nose Throat Mon.*, **43**, 39(1964).
56. "Contact Lens Practice," R. B. Mandell, Ed., Charles C Thomas, Springfield, Ill., 1974, pp. 255-284.
57. H. W. Hind and F. M. Goyan, *J. Am. Pharm. Assoc. Sci. Ed.*, **36**, 33(1947).
58. K. C. Swan, *Am. J. Ophthalmol.*, **27**, 1118(1944).
59. S. Riegelman *et al.*, *J. Am. Pharm. Assoc. Sci. Ed.*, **45**, 93(1956).
60. D. R. McGregor and P. R. Elliker, *Can. J. Microbiol.*, **4**, 499(1958).
61. J. C. Neill and J. J. Hanna, *Contacto*, **7**, 10(1963).
62. C. E. Watkins, *Optometric World*, (Oct. 1964).
63. F. M. Kapetansky *et al.*, *Am. J. Ophthalmol.*, **57**, 255(1964).
64. H. Allen, *Arch. Ophthalmol.*, **67**, 119(1962).
65. J. M. Dixon *et al.*, *Am. J. Ophthalmol.*, **54**, 461(1962).
66. M. F. Obear and F. C. Winter, *Am. J. Ophthalmol.*, **57**, 441(1964).
67. N. C. Hall and J. Z. Krezanoski, *N. Engl. J. Optom.*, **14**, 229(1963).
68. O. H. Dabezies, *Eye Ear Nose Throat Mon.*, **45**, 78-84 (1966).
69. O. H. Dabezies and T. Naugle, *Eye Ear Nose Throat Mon.*, **50(10)**, 378(1971).
70. R. E. Phares, *Contact Lens Soc. Am. J.*, **7(1)**, 37(1973).
71. O. H. Dabezies, *Contact Lens Med. Bull.*, **7(3)**, 45(1974).
72. G. L. Cureton *et al.*, *J. Am. Optom. Assoc.*, **46**, 259(1975).
73. M. J. Sibley and D. E. Lauck, *Contact Lens. J.*, **8(2)**, 10(1974).
74. "Prescription Requirements for First-Quality Contact Lenses," American National Standards Institute, New York, N.Y., 1972.
75. R. E. Phares, *J. Am. Optom. Assoc.*, **43(3)**, 308(1972).
76. G. L. Cureton and N. C. Hall, *Am. J. Optom. Physiol. Optics*, **51**, 406(1974).
77. J. Z. Krezanoski, *Contact Lens. Soc. Am. J.*, **7(4)**, 9(1974).
78. J. A. Baldone, *Contact Lens Med. Bull.*, **4(2)**, 9(1971).
79. J. Z. Krezanoski, *Ont. Optician*, **5(3)**, 9(1974).
80. J. Z. Krezanoski, "Where are We in the Development of Pharmaceutical Products for Soft (Hydrophilic) Lenses?" (unpublished report).
81. J. Z. Krezanoski, *Int. Cont. Clin.*, (to be published).
82. M. S. Favero *et al.*, *Science*, **173**, 836(1971).
83. S. Ericksen, "Cleaning Hydrophilic Contact Lenses: An Overview," (unpublished report).
84. R. E. Phares and N. C. Hall, in "Symposium on the Flexible Lens," J. L. Bitonte and R. H. Keates, Eds., Mosby, St. Louis, Mo., 1972, pp. 205-212.
85. H. A. Knoll, in "Symposium on the Flexible Lens," J. L. Bitonte and R. H. Keates, Eds., Mosby, St. Louis, Mo., 1972, pp. 11-21.
86. W. Sagan and K. N. Schwaderer, *J. Am. Optom. Assoc.*, **45**, 266(1974).
87. H. I. Silverman *et al.*, *J. Am. Optom. Assoc.*, **44**, 1040(1973).
88. J. Z. Krezanoski, *Ophthalmol. Opt.*, **12**, 1035(1972).
89. K. A. Whitman, in "Symposium on the Flexible Lens," J. L. Bitonte and R. H. Keates, Eds., Mosby, St. Louis, Mo., 1972, pp. 66-70.
90. E. D. Varnell and H. E. Kaufman, in "Soft Contact Lens," A. R. Gasset and H. E. Kaufman, Eds., Mosby, St. Louis, Mo., 1972, pp. 244-253.
91. J. V. Aquavella, in "Soft Contact Lens," A. R. Gasset and H. E. Kaufman, Eds., Mosby, St. Louis, Mo., 1972, pp. 99-105.
92. A. R. Gasset and H. E. Kaufman, in "Symposium on the Flexible Lens," J. L. Bitonte and R. H. Keates, Eds., Mosby, St. Louis, Mo., 1972, pp. 52-58.
93. M. G. Harris and L. G. Mock, *Am. J. Optom. Physiol. Optics*, **51**, 457(1974).

Products 21 HARD LENS

roduct (manufacturer)	Suggested use	Viscosity agent	Preservative	Other
ll-In-One (Rexall)	cleaning wetting soaking	—	edetate disodium, 0.1% thimerosal, 0.004%	—
link-N-Clean (Allergan)	cleaning	polyoxyl 40 stearate polyethylene glycol 300	chlorobutanol, 0.5%	—
leaning and Soaking Solution (Barnes-Hind)	cleaning soaking	—	edetate disodium, 0.2% benzalkonium chloride, 0.01%	buffering and cleaning agents [b]
lean-N-Soak (Allergan)	cleaning soaking	—	phenylmercuric nitrate, 0.004%	cleaning agent [b]
ontactisol (Smith, Miller & Patch)	cleaning wetting	hydroxypropyl methylcellulose	benzalkonium chloride, 0.01% edetate disodium, 0.01%	sodium carbonate boric acid potassium chloride

Product (manufacturer)	Suggested use	Viscosity agent	Preservative	Other
Contique Cleaning Solution (Alcon)	cleaning	—	benzalkonium chloride, 0.02%	—
Contique Clean-Tabs[a] (Alcon)	cleaning	—	—	cleaning agents[b]
Contique Soaking Solution (Alcon)	soaking	—	benzalkonium chloride, 0.01% edetate disodium, 0.01%	—
Contique Soak-Tabs[a] (Alcon)	soaking	—	thimerosal, 0.08% benzalkonium chloride, 4%	—
Contique Wetting Solution (Alcon)	wetting	hydroxypropyl methylcellulose	benzalkonium chloride, 0.004% edetate disodium, 0.025%	—
d-Film Gel (Flow)	cleaning	—	—	nonionic detergent[b]
duo-Flow (Flow)	cleaning soaking	—	edetate disodium, 0.25% benzalkonium chloride, 0.013%	—
Gel-Clean (Barnes-Hind)	cleaning	—	thimerosal, 0.004%	nonionic surfactant[b]
hy-Flow (Flow)	wetting	polyvinyl alcohol	edetate disodium, 0.025% benzalkonium chloride, 0.01%	sodium chloride, 1% potassium chloride, 0.2%
LC-65 (Allergan)	cleaning	—	thimerosal, 0.001%	cleaning agents[b]
Lensine (Abbott)	cleaning wetting soaking	hydroxypropyl methylcellulose	edetate disodium, 0.1% benzalkonium chloride, 0.01%	boric acid, 0.7% (but pH is alkaline)
Lens-Mate (Alcon)	cleaning wetting soaking	polyvinyl alcohol hydroxypropyl methylcellulose	benzalkonium chloride, 0.1% edetate disodium, 0.01%	—
Liquifilm Wetting Solution (Allergan)	wetting	hydroxypropyl methylcellulose polyvinyl alcohol	benzalkonium chloride, 0.004%	sodium chloride potassium chloride
One Solution (Barnes-Hind)	cleaning wetting soaking	NS[b]	edetate disodium, 0.1% benzalkonium chloride, 0.01%	cleaning agents[b]
Pre-Sert (Allergan)	wetting	polyvinyl alcohol, 3%	benzalkonium chloride, 0.004%	—
Soakare (Allergan)	soaking	—	edetate disodium, 0.25% benzalkonium chloride, 0.01%	—
Soquette (Barnes-Hind)	soaking	polyvinyl alcohol	chlorobutanol, 0.4% edetate disodium, 0.2% benzalkonium chloride, 0.01%	—
Titan (Barnes-Hind)	cleaning	—	benzalkonium chloride edetate disodium	nonionic cleaner buffers[b]
Total All-in-one Contact Lens Solution (Allergan)	cleaning wetting soaking	polyvinyl alcohol hydroxypropyl methylcellulose	benzalkonium chloride edetate disodium	sodium chloride potassium chloride dextrose
Visalens Soaking/Cleaning (Leeming)	cleaning soaking	—	phenylmercuric nitrate, 0.004%	—
Visalens Wetting Solution (Leeming)	wetting	methylcellulose	benzalkonium chloride, 0.004% edetate disodium	sodium chloride potassium chloride
Wet-Cote (Milroy)	wetting	polyvinyl alcohol hydroxyethylcellulose	edetate disodium, 0.025% benzalkonium chloride, 0.01%	sodium chloride potassium chloride
Wetting Solution (Barnes-Hind)	wetting	polyvinyl alcohol, 2%	edetate disodium, 0.02% benzalkonium chloride, 0.004%	sodium chloride
Wetting Solution (Rexall)	wetting	—	edetate disodium, 0.01% benzalkonium chloride, 0.004%	—

[a] Tablet must be dissolved in water.
[b] Not specified.

Product (manufacturer)	Suggested use, type of lens	Viscosity agent	Preservative	Other
Pliagel (Flow)	cleaning, hydrocurve	—	antimicrobials	surfactants
Preflex (Burton Parsons)	cleaning, hydrocurve	hydroxyethylcellulose polyvinyl alcohol	edetate disodium, 0.02% thimerosal, 0.004%	sodium phosphate sodium chloride tyloxapol
Ren-O-Gel (Flow)	cleaning, hydrocurve	—	—	surfactant
Soflens Tablets (Allergan)	cleaning, polymacon	—	—	papain
Soft Mate (Barnes-Hind)	cleaning, hydrocurve	hydroxyethylcellulose	edetate disodium, 0.2% thimerosal, 0.004%	octoxynol sodium chloride

Dental Products

Robert L. Day

Questions to ask the patient

How long have you been aware of the problem?

Have you consulted a dentist about the condition?

How often do you brush your teeth?

Do you use dental floss or tape regularly?

Do your gums bleed when you brush or floss your teeth?

What kind of toothpaste do you use (regular; for sensitive teeth)?

What style toothbrush do you use (size; hard or soft bristles)?

(For denture wearers) What products do you use with your dentures (e.g., pastes, denture brush, soaking solutions, denture cushions, denture reliners)?

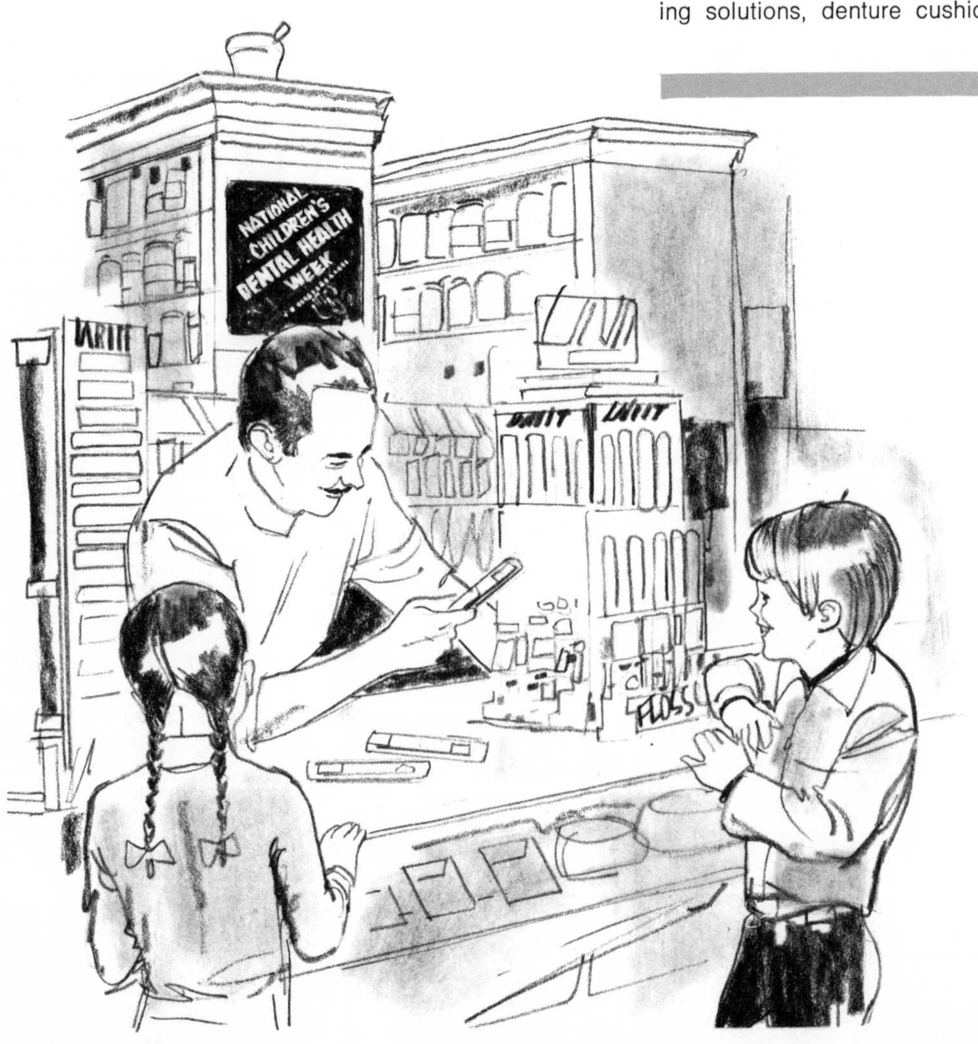

CHAPTER 22

It probably is safe to state that no scientist has ever bothered to compile statistics on the size (volume and surface area) of the average human mouth. So, unscientific as it may be, let us just admit that in contrast to the size and volume of the rest of the body, the mouth is quite small. From a disease/problem point of view, however, it is massive.

The mouth is a primary site for cancer, infection, malocclusion (faulty bite), bone resorption, caries, toothache, periodontal disease, dentures, canker sores, cold sores, and it serves as the major portal through which "bad breath" may be issued into the immediate environment. This small anatomical area has mobilized an army composed of 110,000 dentists (data from Bureau of Economic Research, American Dental Association) and untold numbers of dental assistants and dental hygienists. One need only to survey the dental products inventory of a pharmacy, a supermarket, or a variety store to gain the paraphrased impression that "never has so much been done for so little (an area)."

The mouth—an overview

For all of its faults, the mouth is a remarkable engineering feat. Considering their size, the muscles which activate the jaw are extremely powerful and are capable of delivering a biting pressure that can lift a weight of more than 100 pounds.[1] The salivary glands can spill out as much as 1 liter of saliva a day for the purpose of rinsing the mouth, facilitating swallowing, aiding digestion, neutralizing acidic materials, and holding certain microbes in check.[2] A variety of micro-organisms inhabit the oral cavity, including some of the "Big Ten" pathogens—but these usually are restrained by benign micro-organisms and other protective mechanisms.[3 4]

Anatomy of the tooth and supporting structures

Figure 1 shows a highly simplified cross section of a tooth and its surrounding structures. A tooth can be grossly divided into two areas: 1) the crown—the portion that extends above the gingiva (gums) and is coated with enamel, and 2) the root—the portion that extends below the gingiva into the socket, and is coated with cementum.

Enamel is a light-yellow material composed of calcium compounds (hydroxyapatite); it is the hardest material produced by the human body. Its major function is to resist the wear resulting from a lifetime of grinding hard and soft materials into swallowable particles which threaten neither the lungs nor the digestive tract. It is, therefore, thickest at the points where it comes in contact with foods or with other teeth. Encapsulated between the enamel and the cementum is another calcium-containing material called dentin. Dentin is pronounced yellow and comprises the bulk of the tooth. It is somewhat "softer" than enamel, but nevertheless is the second hardest material produced by the body. The innermost material of the tooth is called dental pulp, a fleshy material consisting mainly of connective tissue, arteries, veins, lymphatics, and nerve endings.

Cementum, which is somewhat softer than human bone, is of major importance because it is the material to which thousands of strong fibers from the periodontal ligament (sometimes called periodontal membrane) attach and thereby hold the tooth in place. Although a varying number of these fibers will detach during normal chewing (or as a result of injury or orthodontic procedures), this is seldom a concern because the cementum constantly regenerates and the fibers will reattach. The root of a normal tooth does not directly attach to the alveolar bone of the jaw; it is attached only by means of the periodontal fibers. The bone serves as a neatly tailored receptacle which, if angered, will withdraw and say "goodbye forever" to the tooth.

Of interest also is the gingiva (or gums) which, in their healthy state, extend above the point where the cementum ends and the enamel begins (the cemento-enamel junction). Collectively, the cementum, the alveolar bone, the periodontal ligament, the gingiva, and the dento-gingival junction (epithelial attachment and connective tissue) are referred to as the periodontium.

Pathophysiology

Plaque, the tooth fairy's friend

Ask almost any person what the number one dental problem is, and you will be told that it is tooth decay (dental caries, or cavities) because, if the decay process is not arrested, the tooth may be lost through disintegration or extraction. Tooth loss, however, is not always related to tooth decay. In fact, beyond a particular age (34 for males, 39 for females) periodontal disease accounts for two to three times as many extractions as dental decay.[5] Although these figures might lead one to believe that periodontal disease is solely a problem of the mature adult, it strikes young and old, although its prevalence and severity increase with age.[6-8] Regardless of the problem—caries or periodontal disease—one factor, dental plaque, has been indisputably linked to both.[9-16] Plaque, therefore, must be considered to be the number one dental problem.

Plaque is a tenacious, soft deposit which forms over the tooth surface and consists chiefly of bacteria and bacterial products.[17] It begins to form within minutes of the time a tooth is cleaned, professionally or otherwise. As a first step, a film composed of salivary protein is deposited which shortly becomes insoluble, to form what is called the "acquired pellicle."[2 18] Following this, micro-organisms (chiefly *Streptococcus mutans* and *S. sanguis*) adhere to the pellicle and begin to multiply.[2] Eventually, these are glued together by dextrans, glycoproteins, etc. The process continues, and plaque has been formed.

If the conditions are right, dental plaque may slowly evolve into a hard, calcified material called dental calculus. Although there are many theories concerning its formation (e.g., calcium salts from the saliva impregnate plaque and are precipitated, or the enzyme enterase may initiate calcification by hydrolyzing fatty esters into fatty acids), some researchers do not believe that dental calculus (tartar) is a primary or essential factor in the etiology of periodontal disease. Nevertheless, its removal is considered advisable.[19]

Dental caries

Dental caries (cavities) are formed when "sugar" diffuses into the plaque and is metabolized by resident micro-organisms into acids which, over a period of time, erode the enamel of the tooth.

Sugars. If the human diet were devoid of sugar (or various sugar-forming carbohydrates), there would probably be no such thing as dental caries because some studies have revealed that a reduction of sugar intake corresponds with a reduction in caries rate.[20 21] Unfortunately, the human diet relies upon the intake of carbohydrates, and some attention has been directed toward identifying the biggest villains. Sucrose is probably the most cariogenic of the sugars, followed by fructose, lactose, and glucose.[22] On a different scale, one investigator identifies sucrose as the major dietary cariogenic factor, and starch as the least cariogenic.[23] Sticky sources appear to cause more caries than liquid sources, and frequency of eating appears to have an effect as well.[24-26] One study, for example, reveals that 10 g of caramel (obviously sticky) eaten four times a day will—over a period of time—give rise to twice as many caries as 20 g of caramel eaten twice a day.[27] Chewing gum is also an excellent source of sugar and, as might be expected, has been implicated in at least one study as a causative factor in increased caries rate.[28] For reasons such as these, many chewing gum manufacturers openly cite the fact that their product is sugarless. However, there is room for controversy in the affairs of the gum chewing world: one well-controlled study showed that a group of children chewing a sugared gum (Wrigley's Spearmint) did not have a significantly higher incidence of dental caries than the non-gum-chewing group.[29]

Regardless, the message conveyed by the vast majority of all studies is quite clear: caries correlate well with sugar intake.

Plaque. Plaque is an insidious material for a number of reasons. First, it is the home of the acid-producing micro-organisms (perhaps *S. mutans* and lactobacilli).[17 30] Secondly, its structure may actually hold the produced acids in contact with the tooth surface. Its thickness is somewhat important, therefore, because it is directly related to the amount of microbes present; the more microbes, the faster that acid is produced. Also, the thicker the plaque, the slower the diffusion of the acid out of the plaque.[2] Although lactic acid usually is identified as the offender, pyruvic, acetic, proprionic, and butyric acids have been detected as well.[31]

The tooth. One of the greatest enigmas in dental science is the fickle nature of caries. Some individuals have plaque-laden teeth, yet seldom develop caries. This phenomenon may be explained partially by nutrition because the resistance of a tooth to decay may be affected by nutrients (notably calcium, phosphorus, vitamin D, fluoride, and protein) at the time the tooth is forming and erupting.[24] This theory does not exactly explain why different teeth in the same mouth undergo varying decay rates. It may have something to do with the fact that some plaque is cariogenic, and some is not; the nutritional state which existed at the time each tooth was forming and erupting was different for different teeth; that some teeth, because of their location, have greater exposure to the rinsing action of saliva or the bristles of a toothbrush; or all of these factors.[2 24] Whatever the cause, the matter awaits resolution.

Periodontal disease

As stated earlier, plaque is a source not only of caries but also of periodontal disease. The problem appears to start at the interface between the plaque and gingiva.[32] In the process of growth, plaque micro-organisms produce a wide variety of chemical substances that appear to be capable of inciting gingival inflammation (the gingiva become red and swollen). Within the gingiva, the inflammation results in the localization of a battalion of biochemicals that may destroy the host tissues at the same time they are destroying invading bacteria. After many months and years, the fibers making up the structural framework of the gingiva and the periodontal fibers that hold the tooth in place—as well as the supporting alveolar bone itself—begin to melt away. As a result, the tooth becomes loose in its socket and eventually may be lost.[33-37]

There are still some unanswered questions. Why, for example, do the extent and severity of periodontal disease increase with age? It has been noted that in individuals over age 75, advanced tissue destruction is apparent in 50 to 60 percent of the patients.[38] (Is this due to an accumulation of effects over a period of years, or to another unidentified factor?) What role does nutrition play?[39-41] Numerous studies and statements will leave this question unanswered, although vitamin C and multivitamins do not appear to be effective in the treatment of the active disease.[23 24 42 43]

Until such time as the etiology of the disease is better understood (and maybe not even then), the major thrust of treatment will continue to be directed at minimizing (or eliminating) the most visible and accessible portion of the periodontal puzzle: dental plaque. It has been demonstrated that lack of oral hygiene (brushing, etc.) accelerates periodontal disease and that programs aimed at the improvement of oral hygiene can slow its progress.[10 44-47]

Plaque removal

Toothbrushing technique

Toothbrushing has been shown to be effective in minimizing the progression of periodontal disease perhaps because of the simple removal of plaque and perhaps for other reasons.[45] The question is how should one brush? There are at least two schools of thought on toothbrushing technique. One advocates the horizontal (scrub) method, where the brush is moved back and forth horizontally with a scrubbing motion, covering segments of two or more teeth at a time. The other advocates the vertical (roll) method in which the brush is rotated up and down, brushing upper and lower teeth with the same sweep.

Although there have been a considerable number of studies that compare the plaque-removing abilities of each method, and the horizontal method has continually been declared the winner, one well-controlled study noted that there was no substantial difference between the two.[48-53] In an election, a ratio of five votes to one would win—scientific issues, however, are not always decided on the basis of popularity. In evaluating the studies in which the horizontal method appeared to be the better method, the variability between the scientific methods becomes apparent immediately. Patient instruction varied from study to study. Specific technique varied, and in some cases trained professionals were used to brush the patients' teeth. Therefore, the results of these comparative studies are inconclusive and, in the long run, it is highly probable that specific brushing technique (horizontal or vertical) does not matter as much as the thoroughness of brushing.[54]

How often should the teeth be brushed? Once a day, twice a day, or more? From a periodontal disease point of view, one large study showed that twice-a-day brushing is no better than once-a-day brushing, and that neither is better than brushing every other day.[55] However, one dental authority cautions that, although complete removal of plaque every second day may be compatible with good periodontal health, it is not known if this interval is sufficient for the control of caries.[56] Until further information is forthcoming, it is perhaps best to advise careful and thorough brushing at least twice a day, preferably after meals.

Manual toothbrushes. The dental literature abounds with short and lengthy studies on the pros and cons of various types of toothbrushes (and bristles) with regard to their relative plaque-removing ability and their ability to control periodontal disease.[57-65] Based on research to date, no specific toothbrush can be recommended as superior for all persons.[66] The reason for this not-very-helpful statement is that a number of variables will influence the results of any study that attempts to evaluate toothbrushes, including bristle size and shape, the brushing method used, and the motivation of the patient. The Council on Dental Therapeutics of the American Dental Association has recognized this by noting that "The type of toothbrushes to be selected may depend to some extent on the method of toothbrushing to be employed and on the specific anatomic and manipulative skills of the individual. It must therefore conform to individual requirements in size, shape and texture." [66] There are some practical considerations that appear between the lines of this statement. It makes little sense to recommend a large, long-bristled toothbrush for a small mouth. The angles of the mouth are not square, and therefore, toothbrushes with sharp angles should be avoided because they might injure the mucosa. In addition, natural bristles do not wear as well as synthetic bristles, and "hard" bristles are stiff, do not easily reach the plaque that has collected below the gingiva, and can actually mutilate the gums in the process.[67 68]

Powered toothbrushes. The 1960's may well have earned themselves the title of "The Age of Electrical Gadgetry," for it was then that all sorts of manually operated devices became motorized. Parents, for example, learned that certain toys were immobile unless short-lived and expensive batteries were installed. A seemingly endless parade of electrified devices spilled onto the marketplace including electric shot glasses, electric manicure sets, electric swizzle sticks, electric backscratchers, and yes, the electric toothbrush. It was tempting to group all of these byproducts of vivid marketing imagination into one category: gimmicks for the affluent or the lazy (or both). Time, however, has shown that the electric toothbrush does not belong to this group; it is an effective and efficient cleaning device.[69-84]

As might be expected, electric toothbrushes have been developed which attempt to mimic the bristle movement of one of the manual methods. They are available with arcuate action (up and down movement), reciprocating action (back and forth movement), combined (dual) arcuate and reciprocating action, or rotating action. There is no conclusive evidence that any one "action" is better than another, probably because no powered toothbrush can realistically duplicate the actions of a manual procedure and, as stated earlier, there is no conclusive evidence that any one manual method (or action) is superior to another.[54 85] The Council on Dental Therapeutics questions whether the electric toothbrush is superior to the manual toothbrush.[86] Nevertheless, the electric toothbrush is an effective cleaning device which, because of its sheer novelty (it buzzes and hums), may motivate a child or even an adult to brush regularly. It is, without question, of greatest benefit to the mentally or physically disadvantaged who are incapable of properly brushing their teeth manually.[74 76]

As of January 1, 1975, the Council classified the following powered toothbrushes as "Acceptable": Broxident Automatic; General Electric Automatic (arcuate, reciprocating, or dual; corded); J. C. Penney Automatic (dual); Presto Cordless Automatic; Sunbeam Cordless Hygienic; and Touch Tronic.[87]

Dentifrices. All dentifrices—powders, pastes, and gels—contain at least four types of ingredients: abrasives, surface-active agents, flavoring agents, and sweetening agents.

A wide variety of abrasives is used, including dibasic calcium phosphate, insoluble sodium metaphosphate, calcium pyrophospate, calcium orthophosphate, calcium carbonate, magnesium carbonate, hydrated aluminum oxides, silicates, and silica gels.[88]

The most commonly used surface-active agents are sodium lauryl sulfate and sodium *N*-lauroyl sarcosinate. At one time, the latter agent was claimed by the manufacturers of Colgate Toothpaste (nonfluoride) to have anticaries activity (the "Invisible Shield"). At least one large study has shown that it is no better in caries control than a dentifrice containing another surface-active agent.[89]

Flavoring agents are used in the various products and are significant only as far as individual taste preferences. A few allergic responses to a cinnamon-flavored dentifrice (Close-up) have been noted in Great Britain.[90]

Saccharin is the most commonly used sweetening agent, if only because dental authorities discourage the use of sugar-containing dentifrices.[88]

Pastes differ from powder dentifrices in that they contain thickening agents (tragacanth, karaya, sodium alginate, methylcellulose, carboxymethylcellulose sodium, bentonite, aluminum magnesium silicate), humectants (sorbitol, glycerin, propylene glycol), and water, in addition to the previously listed ingredients.

The decision as to which of the many nonfluoride dentifrices should be recommended is seldom a crucial one. Some products are more abrasive than others—indeed, so-called tooth "whitening" or "brightening" products simply are dentifrices that contain harsher abrasives.[88] These products probably should not be recommended for persons with exposed cementum or dentin or for those who have had tooth surfaces restored with synthetic materials.[88]

The Council on Dental Therapeutics notes that it is unlikely that significant amounts of dental enamel will be lost by "judicious" use of most of the available dentifrices, but adds that there appears "to be no valid reason for the use of a dentifrice of greater abrasiveness than is necessary to prevent residual accumulation on the teeth." [88] The term "judicious" suggests that highly abrasive products should not be used by persons who brush their teeth harshly for relatively long periods. At least two researchers have questioned whether nonfluoride dentifrices have any effect in reducing the rate of caries formation.[91 92]

Dentifrices with fluorides. There is an overwhelming amount of evidence to indicate that routine use of dentifrices that contain either sodium monofluorophosphate or stannous fluoride will significantly reduce the rate of caries formation (between 17 and 34 percent) in young and old alike even in regions where the local water supply is fluoridated.[92-116] Neither ingredient has been shown conclusively to be superior.[99 100] Although some dentifrices also contain sodium fluoride, the topical efficacy of these products is still questionable.[117-121] Early investigations of sodium fluoride dentifrices have inconclusive results, and perhaps this is the reason why the Council on Dental Therapeutics considers this ingredient "Unacceptable." [117-119] Later evidence suggests, however, that the "inefficacy" of products containing sodium fluoride may be related to incompatibilities of sodium fluoride with other dentifrice ingredients because subsequent formulation modifications result in products that reduce the incidence of caries.[114 120 121] The question of the efficacy of sodium fluoride, like other questions, awaits resolution.

Theory has it that, under given conditions, fluoride (in stannous fluoride or sodium monofluorophosphate dentifrices) reacts with hydroxyapatite (enamel substance) to form fluoroapatite and/or calcium fluoride, which renders the surface less soluble to the acids created by the plaque micro-organisms.[122-124] Regardless of the mechanism, the message is quite clear: fluoride dentifrices are undeniably superior to nonfluoride dentifrices and should be recommended whenever possible.

Dentifrices for sensitive teeth. Several dentifrices on the market are claimed to be effective in the treatment of sensitive teeth (those that register pain upon exposure to certain stimuli, e.g., heat, cold, sugar). One of these products (Thermodent) contains formaldehyde (1.4 percent) and has been the subject of several published studies, all of which are best summarized by the 1973 statement of the Council on Dental Therapeutics that although ". . . formaldehyde solution has been used for relieving pain due to hypersensitive dentin . . . its effectiveness in a dentifrice for desensitizing has not been established." [125-129] Prior to 1976, the Council classified Thermodent as "Unacceptable." [119]

Another product, Sensodyne, contains strontium nitrate (10 percent) and has also been the subject of a number of studies, some of which are uncontrolled (therefore, unreliable) and some of which are controlled (i.e., Sensodyne compared to dentifrices not containing strontium nitrate).[130-138] None of the studies provide convincing evidence that Sensodyne is more effective than placebo dentifrices. In two of the aforementioned studies, a sodium monofluorophosphate dentifrice was superior or equivalent to Sensodyne in decreasing tooth sensitivity.[136 138] This effect is perhaps not very surprising because other observers have suggested that fluorides, in general, may be desensitizing agents.[139-142] [There have been other studies (although not totally reliable) that indicate that sodium monofluorophosphate dentifrices are desensitizing.[143-145]] If fluoride dentifrices match or exceed the desensitizing effect of Sensodyne, they—and not Sensodyne—would be the products of choice because Sensodyne does not have the demonstrated added anticaries activity of the fluoride dentifrices.

At least one uncontrolled study has suggested that a dentifrice containing potassium nitrate (10 percent) is also effective as a desensitizing agent.[146] No conclusions can be drawn.

Dental floss or tape? (waxed or unwaxed?)

A number of investigators and an increasing number of dentists have recommended the use of dental floss or tape for the removal of interdental (between the teeth) plaque—the general feeling being that a brush does not easily reach this area.[147-153] A patient is advised to hold approximately 18 inches of floss or tape firmly between the fingers and to insert it at each interdental area by gently sawing it back and forth until it slips through the contact point. It is then to be carried to slightly below the gingival margin (until resistance is met) and activated by moving it up and down the tooth surface to break up the accumulated plaque.[154]

Which is better, floss or tape? There is no evidence to indicate that one is superior to the other.[154] Should one use a waxed or unwaxed product? Some authorities have expressed preference for unwaxed floss.[148 150 152] Others have noted that it does not seem to make a difference whether a waxed or unwaxed product is used; the Council on Dental Materials and Devices of the American Dental Association agrees and has stated that there is no conclusive evidence that one form is superior to the other.[53 154 155] Until other evidence is presented, it appears that it is not so important which product is used (floss or tape; waxed or unwaxed), as long as one of them is used.[86]

There is some evidence to indicate that flossing skills are not automatically acquired and that patients who are simply told to use floss (or to follow the directions on the package) will receive only marginal benefits. One investigator, for example, has demonstrated that personalized instruction (one to one and/or use of visual aids) is necessary if maximum flossing proficiency is to be achieved.[156] Another author states that periodic reinstruction (for elementary school children) is a must if proper flossing habits are to be established.[157] Furthermore, overzealous or improper flossing can result in abrasion of the teeth or damage to the periodontal structures.[158 159] One authority points out that the interdental space in many young children with normal dentition is completely filled in with gingiva, and cautions that "[insertion of] floss or toothpicks will almost certainly result in damage to the junctional [attachment] epithelium." [160] A pharmacist can be of service if she or he will take the time to determine if a patient who purchases a flossing product actually knows how to use it. Assuming that she or he has received training from a dental hygienist or dentist, a pharmacist can instruct the patient or reinforce previously received instruction.

Toothpicks and rubber tips

There are numerous little devices on the market which are claimed to be useful for cleaning the interdental spaces or for massaging (stimulating) the gingiva. They are made from various materials, i.e., wood (toothpicks), balsa (Stimudent), flexible plastic (Pic-A-Dent), and rubber (Lactona or Pycopay tip). About the best that can be said about them all is that they are possibly beneficial in the removal of interdental plaque, although quite possibly no more beneficial than conscientious toothbrushing.[86 161] With regards to "gingival massage," it has not been shown that such treatment has anything whatsoever to do with the prevention or control of periodontal disease.[40 152] Toothpicks and rubber tips also are capable of damaging the interdental gingiva of children and probably are undesirable products for these individuals.[160]

Water jet devices

There are several different types of devices on the market that enable the user to direct a fine, high-velocity stream of water at the teeth for the purpose of dislodging relatively loose plaque. One type fits on a faucet and uses existing water pressure as its propelling force (e.g., Pulsar). Another contains a self-enclosed motor-driven pump (e.g., Water-Pik). Both appear to do the same job. There is some question, however, as to what job it is that they do. Various studies have been published which allude to the plaque-removing "effectiveness" of these devices, or their beneficial effects in the prevention or treatment of periodontal disease.[87 162-172] Although these studies vary in character and quality, several conclusions may be drawn. Water jet devices are not a replacement for a toothbrush—in fact, they appear to be incapable of removing very much plaque unless preceded by toothbrushing.[173] Furthermore, any suggestion that these devices are beneficial in the treatment or prevention of periodontal disease on the basis of their gingival stimulating "activity" is speculative because, as stated earlier, gum stimulation has not been shown to relate to the prevention or treatment of periodontal disease.[40 154 163]

Patients who purchase water jet devices should do so only on the advice of a dentist and should be carefully instructed in their use (or at the very least should be cautioned to carefully read the instructions for use) because careless or improper use can result in tissue damage.[174 175] The Council on Dental Materials and Devices considers the water jets to be useful only "as an adjunctive device to toothbrush and interdental cleaning agents . . ." and restricts the manufacturers of "Acceptable" products from making "any claim as to treatment or prevention of any oral disease . . ."[176] As of January 1, 1975, Dento Spray, Hydro Dent, and Pulsar have been classified as "Acceptable."[177] Water-Pik had been previously classified "Acceptable," but the manufacturer voluntarily withdrew the product from the Council's "acceptance" program.[178]

Plaque disclosing agents

Regardless of the device used to remove it, plaque is not readily apparent to the untrained eye. Significant amounts may remain behind following what the patient thought to be a conscientious, self-administered cleaning procedure (brushing, flossing, etc.). A number of materials, usually dyes, have been cited as being useful as plaque disclosing (revealing) agents, including iodine, merbromin, basic fuchsin, and erythrosine sodium (FD & C Red No. 3).[179-181] These materials are either painted on the teeth or chewed and are supposed to selectively stain the plaque. The resultant mess is so ghastly in appearance that one wants only to get it off. For this reason, these agents are considered to be useful not only in teaching proper cleaning technique, but also as suitable stimuli for the continuation of such behavior.[182]

Erythrosine sodium, the most commonly used agent in products for home use, is available as a chewable tablet from various manufacturers.[183] It is not an ideal material, however, because it does not differentiate the plaque at the gum margin as closely as might be desired.[182] Furthermore, it will stain the pellicle, the gums, the tongue, and the lips for many hours.[184 185] Such unsettling cosmetic disadvantages of these products have encouraged dental researchers to seek another disclosing agent.[185 186] Fluorescein sodium produces a plaque "stain" which becomes visible only when exposed to U.V. light. An obvious disadvantage is that a U.V. light source is required which raises certain safety questions (shock, eye damage, etc.).

Plaque removal—an overview

On the basis of the devices and products mentioned thus far, it is not too difficult for one to conjure up an image of erythrosine stained, fluoride lathered teeth being compulsively brushed up and down and back and forth, then flossed, then toothpicked, then rubber pronged, then water jetted in a frenzied search for everlasting periodontal happiness. A logical question follows: how much is too much (or too little)? Isn't for example, flossing really enough in addition to toothbrushing? The question is not as easy to answer as it appears—if only because of the widespread controversy cited in nearly every one of the preceding sections. It may be that flossing in addition to toothbrushing is enough for some but not for others. It may be that thorough cleaning has not so much to do with the material (*the* brush, *the* floss, *the* toothpick, etc.), but with *the* person. A term constantly encountered throughout the dental literature is "patient motivation"; if a patient

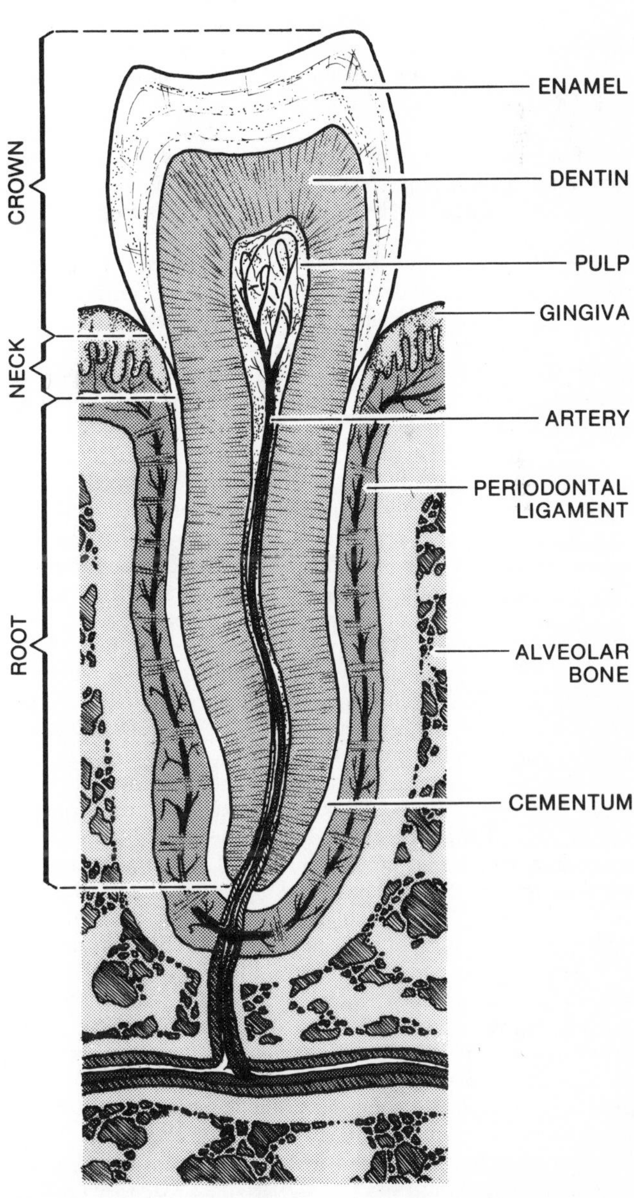

Figure 1. Anatomy of the tooth and its environment.

isn't motivated, the most bizarre collection of devices and materials will fail to affect caries or periodontal disease.[176 187-189] Perhaps there is a clue here. Perhaps an ordinary toothbrush is all that is necessary if it is propelled by a well-motivated hand. Perhaps the addition of floss (or another interdental cleaning material) forces the less motivated to make up for unmotivated brushing efforts.

No one denies that the majority of the plaque-removing gimmicks (yes, let us finally call them that) actually remove plaque; the question is: do they really contribute that much? Maybe they do, and will continue to do so until pharmacists, dental hygienists, dentists, and patients team up in an all-out effort to educate and thereby motivate the population to correct oral hygiene habits.

Products for toothache

Very few living persons will register surprise upon being told that a tooth that is chipped, cracked, or eroded by caries is capable of registering a rather high level of pain. Sometimes overlooked, however, is the fact that there are some serious conditions (e.g., impacted tooth infections, root canal infections) other than those listed above that are equally capable of causing pain and that may be confused with simple toothache. These may or may not be attended by an increase in body temperature.

For reasons such as these, it is always advisable to question a patient requesting a toothache product as to the nature and source of the pain. Is it truly caused by an exposed caries? Is it actually originating from a tooth—as opposed to the gums? Beyond that, a patient should be encouraged to see a dentist without delay. If one is not immediately available, some relief may be obtained through use of a toothache product if the offender is an exposed caries. The patient should be advised that the pain response is, in all probability, due to a problem which may continue even if the pain is relieved.

Eugenol (clove oil). Eugenol is a common ingredient of toothache drops. It has been described as a germicide, and it is not known if its action is due to an anesthetic effect *per se* or the fact that it is an irritant.[190] Other products that contain demonstrated anesthetics (benzocaine, butacaine sulfate) may be helpful if the pain site is exposed and/or accessible to penetration of the active ingredient(s). One product, Poloris Poultice, has not been shown to be effective when compared to a placebo poultice and has been declared "Unacceptable" by the Council on Dental Therapeutics.[119 191 192] (Dent's Dental Poultice has a similar composition.)

Aspirin. Aspirin may also be helpful, but only if taken internally. It should never be packed into a caries site or tucked into the cheek beside the cavity because it is an acid which can erode the enamel, traumatize nerve endings, or burn the oral mucosa.[193 194] This, coupled with the fact that aspirin has no demonstrated topical activity, makes the procedure, at best, an exercise in self-destruction.

Teething products. Teething lotions basically are toothache preparations traveling under another name. Indeed, many products list the dual use. Teething pain originates for the most part in the area below the gum surface and is caused by the cutting action of a tooth as it is erupting. A topically applied anesthetic cannot realistically be expected to penetrate to the source of the pain. This, and the fact that anesthetics are potential sensitizers, suggests that they should not be used at all. Frozen or cooled teething rings have not been evaluated in the literature.[195]

Denture products

It is a little known fact (and maybe it is just as well) that as the Duke of Wellington rode into history at Waterloo, he wore a full set of dentures.[196] This seemingly insignificant piece of trivia might have altered the course of British history had the Duke not assumed command because of his Royal connections. Had he attempted to rise through the ranks, he would never have made it because soldiers were required to have their own teeth to bite open the packets containing shot. Although dentures were not common in those days, it is estimated that more than 37 million U.S. citizens now wear full or partial dentures.[197]

Dentures, from the day they are installed, create a number of problems for the wearer. Speech is affected, although individuals readily adjust. Sneezing, coughing, or athletic exercise may dislodge dentures at inopportune moments. Dentures need to be cleaned differently from teeth, and may be the cause of a TV phenomenon called "denture breath." The greatest problem is that dentures almost never live up to patient expectations.[198] The patient instantly learns that new chewing habits must be established because dentures in no way match the flexibility of the natural chewing process. Some, perhaps many, patients may resist or may confuse these difficulties with the "fit" of the denture and may seek the assistance of products that are claimed to hold the dentures in place.

Denture adhesives

It should be understood at the outset that the Council on Dental Materials and Devices is not particularly enamored with the casual use of denture adhesives. Although it agrees that, subject to "continued professional scrutiny," such products may be effective for patients with flat ridges, elderly patients, cleft palate patients, or post-cancer prostheses, they are particularly critical of self-treatment, feeling that denture adhesives:

- ☐ Encourage the patient to wear dentures which should be adjusted, rebased, or reconstructed.
- ☐ Create false retention, thereby discouraging the development of habits that keep the denture in place.
- ☐ May be excessively used, causing uneven support which may accelerate alveolar bone resorption and may make the construction of new dentures very difficult due to lack of supporting bone structures.[176]

There is some evidence that denture adhesives do not work as well for newly fitted dentures as they do for older, distorted dentures—a somewhat ominous correlation—because, as stated, unevenly fitted dentures may lead to destruction of the bone they rely upon for support.[199] It would be advisable for the pharmacist to ascertain if a patient requesting a denture adhesive product is doing so at the direction of, or under the supervision of, a dentist. If not, the patient should be encouraged to see a dentist immediately for denture readjustment or refitting.

Denture adhesive powders usually contain karaya or another water-soluble gum such as cellulose derivatives or polymers of ethylene oxide. Denture adhesive pastes also contain petrolatum. There is no evidence that one form is superior to the other.[176] The Council on Dental Materials and Devices has placed a number of dental adhesives in its "Acceptable" category, but requires as a condition of acceptance that the manufacturers publish the following message on the trade package: "(Name of Product) is acceptable as a temporary measure to provide increased retention of dentures. However, an ill-fitting denture may impair your health—consult your dentist for periodic examination." [176]

Denture reliners and cushions

A number of patients, feeling perhaps that their dentures are not fitting well or are causing irritation, will resort to the use of denture reliners or cushions; they do so at great risk. A series of articles has appeared in the dental and medical literature pointing out that long-term use of such products will distort dentures, causing bite problems and jaw-joint pain.[200-210] Furthermore, an unevenly fitting denture will cause excessive pressure in many areas of the jaw bone, resulting in eventual bone resorption, and in some cases may actually obliterate the ridge of bone upon which the denture rests. If this should happen, some drastic and expensive dental procedures will be required to remedy the situation. The following products were specifically cited in the aforementioned studies: Cushion Grip, Dentyte, Ezo Dento Cushions, and Brimms' Plasti-Liner.

One investigator has stated that anyone who finds it ncessary to use an OTC denture reliner actually needs new dentures, and that these products should be totally discouraged, perhaps by making them prescription-only items.[206] To discourage the home use of reliners, etc., the Bureau of Dental Health Education of the American Dental Association has published a consumer pamphlet entitled, "Don't Do It Yourself." The Food and Drug Administration (FDA) now requires that the following labeling appear on denture reliners, pads, and cushions: "Warning. For temporary use only. Long-term use of this product may lead to faster bone loss, continuing irritation, sores, and tumors. For use only until a dentist can be seen." [211]

Denture repair kits

A denture repair kit is another potentially dangerous OTC denture accessory. Composed of special glues and supporting materials, these items are indicated as useful in the repair of cracked or broken dentures. Winter,[209] however, noted that careful measurements by skilled professionals are required to properly align a new denture, and points out that home-repaired dentures are always misaligned, a factor leading to poor fit and bone resorption. If items such as these are to be sold, the pharmacist should caution the patient that these products are for temporary (e.g., over the weekend) repairs only and should make certain that the patient fully understands the meaning of the following message which FDA requires be published on the kit label: "Warning. For emergency repairs only. Long-term use of home-repaired dentures may cause faster bone loss, continuing irritation, sores, and tumors. See your dentist without delay." [211]

Denture cleansers

Although dentures are usually made of acrylic resins, they do collect plaque, calculus, and stains. A series of different types of products has been developed to clean these appliances.

Soaking solutions. It generally is recommended that dentures be removed at least 8 hours a day to permit the gums to "rest." [198] Because patients with dentures usually will elect to do this at night, this also provides them with a convenient time to clean their dentures in a soaking solution. These products contain ingredients such as surface-active agents, alkaline perborates and peroxides (oxygen generating), alkaline hypochlorites (bleaches) and chelating agents. In one study involving 546 persons, there was no general agreement as to which product was best.[212] This perhaps is explained by the results of a study cited by Beck [197] in which 11 soak-type cleansers were tested and only one, a sodium hypochlorite–tribasic sodium phosphate solution, removed all of the daily accumulation of plaque after a 9-hour soaking. Results such as these do not reflect favorably on those various advertisements for soak-type preparations that infer that dentures can be cleaned rapidly. This study also supports the statement of the Council on Dental Materials and Devices that a denture brush "is an essential instrument" for the cleaning of a denture.[176] In other words, a patient who purchases a commercial soak-type preparation should be informed that the dentures should be immersed at least overnight, and they also should be scrubbed with a denture brush.

Mechanical cleaning devices. There are a number of electrically powered devices on the market that agitate soaking solutions and therefore—in theory—efficiently clean the denture. The simplest of these is the type that vibrates and, although some representatives of this class have ultrasonic sounding names (Prosonic, Sonak), they are not ultrasonic. Then, there's the magnetic stirring device (Sonic Action, Whirlpool Action, Whirl-A-Dent), and finally, some truly ultrasonic devices (Branson Ultrasonic, E/MC Ultrasonic, Shick Ultrasonic). In evaluating these devices, the Council on Dental Materials and Devices has ranked the ultrasonic as first, the magnetic stirrers as second, followed by the vibrating type.[176] They are, however, somewhat unenthusiastic as revealed by their comment that mechanical cleaners are only "slightly more effective" than the soak solution alone and their additional observation that none of these devices can remove all stain and debris from the denture without some brushing.[176]

Denture brushes and pastes. A denture brush is larger than an ordinary toothbrush, and ideally, should conform with the contour of the denture. As stated earlier, the denture brush is indispensable if the patient wishes to have thoroughly cleaned dentures. Denture cleaning pastes are similar to ordinary dentifrices in almost every regard, except that extremely abrasive materials are avoided. Generally speaking, denture wearers should be cautioned against using regular dentifrices because such products may etch the surfaces of the acrylic resins used in making the dentures.

Mouthwashes

OTC mouthwashes basically are dilute solutions of aromatic substances which may be sweetened with saccharin and colored with hues selected from the rainbow. They also may contain ethanol and astringents (e.g., zinc salts)—neither of which has any demonstrated efficacy. In addition, they may contain surface-active agents which do little more than foam and quaternary ammonium halides (antiseptic agents), which have no demonstrated ability to kill "germs" in the time span of the average gargle, and even if they could kill them under test tube conditions, would probably not be able to do so in the mouth because such agents are absorbed and partially deactivated by protein (e.g., oral mucosa, salivary protein).[2, 213, 214] Even if these ingredients could kill "germs" under conditions of use—there is no conclusive evidence to indicate that their slaughter would result in a positive contribution to oral health or treatment of systemic disease.[185, 213]

Furthermore, a survey of the literature of the last 30 years did not reveal an incident of a saved marriage, an improved working relationship, that second kiss, or evidence that onion eaters are better loved on crowded buses following a gargle in time. However, mouthwashes are fairly popular and as such are "living" testimonials to the impact of those advertisements which have made the populace "bad breath" conscious.

What about good old offensive, socially debilitating "bad breath"? It can be godawful in the morning because various foodstuffs, decaying protein, etc., have had the opportunity to stew overnight—but this is one time when one brushes his or her teeth and it should be kept in mind that dentifrices contain sweet-smelling substances that instantly manufacture an inexpensive "mouthwash" during the brushing process. During the day the lungs may also contribute their first share to "bad" breath—especially following smoking or an onion and/or garlic meal (or as a result of some systemic disease process)—but this odor may not necessarily be masked by the pleasant odor the expired lung air will pick up while transversing through the mouthwashed mouth.[215] In the long run, mouthwashes make little sense when contrasted to toothpastes, if only because toothbrushing—although it leaves the breath "kissing sweet"—also provides protection against caries (assuming that a fluoride dentifrice is used) and periodontal disease. OTC mouthwashes do not.[161 185 213] Experimental fluoride rinses may have anticaries activity, and chlorhexidine gluconate rinses appear to prevent plaque formation.[56 216-219]

Oral ulcers

The mouth and the lips are sites for a number of major ulcerations of different etiology, some of which are cancerous. As a general rule, any patient exhibiting an oral ulcer which persists for 3 weeks or more should be dispatched to a dentist. OTC products are available for only three types of ulcers: herpes labialis, recurrent intraoral herpes, and recurrent aphthous stomatitis.

Herpes labialis. Do not be alarmed if you do not recognize the term. It has many names, including herpes facialis, fever blister, cold sore. It is caused by herpes simplex virus, more formally classified as *Herpesvirus hominis,* and appears—after being announced by a burning sensation—on the lips as a small red papule which quickly turns into a vesicle (blister).[220 221] The vesicles usually appear in groups, usually fill with pus and usually rupture, forming shallow ulcers with a yellow crust. The process subsides within a few days and healing usually proceeds without scarring in 7 to 14 days. These lesions may appear in only a small area of the lip, or may involve the whole lip. Concurrent lesions may appear on the skin around the nostrils or the chin.[222]

Recurrent intraoral herpes. Also caused by herpes simplex, these lesions appear most commonly on the hard palate, the alveolar ridges, or the attached gingiva. They appear less commonly on the mucosa of the cheek and lips. They follow the same pattern as herpes labialis (i.e., burning sensation-vesicle-rupture) except that the lesion formed has a red center.[222]

Recurrent aphthous stomatitis. Science has a way with words, and lay people have a way of doing away with them. Lesions that clinicians may call recurrent aphthous stomatitis, aphthous ulcers, or recurrent oral aphthae are called canker sores by the public. Although it is not known what causes a canker sore, herpes simplex has been ruled out.[221-223] A canker sore is perhaps the most common of oral lesions, and it can arise on the mucosa of the cheeks and lips, the tongue, or on the soft palate.[222] It starts as a small raised, whitish papule which eventually ulcerates.[224 225] The lesion that forms may have a yellow or gray center bordered by an erythematous halo. It heals in 10 to 14 days without scarring.

Treatment of oral ulcers

Lotions. There are a few "specialized" liquid products for oral ulcers which may contain astringents, anesthetics, menthol, camphor, or benzoin. (The labels of most toothache products also suggest that they are helpful for cold sores and canker sores.) These products have not been evaluated in the literature and, therefore, nothing positive can be said of their efficacy.

Silver nitrate. Silver nitrate in various forms occasionally is used to cauterize lesions inside the mouth but is seldom used outside because it causes a black stain; it is specifically contraindicated for herpes labialis.[226] There is no evidence that this product is useful. In fact, application of an excessive amount can lead to severe irritation of the surrounding mucosa.[193] A careless patient will discover that silver nitrate also has the ability to stain the teeth.

Orabase and denture adhesives. It is likely that some of the pain associated with an oral lesion arises from the simple mechanical irritation of a tooth (or adjacent tissue) rubbing against it. Orabase or an ordinary denture adhesive may be helpful.[226] Both products firmly adhere to the lesion, forming a protective coat with a slippery outer layer. Theoretically, the friction between the lesion and the offending structure is diminished.

Lactobacillus preparations. There are at least two products on the market that contain viable strains of *Lactobacillus acidophilus* and *L. bulgaricus* and that have, at one time or another, been claimed by their manufacturers to be useful in the treatment of cold sores or canker sores.[227] Although the manufacturer of one of these products (Bacid) appears to have discontinued such claims, the manufacturer of Lactinex still claims that the product "has been found to be useful in the treatment of . . . acute fever blisters and canker sores of herpetic origin."[228 229] The latter portion of this claim ("canker sores of herpetic origin") is extremely interesting in light of the fact that these lesions are not caused by herpes.[221 222] In addition, these claims of usefulness appear to be based on four favorable reports which have appeared in the literature, all of which involved small numbers of patients (ranging from 6 to 46) and all of which were uncontrolled studies (no placebo used, no comparison to an untreated group).[230-233] One investigator actually biased patients by telling them that they were being given the product in the "hope that [it] would clear up or at least lessen the discomfort caused by their oral lesions."[233] Until such time as well-designed, controlled studies are undertaken, usefulness claims for *Lactobacillus* preparations are mere speculation. The Council on Dental Therapeutics has stated that therapeutic usefulness of these products has not been established.[227]

Summary

If there is anything to be learned from reading (and hopefully studying) the material contained within this chapter, it is that dental products—like many other OTC products—are subject to quackery and controversy as well as demonstrated proof of efficacy. Although the reader may not have heard it all here first, a good question is "Where are you going to hear it the next time?" In other words, although the products mentioned in this chapter are sold primarily through pharmacies, the majority of the studies that pick them apart appear in the dental, not pharmaceutical, literature. Even then, there is the lingo used in the dental literature (DMFT, DMFS, Plaque Index, Incremental Caries Scores, etc.) which is not easily understood. If there is a desire on the part of the reader to continue her or his education in the affairs of the subject matter of this chapter, one way of resolving this impasse might be to stimulate the local pharmaceutical association to form a liaison with the local dental unit for the purpose of mutual education and action. As a good beginning every pharmacy in the nation could benefit by the addition to the pharmacy library of current editions of *Accepted Dental Therapeutics* and *Guide to Dental Materials and Devices.*

References

1. M. Klatsky, *J. Dent. Res.,* **21,** 389(1942).
2. I. D. Mandel, *J. Dent. Res.,* **53,** 246(1974).
3. E. Jawetz *et al.,* "Review of Medical Microbiology," 11th ed., Lange Medical Publications, Los Altos, Calif., 1974, p. 256.
4. R. C. Darlington, in "Handbook of Non-Prescription Drugs," American Pharmaceutical Association, Washington, D.C., 1973, pp. 62-76.
5. Bureau of Economic Research and Statistics, *J. Am. Dent. Assoc.,* **46,** 200(1953).
6. P. N. Baer and S. D. Benjamin, "Periodontal Disease in Children and Adolescents," Lippincott, Philadelphia, Pa., 1974.
7. A. L. Russell, *Int. Dent. J.,* **17,** 282(1967).
8. G. C. Hansen, *J. Periodontol.,* **44,** 269(1973).
9. H. V. Jordan and P. H. Keyes, *Arch. Oral Biol.,* **9,** 401(1964).
10. H. E. Löe *et al., J. Periodontol,* **36,** 177(1965).
11. "Periodontal Disease: Report of An Expert Committee on Dental Health," *WHO Tech. Rep. Ser.,* **207,** 10(1961).
12. M. M. Ash *et al., J. Periodontol.,* **35,** 424(1964).
13. I. D. Mandel, *J. Periodontol.,* **37,** 537(1966).
14. F. J. Orland *et al., J. Dent. Res.,* **33,** 147(1954).
15. R. J. Fitzgerald and P. H. Keyes, *J. Am. Dent. Assoc.,* **61,** 9(1960).
16. "Thos' Oral Pathology," R. J. Gorlin and H. M. Goldman, Eds., Mosby, St. Louis, Mo., 1970, p. 283.
17. Council on Dental Therapeutics, "Accepted Dental Therapeutics," American Dental Association, Chicago, Ill., 1973, p. 228.
18. I. D. Mandel, *Ala. J. Med. Sci.,* **5,** 313(1968).
19. J. F. Prichard, "Advanced Peridontal Disease," 2d ed., Saunders, Philadelphia, Pa., 1972, pp. 6-10.
20. H. Becks *et al., J. Am. Dent. Assoc.,* **31,** 189(1944).
21. P. Jay, *Am. J. Orthod. Oral Surg.,* **33,** 162(1947).
22. R. G. Campbell and D. D. Zinner, *J. Nutr.,* **100,** 11(1970).
23. L. D. McBean and E. W. Speckmann, *J. Am. Dent. Assoc.,* **89,** 109(1974).
24. A. E. Nizel, "Nutrition in Preventive Dentistry: Science and Practice," Saunders, Philadelphia, Pa., 1972.
25. A. E. Nizel, *World Rev. Nutr. Diet.,* **16,** 25(1973).
26. A. D. Steinberg *et al., J. Am. Dent. Assoc.,* **85,** 81(1972).
27. B. E. Gustafsson *et al., Acta. Odontol. Scand.,* **11,** 232(1952).
28. S. B. Finn and H. C. Jamison, *J. Am. Dent. Assoc.,* **74,** 987(1967).
29. G. L. Slack *et al., Br. Dent. J.,* **133,** 371(1972).
30. D. H. Bowen, *Arch. Dis. Child,* **47,** 849(1972).
31. D. A. M. Geddes, *Arch. Oral Biol.,* **17,** 537(1972).
32. A. A. Rizzo, *J. Am. Dent. Assoc. (Special Issue),* **87,** 1019(1973).
33. R. Snyderman, *J. Am. Dent. Assoc. (Special Issue),* **87,** 1020(1973).
34. P. Goldhaber *et al., J. Am. Dent. Assoc., (Special Issue),* **87,** 1027(1973).
35. D. C. Klein and L. G. Raisz, *Endocrinology,* **86,** 1436(1970).
36. J. M. Goodson *et al., J. Dent. Res. (Special Issue),* **52,** 496(1973).
37. D. L. Dreier, *J. Am. Dent. Assoc.,* **88,** 698(1974).
38. H. M. Goldman and D. W. Cohen, "Periodontal Therapy," Mosby, St. Louis, Mo., 1968, p. 66.
39. L. N. Peterson, *J. Appl. Nutr.,* **24,** 87(1972).
40. J. D. Suomi, *J. Am. Dent. Assoc.,* **83,** 1271(1971).
41. S. S. Stahl, *World Rev. Nutr. Diet,* **13,** 277(1971).
42. C. D. M. Day and L. Shouriek, *Indian J. Med. Res.,* **31,** 153(1953).
43. S. E. Keller *et al., J. Periodontol.* **34,** 259(1963).
44. D. R. Hoover, *J. Periodontol.,* **36,** 193(1965).
45. J. D. Suomi *et al., J. Periodontol.,* **42,** 152(1971).
46. A. Lovdal *et al., J. Am. Dent. Assoc.,* **56,** 21(1958).
47. J. C. Green, *Am. J. Public Health,* **53,** 913(1963).
48. D. B. McClure, *J. Dent. Child.,* **33,** 205(1966).
49. B. B. Kimmelman and G. C. Tassmann, *J. Dent. Child.,* **27,** 60(1960).
50. A. M. Frandsen *et al., Scand. J. Dent. Res.,* **78,** 459(1970).
51. F. Hansen and P. Gjermo, *Scand. J. Dent. Res.* **79,** 502-506(1971).
52. G. Sangnes *et al., J. Dent. Child.,* **39,** 94(1972).
53. T. J. O'Leary, *J. Periodontol.,* **41,** 625(1970).
54. Council on Dental Therapeutics, "Accepted Dental Therapeutics," American Dental Association, Chicago, Ill., 1973, p. 230.
55. J. Berenie *et al., J. Public Health Dent.,* **33,** 160(1973).
56. H. Löe, *J. Am. Dent. Assoc. (Special Issue),* **87,** 1034-1036(1973).
57. I. Hirschfeld, *J. Am. Dent. Assoc.,* **32,** 80(1945).
58. H. B. McCauley, *J. Am. Dent. Assoc.,* **33,** 283(1946).
59. A. O. Gruebbel and J. M. Wisan, *J. Am. Dent. Assoc.,* **37,** 346(1948).
60. J. M. Wisan and A. O. Gruebbel, *J. Am. Dent. Assoc.,* **38,** 19(1949).
61. C. G. Maurice and D. A. Wallace, *Ill. Dent. J.,* **26,** 286(1957).
62. I. Bay *et al., J. Periodontol.,* **36,** 526(1967).
63. C. M. Scully and A. B. Wade, *Dent. Pract. (Bristol),* **20,** 244(1970).
64. N. A. E. Robertson and A. B. Wade, *J. Periodontol. Res.* **7,** 346(1972).
65. I. Bay *et al., R. Soc. Health J.,* **92,** 218(1973).
66. Council on Dental Therapeutics, "Accepted Dental Therapeutics," American Dental Association, Chicago, Ill., 1973, p. 231.
67. A. B. Wade, *Br. Dent. J.,* **94,** 260(1953).
68. H. M. Goldman *et al.,* "Current Therapy in Dentistry," vol. 2, Mosby, St. Louis, Mo., 1967.
69. P. D. Toto and A. Franchione, *J. Periodontol.,* **32,** 249(1961).
70. N. W. Chilton *et al., J. Am. Dent. Assoc.,* **64,** 777(1962)
71. E. A. Phaneuf *et al., J. Am. Dent. Assoc.,* **65,** 12(1962).
72. D. R. Hoover *et al., J. Am. Dent. Assoc.,* **65,** 136(1962).
73. G. A. Quigley and J. W. Hein, *J. Am. Dent. Assoc.,* **65,** 26(1962).
74. A. Green *et al., J. Dent. Child.,* **29,** 169(1962).
75. W. Lefkowitz and H. B. G. Robinson, *J. Am. Dent. Assoc.,* **65,** 351(1962).
76. M. Kelner, *Pa. Dent. J.,* **30,** 102(1963).
77. P. M. Soparkar and G. A. Quigley, *J. Am. Dent. Assoc.,* **68,** 182(1964).
78. A. E. Iwersen *et al., J. Am. Dent. Assoc.,* **68,** 178(1964).
79. R. R. Lobene, *J. Periodontol.,* **35,** 137(1964).
80. W. A. Smith and M. M. Ash, Jr., *J. Periodontol.,* **35,** 127(1964).
81. J. C. Derbyshire *et al., J. Am. Dent. Assoc.,* **69,** 317(1964).
82. M. M. Ash, Jr. *et al., J. Am. Dent. Assoc.,* **69,** 317(1964).
83. C. M. Fraleigh, *J. Am. Dent. Assoc.,* **70,** 380(1965).
84. B. S. Chaikin *et al., Periodontics,* **3,** 200(1965).
85. Council on Dental Materials and Devices, "Guide to Dental Materials and Devices," 7th ed., American Dental Association, Chicago, Ill., 1974-75, p. 150.

86. Council on Dental Therapeutics, "Accepted Dental Therapeutics," American Dental Association, Chicago, Ill., 1973, p. 232.
87. O. P. Gupta *et al.*, *J. Periodontol.*, **44**, 294(1973).
88. Council on Dental Therapeutics, "Accepted Dental Therapeutics," American Dental Association, Chicago, Ill., 1973, p. 253.
89. W. A. Zacherl, *J. Dent. Child.*, **40**, 451(1973).
90. L. Millard, *J. Dent.*, **1**, 168(1970).
91. J. W. Dale, *Aust. Dent. J.*, **14**, 121(1969).
92. H. S. Horowitz *et al.*, *J. Am. Dent. Assoc.*, **72**, 408(1966).
93. E. A. Fanning *et al.*, *Aust. Dent. J.*, **13**, 201(1968).
94. M. N. Naylor and R. D. Emslie, *Br. Dent. J.*, **123**, 17(1967).
95. I. J. Moller *et al.*, *Br. Dent. J.*, **124**, 209(1968).
96. A. Thomas and H. Jamison, *Acad. Med. N.J. Bull.*, **14**, 241(1968).
97. M. Mergele, *Acad. Med. N.J. Bull.*, **14**, 247(1968).
98. M. Mergele, *Acad. Med., N.J. Bull.*, **14**, 251(1968).
99. S. B. Finn and H. C. Jamison, *J. Dent. Child.*, **30**, 17(1963).
100. A. N. Frankl and J. E. Altman, *J. Oral Ther.*, **4**, 443(1968).
101. J. C. Muhler *et al.*, *J. Dent. Res.*, **33**, 606(1954).
102. J. C. Muhler *et al.*, *J. Am. Dent. Assoc.*, **50**, 163(1955).
103. J. C. Muhler *et al.*, *J. Am. Dent. Assoc.*, **51**, 556(1955).
104. J. C. Muhler *et al.*, *J. Dent. Res.*, **35**, 49(1956).
105. J. C. Muhler and A. W. Radike, *J. Am. Dent. Assoc.*, **55**, 196(1957).
106. W. A. Jordan and J. K. Peterson, *J. Am. Dent. Assoc.*, **54**, 589(1957).
107. W. A. Jordan and J. K. Peterson, *J. Am. Dent. Assoc.*, **58**, 42(1959).
108. G. E. Peffley and J. C. Muhler, *J. Dent. Res.*, **39**, 871(1960).
109. J. C. Muhler, *J. Dent. Res.*, **38**, 994(1959).
110. J. C. Muhler, *J. Dent. Res.*, **39**, 955(1960).
111. T. J. Hill, *J. Am. Dent. Assoc.*, **59**, 1121(1959).
112. J. C. Muhler, *J. Am. Dent. Assoc.*, **64**, 216(1962).
113. W. A. Zacherl and C. W. B. McPhail, *J. Can. Dent. Assoc.*, **36**, 262(1970).
114. F. Brudevold and N. W. Chilton, *J. Am. Dent. Assoc.*, **72**, 889(1966).
115. A. H. Segal *et al.*, *J. Oral Ther.*, **4**, 175(1967).
116. C. W. Gish and J. C. Muhler, *J. Am. Dent. Assoc.*, **73**, 853(1966).
117. B. G. Bibby, *J. Dent. Res.*, **24**, 297(1945).
118. E. O. Shaner and R. R. Smith, *J. Dent. Res.*, **25**, 121(1946).
119. Council on Dental Therapeutics, "Accepted Dental Therapeutics," American Dental Association, Chicago, Ill., 1973, p. 313.
120. G. Koch, *Caries Res.*, **4**, 149(1970).
121. M. W. Reed, *J. Am. Dent. Assoc.*, **87**, 1401(1973).
122. W. F. Neuman *et al.*, *J. Biol. Chem.*, **187**, 655(1950).
123. H. C. McCann and F. A. Bullock, *J. Dent. Res.*, **34**, 59(1955).
124. J. A. Gray *et al.*, *J. Dent. Res.*, **37**, 638(1958).
125. G. Fitzgerald, *Dent. Dig.*, **62**, 494(1956).
126. P. D. Toto *et al.*, *J. Periodontol.*, **29**, 192(1958).
127. J. O. Forrest, *Br. Dent. J.*, **114**, 103(1963).
128. B. B. Kimmelman *et al.*, *J. N.J. State Dent. Soc.*, **41**, 101(1969).
129. Council on Dental Therapeutics, "Accepted Dental Therapeutics," American Dental Association, Chicago, Ill., 1973, p. 182.
130. A. Cohen, *Oral Surg. Oral Med. Oral Pathol.*, **14**, 1046(1961).
131. H. Zelman, *N.Y. J. Dent.*, **33**, 259(1963).
132. H. Skurnik, *J. Periodontol.*, **34**, 183(1963).
133. M. R. Ross, *J. Periodontol.*, **32**, 49(1961).
134. L. M. Nevins, *N.Y. State Dent. J.*, **30**, 157(1964).
135. B. Blitzer, *Periodontics*, **5**, 318(1967).
136. W. B. Shapiro *et al.*, *J. Periodontol.*, **41**, 702(1970).
137. H. P. Carrasco, *Pharmacol. Ther. Dent.*, **1**, 209(1971).
138. F. Hernandez *et al.*, *J. Periodontol.*, **43**, 367(1972).
139. W. H. Hoyt and B. G. Bibby, *J. Am. Dent. Assoc.*, **30**, 1372(1943).
140. Council on Dental Therapeutics, *J. Am. Dent. Assoc.*, **38**, 762(1949).
141. M. Masler, *J. Dent. Res.*, **34**, 761(1955).
142. G. C. Hunter, Jr. *et al.*, *J. Periodontol.*, **32**, 333(1961).
143. T. E. Bolden *et al.*, *Periodontics*, **6**, 112(1968).
144. S. P. Hazen *et al.*, *Periodontics*, **6**, 230(1968).
145. M. C. Kanouse and M. M. Ash, *J. Periodontol. Periodontics*, **40**, 38(1969).
146. M. Hodosh, *J. Am. Dent. Assoc.*, **88**, 831(1974).
147. C. C. Bass, *J. La. State Med. Soc.*, **106**, 100(1954).
148. C. C. Bass, *D. Items Interest*, **70**, 697(1948).
149. D. H. Masters, *Dent. Clin. North Am.*, **13**, 3(1969).
150. S. S. Arnim, *Northwest Dent.*, **45**, 3(1966).
151. S. I. Gold, *N.Y. State Dent. J.*, **37**, 281(1971).
152. R. F. Barkley, *Dent. Clin. North Am.*, **15**, 569(1971).
153. P. E. Jaffe, *N.Y. J. Dent.*, **43**, 245(1973).
154. Council on Dental Materials and Devices, "Guide to Dental Materials and Devices," 7th ed., American Dental Association, Chicago, Ill., 1974-75, p. 151.
155. H. C. Hill *et al.*, *J. Periodontol.*, **44**, 411(1973).
156. W. H. Radentz *et al.*, *J. Periodontol.*, **44**, 177(1973).
157. J. A. Terhune, *J. Am. Dent. Assoc.*, **86**, 1332(1973).
158. F. G. Everett and P. W. Kunkel, Sr., *J. Periodontol.*, **24**, 186(1953).
159. R. M. Leggett and L. N. Peterson, *Acad. Rev.*, **6**, 93(1958).
160. M. A. Listgarten, *J. Dent. Child.*, **39**, 347(1972).
161. J. L. Bernier *et al.*, *J. Periodontol.*, **37**, 267(1966).
162. J. J. Krajewski *et al.*, *J. Periodontol.*, **2**, 76(1964).
163. P. J. Crumley and C. F. Summer, *Periodontics*, **3**, 193(1965).
164. S. S. Arnim, *J. Tenn. Dent. Assoc.*, **47**, 65(1967).
165. M. T. Cantor and S. S. Stahl, *J. Periodontol.*, **39**, 292(1968).
166. P. D. Toto *et al.*, *J. Periodontol.*, **39**, 296(1968).
167. W. A. Peterson and W. R. Shiller, *J. Periodontol.*, **39**, 335(1968).
168. D. R. Hoover and H. B. G. Robinson, *J. Periodontol.*, **39**, 43(1968).
169. H. M. Goldman and D. Cohen, "Periodontal Therapy," Mosby, St. Louis, Mo., 1968, p. 467.
170. R. Lobene, *J. Periodontol.*, **40**, 667(1969).
171. J. Derbyshire, *Dent. Clin. North Am.*, **242**, (1964).
172. D. R. Hoover and H. G. B. Robinson, *J. Periodontol.*, **42**, 37(1971).
173. N. R. Covin *et al.*, *J. Periodontol.*, **44**, 286(1973).
174. S. N. Bhaskar *et al.*, *J. Periodontol.*, **40**, 593(1969).
175. Council on Dental Materials and Devices, *J. Am. Dent. Assoc.*, **78**, 347(1969).
176. Council on Dental Materials and Devices, "Guide to Dental Materials and Devices," 7th ed., American Dental Association, Chicago, Ill., 1974-75, p. 152.
177. Council on Dental Materials and Devices, *J. Am. Dent. Assoc.*, **90**, 181(1975).
178. Council on Dental Materials and Devices, *J. Am. Dent. Assoc.*, **80**, 1178(1974).
179. F. H. Skinner, *Dent. Cosmos*, **56**, 299(1914).
180. R. M. King, *J. Dent. Res.*, **30**, 399(1951).
181. G. L. M. Williams, *Dent. Pract.*, **6**, 202(1966).
182. Council on Dental Therapeutics, "Accepted Dental Therapeutics," American Dental Association, Chicago, Ill., 1973, p. 233.
183. S. S. Arnim, *J. Periodontol.*, **34**, 227(1973).
184. H. Björn and J. Carlsson, *Odontol. Revy*, **15**, 23(1964).
185. N. P. Lang *et al.*, *J. Periodontol. Res.*, **7**, 59(1972).
186. D. W. Cohen *et al.*, *J. Periodontol Res.*, **43**, 333(1972).
187. J. C. Green and J. R. Vermillion, *J. Dent. Res.*, **50**, 184(1971).
188. J. Waerhaug, *J. Periodontol.*, **40**, 155(1969).
189. F. M. Wentz, *J. Am. Dent. Assoc.*, **85**, 887-891(1972)
190. "U.S. Dispensatory," 25th ed., A. Osol and C. E. Farrar, Eds., Lippincott, Philadelphia, Pa. 1955.
191. Council on Dental Therapeutics, *J. Am. Dent. Assoc.*, **23**, 2174(1936).
192. Council on Dental Therapeutics, *J. Am. Dent. Assoc.*, **38**, 370(1949).

193. S. Silverman, "Dental Health and the Profession of Pharmacy, a Symposium," presented at the University of California, January 12, 1967.
194. H. M. Clarman, *J. Am. Med. Assoc.*, **202,** 651(1967).
195. H. R. Morse, *Pa. Med. J.*, **68,** 39(1965).
196. C. B. Henry, *Br. Dent. J.*, **125,** 354(1968).
197. H. O. Beck, *J. Am. Pharm. Assoc.*, **NS13,** 246(1973).
198. C. M. Heartwell and A. O. Rahn, "Syllabus of Complete Dentures," 2d ed., Lea and Febiger, Philadelphia, Pa., 1974, p. 81.
199. D. J. Neill and B. J. Roberts, *J. Dent.*, **1,** 219(1973).
200. R. B. Lytle, *Dent. Prog.*, **1,** 221(1961).
201. J. B. Woelfel *et al., J. Am. Dent. Assoc.*, **64,** 763(1962).
202. J. D. Larkin, *Tex. Dent. J.*, **82,** 9(1964).
203. C. R. Means, *J. Prosthet. Dent.*, **14,** 623(1964).
204. C. R. Means, *J. Prosthet. Dent.*, **14,** 935(1964).
205. C. R. Means, *J. Prosthet. Dent.*, **14,** 1086(1964).
206. J. B. Woelfel *et al., J. Am. Dent. Assoc.*, **71,** 603(1965).
207. J. B. Woelfel *et al., J. Am. Dent. Assoc.*, **71,** 23(1965).
208. Questions and Answers, *J. Am. Med. Assoc.*, **191,** 962(1965).
209. C. M. Winter, *Ohio Dent. J.*, **40,** 227(1966).
210. Council on Dental Research–Council on Dental Therapeutics, *J. Am. Dent. Assoc.*, **47,** 214(1953).
211. *Fed. Regist.*, **34,** 14167(1969).
212. D. J. Neill, *Br. Dent. J.*, **124,** 107(1968).
213. Council on Dental Therapeutics, "Accepted Dental Therapeutics," American Dental Association, Chicago, Ill., 1973, p. 256.
214. C. A. Lawrence, "Surface Active Quaternary Ammonium Germicides," Academic Press, New York, N.Y., 1950, p. 227.
215. W. A. Corby, *J. Soc. Cosmet. Chem.*, **15,** 541(1964).
216. F. Rosenkranz, *Odontol. Tidskr.*, **75,** 528(1967).
217. P. Torell and A. Silberg, *Odontol. Revy*, **13,** 62(1962).
218. S. B. Heifetz *et al., J. Am. Dent. Assoc.*, **87,** 364(1973).
219. L. P. Cancro *et al., J. Periodontol.*, **43,** 687(1972).
220. F. L. Horsfall and T. Tamm, "Viral and Rickettsial Infections of Man," 4th ed., Lippincott, Philadelphia, Pa., 1965, p. 892.
221. P. N. Baer and S. B. Benjamin, "Periodontal Disease in Children and Adolescents," Lippincott, Philadelphia, Pa., 1974, p. 37.
222. E. H. Lennette and R. L. Magoffin, *J. Am. Dent. Assoc.*, **87,** 1055(1973).
223. S. Rovin, *Dent. Clin. North Am.*, **10,** 3(1966).
224. D. R. Weathers and J. W. Griffin, *J. Am. Dent. Assoc.*, **81,** 81(1970).
225. T. C. Francis, *Oral Surg.*, **30,** 476(1970).
226. Council on Dental Therapeutics, "Accepted Dental Therapeutics," American Dental Association, Chicago, Ill., 1973, p. 283.
227. Council on Dental Therapeutics, "Accepted Dental Therapeutics," American Dental Association, Chicago, Ill., 1973, p. 308.
228. "Physicians' Desk Reference," 29th ed., Medical Economics, Oradell, N.J., 1975, p. 785.
229. "Physicians' Desk Reference," 29th ed., Medical Economics, Oradell, N.J., 1975, p. 823.
230. J. Lichtenstein *et al., J. Oral Ther. Pharmacol.*, **1,** 308(1964).
231. P. L. Abbott, *J. Oral Surg.*, **19,** 310(1961).
232. D. L. Weeks, *N.Y. State J. Med.*, **58,** 2672(1958).
233. L. Rapoport *et al., Oral Surg. Oral Med. Oral Pathol.*, **20,** 591(1965).

Products 22 TOOTHPASTE

Product (manufacturer)	Ingredients
Aim (Lever Bros)	stannous fluoride, 0.4%; alcohol; sorbitol; glycerin; hydrated silica; polyethylene glycol 32; sodium lauryl sulfate; sodium and potassium carrageenans; saccharin sodium; sodium benzoate; flavor
Amosan (Cooper)	sodium peroxyborate monohydrate, sodium bitartrate
Caroid Tooth Powder (Breon)	papain
Chloresium (Rystan)	chlorophyll
Close-up (Lever Bros)	sorbitol, hydrated silica, glycerin, polyethylene glycol 32, sodium lauryl sulfate, alcohol, saccharin sodium, cellulose gum, sodium benzoate, sodium phosphate, disodium phosphate, flavor
Colgate with MFP (Colgate-Palmolive)	sarcosinate, sodium monofluorophosphate
Crest (Procter & Gamble)	stannous fluoride, 0.40%; calcium pyrophosphate; cellulose gum; glycerin; sorbitol; stannous pyrophosphate; flavor
Depend (Warner-Lambert)	alcohol, 23.8%; sorbitol; glycerin; polysorbate 80; saccharin sodium; sodium phosphate; caramel; disodium phosphate; flavor
Extar (Extar)	sodium polymetaphosphate, extra heavy mineral oil, magnesium oxide, tragacanth, sodium lauryl sulfate, saccharin sodium, spralene mint, silica gel, calcium carbonate, mint oil flavor
Gleem II (Procter & Gamble)	sodium fluoride, 0.22%; calcium pyrophosphate; glycerin; sorbitol; blend of anionic surfactants; cellulose gum; flavor
Ipana (La Maur)	stannous fluoride
Listerine (Warner-Lambert)	dicalcium phosphate

PRODUCTS **22** TOOTHPASTE

Product (manufacturer)	Ingredients
Listermint (Warner-Lambert)	alcohol, 12.8%; glycerin; poloxamer 407; polysorbate 80; saccharin sodium; zinc chloride; saccharin; flavoring
Macleans (Beecham Products)	dicalcium phosphate dihydrate, glycerin, calcium carbonate
Macleans Fluoride Toothpaste (Beecham Products)	sodium monofluorophosphate, 0.76%; calcium carbonate, 38%; glycerin, 26%; sodium lauryl sulfate, 1.15%
NDK Liquid (NDK Co.)	fluorophosphate, benzethonium chloride
Pearl Drops Liquid (Carter)	dicalcium phosphate, aluminum hydroxide, sorbitol, carboxymethylcellulose
Pepsodent (Lever Bros)	sorbitol, alumina, hydrated silica, glycerin, polyethylene glycol 32, sodium lauryl sulfate, dicalcium phosphate, cellulose gum, titanium dioxide, saccharin sodium, sodium benzoate, flavor
Pepsodent Ammoniated Tooth Powder (Lever Bros)	sodium metaphosphate, tricalcium phosphate, diammonium phosphate, urea, sodium lauryl sulfate, polyethylene glycol, carrageenan, saccharin, flavor
Pepsodent Tooth Powder (Lever Bros)	sodium metaphosphate, dicalcium phosphate, magnesium trisilicate, sodium lauryl sulfate, polyethylene glycol, carrageenan, saccharin, flavor
Pycopay Tooth Powder (Block)	sodium chloride, sodium bicarbonate, calcium carbonate, magnesium carbonate, tricalcium phosphate, flavor
Revelation Tooth Powder (Alvin Last)	calcium carbonate, soap, sodium bicarbonate, sodium chloride, menthol, methyl salicylate
Sensodyne (Block)	strontium chloride
Thermodent (Leeming)	magnesium carbonate, calcium carbonate, sodium chloride, potassium sulfate, formaldehyde

Products 22 DENTURE CLEANER

Product (manufacturer)	Ingredients
Denalan (Whitehall)	sodium peroxide, 9.5%; sodium chloride, 90%
Efferdent Tablets (Warner-Lambert)	potassium monopersulfate, 960 mg; sodium borate perhydrate, 480 mg; sodium carbonate; sodium lauryl sulfoacetate; sodium bicarbonate, 1.116 g; citric acid, 362 mg; magnesium stearate; simethicone
Effervescent Denture Tablets (Rexall)	sodium bicarbonate, citric acid, sodium perborate, sodium acid pyrophosphate, sodium benzoate, trisodium phosphate, sodium lauryl sulfate, poloxamer 188, sorbitol, silica, peppermint oil, povidone
K.I.K. (K.I.K. Co.)	sodium perborate, 25%; trisodium phosphate, 75%
Mersene Dental Cleaner (Hoyt)	troclosene potassium, sodium perborate, trisodium phosphate
Polident Denture Cleanser Powder (Block)	sodium perborate, potassium monopersulfate, sodium carbonate, sodium tripoly-phosphate, surfactant, sodium bicarbonate, flavor
Polident Tablets (Block)	potassium monopersulfate, sodium perborate, sodium carbonate, surfactant, sodium bicarbonate, citric acid, flavor

Products 22 TOOTHACHE/COLD SORE/CANKER SORE

Product (manufacturer)	Ingredients
Baby Orajel (Commerce)	benzocaine, viscous water-soluble base
Benzodent (Vick)	benzocaine, 20%; eugenol, 0.4%; 8-hydroxyquinoline sulfate, 0.1%; denture adhesive-like base
Betadine Mouthwash/Gargle (Purdue Frederick)	povidone-iodine, 0.5%; alcohol, 8.8%
Blistex Ointment (Blistex)	phenol, 0.4%; camphor, 1%; ammonia; mineral oil; lanolin; petrolatum; paraffin; alcohol; sorbitan sesquioleate; peppermint oil; lanolin alcohol; soya sterol; ammonium carbonate; fragrance
Cold Sore Lotion (DeWitt)	camphor, 3.6%; tincture of benzoin, 4.2%; phenol, 0.3%; menthol, 0.3%; alcohol, 90%
Dalidyne (Dalin)	methylbenzethonium chloride; benzocaine; tannic acid; camphor; chlorothymol; menthol; benzyl alcohol; alcohol, 61%; aromatic base
Dr. Hands Teething Gel (Roberts)	tincture of pellitory; menthol; clove oil; hamamelis water; alcohol, 10%
Dr. Hands Teething Lotion (Roberts)	tincture of pellitory; menthol; clove oil; hamamelis water; alcohol, 10%
Jiffy (Block)	benzocaine; eugenol; alcohol, 56.5%
Numzident (PurePac)	benzocaine, eugenol, peppermint oil, polyethylene glycol-like base
Numzit (PurePac)	glycerin; alcohol, 10%; gel vehicle
Orabase (Hoyt)	benzocaine
Orajel (Commerce)	benzocaine, polyethylene glycol-like base
Ora-Jel-d (Commerce)	benzocaine, clove oil, benzyl alcohol, adhesive base
Pain-A-Lay (Roberts)	boric acid, cresol
Proxigel (Reed & Carnrick)	urea carbamide, gel vehicle
Rexall Cold Sore Lotion (Rexall)	phenol; benzoin; camphor; menthol; alcohol, 90%
Rexall Cold Sore Ointment (Rexall)	phenol; benzoin; camphor; menthol; alcohol, 30%; viscous base
Tanac (Commerce)	benzalkonium chloride, tannic acid
Teething Lotion (DeWitt)	propylene glycol, 44%; glycerin, 29%; benzocaine, 5.6%; benzyl alcohol, 2.5%; tincture of myrrh, 4.5%; alcohol
Toothache Drops (DeWitt)	clove oil, 9.98%; benzocaine, 5.01%; creosote beechwood, 4.83%; flexible collodion (base); alcohol, 20%

Products 22 DENTURE ADHESIVE

Product (manufacturer)	Ingredients
Brace (Norcliff-Thayer)	cellulose gum, 2.5%; methyl vinyl ether–maleic anhydride and/or acid copolymer, 1.5%; povidone, 1%; petrolatum, 3.5%; mineral oil, 1.5%; flavor, 0.02%
Confident (Block)	carboxymethylcellulose gum, 32%; ethylene oxide polymer, 13%; petrolatum, 42%; liquid petrolatum, 12%; propylparaben, 0.05%
Corega Powder (Block)	karaya gum, 94.6%; water-soluble ethylene oxide polymer, 4.76%; calcium silicate, 0.07%; flavor, 0.4%

PRODUCTS 22 DENTURE ADHESIVE

Product (manufacturer)	Ingredients
Effergrip Denture Adhesive Cream (Warner-Lambert)	carboxymethylcellulose sodium, 39%; cationic polyacrylamide polymer, 10%
Effergrip Denture Adhesive Powder (Warner-Lambert)	carboxymethylcellulose sodium, 40%; cationic polyacrylamide polymer, 10%
Fasteeth (Vick)	karaya gum, sodium borate
Firmdent (Moyco)	karaya gum, 90.91%; sodium tetraborate, 9.05%; powdered flavor essence of peppermint, 0.04%
Fixodent (Vick)	calcium, sodium, polyvinyl methyl ether maleate, petrolatum base
Orafix (Norcliff-Thayer)	karaya gum, 51%; petrolatum, 30%; mineral oil, 13%; peppermint oil, 0.08%
Orafix M (Norcliff-Thayer)	karaya gum, 51%; benzocaine, 2%; allantoin, 0.2%; petrolatum, 28%; mineral oil, 13%; peppermint oil, 0.08%
Orahesive Powder (Hoyt)	gelatin, 33.3%; pectin, 33.3%; carboxymethylcellulose sodium, 33.3%
Perma-Grip Powder (Lactona)	polyethylene wax, 50.9%; carboxymethylcellulose sodium, 39.0%; cationic acrylic polymer, 10.0%; flavor
Polident Dentu-Grip (Block)	carboxymethylcellulose gum, 49%; ethylene oxide polymer, 21%; flavor, 0.4%
Poli-Grip (Block)	karaya gum, 51% petrolatum, 36.7%; liquid petrolatum, 9.4%; magnesium oxide 2.7%; propylparaben; flavor
Wernet's Cream (Block)	carboxymethylcellulose gum, 32%; petrolatum, 42%; liquid petrolatum, 12%; ethylene oxide polymer, 13%; propylparaben, 0.05%; flavor, 0.5%
Wernet's Powder (Block)	karaya gum, 94.6%; water-soluble ethylene oxide polymer, 4.76%; calcium silicate, 0.07%; flavor, 0.4%

Products 22 MOUTHWASH

Product (manufacturer)	Ingredients
Astring-O-Sol (Breon)	tincture of myrrh; methyl salicylate; alcohol, 70%; zinc chloride
Cherry Chloraseptic Mouthwash and Gargle (Eaton)	phenol, sodium phenolate
Chloraseptic (liquid) (Eaton)	phenol, sodium phenolate
Chlorazene Aromatic Powder (for solution) (Wisconsin Pharmacal)	chloramine-T, 5%; sodium chloride, 88%; sodium bicarbonate, 5%; eucalyptol; saccharin sodium
Colgate 100 (Colgate-Palmolive)	benzethonium chloride, 0.075%; alcohol, 15%
Forma-Zincol Concentrate (Ingram)	formaldehyde, zinc chloride, anise oil, menthol
Gly-Oxide (International Pharmaceutical)	carbamide peroxide, 10%; anhydrous glycerin; flavor
Greenmint Mouthwash (Block)	chlorophyll
Isodine Mouthwash/Gargle Concentrate (Blair)	povidone-iodine, 7.5%; alcohol, 35%
Kasdenol Powder (Kasdenol)	available chlorine 5-6% (as oxychlorosene)

Product (manufacturer)	Ingredients
Lavoris (Vick)	zinc chloride, 0.22%; alcohol, 5%; cinnamaldehyde and clove oil, 0.06%
Listerine (Warner-Lambert)	menthol; boric acid; thymol; eucalyptol; methyl salicylate; benzoic acid; alcohol, 25%
Micrin Plus Gargle & Rinse (Johnson & Johnson)	alcohol, glycerin, poloxamer 407, flavor, saccharin sodium, monosodium glutamate–glutamic acid buffer, cetylpyridinium chloride
Mouthwash and Gargle (McKesson)	cetylpyridinium chloride; alcohol, 14%
Odara (Lorvic)	phenol (less than 2%); zinc chloride; glycerin; potassium iodide; methyl salicylate; eucalyptus oil; myrrh tincture; alcohol, 48%
Oral Pentacresol (Upjohn)	secondary amyltricresols, 100 mg/100 ml; alcohol, 30%; sodium chloride, 861 mg/100 ml; calcium chloride, 33 mg/100 ml; potassium chloride, 29.9 mg/100 ml
Proxigel (Block)	carbamide peroxide, 11%; anhydrous glycerin; thickeners; flavor
Scope (Procter & Gamble)	cetylpyridinium chloride; domiphen bromide, 0.005%; alcohol, 18.5%; glycerin; saccharin; polisorbate 80; flavor
S.T. 37 (Calgon)	hexylresorcinol, 0.1%; glycerin

Insect Sting and Bite Products

Farid Sadik

Questions to ask the patient

Do you have a personal or family history of allergic reactions such as hay fever?

Have you previously had severe reactions to insect stings or bites?

How extensive are the stings or bites on your body?

If the patient is not an adult, what is the age and approximate weight of the patient?

Are your symptoms mild or severe?

Have you ever had adverse reactions to topically applied products?

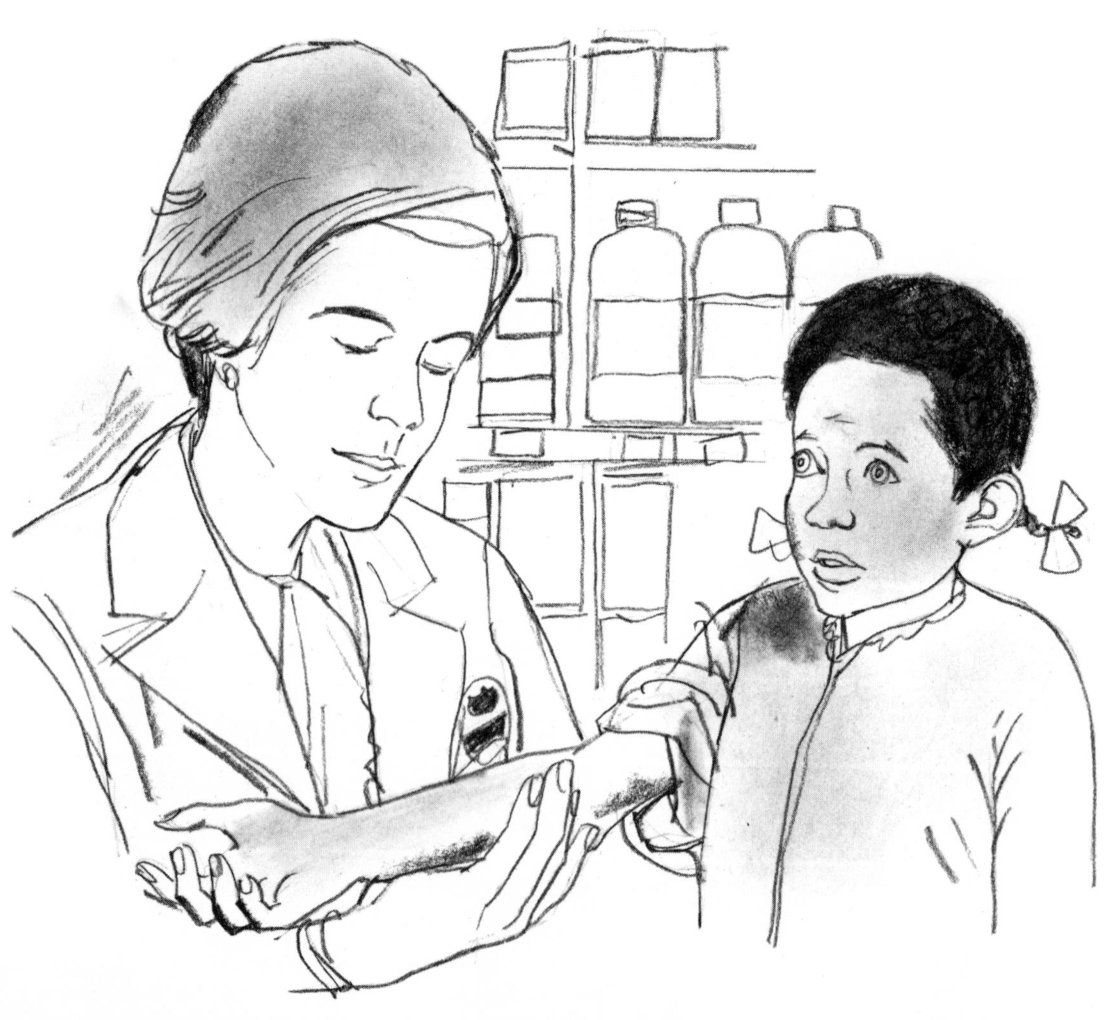

CHAPTER 23

An insect sting or bite is an injury to the skin caused by penetration of the stinging or biting organs of an insect. (See Chapter 27 for a complete discussion of the skin.) The reactions that follow are produced mainly by substances contained in the venom of stinging insects or in the saliva of biting insects. The literature is replete with articles on allergic reactions to insect stings and bites. Although the pain associated with the penetration of the skin by the stinging or biting organ is brief, the aftereffects vary considerably. Reactions in nonallergic individuals are usually confined to the site of the sting or bite. Occasionally, people die as a result of insect stings and bites, and others, who are hypersensitive, require treatment for severe systemic reactions. Information on 460 deaths from venomous animals and insects shows that 229 were caused by Hymenoptera, 138 by snakes, 65 by spiders, and 28 by miscellaneous animals.[1]

Stinging Insects

Stinging insects, which include bees, wasps, hornets, yellow jackets, and ants, belong to the order Hymenoptera (membranous wings). Although they are small, these insects have a venom that is, drop for drop, as potent as that of snakes. They inject the venom into the bodies of their victims through a piercing organ (stinger), a specialized ovipositor delicately attached to the rear of the abdomen of the female. Males do not have an ovipositor and consequently are stingless. The stinger consists of two lancets, made of highly chitinous material, that are separated by the poison canal. The venom flows through the canal from the venom sac which is attached to the dorsal section of the stinger. The tip of the stinger, which is directed posteriorly, has sharp barbs, and the base enlarges into a bulblike structure. Most species of bees and wasps have two types of venom glands under the last segment of the abdomen. The larger gland secretes an acidic toxin directly into the venom sac; the smaller one, at the base of the sac, secretes an alkaline toxin which is less potent than the acidic one.

Honeybee. When the honeybee attacks, it first attaches firmly to the skin with tiny, sharp claws at the tip of each foot; then, it arches its abdomen and immediately jabs the barbed stinger into the skin. Because of the barbs, the stinger remains firmly embedded, and when the honeybee pulls away or is brushed off, the entire stinging apparatus (stinger, appendages, venom sac, and glands) is detached from the bee's abdomen. The disemboweled bee later dies. The abandoned stinger is driven deeper into the skin by rhythmic contractions of the smooth muscle wall of the venom sac and continues to inject venom.

Wasps and bumblebees. The stinging mechanism of wasps and bumblebees is basically the same as that of the honeybee. The main difference is that their stingers are not barbed. The stingers can be withdrawn easily after injecting the venom, enabling these insects to survive and sting repeatedly.

Ants. Ants use their mandibles to cling to the skin of their prey, then bend their abdomen, sting the flesh, and empty the contents of their poison vesicle into the wound.[2] Because they use their mandibles, it is often believed that the bite causes the reaction.

Biting insects

Insects such as mosquitoes, fleas, lice, bedbugs, ticks, and chiggers bite their prey. They insert their biting organs into the skin to feed by sucking blood from their hosts.

Mosquitoes. Mosquitoes usually attack exposed parts of the body—face, neck, forearms, and legs—but can also bite through thin clothing. When a mosquito alights on the skin, it starts to feed by cutting the skin with its mandibles and maxillae. A fine, hollow, needlelike, flexible structure (proboscis) is introduced into the cut and probes the tissue for a blood vessel. Blood is sucked directly from the lumen of a capillary or from previously lacerated capillaries with extravasated blood.[3] During feeding, the mosquito injects a salivary secretion containing antigenic components into the wound.

Fleas. Fleas are tiny (1.5 to 4 mm long), bloodsucking, wingless parasites that have strongly developed posterior legs used for jumping. They are found throughout the world but breed best in warm areas with relatively high humidity. Fleas bite covered parts of the body; their bites usually are multiple and grouped and cause intense itching. Each lesion is characterized by an erythematous region around the puncture. Fleas are not only annoying, but they are also responsible for transmitting a variety of diseases such as bubonic plague and endemic typhus. They can be carried into the home on pets or on clothing from flea-infested places. They can survive and multiply without food for several weeks. In many cases, places that have been vacant for weeks are heavily infested.

Lice. Lice are wingless parasites with well-developed legs. Each leg has a claw which helps the louse cling firmly to the skin while sucking blood. Three types of lice attack humans—head lice, body lice, and pubic lice. Head lice usually infest the head but are found on other hairy parts of the body as well. The female deposits 50 to 150 eggs (nits) which become glued to the hair and hatch in 5 to 10 days. Body lice live, hide, and lay their eggs in clothing, particularly in seams and folds of underclothing. They infest crowded, impoverished environments. Pubic lice are commonly called crab lice because of their crablike appearance. They infest the pubic area, armpits, and occasionally, eyelashes, mustaches, beards, and eyebrows.

Bedbugs. Bedbugs are 4 to 5 mm long and 3 mm wide. They have a short head and a broad, flat body. Their mouth parts consist of two pairs of stylets which are used to pierce the skin. The outer pair has barbs which saw the skin, and the inner pair is used to suck blood and to allow salivary secretions to flow into the wound.

Ticks. Ticks are parasites that attack people and domestic animals. They feed on the blood of their hosts. During feeding, the tick's mouth parts are introduced into the skin, enabling it to hold firmly. If the tick is removed, the parts of the mouth are torn from the body of the tick and remain embedded, causing intense itching and nodules. If the tick is left attached to the skin, it becomes fully engorged with blood and remains as long as 10 days before it drops off.

Chiggers. Chiggers (red bugs) are prevalent in the southern part of the U.S., mainly during summer and fall. Only the larvae, which are nearly microscopic, attack the host by attaching to the skin and sucking blood. Once in contact with the skin, the larvae insert their mouth parts into the skin and secrete a digestive fluid which causes disintegration of the cells of the affected area.

Parasitic infestation

Scabies. The mite causing scabies does not bite or sting. Also called "the itch," scabies is a contagious parasitic skin infestation which is caused by the mite *Sarcoptes scabiei.* It is characterized by secondary inflammation, intense itching, and burrows beneath the stratum corneum. This infestation is associated with poor hygiene and crowded conditions. The female mite, which is responsible for causing scabies, is readily transmitted by close personal contact with an infected person. Once on the skin, the impregnated female burrows into the stratum corneum with her jaws and the first two pairs of legs, forming tunnels in which she lays eggs and excretes fecal matter. In a few days the hatched larvae form their own burrows and develop into adults. They copulate, and the impregnated females burrow into the stratum corneum to start a new life cycle. The most common sites of infestation are the interdigital spaces of the fingers, the flexor surface of the wrists, the external genitalia in men, the buttocks, and the anterior axillary folds. The head and neck are not affected, except in infants.

Allergic reactions to stings/bites

Antigens

Allergic reactions to insect stings and bites are caused by antigenic proteins in the venom of the stinging insects and in the salivary secretions of the biting insects.

Bee venom is a combination of acidic and alkaline venom gland secretions. The secretions, which flow separately from each gland, are mixed in the venom canal of the stinger before they are injected. Bee venom contains histamine and three protein fractions.[4] Apamin, a basic peptide, has also been found in bee venom.[5]

Wasp venom contains histamine, 5-hydroxytryptamine, and hyaluronidase, a substance which dissolves intracellular cement to allow greater penetration of venom.[6] Hornet venom contains 5-hydroxytryptamine, histamine, and acetylcholine.[4] The poison of ants of the Formica family contains formic acid and 17 free amino acids.

Some species of mosquitoes have agglutinin and anticoagulant agents in their salivary secretions; others have neither.[7] Many attempts have been made to identify the antigenic factors in mosquito bites by studying whole mosquito extracts. McKiel and Clunie [8] have shown by paper chromatography that extracts from *Aedes aegypti* contain at least four fractions that can produce skin reactions. Chromatographic fractionation of whole extracts showed that the antigenic principle contained four constituents. Eluates of each constituent have caused positive reactions in sensitized individuals.[9] Eighteen amino acids have been identified in the extracts of all species of mosquitoes.[10]

Sensitization

There are definite stages in acquiring sensitization to mosquito bites. Mellanby,[11] in an experiment with 25 volunteers who previously had not been bitten by the species *A. aegypti,* divided the subjects' reactions into four stages:

Stage	Immediate reaction	Delayed reaction
I	−	+
II	+	+
III	+	−
IV	−	−

The degree and kind of reaction depend mainly on the history of exposure to bites and on the present stage of sensitization. The first stage (incubation) begins after the first bite. The bite does not cause an immediate, cutaneous reaction or itching because no previous sensitization has occurred. However, in about 24 hours, a papular reaction accompanied by itching occurs at the site of the sting. As biting continues over time, sensitization increases. An allergic state now exists. In the second stage, a reaction occurs during or immediately after the mosquito has fed. It is characterized by a wheal surrounded by erythema and is accompanied by itching, heat, and pain. These symptoms usually subside within 2 hours. A delayed papular reaction occurs about 24 hours later. With regular exposure to bites, the delayed reaction gradually starts to diminish (the third stage) and eventually disappears; the immediate reaction continues during or after each bite. The fourth stage, which is uncommon, is marked by the absence of the immediate and delayed reactions following a bite. This stage occurs only after regular exposure to many bites over a period of years. Because desentization is transient, the fourth stage is replaced by the third if exposure to bites is irregular.

The reactions to other biting insects, such as fleas, bedbugs, ticks, and chiggers, are similar to those of mosquito bites.

Signs and symptoms

The intensity of the reactions to stings of venomous insects varies significantly. The thrust of the stinger into the flesh causes a sharp pain. The reaction that follows can be one or more of the following: localized irritation, itching, swelling, generalized urticaria, feeling of heat and flushing of the skin, excessive perspiration, vomiting, fainting, respiratory distress, choking sensation, and loss of consciousness or death from anaphylactic shock. Temporary paralysis has occurred following tick bites.[12]

The systemic reaction to injected venom occurs quickly. It starts immediately after stinging or within 20 minutes. The intensity of the reaction reaches a peak within 30 minutes. Although the pain may be acute for 1 hour or more, symptoms start to resolve and usually disappear within 3 to 4 hours.[6]

Systemic and local allergic manifestations usually occur in individuals who previously have been stung or bitten.[13] Each succeeding sting precipitates a reaction more severe than the preceding one. Cross-sensitization may occur in individuals who have been sensitized by a member of the order Hymenoptera (bees).[13,14] For example, a severe reaction may occur after the first sting of ants or wasps in individuals sensitized to bee venom.

The reaction to ant stings generally is limited to the area surrounding the site of the sting. Immediately after a sting, the skin flares and forms a wheal that lasts for about an hour. Swelling, pruritus, papular urticaria, eczematoid dermatitis, and, in some cases, allergic systemic reactions may occur. In one report, a patient experienced large, white blotches surrounded by reddened areas accompanied by intense body itching, difficulty in breathing, profuse sweating, and semiconsciousness a few minutes after stinging by not more than 10 fire ants.[15] Morhouse [16] reported a case following an ant sting in which there was a urticarial rash over the entire body, swollen eyes, stertorous breathing, frothy mucus expectoration from the mouth, and a near state of shock. In one study, biopsy specimens were obtained at 6 and 30 minutes and 24 and 72 hours after volunteers were stung by ants and the specimens were studied histopathologically.[15] Epidermal intracellular edema and dermal necrosis occurred early. Pustules developed consistently at the site of the sting and were accompanied by severe, deep necrosis. Brown [17] reported anaphylactic reactions following fire ant stings.

Allergic reactions to mosquito bites vary in intensity. The formation of a wheal, erythema, papular reaction, and itching are characteristic. Unrestrained scratching can cause the formation of papules and nodules which may persist for a long time and may lead to secondary infections such as impetigo, furunculosis, or infectious eczematoid dermatitis. The site of the sting can influence the intensity of reaction; bites are more severe on ankles and legs than on other parts of the body because of the relative circulatory stasis in the legs. Consequently, the tendency toward vesiculation, hemorrhage, eczematization, and ulceration is greater in these areas.[18] Systemic reactions such as fever and malaise are also common.

Symptoms of scabies usually appear following the formation of the first burrow. Intense itching, especially at night, always occurs at the site of infestation. The burrow (less than 1 cm long) can be seen by the naked eye and appears as a narrow, slightly raised dark line. Unrestrained scratching can result in secondary bacterial infections (impetigo, furuncles, cellulitis, etc.) and excoriation. Scabies may be diagnosed by identification of the mite by microscopic examination and by burrows in the skin.

When death ensues from an insect sting or bite, it is caused by anaphylactic shock—a result of hypersensitivity to certain proteins in the venom—rather than to the "toxicity" of the venom. A person would have to sustain approximately 500 stings simultaneously to be killed by the toxicity of the venom. Swinny [19] postulated that the severity of anaphylactic symptoms depends on the amount of the substance injected, the antigenicity of the substance, and the individual's degree of sensitivity. Thomas [20] stated that "anaphylactic shock from insects is not generally known to the medical profession nor to the coroners, and cases listed as heart disease, cerebral accidents and a number of sudden deaths are sometimes due to insects."

The pathological findings in fatal cases of insect stings and bites include laryngeal obstruction and edema, pulmonary emphysema, pulmonary edema, dilation of the heart, epicardial hemorrhage, cerebral edema, and visceral congestion. Localized necrosis, edema, and cellular infiltration at the site of the bee sting occur in unsensitized tissue. Wasp venom can also cause necrosis of sweat glands.[6]

Treatment of stings and bites

Body defenses are important in determining the intensity and kind of reaction to insect stings and bites. Some individuals acquire hypersensitivity after repeated stings or bites; others develop a tolerance. Beekeepers may stop developing reactions to the stings of bees and other insects of the order Hymenoptera. Allington and Allington [18] reported that adults who are initially bothered by fleas stop reacting within 1 or 2 years after regular exposure. Whether or not this is caused by a specific immunologic mechanism which blocks the reaction to an injected antigen is not known.

Sensitivity to insect stings can be treated prophylactically by desensitization. Successful attempts have been made at desensitization by inoculations of diluted extracts from the responsible insect over a long period.[21-23] Loveless and Fackler [24] used venom from the sacs of live wasps to diagnose and immunize against allergies to wasps. Torsney [25] reported, however, that several fatalities have occurred following insect stings, despite previous desensitization therapy.

Because of the wide range of reactions to insect stings and bites, treatment usually depends on the symptoms. Nonprescription drugs are of no value in systemic reactions; such cases need the prompt attention of a physician. For locally confined reactions, an OTC product that minimizes scratching by relieving discomfort, itching, and pain can be recommended. Prophylactic products, such as insect repellents, are also available.

Physician-directed medical treatment (acute or prophylactic) is important in many cases. Because hypersensitive reactions to insect stings and bites occur rapidly and are usually severe, the faster that medical attention is given, the better the chances are for recovery. Systemic reactions caused by insect stings and bites are considered emergencies and are usually treated with one or more of the following drugs: epinephrine hydrochloride, isoproterenol, corticosteroids, and antihistamines. Oxygen respiratory support should be available, if needed; in severe cases, a tracheostomy may be necessary.[26]

First aid

Basic first aid measures are helpful until medical help is available. Promptly applying ice packs on the sting site helps to slow the absorption of venom and reduce itching, swelling, and pain.[27] Removing the honeybee's stinger and venom sac, which are usually left in the skin, is another measure that should be offered or explained, particularly to allergic individuals. The stinger should be removed before all the venom is injected; it takes about 2 to 3 minutes to empty all the contents from the venom sac of the honeybee. The sac should not be squeezed, because rubbing, scratching, or grasping it releases more venom.[27] Scraping the stinger with tweezers or a fingernail minimizes the flow of venom. After removing the stinger, an antiseptic should be applied.

Emergency kits

Insect-sting emergency kits for hypersensitive individuals should be available. The directions and the benefits to be gained from using the kit should be carefully explained. The typical kit includes:

Epinephrine hydrochloride 1:1000 injection.[28] This medication is preferred because of its potent and rapid action. It should be administered immediately after stinging. Some insect-sting emergency kits have a preloaded (0.3 ml), sterile syringe. For people who have cardiovascular disease, diabetes, hypertension, or hyperthyroidism, the injection should be administered carefully.

Isoproterenol tablets, 10 mg, sublingual. The tablets replace or complement epinephrine hydrochloride. Initially, one tablet should be dissolved under the tongue. If symptoms persist for 5 to 10 minutes, another tablet should be used.

Epinephrine hydrochloride aerosol.[28] Inhalation of the drug relieves difficulty in breathing.

Antihistamines. Although they are slow in onset of action and are often ineffective in severe reactions, antihistamines are often used in conjunction with epinephrine hydrochloride. They are administered orally or parenterally.

Steroids. Steroids are slow in combating acute systemic symptoms. They usually are administered orally or parenterally with epinephrine hydrochloride.

Tweezers. Tweezers are used to remove the honeybee stinger.

Ingredients in OTC products

Most OTC products which are used for symptomatic relief of insect stings and bites contain one or more of the following pharmacologic agents: zinc oxide, calamine, zirconium oxide, menthol, camphor, phenol, local anesthetics, antibacterials, and antihistamines. A strong household ammonia solution or sodium bicarbonate paste applied at the site of the sting of a bee or wasp to relieve pain and discomfort is of little value. The treatment is based on the erroneous theory that ammonia solution and bicarbonate neutralize formic acid, mistakenly believed to be the toxic component of the venom of bees and wasps.

Zinc oxide, calamine, and zirconium oxide. These ingredients are used in lotions, ointments, creams, and sprays for their protective and astringent properties. Zinc oxide and calamine tend to toughen the skin, reducing inflammation and oozing. Although these two compounds have been used widely, their effectiveness has not been substantiated. Zirconium oxide causes side effects when applied to the skin; deodorant-antiperspirants that contain zirconium oxide have caused axillary granulomas (papular lesions). This condition can occur as a result of sensitivity to zirconium salts.

Menthol, camphor, and phenol. These agents temporarily relieve itching. They are used empirically for their mild, local anesthetic, antipruritic, and counterirritant properties.

Benzocaine. This and other local anesthetics are used to relieve itching and pain. However, they are of little value in the concentration available in most OTC products (1 to 2 percent). Some of these compounds can themselves be sensitizing if they are used for a long period.

Antibacterials. Benzethonium chloride and benzalkonium chloride are antibacterial agents that are used to prevent and treat secondary infections that can result from scratching .

Antihistamines. Antihistamines have mild, local anesthetic properties. When they are used locally, they can relieve pruritus. These compounds should be used with caution because they can cause sensitization, especially if they are applied regularly for a long period. Antihistamines are of greater value if taken orally.

Benzyl benzoate and gamma benzene hexachloride. These are the drugs of choice for scabies, and are available by prescription only. The patient should bathe, vigorously scrubbing the infested area. Then, a 25-percent emulsion of benzyl benzoate or 0.5- to 1-percent cream of gamma benzene hexachloride is applied to the entire body except the face. It should remain on the skin for 24 hours, after which the patient may bathe. A second application is recommended 1 week after the first one to destroy the hatched eggs. Additional applications should be avoided because contact dermatitis may occur. If itching is not relieved immediately after treatment, a soothing lotion such as calamine lotion with menthol and camphor may be used.

Product selection

Medication is often requested after symptoms have appeared, and it is important to determine the nature of symptoms following the sting or bite, how soon the symptoms appeared, the severity of the symptoms, and other drugs which are presently used. Personal or family history of hay fever, asthma, or contact dermatitis is also important in recommending medication for severe reactions to stings and bites. Cases of severe local reactions and systemic reactions should be referred to a physician. OTC products are of minimal value to hypersensitive people.

The pharmacist should record all information on hypersensitive individuals and should recommend that the person wear a tag or carry a card showing the nature of the allergy.

If the symptoms are minor, such as localized irritation, itching, or swelling, and there is no history of allergies, an appropriate nonprescription product can be recommended. Topical lotions, creams, ointments, and sprays are the main OTC products used for symptomatic relief of local reactions to insect stings and bites. The main considerations in product selection are reducing the possibility of additional stings or bites, providing proper protection to the affected skin, preventing secondary infection in the affected area, and relieving itching and irritation. Greasy ointments should be avoided because they can facilitate skin maceration. The best results can be obtained with lotions and sprays. OTC preparations for stings and bites should not be used excessively; local anesthetics and antihistamines can cause sensitivity.

Insect repellents

Insect repellents are chemicals that do not kill insects but keep them away from treated areas. When they are applied to the skin, repellents discourage the approach of insects and, as a result, protect the skin from insect bites. Most repellents are volatile, and when they are applied to skin or clothing, their vapor tends to prevent insects from alighting. However, a decrease in concentration of the repellent allows insects to alight momentarily.

Oils of citronella, turpentine, pennyroyal, cedarwood, eucalyptus, and wintergreen had been used for many years in insect repellent formulations. However, during and after World War II, investigations showed that these were relatively ineffective. Although more than 15,000 compounds have been tested as insect repellents, only a few have proved effective and safe enough to use on the skin. An insect repellent should be nontoxic, nonirritating, nonallergenic, and harmless to clothing. It should have an inoffensive odor, protect for several hours, be effective against as wide a variety of insects as possible, be able to withstand all conditions of weather, and have an esthetic feel and appearance.

The best all-purpose repellent is diethyltoluamide (NF) (*N*,*N*-diethyl-*m*-toluamide). Ethohexadiol (USP XVIII) (ethylhexanediol, Rutgers 612), dimethyl phthalate, dimethyl carbate, and butopyronoxyl (*N*-butyl 3,-4-dihydro-2, 2-dimethyl-4-oxo-1, 2*H*-pyran-6-carboxylate) are effective repellents, but they are not as effective against as wide a variety of insects as diethyltoluamide. However, a mixture of two or more of these repellents is more effective against a greater variety of insects than any one repellent. Repellents can be toxic if they are taken internally. People who are sensitive to these chemicals may develop skin reactions such as itching, burning, and swelling. These repellents cause smarting when they are applied to broken skin or mucous membranes. They should be applied carefully around the eyes because they may cause a temporary burning sensation.

Summary

Stings of honeybees, bumblebees, yellow jackets, hornets, wasps, and ants can cause pain, discomfort, illness, and severe local and systemic reactions. In normal individuals, stinging and biting insects cause local irritation, inflammation, swelling, and itching which provoke rubbing and scratching. Papules or nodules can form and persist for months. Secondary infections can occur and can lead to impetigo, furunculosis, or eczematoid dermatitis. Topical OTC products which include zinc oxide, calamine, benzocaine, antihistamines, benzalkonium chloride, benzethonium chloride, camphor, and menthol can relieve or prevent these symptoms.

The pharmacist should advise hypersensitive individuals on emergency procedures for insect stings and bites:

☐ The victim must seek medical attention immediately after an insect sting or bite.

☐ Basic first aid measures such as application of ice to the sting and removal of the stinger are helpful.

☐ The benefits gained from using the insect-sting emergency kit must be explained. It must be emphasized that epinephrine is the drug of choice for anaphylactic reactions.

People who are sensitized to the venom of these insects can react violently when they are stung. They need immediate, active treatment such as the administration of epinephrine hydrochloride, corticosteroids, or antihistamines. Desensitization is accomplished by inoculating with an extract of the whole body of the responsible insect.

References

1. S. E. Barr, *Ann. Allergy*, **29**, 49(1971).
2. N. A. Weber, *Am. J. Trop. Med.*, **17**, 765(1937).
3. R. M. Gordan and W. Crewe, *Ann. Trop. Med. Parasitol.*, **42**, 334(1948).
4. E. E. Buckley and N. Porges, Publication No. 44, Washington, D. C., AAAS, 1956, p. 171.
5. E. Habermann and K. G. Reiz, *Biochem. Z.*, **343(2)**, 192(1965).
6. T. K. Marshal, *Practitioner*, **178**, 712(1957).
7. W. R. Horsfall, "Medical Entomology," Ronald Press, New York, N.Y., 1962, p. 182.
8. J. A. McKiel and J. C. Clunie, *Can. J. Zool.*, **38**, 479(1960).
9. A. Hudson *et al.*, *Mosq. News*, **18**, 249(1958).
10. D. W. Micks and J. P. Ellis, *Proc. Soc. Exp. Biol. Med.*, **78**, 69(1951).
11. K. Mellanby, *Nature*, **158**, 554(1946).
12. D. S. Sax and J. Mejlszenkier, *N. Engl. J. Med.*, **285**, 293(1971).
13. J. R. Schenken *et al.*, *Am. J. Clin. Pathol.*, **23**, 1216(1953).
14. H. L. Meuller and L. W. Hill, *N. Engl. J. Med.*, **249**, 726(1953).
15. M. R. Caro *et al.*, *Arch. Dermatol.*, **75**, 475(1957).
16. C. H. Morhouse, *J. Am. Med. Assoc.*, **141**, 193(1949).
17. L. L. Brown, *South. Med. J.*, **65**, 273(1972).
18. H. V. Allington and R. R. Allington, *J. Am. Med. Assoc.*, **155**, 240(1954).
19. B. Swinny, *Tex. State J. Med.*, **46**, 12(1950).
20. J. W. Thomas, *W. V. Med. J.*, **55**, 115(1959).
21. H. R. Prince and P. G. Secrest, *J. Allergy*, **10**, 379(1939).
22. L. L. Henderson, *Postgrad. Med.*, **49**, 191(1971).
23. M. I. Levine, *J. Am. Med. Assoc.*, **217**, 964(1971).
24. M. J. Loveless and W. R. Fackler, *Ann. Allergy*, **14**, 347(1956).
25. P. J. Torsney, *J. Allergy Clin. Immunol.*, **52**, 303(1973).
26. M. D. Ellis, "Dangerous Plants, Snakes, Arthropods and Marine Life of Texas," U.S. Department of Health, Education, and Welfare, 1975, p. 175.
27. R. E. Arnold, "What to Do About Bites and Stings of Venomous Animals," Collier Books, Division of Macmillan, New York, N.Y., 1973, p. 9.
28. M. A. Passerro and S. C. Dees, *Am. Physician*, **7**, 74(1973).

Products 23 INSECT STING AND BITE

Product (manufacturer)	Application form	Ingredients
Bactine (Miles)	liquid	alcohol, 3.17%; methylbenzethonium chloride, 0.5%; octoxynol, 0.35%; chlorothymol, 0.1%
Benadex (Fuller)	ointment	benzocaine, 2%; aluminum acetate, 2%; phenol, 1%; petrolatum
Bevill's Lotion (Bevill)	lotion	alcohol, 68%; ether, 8%; methyl salicylate, 1%; salicylic acid
Chiggerex (First Texas)	ointment	benzocaine, 2.0%; camphor, 0.008%; olive oil, 0.008%; menthol, 0.005%; peppermint oil, 0.005%; methylparaben, 0.002%; clove oil, 0.002%
Chiggertox Liquid (First Texas)	liquid	isopropyl alcohol, 53%; benzyl benzoate, 21.4%; soft soap, 21.4%; benzocaine, 2.1%
Derma Medicone (Medicone)	ointment	zinc oxide, 137.0 mg/g; benzocaine, 20.0 mg/g; 8-hydroxyquinoline sulfate, 10.5 mg/g; ichthammol, 10.0 mg/g; menthol, 4.8 mg/g; petrolatum; lanolin; perfume
Dermoplast (Ayerst)	spray	benzocaine, 4.5%; methylparaben, 2%; isopropyl alcohol, 1.9%; menthol, 0.5%; benzethonium chloride, 0.1%
Mediconet (Medicone)	saturated medical pads	hamamelis water, 50%; glycerin, 10%; ethoxylated lanolin, 0.5%; methylparaben, 0.15%; benzalkonium chloride, 0.02%; perfume
Nupercainal Cream (Ciba)	cream	dibucaine, 0.5%; acetone sodium bisulfite, 0.37%; water-washable base
Nupercainal Ointment (Ciba)	ointment	dibucaine, 1%; acetone sodium bisulfite, 0.5%
Nupercainal Spray (Ciba)	spray	dibucaine, 0.25%; alcohol, 46%
Pyribenzamine (Ciba)	cream ointment	tripelennamine, 2%; water-washable base (cream); petrolatum base (ointment)
Rexall First Aid Spray (Rexall)	spray	benzocaine; methylbenzethonium chloride; tyloxapol; chlorothymol; isopropyl alcohol, 4%; camphor
Surfadil (Lilly)	cream lotion	methapyrilene hydrochloride, 2%; cyclomethycaine, 0.5%; titanium dioxide, 5% (lotion)
Tucks and Tucks Take-Alongs (Fuller)	saturated medical pads	hamamelis water, 50%; glycerin, 10%; methylparaben, 0.1%; benzalkonium chloride, 0.003%

Burn and Sunburn Products

Nathan A. Hall
James W. McFadden

Questions to ask the patient

How old is the person who will be using the product?

What caused the burn—chemicals, sun exposure, or heat?

How severe is the burn? Is the skin broken and/or blistered?

Where is the burn? How large is the burned area?

Is the burn painful?

Which treatments have been used?

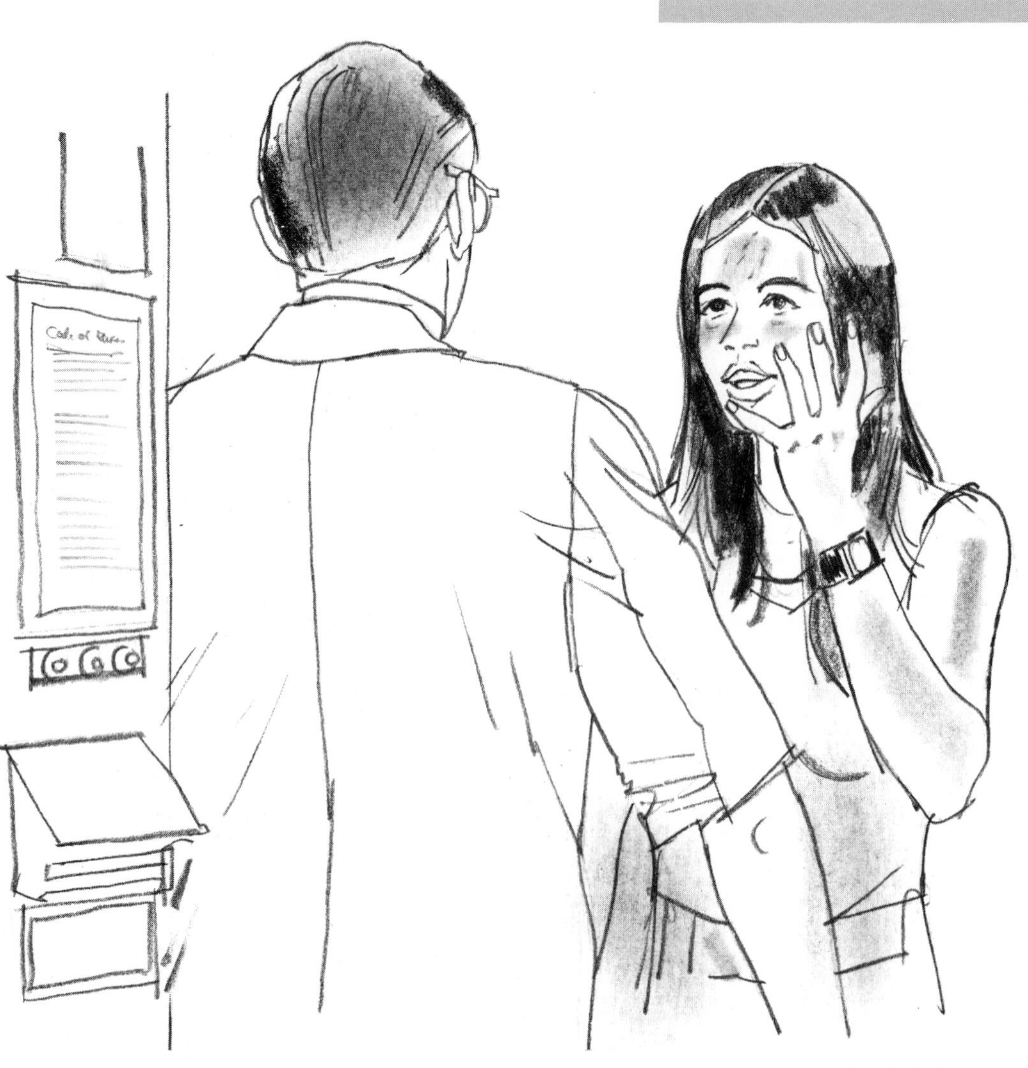

CHAPTER 24

Few bodily injuries are more traumatic than major burns. By scorching through skin and muscle, destroying nerves and blood vessels, and setting the stage for a fertile culture medium for infectious microbes, burns can cripple, disfigure, and kill. Approximately 2 million different burn cases occur annually in the U.S., and 7,500 people die as a result of burn injuries. Of the 7,500, 1,800 are under age 15.[1] Although these figures are high, the annual number of burn deaths has remained relatively constant while the population has increased, and the recovery rate from serious burns has improved significantly. The improvement in care of the burned patient has resulted from a better understanding of the pathophysiology of the burn wound, better methods of local treatment for controlling infection, and the establishment of specialized burn centers for the care of the seriously burned. Hopefully, the enforcement of recently passed Federal garment flameproofing legislation will markedly reduce burn morbidity and mortality in the future.

Etiology of burns

Burns can result from several causes and, depending on their severity, can inflict minor to extensive damage to the skin or underlying organs. Thermal trauma from flame, hot or scalding liquid, or hot objects are the most common causes. Chemicals, high voltage current, and radioactive materials can also cause burns. Sunburn is also common. Although sunlight includes radiation with wavelengths ranging from 2,900 to 18,500 Å, only the U.V. radiation of less than 3,000 Å can produce sunburn.[2]

The very young, the elderly, and those with chronic illnesses such as diabetes, alcoholism, obesity, or arteriosclerotic heart disease tolerate burn traumas poorly. Generally, a burn of more than 2 percent of the body surface should be treated by a physician.

Pathophysiology of burns

The skin is the largest organ of the human body, comprising about one-sixth of the body weight. (See Chapter 27 for a complete discussion of the skin.) Almost one-third of the circulative blood is housed in the skin. There is constant interflow of fluid and electrolytes between the components of the skin and the blood. The main functions of the skin are protection for the underlying structures (e.g., preventing the ingress of microbes), temperature regulation, as a reservoir of fat and vitamin D, sensation, and secretion.

Burns are usually described and evaluated on the basis of the area of the body affected and the depth of penetration of the burn into the skin. This helps determine the necessary treatment regimen and whether self-treatment, physician outpatient treatment, or hospitalization is required.

Assessing the area and degree of the burn

The "rule of nines" is a rapid method of estimating the percentage of body surface involved in a burn wound. The body surface is divided into 11 areas, each representing about 9 percent of the total. Nine percent is assigned to the head and neck area and to each arm and hand area; 18 percent is assigned to the anterior trunk, the posterior trunk, and each leg and foot area. Estimates are fairly good for adults but are less accurate for children and infants (Table 1). Special rapid estimating procedures have been advocated for children.

Determination of the depth of a burn is a clinical judgment. Distinctions of first, second, third, and fourth degree are clear theoretically, but the nature of the burning agent, the duration of its application, and the circumstances of the burn produce different characteristics, making experience the best guide. Table 2 describes the depth classifications of burns by degree. A burn wound usually has characteristics of less severe burns on its periphery.

Reepithelialization following burns depends on the depth of injury. Partial-thickness, cutaneous damage often leaves intact a viable number of appendages from which resurfacing can occur; it takes 2 to 3 days for superficial, second-degree burns and as long as 6 weeks for a deep, second-degree burn. Full-thickness damage causes irreversible destruction of all the skin layers and appendages so that regeneration occurs only at the wound edges (Fig. 1). A uniform burn, such as that caused by scalding, may result in an injury of variable depth because of differences in skin thickness between individuals and age groups, regional differences in thickness, and the distribution and depth of skin appendages in the burned area.[3] In a large deep burn (e.g., 50 percent, third degree), hospitalization with massive intravenous fluid administration is necessary to correct severe shock and prevent death secondary to leakage of fluid and protein from the vascular compartment into the burn wound, effectively reducing blood volume.[1,4]

Minor burns include partial-thickness burns of less than 15 percent of the body surface and full-thickness burns of less than 2 percent of the body surface. These may be treated on an outpatient basis. Most patients with a small superficial burn complain of pain. Third-degree burns are anesthetic because the sensory nerves are destroyed. Blisters are lacking because the small blood vessels are coagulated.[1]

Infection

Burn-wound infection was at one time responsible for much late mortality in severe burns.[3] Early colonization of the burn wound by gram-positive bacteria *(Staphylococcus, Streptococcus)* occurs during the first day. After the third day, gram-negative bacteria (mainly *Pseudomonas*) predominate and can convert a second-degree burn to third degree. The area is a luxuriant culture medium for microorganisms because there is much necrotic tissue and normal body defense mechanisms are impaired by the occluded vascular circulation. Thus, topical therapy is essential and should be active against *Pseudomonas*. Silver sulfadiazine, silver nitrate, and mafenide acetate (prescription only) are commonly used topically for severe burns.[5]

Table 1. Percent Surface Area of Various Body Parts[a]

Surface	Birth	Years 1	5	10	15	Adult
Head	19	17	13	11	9	7
Neck	2	2	2	2	2	2
Anterior trunk	13	13	13	13	13	13
Posterior trunk	13	13	13	13	13	13
Buttocks	5	5	5	5	5	5
Genitalia	1	1	1	1	1	1
Upper arms	8	8	8	8	8	8
Forearms	6	6	6	6	6	6
Hands	5	5	5	5	5	5
Thighs	11	13	16	17	18	19
Legs	10	10	11	12	13	14
Feet	7	7	7	7	7	7

[a]Adapted from *Skin Xenografts*, Burn Treatment Skin Bank, Phoenix, Ariz.

Sunburn

Dermatitis actinica is an acute inflammatory skin reaction resulting from sunburn, drug photosensitization, contact photosensitivity caused by chemicals, or unusual sensitivity to actinic rays.[6] Different reactions to sunlight are caused mainly by differences in skin pigmentation. The progress of skin coloration during sun exposure seems to follow a pattern. Within the first 20 minutes, initial reddening appears caused by oxidation of the bleached melanin; this pigmentation rapidly disappears. True sunburn erythema begins within 2 to 8 hours and persists for several days. Tanning usually occurs in about 2 days. Discomfort, pain, and blistering result from excessive exposure to U.V. radiation. If the affected area is large, malaise, nausea and vomiting, chills, and fever can occur.[7]

The delayed reaction of sunburn has puzzled researchers for years. Some evidence indicates that prostaglandins are involved because prostaglandin inhibitors can prevent the erythema or even blanch the reddening already present.[8, 9] A 2.5-percent indomethacin solution (prostaglandin inhibitor) can cause blanching when applied 1.5 hours after redness is first noted. Blanched areas are cooler than the reddened areas. A fluoridated steroid preparation applied similarly has no better effect than the control vehicle. Further studies of the inflammatory consequence of sunburn may provide therapeutic prostaglandin inhibitors that can be used after excessive sun exposure and before suffering.

Table 2. Depth Classification of Burns

Type	Tissue affected	Characteristics
First degree	Epidermis	Erythema, pain, no blistering
Second degree	Epidermis, some dermis	Blisters, pain, skin regenerates
Third degree	Full skin thickness	No blisters, leathery appearance, less pain, skin grafting required
Fourth degree and char burn	Full skin thickness and underlying tissue	Blackened appearance, dryness, pain, danger of deep infection

Sunburn is usually benign and self-limiting unless the burn is severe or occurs as an associated finding in a more serious disorder (e.g., porphyria, lupus, or pellagra).[6] In some patients, the severity of sunburn is greater than normal for the amount of exposure. The problem may be due to drug photosensitivity. The distribution of the sunburn can be a clue; distinct boundaries of exposed areas may imply photosensitivity. Drug photosensitivity is often manifested as a phototoxic or photoallergic reaction. Phototoxic reactions are those that can be elicited in nearly everyone, if enough light energy of the appropriate wavelength is received or if appropriate concentrations of the phototoxic compound are applied topically or are ingested. The reaction is characterized by an exaggerated sunburn with or without painful edema. It occurs within a few hours after exposure. Photoallergy to drugs is an acquired and altered capacity of the skin to respond to light energy in the presence of a photosensitizer. It is presumed that the reaction depends on an antigen-antibody relationship or a cell-mediated, delayed, hypersensitivity response.

The clinical patterns in drug-induced, photoallergic reactions may range from eczematous or papular lesions, appearing 24 hours or more after sun exposure, to acute urticarial lesions, developing within a few minutes after exposure. The eruption is not exclusively localized at the sites of sun exposure but frequently extends beyond the areas of exposure.

Many different classes of systemic and contact chemicals and drugs may cause photosensitivity reactions.[10] They include bacteriostatic agents in soaps, antiseptics such as hexachlorophene and bithionol, and sunscreens such as esters of aminobenzoic acid. Brightening agents for cellulose, nylon, or wool fibers; cadmium sulfide in tattoos; essential oils in cosmetics and beauty aids; various plants used in perfumery, as flavorings, or as spices; various dyes; many drugs (Table 3); and cyclamates formerly allowed as artificial sweeteners may also cause photosensitivity reactions.

Treatment of burns

When a small burn occurs on the hand or arm, immediate immersion in cold water of the burned area or the application of towels soaked in ice water usually brings immediate pain relief. The affected part should be cooled continuously for several minutes; the cooling may have some value in arresting heat damage to the tissues.[1] A minor burn may repair itself with or without treatment. A serious burn needs expert medical attention to prevent complications and to minimize scarring. Initial self-medication is actually first aid generally aimed at the intense but short-lived pain.

The judgment of whether a burn is minor or serious is not easy. Immediately following the burn, an estimate of the extent of the burn may be made from the nature of the cause of the injury, the painful area, and the appearance of the skin. Judgment of depth is much more difficult. Even burn surgeons with considerable experience have problems in judging differences between second- and third-degree burns soon after the injury. As the wound ages, the extent and the depth of the traumatized area become more apparent.

If there is doubt as to the severity of the burn, it is probably better to recommend physician referral than self-treatment. Patients with obviously extensive and deep burns should be sent to an expert burn service of a hospital or medical center as soon as possible (Table 4). The treatment of serious and extensive burns often requires a highly skilled team of specialists with intensive training in caring for the burned patient.

Resuscitation and treatment of shock and secondary complications with large amounts of fluids and electrolytes are primary concerns. Next, an attempt should be made to control microbial invasion of the burned area, where the vascular supply is occluded and necrotic tissue is an excellent culture medium. Topical applications of silver nitrate, silver sulfadiazine, mafenide acetate, or antibiotics may be used. When the immediate danger has passed, the treatment of secondary problems such as hypertension and stress (Curling's) ulcer is undertaken. Simultaneously, the burned surface must be kept viable so that skin grafting will be successful. Wound closures with homograft (cadaver skin) or heterograft (blond pig skin) are used.[5] The final stage of treatment is dealing with emotional problems and rehabilitation of the patient.

As with other traumas, overtreatment of burns is a danger. Surgeons have often complained of having to remove the contamination applied to the burn by well-meaning friends, causing increased stress to an already distressed patient. If they are used appropriately on minor burns, burn remedies in self-medication may be of some help. However, they may not be as valuable as the simple, readily available, nonpharmaceutical measure for minor or serious burns—cool water. Burn remedies containing a mixture of chemicals always involve a certain amount of risk. A burn may destroy the barrier layer of the skin which prevents invasion by external chemicals, and potentially toxic chemicals may be absorbed. Many chemicals applied to injured skin also increase the hazard of allergic hypersensitivity reactions. If a burn is serious, the residue from the remedy may capture and protect environmental micro-organisms, increasing the danger of infection. Also, the residue will have to be removed by painful procedures if a viable surface is needed for skin grafting. Water has none of these disadvantages.

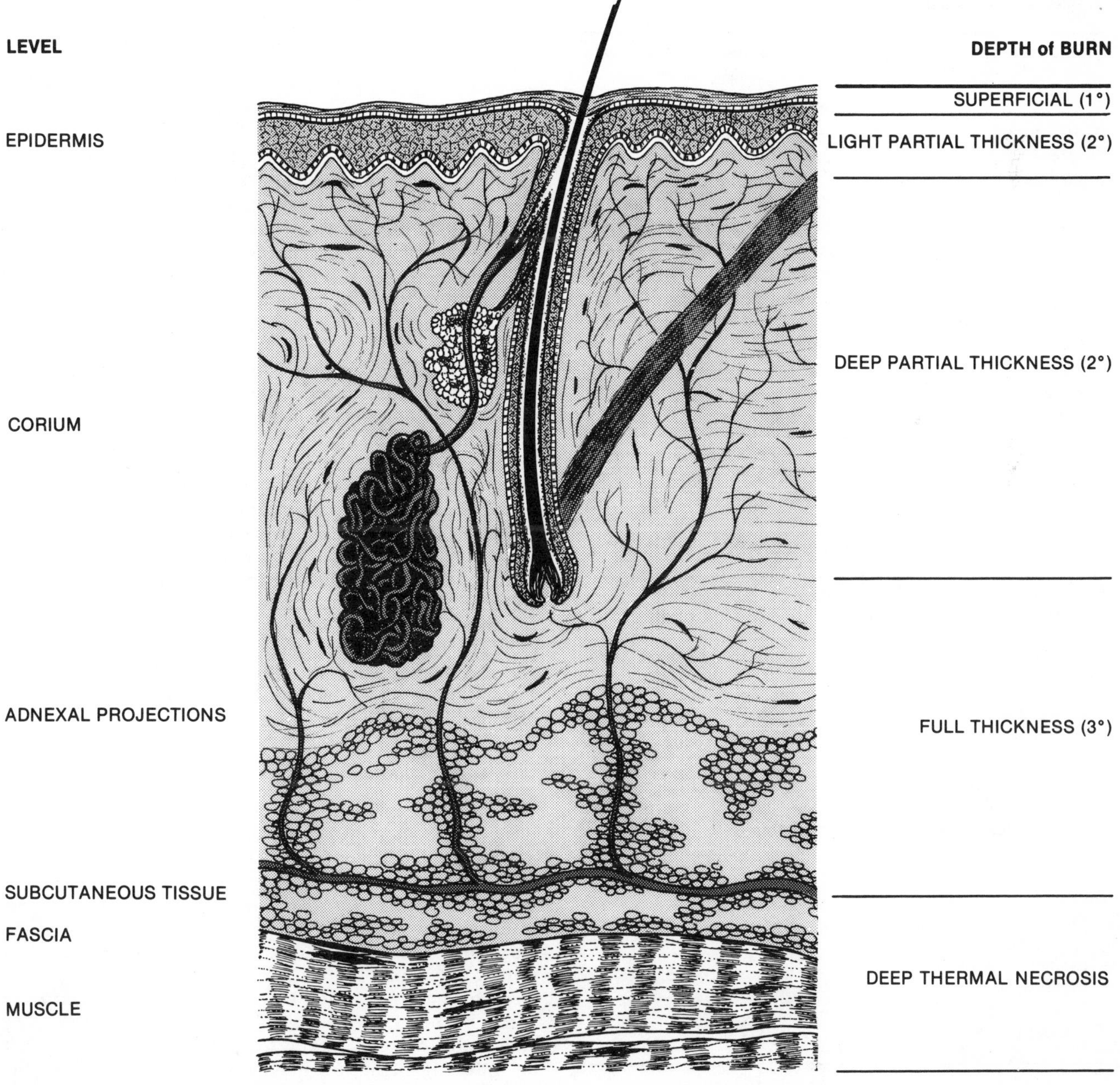

Figure 1. Cross section of skin showing depth of burns.

Table 3. Classes of Drugs with Photosensitizing Potential[a]

Anticonvulsants
Antihistamines
Antineoplastics
Barbiturates
Dyes
Gold and silver salts
Griseofulvin
Local anesthetics (procaine-related)
Nonsteroidal anti-inflammatories
Phenothiazine antipsychotics
Psoralen dermatologicals
Salicylates
Sex hormones
Sulfonamides
Sulfonylurea antidiabetics
Tetracycline antibiotics
Thiazide diuretics
Topical antimicrobials

[a]Adapted from E. Stempel and R. Stempel, *J. Am. Pharm. Assoc.*, **NS13**, 200(1973).

Cool water applications are often advised in the initial treatment of serious burns. Early cooling may mean the difference between an extensive deep burn and one that is superficial by preventing the extension of coagulation necrosis.[11] Local edema may be reduced even if as long as 45 minutes has elapsed before cooling is begun.[12] However, the evidence for physiological benefit of cooling in serious burns is less than conclusive, and the lack of standardized experimental conditions make critical clinical evaluation difficult.[13] Nevertheless, the subjective relief of pain by cooling is well accepted.[14-16]

Local anesthetics

The advantage of the poorly soluble, local anesthetic agents, e.g., benzocaine (ethyl aminobenzoate) and butamben picrate (butyl aminobenzoate picrate) over the soluble ones is the lessened danger of absorption to produce systemic toxicity. Penetration of benzocaine through the intact skin to nerve endings is slow, but concentrations as low as 5 percent in appropriate solution can produce local anesthesia. Commercial preparations below 20-percent concentration may fail to have an effect on intact or mildly sunburned skin.[17] Concentrations of benzocaine in these products range from 0.5 to 20 percent. In burns that disrupt the skin barrier, an effect comparable to that on mucous membranes is expected, and lower concentrations may be active.

Local anesthetics in their salt forms are water soluble; in their free base form, water solubility is low. It is the free base form that possesses local anesthetic activity. When the salt form encounters buffering body fluids, a proportion is converted to the active free base form, depending on the pKa of the base and relative buffer capacity. It was found that, clinically, aqueous solutions of salts are inactive on intact skin, but solutions of the free bases at similar concentrations show activity. Common water-soluble agents in burn remedies include dibucaine, lidocaine, tetracaine, and pramoxine in both salt and free base forms. A study of commercial preparations containing water-soluble agents shows no objective response on intact or sunburned skin but shows some subjective effect in sunburn.[17] More effectiveness is expected on burns that destroy the barrier layer.

Acute toxicity from applied local anesthetics is rare because the short-term use in minor burns makes a systemic buildup resulting in elevated blood levels unlikely. Highly concentrated products used inappropriately on large area, second- and third-degree burns may elicit toxic reactions, but these remedies generally contain low concentrations of the more toxic local anesthetics. Benzocaine has been implicated in producing methemoglobinemia in infants.[18 19] It also seems to be a major offender in sensitization and subsequent allergic reaction. Epstein[20] reports that 6 of 413 patients with contact dermatitis were allergic to benzocaine as detected by patch tests. Because lidocaine is an amide rather than an ester type of local anesthetic, it sometimes may be substituted for other agents to which the patient is allergic; however, allergy to lidocaine is also encountered. With the short-term use of burn preparations, the development of allergic reactions is less probable than with preparations applied to more persistent dermatitis. Because the skin is abraded in many burns, sensitization followed by an allergic reaction to the local anesthetic is possible if the preparation is used at a later time.

The final report of the FDA Panel on Topical Analgesic, Antirheumatic, Otic, Burn, Sunburn Treatment and Prevention OTC Products will list the safety and efficacy of topically applied local anesthetics.[21]

Table 4. Health Care Requirements of Burns[a]

General hospital	Community hospital	Local
Critical burns	*Moderate burns*	*Minor burns*
Second-degree burns of more than 30%.[b]	Second-degree burns of 15-30%.	Second-degree burns of less than 15%.
Third-degree burns of face, hands, or of more than 10%.	Third-degree burns of less than 10%, except face, hands, or feet.	Third-degree burns of less than 2%.
Burns complicated by respiratory tract injury, major soft-tissue injury, or fractures.		
Electrical burns.		

[a]Adapted from C. P. Artz, *Drug Ther.*, **5**, 127 (1975).
[b]Percentages refer to the extent of body surface burned.

Antimicrobials

Antimicrobials include quaternary ammonium compounds, iodophors, organic mercurials, phenols, and antibiotics. (See Chapter 27 for further discussion of topical anti-infectives.)

Their spectra of action are variable, although most of them show activity against gram-positive bacteria in the laboratory. As with other skin infections, burn infections usually contain more than one kind of organism. The primary offenders in major burn sepses are *Staphylococcus* (gram positive) and *Pseudomonas* (gram negative). The undesirable consequences of topical antimicrobials are that the infecting organisms may acquire a resistance to the agent or the agent may upset the ecological balance of the normal flora so that nonsensitive, resistant, and possibly more dangerous organisms predominate in the microbial population. Unless the prophylactic or therapeutic agent is specific and effective, more harm than good can result.

A group of specific topical agents that are essential in treating major burns are restricted to physician use. The nonprescription burn remedies generally lack the specificity and effectiveness to be recommended. Few of them are effective against *Pseudomonas*. The activity of the nonprescription antimicrobials against gram-positive organisms may even favor early invasion by *Pseudomonas*.

The final report of the first FDA Panel on OTC Antimicrobials (Antimicrobial I) presents much useful information for understanding the antimicrobial ingredients in burn remedies.[22] [The review process for antimicrobial products is being continued by a second Panel (Antimicrobial II)]. For many topical antimicrobials, insufficient evidence was at hand to evaluate them under the Panel guidelines as "generally recognized as safe and effective." To make definitive judgments, the Panel created seven new classes of antimicrobial products, three of which are potentially applicable to burn remedies:

Skin antiseptic. "A safe, non-irritating antimicrobial-containing preparation which prevents overt skin infection." This class of preparations is especially applicable to burn remedies. Claims must be supported by clinical studies demonstrating effectiveness. None of the examined ingredients qualified for approval. The quaternary ammonium compounds, hexylresorcinol, iodophors, phenol (1.5 percent or less), chloroxylenol, and triclosan were among the active ingredients for which more data were needed. Hexachlorophene, halogenated salicylanilides, phenol (more than 1.5 percent), and tincture of iodine were judged not safe and/or effective.

Skin wound cleanser. "A safe, non-irritating liquid preparation (or product to be used with water) which assists in the removal of foreign material from small superficial wounds and does not delay wound healing." These products would have limited use in burn wounds. They may or may not contain antimicrobials, but they must help cleanse the wound. The quaternary ammonium compounds and hexylresorcinol were judged as safe and effective ingredients. Except for these, the ingredients requiring more data were the same as those under skin antiseptics, and active ingredients that were not safe and effective were the same.

Skin wound protectant. "A safe, non-irritating preparation applied to small cleansed wounds which provides a protective (physical and/or chemical) barrier and neither delays healing nor favors the growth of microorganisms." This class of products might be useful as a first aid measure in preventing wound contamination. For antimicrobials in nonprescription remedies, evaluation of suitability must be based on efficacy and possible toxicity. Specific toxicity of supposedly innocuous, topical antimicrobial agents was given only minor attention prior to recent experiences with hexachlorophene. It is now recognized that absorption from topical preparations often occurs, and toxic or potentially harmful blood levels of the antimicrobial agents may be reached when the preparation is used routinely or when sufficient skin destruction has taken place for absorption to occur.[23,24]

Hexachlorophene has been removed from nonprescription availability largely because of its toxic effect on brain tissue when it is absorbed. Because of the production of severe, disabling photosensitivity caused by halogenated salicylanilides (e.g., tribromsalan), these ingredients have been judged unsafe for all drug and cosmetic purposes. Topical application of phenol in concentrations of 2 percent or more can cause CNS toxicity and gangrene.[25] Accordingly, phenol concentrations of more than 1.5 percent (aqueous or alcoholic solution) have been judged unsafe for general use as a nonprescription, topical antimicrobial. Iodine tincture is irritating to broken skin and delays wound healing. Therefore, for other than preparation of intact skin for surgery, it is not a safe antimicrobial, according to the Panel.

Nonprescription antibiotic preparations were not evaluated by the Antimicrobial I Panel; they will be reviewed by the Antimicrobial II Panel. The mixture of neomycin, polymyxin B sulfate, and bacitracin is widely used, but evaluations of the mixture have been equivocal in spite of the broad spectrum of activity and the specificity of polymyxin B sulfate against *Pseudomonas in vitro*. The absorption of toxic amounts from misuse of neomycin on large area burns and allergic hypersensitivity reactions to neomycin have occurred.[20]

Many preparations contain low concentrations of antimicrobials as preservatives against spoilage. The name of an antimicrobial on the label may infer therapeutic or suppressant action. Unfortunately, only the names (not the amounts or concentrations) of active ingredients have been required on the labels of nonprescription products. Preservative ingredients also will be reviewed by the Antimicrobial II Panel.

Product formulation

Few, if any, of the products claimed as useful in minor burns contain only one ingredient. Other components of a formulation may affect the action or toxicity of the active ingredient. The policy of the Antimicrobial I Panel states that combinations of nonantimicrobial ingredients with antimicrobials are suitable if:

- ☐ The antimicrobial remains safe and effective.
- ☐ The nonantimicrobial ingredient is safe and effective.
- ☐ The labeling indicates pharmacologic effects of all active ingredients.
- ☐ The combination provides rational concurrent therapy for a significant part of the target population.
- ☐ The combination meets the requirement of the definitions for the antimicrobial product category.

Burn remedies have not been subjected to this kind of examination in the past. Secondary ingredients such as volatile oils, menthol, eugenol, thymol, vitamin A, and zinc compounds will be examined to determine whether they contribute to or interfere with a claim made for a product.

In using nonprescription products for the treatment of burns, consideration must be given to the placebo effect of the application. Aromatic ingredients may reinforce the idea that something is being done to help this very painful condition. One surgeon has reported excellent pain relief from aerosol foam shaving cream applied to the burn when the can was labeled "Special Burn Cream." If the patient saw that it was shaving cream, little relief was reported.[26]

Dosage forms

Ointments, because of their usually greasy base, are probably the least desirable form of burn treatment. Their possible misuse on serious burns can facilitate microbial contamination, and they require removal before further local treatment can be given. Creams, solutions, and sprays are easier to remove and may, by cooling, assist other ingredients in deadening the pain. Sprays and aerosols deliver the medication in the least traumatizing manner, but there may be danger from inhalation of the suspended particles.

Patient consultation

If the burn is minor and if the early painful phase has passed, an unmedicated emollient preparation probably is as effective as a special burn remedy. If the patient has suffered a minor but painful sunburn, only preparations containing fairly high concentrations of lipid-soluble, local anesthetics can provide adequate pain relief. Creams or rapidly evaporating solutions or sprays may relieve pain by cooling. However, cool water applications may be as effective.

If the burn is extensive and deep (second or third degree), the patient should be referred to a physician immediately. Temporary relief of pain can be controlled with cool water immersion or, where immersion is impractical, with moist, cool, clean coverings. If a large area of skin has been burned severely, the patient should be taken to the hospital (preferably one with a burn unit) as quickly as possible.

If a burn preparation is for part of a first aid supply, the pharmacist should explain first aid for serious burns and point out the label caution that the burn remedy should not be used for serious burns. The guidelines recommended by a British first aid manual for treatment of burns may be appropriate: [27]

- ☐ Extinguish fire on the clothing and rapidly cool the burn with water.
- ☐ For scalds, hold the extremity under running cold water or pour cold water on the area.
- ☐ Lay the victim flat. Remove obstructions and compress the burned area with cool moist dressings. Soak extremities in cold water.
- ☐ Quickly transport the victim to the hospital while maintaining the moisture of the cool compresses.
- ☐ Prevent systemic hypothermia by wrapping the victim in clean, warm blankets and allowing sips of warm liquids by mouth.

Severe sunburn can occur when a patient is taking certain prescription medications. Whenever medication is dispensed that has photosensitizing potential, the pharmacist should warn the patient. Warnings are particularly important when the patient is likely to be outdoors in the sunshine such as in summer or during the skiing season.

Summary

Burn remedies should be used only on minor burns. Pharmacists should try to ensure proper use by appropriate counseling of those seeking burn remedies. As indicated, there is little firm scientific basis for selecting one remedy over another. A burn surgeon has advised, "Minor or trivial burns do well with almost any reasonable form of local treatment which has as its object the protection of the damaged area and prevention of infection." [28] Cool water and clean, moist dressings would seem to meet these criteria as well as nonprescription burn products, and they involve less potential chemical hazard and carry less risk of getting in the way of treatment should the burn turn out to be serious.

References

1. C. P. Artz, *Drug Ther.*, **5**, 127(1975).
2. "The Merck Manual of Diagnosis and Therapy," 12th ed., D. N. Holvey, Ed., Merck, Sharp and Dohme, Rahway, N.J., 1972, p. 1492.
3. F. D. Foley, *Surg. Clin. North Am.*, **50**, 1201(1970).
4. B. Cosman, *Hosp. Med.*, **7**, 55(1971).
5. J. A. Moncrief, *N. Engl. J. Med.*, **288**, 444(1973).
6. "Current Diagnosis and Treatment," M. A. Krupp *et al.*, Eds., Lange Medical Publications, Los Altos, Calif., 1971, p. 49.
7. Editorial, *Lancet*, **2**, 30(1973).
8. D. S. Snyder and W. H. Eaglstein, *J. Invest. Dermatol.*, **60**, 110(1973).
9. D. S. Snyder and W. H. Eaglstein, *Br. J. Dermatol.*, **90**, 91(1974).
10. E. Stempel and R. Stempel, *J. Am. Pharm. Assoc.*, **NS13**, 200(1973).
11. M. F. Epstein and J. D. Crawford, *Pediatrics*, **52**, 430(1973).
12. O. J. Ofeigsson *et al.*, *J. Pathol.*, **108**, 145(1972).
13. J. A. Moncrief, *N. Engl. J. Med.*, **290**, 59(1974).
14. H. Kravitz, *Pediatrics*, **53**, 766(1974).
15. A. Blumefeld, *N. Engl. J. Med.*, **290**, 58(1974).
16. J. G. Appleyard, *Lancet*, **2**, 1370(1972).
17. H. Dalili and J. Adriani, *Clin. Pharmacol. Ther.*, **12**, 913(1971).
18. H. Peterson, *N. Engl. J. Med.*, **263**, 454(1960).
19. N. Goluboff and D. S. Macfayden, *J. Pediatr.*, **47**, 222(1955).
20. E. Epstein, *J. Am. Med. Assoc.*, **198**, 517(1966).
21. *Fed. Regist.*, **37**, 9464(1972).
22. *Fed. Regist.*, **39**, 33103(1974).
23. D. L. Larson, *J. Am. Hosp. Assoc.*, **42**, 63(1968).
24. K. J. LaVelle *et al.*, *Clin. Pharmacol. Ther.*, **17**, 365(1975).
25. W. B. Deichman and M. L. Keplinger, in "Industrial Hygiene and Toxicology," vol. 2, 2d ed., Interscience Publishers, New York, N.Y., 1963.
26. R. F. Hogarty, in "Burns: A Symposium," Charles C Thomas, Springfield, Ill., 1964, p. 74.
27. "First Aid," Authorized Manual of St. John Ambulance Association, St. Andrews Ambulance Association and British Red Cross, 3d ed., London, England, 1972.
28. R. H. B. Elliott, Jr., in "Trauma," H. L. McLaughlin, Ed., Saunders, Philadelphia, Pa., 1959, p. 79.

Product (manufacturer)	Dosage form	Anesthetic	Antimicrobial	Other
Aerosept (Dalin)	aerosol	lidocaine	cetyltrimethylammonium bromide chloroxylenol	aromatic base
Americaine (Arnar-Stone)	aerosol ointment	benzocaine, 20%	benzethonium chloride, 0.1% (ointment)	polyethylene glycols (ointment), water-dispersible base (aerosol)
Bactine (Miles)	liquid	—	methylbenzethonium chloride, 0.5% chlorothymol, 0.1%	alcohol, 3.17%; octoxynol, 0.35%
Betadine (Purdue Frederick)	aerosol ointment	—	povidone-iodine, 5% (aerosol) 10% (ointment)	aqueous base (aerosol), water-miscible base (ointment)
Biotres (Central)	ointment	—	polymyxin B sulfate, 10,000 units/g bacitracin zinc, 500 units/g	—
Burn-a-lay (Colgate-Palmolive)	cream	benzocaine, 1.25%	chlorobutanol, 0.75% benzoxiquine, 0.025%	zinc oxide, 2%; thymol, 0.5%
Burn Relief Spray (Rexall)	spray	benzocaine	chlorobutanol, 0.3% benzethonium chloride	polyalkylene glycol; menthol; isopropyl alcohol, 11%
Burntame Spray (Otis Clapp)	spray	benzocaine, 20%	8-hydroxyquinoline	—
Butesin Picrate (Abbott)	ointment	butamben picrate, 1%	—	—
Dermoplast (Ayerst)	spray	benzocaine, 4.5%	benzethonium chloride, 0.1%	methylparaben, 2%; isopropyl alcohol, 1.9%; menthol, 0.5%
Foille (Carbisulphoil)	liquid ointment aerosol	benzocaine, 2%	benzyl alcohol, 4% 8-hydroxyquinoline	sulfur, bland vegetable oil
Gebauer's Tannic Spray (Gebauer)	spray	ethyl chloride, 33.3% benzocaine, 0.5%	chlorobutanol, 1.2%	tannic acid, 3.9%; menthol, 0.1%
Hist-A-Balm Medicated Lotion (Columbia Medical)	lotion	diperodon hydrochloride, 0.25%	benzalkonium chloride, 0.1%	phenyltoloxamine dihydrogen citrate, 0.75%; menthol; camphor
Hyrocain (Amer. Pharm.)	cream	benzocaine dibucaine tetracaine	—	—
Kip First Aid Spray (Young's)	aerosol lotion	benzocaine, 3% *o*-phenylphenol, 0.5%	—	bay oil, spearmint oil, sesame oil, thyme oil, cottonseed oil, castor oil, methyl salicylate, salicylic acid, propellants
Kip for Burns (Young's)	ointment	*o*-phenylphenol, 0.5%	phenol, 0.5%	spearmint oil, bay oil, methyl salicylate, salicylic acid, zinc oxide, petrolatum, paraffin, lanolin
Kip Moisturizing Lotion (Young's)	lotion	benzocaine, 2%	benzalkonium chloride	salicylic acid, stearic acid, glyceryl monostearate, castor oil, sesame oil, cottonseed oil, isopropyl myristate, propylene glycol, triethanolamine, methylparaben, butylated hydroxyanisole, perfume
Kip Sunburn Spray (Young's)	aerosol	benzocaine, 10%	benzalkonium chloride	menthol; lanolin; propylene glycol; isopropyl alcohol, 7%; hexadecyl alcohol; propellants

Product (manufacturer)	Dosage form	Anesthetic	Antimicrobial	Other
Medicone Dressing Cream (Medicone)	cream	benzocaine, 5 mg/g	8-hydroxyquinoline sulfate, 0.5 mg/g	cod liver oil, 125 mg/g; zinc oxide, 125 mg/g; menthol, 1.8 mg/g; petrolatum; lanolin; paraffin; talc; perfume
Mediconet (Medicone)	cloth wipe	—	benzalkonium chloride, 0.02%	hamamelis water, 50%; glycerin, 10%; ethoxylated lanolin, 0.5%; methylparaben, 0.15%; perfume
Medi-Quik (Lehn & Fink)	aerosol pump spray	lidocaine	benzalkonium chloride	isopropyl alcohol, 12% (aerosol), 79% (pump)
Morusan (Beecham Labs)	ointment	benzocaine, 2%	—	cod liver oil concentrate, lanolin, petrolatum
Noxzema Medicated (Noxell)	cream lotion	—	phenol, <0.5%	menthol, camphor, clove oil, eucalyptus oil, lime water, water-dispersible base
Noxzema Sunburn Spray (Noxell)	aerosol	benzocaine, 1%	benzalkonium chloride, 0.1%	menthol, 0.1%; alcohol, 7%; emollient
Nupercainal Cream (Ciba)	cream	dibucaine, 0.5%	—	acetone sodium bisulfite, 0.37%; water-washable base
Nupercainal Ointment (Ciba)	ointment	dibucaine, 1%	—	acetone sodium bisulfite, 0.5%
Nupercainal Spray (Ciba)	spray	dibucaine, 0.25%	—	alcohol, 46%
Obtundia Cream (Otis Clapp)	cream	—	—	cresol–camphor complex
Panthoderm Cream (USV)	cream	—	—	dexpanthenol, 2%; water-miscible base
Pontocaine (Winthrop)	cream ointment	tetracaine hydrochloride (equivalent to 1% base) (cream); base, 0.5% (ointment)	—	methylparaben (cream); sodium bisulfite (cream); menthol, 0.5% (ointment); white petrolatum (ointment); white wax (ointment)
Pyribenzamine (Ciba)	cream ointment	—	—	tripelennamine, 2%; water-washable base (cream); petrolatum base (ointment)
Rexall First Aid Spray (Rexall)	spray	benzocaine	chlorothymol methylbenzethonium chloride	isopropyl alcohol, 4%; tyloxapol; camphor
Solarcaine Cream (Plough)	cream	benzocaine, 1%	triclosan	menthol, camphor
Solarcaine Foam (Plough)	foam	benzocaine, 0.5%	triclosan	menthol, camphor
Solarcaine Lotion (Plough)	lotion	benzocaine, 0.5%	triclosan	menthol, camphor
Solarcaine Spray (Plough)	spray	benzocaine, 5%	triclosan	—
Tanurol (O'Neal, Jones & Feldman)	ointment	tannic acid, 3% benzocaine, 1%	phenol, 0.75%	—
Tega Caine (Ortega)	aerosol	benzocaine, 20%	benzyl alcohol, 2.3% chloroxylenol, 0.51%	urea, 5.38%; propylene glycol

Product (manufacturer)	Dosage form	Anesthetic	Antimicrobial	Other
Unguentine (Norwich)	cream aerosol spray	benzocaine (spray)	parahydracin (cream) benzalkonium chloride (spray) chloroxylenol (spray)	phenol, 1%; aluminum hydroxide; zinc carbonate; zinc acetate; zinc oxide; eucalyptus oil; thyme oil; menthol; eugenol (cream only); menthol; alcohol, 7% (spray only)
Unguentine Plus (Norwich)	cream	lidocaine hydrochloride	chloroxylenol	aluminum hydroxide, zinc carbonate, zinc acetate, zinc oxide, phenol, eucalyptus oil, thyme oil, menthol, eugenol
Utesin Picrate (Abbott)	ointment	butamben picrate, 1%	—	—
Vaseline First-Aid Carbolated Petroleum Jelly [a] (Chesebrough-Pond)	ointment	—	chloroxylenol, 0.5%	petroleum jelly; lanolin; phenol, 0.2%
Vaseline Pure Petroleum Jelly (Chesebrough-Pond)	gel	—	—	white petrolatum, 100%
Xylocaine (Astra)	ointment	lidocaine, 2.5%	—	polyethylene glycols, propylene glycol

[a] Not meant for use over extensive body areas (e.g. sunburn).

Sunscreen and Suntan Products

George Torosian
Max A. Lemberger

Questions to ask the patient

Is your skin extremely sensitive to the sun?
Is it difficult for you to tan?
Have you had much exposure to the sun?
Have you ever had a reaction to topical products?
Which products are you currently using?

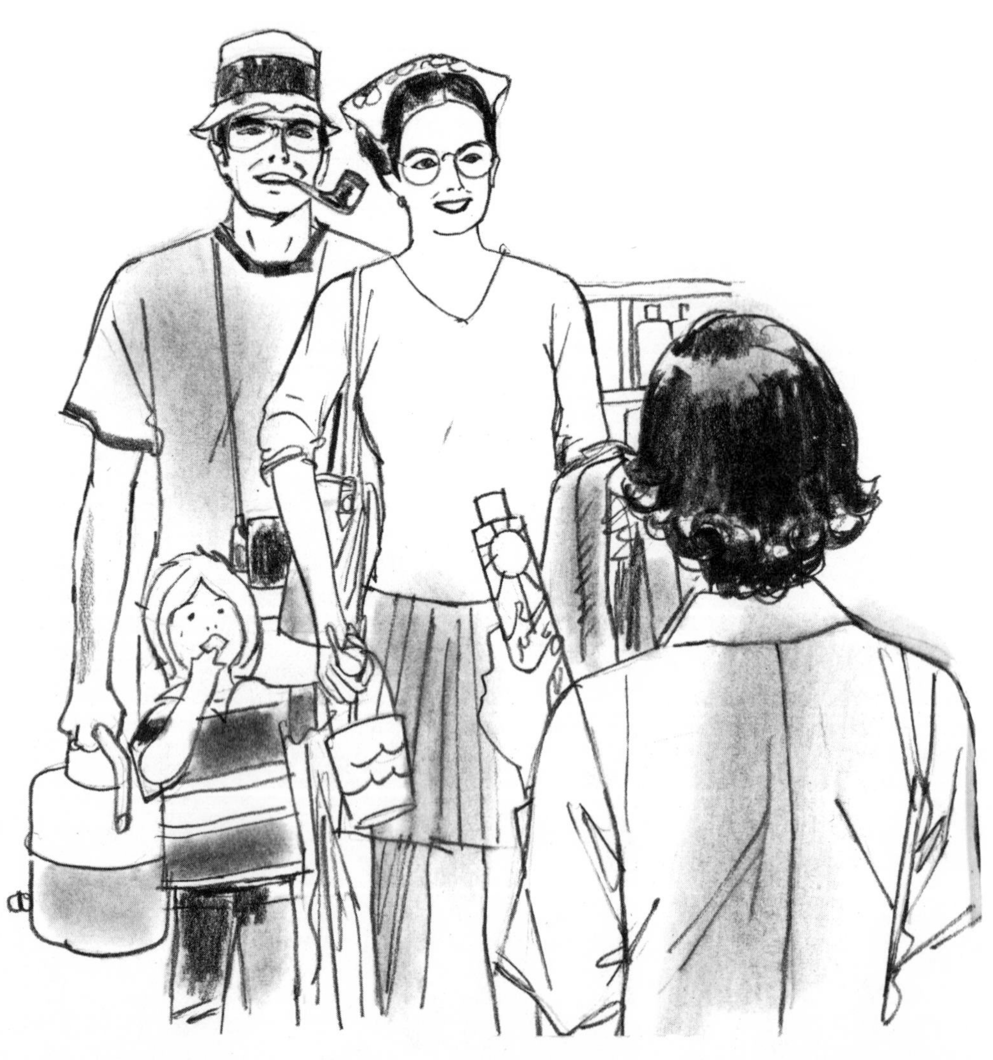

CHAPTER 25

The objectives of sunscreen and suntan products are to prevent sunburn and/or to "promote" suntan. Virtually everyone has experienced sunburn. It can be prevented, however, by using a sunscreen prior to exposure.

Sunburn appears to be a minor problem, but the consequences of continued exposure to the sun are not minor. Long-term exposure leads to premature aging of the skin (loss of elasticity, thinning, wrinkling, and drying). The cumulative exposure to the sun from childhood to adulthood can cause precancerous skin conditions which may lead to skin cancer.

A sunburn is characterized by erythema, edema, tenderness, and, in more severe cases, the formation of vesicles or bullae. The reactions mainly affect the epidermis. (See Chapter 27 for a discussion of skin anatomy.) They are similar to first-degree burns and, when blistering occurs, to second-degree burns. The burns usually are minor but may be serious if large areas blister. Sunburn is not apparent immediately. The onset of symptoms usually occurs within 1 to 24 hours but can be delayed for as long as 72 hours after exposure.

The ultraviolet (U.V.) radiation which causes sunburn and suntan is in the 290- to 320-nanometer (nm) range. Wavelengths above this range can stimulate a short-lived tan by oxidizing (darkening) melanin in the skin. Wavelengths below 290 nm are filtered out by ozone in the atmosphere.[1]

The U.V. light alters the keratinocytes in the basal layer of the epidermis. A slight alteration results in erythema, and a severe alteration results in the formation of bullae from the collection of fluid in the epidermis. To produce a suntan, U.V. light (290 to 320 nm) stimulates the melanocytes in the germinating layer to generate more melanin (a pigment that determines skin color) and oxidizes melanin already in the epidermis. This darkening of the skin is a normal body function which protects against further damage from sun exposure.

Sunburn: long-term effects

Skin cancer

Basal- and squamous-cell epitheliomas are common malignancies which involve alterations in growth of keratinocytes. Premalignant growth of keratinocytes is also common. It is called senile, or actinic, keratosis. Sanderson [2] presents a convincing statistical case implicating sunlight as the major cause of skin cancer. The relative incidence of actinic keratosis and squamous-cell carcinomas increases with increased exposure to damaging rays of the sun. However, the incidence of basal-cell carcinomas seems to be dependent on factors other than sunlight.[2]

Sunlight, as pointed out above, is considered the major factor contributing to skin cancer.[2-5] Skin cancer is more common in fair-skinned people, less likely in dark-skinned Caucasians who are not overly exposed, and rare in the Negroid population. The frequency of skin cancer is higher in farmers, sailors, construction workers, etc., whose occupations require many hours of exposure to the sun every day.[2-6] The incidence of skin cancer is greater in tropical and subtropical climates than in moderate ones because the quantity of harmful light that reaches the earth's surface is increased as the angle and distance of the sun to the earth decrease.[2,5,7-10] Auerbach [11] showed a constant rate of increase in the incidence of skin cancer approaching the equator from north to south; the incidence approximately doubled for every 3°48′ reduction in latitude.

Incidence. The incidence of skin cancer (for whites in the U.S.) increases from north to south (Table 1). The incidence is higher in males than in females, who traditionally have not experienced the occupational hazard of long exposure in the sun. It is higher on the face, head, and neck areas than on sites which usually are covered. This again suggests that sunlight is a main causative factor of skin cancer. The nonwhite population shows a much lower incidence than the white population because of the natural protection afforded by darker skin. Sanderson [2] states that the incidence of skin cancer will increase as the desirability of becoming tan continues to be popular. He uses the observations of McDonald and Bubendorf,[12] who showed that the incidence of skin cancer in El Paso per 100,000 Anglo-Americans increased from 126 in 1944 to 290 in 1960 in males and from 50 to 175 in females.

Additional studies also implicate exposure to the sun as a causative factor of skin cancer. Movshovitz and Modan [13] found a mean annual incidence of malignant melanomas of 2.0 per 100,000 in males and 2.9 per 100,000 in females. The incidence rates appeared to increase with age. This study corroborated evidence for the cumulative effect of exposure to the sun on the development of tumors; the protective properties of darkly pigmented skin; and the influence of environmental factors, such as geographic location, national origin, etc., on the incidence of melanomas.[13] Zagula-Mally *et al.*[6] studied the frequency of skin cancer in Caucasian adults in a rural county of Tennessee. They documented that the rate of cancer increases with age—from 0.7 per 100 (to age 44) to 13.6 per 100 (between 65 and 74 years) for males; corresponding figures for females were 0.4 and 6.8.

These studies not only implicate sunlight as the causative agent but also point to its cumulative effects on the skin. A journal editorial has summarized this effect: "The skin never forgets an injury. . . . The eventual condition of the skin results from a summation of all the injuries it has received." [14]

How sunscreens work and are evaluated

Sunscreens act either physically or chemically. Physical sunscreens provide a mechanical barrier to sunlight. Examples are zinc oxide paste and titanium dioxide which scatter U.V. light. Clothing and beach umbrellas are also effective as physical sunscreens, but U.V. light can be reflected from sand and water to reach under a beach umbrella and cause burning.

Chemical sunscreens absorb a specific portion of the U.V. light spectrum. When the light is absorbed by the sunscreen several changes can occur in the absorbing compound:[15]

- ☐ Light energy is converted into heat.
- ☐ The sunscreen molecule can dissociate into atoms or radicals.
- ☐ The molecule can be excited to higher energy levels and its energy transferred through collision with another molecule, followed by a chemical reaction.
- ☐ The compound can become excited and lose its energy immediately by fluorescence or, at a later time, by phosphorescence.

Criteria are needed to judge the effectiveness of sunscreen agents. Testing the agents in humans is difficult because individuals react in varying degrees to sunlight. The minimal erythemal dose (MED) is the amount of sunlight needed for a minimum perceptible erythema (redness) and is used to gauge the degree of sensitivity of the skin to sunlight. The MED can be used for protected and unprotected skin. The protection factor (PF) is the ratio of the MED for protected skin to the MED for unprotected skin. The PF is used to measure the relative effectiveness of sunscreen agents or products (the larger the PF value, the greater the protection).

In addition to the PF, other criteria are used to judge the effectiveness of a sunscreen agent:

- ☐ Its ability to absorb in the 290- to 320-nm U.V. light range. (320 to 500 nm for protection from photosensitizing drugs).[16]
- ☐ Its molar absorptivity in the U.V. range for sunburn or photosensitization. (Molar absorptivity is the ability of a compound to absorb U.V. light—the larger the value at a specified wavelength, the better the absorption.)
- ☐ Its concentration on the skin needed to absorb a desired amount of light without irritation. Not all compounds that absorb in the 290- to 320-nm U.V. light range can be used as sunscreens. For example, salicylic acid absorbs light in this range. However, at its effective concentration of 5 percent, it is keratolytic and may be quite irritating.

Table 2 shows some of the more common compounds used as sunscreen agents and their molar absorptivities. The molar absorptivity values are obtained in identical solvents and conditions that allow the compounds to be compared and ranked as to their efficacy. The larger the number, the greater its ability to absorb light. The position of maximum absorbance, λ_{max}, is also important. To be most effective, the range of maximum absorption for the sunscreen agent must overlap the U.V. range of sunlight that produces sunburn.

Table 1. Incidence of Epidermal Cancer per 100,000[a]

Skin color and region	Male		Female	
	Face, head, and neck	*Other sites*	*Face, head, and neck*	*Other sites*
White				
North[b]	26.8	6.6	20.5	4.9
South	120.6	22.7	72.2	15.8
Nonwhite				
South[c]	2.5	2.9	4.2	4.3

[a] K. V. Sanderson, in "Comparative Physiology and Pathology of the Skin," A. J. Rook and G. S. Walton, Eds., Davis, Philadelphia, Pa., 1965, p. 637.

[b] Geographical regions studied were Chicago, Detroit, Philadelphia, and Pittsburgh in the North and Atlanta, Birmingham, New Orleans, and Dallas in the South.

[c] Figures for the nonwhite population were similar, but smaller, in each category for the northern region.

Table 2. Spectrophotometric Parameters for Sunscreen Agents[a]

Compound	Molar absorptivity	λ_{max}, nanometers
Aminobenzoic acid (*para*-isomer)	18,300	290
Cinoxate (2-ethoxyethyl *p*-methoxycinnamate)	19,400	306
Dioxybenzone (2,2′-dihydroxy-4-methoxybenzophenone)	11,951	282[c]
Glyceryl *p*-aminobenzoate	17,197	298
Homosalate (homomenthyl salicylate)	6,720[b]	310[b]
Isoamyl *p*-*N*,*N*-dimethylaminobenzoate	28,083	312
Menthyl anthranilate	941[b]	315[b]
Oxybenzone (2-hydroxy-4-methoxybenzophenone)	20,381	287[c]
Sulisobenzone (2-hydroxy-4-methoxybenzophenone-5-sulfonic acid)	5,580	287[c]

[a] Obtained in ethanol.

[b] Values from A. C. Giese *et al.*, *J. Am. Pharm. Assoc., Sci. Ed.*, **39**, 30 (1950).

[c] These compounds absorb throughout the U.V. range.

Indications for the use of sunscreens

In addition to preventing sunburn and premature aging of the skin and probably reducing actinic or solar keratosis and some types of skin cancer, sunscreen agents should be considered for protection against photosensitivity caused by certain drugs. Goldman and Epstein[17] described the reaction as phototoxic or photoallergic: "A phototoxic reaction is one in which (1) the chemical absorbs ultraviolet energy, (2) the absorbed energy is transferred from the photoactivated chemical to the vulnerable cellular constituents, and (3) cellular damage results usually with a more or less severe sunburnlike reaction.

"The photoallergic reactions presumably involve an immunologic mechanism in which (1) absorption of energy by the photosensitizing chemical results in the formation of a new haptene, (2) the haptene combines with a skin protein, and (3) this complex of the agent with the 'carrier' protein initiates a hypersensitivity reaction from antigen-antibody activity in the skin. The usual clinical picture is one of an eczematous or polymorphic dermatitis of delayed onset."

A phototoxic reaction, or primary photosensitivity, to a given compound implies susceptibility on first exposure. A photoallergic response is characterized by a delayed onset, occurs in sensitized skin, and recurs with subsequent exposures to U.V. light.[16 17] U.V. light above 320 nm can elicit a photoallergic response.[16-18] The chemically induced sensitivity occurs with compounds such as sulfas, barbiturates, quinine, quinidine, psoralens, erythromycin, tetracycline, demeclocycline, chlorothiazide, chlorpromazine, promethazine, and phenylsulfonylurea.[4 16 19]

The literature shows disagreement on the value of protection of sunscreen agents.[19] However, there is sufficient evidence that these products provide some protection, depending on the degree of photosensitization.[4] Dahlen *et al.*[18] have shown the effectiveness of a 10-percent sulisobenzone lotion as a sunscreen agent in skin that was photosensitized by demeclocycline. Dihydroxyacetone/naphthaquinone (Duoshield) was found to be effective in individuals photosensitized by chlorpromazine reacting to U.V. light between 330 and 400 nm.[20] This combination also protected individuals with erythropoietic protoporphyria which has an action band at 400 nm. It is expected that compounds that absorb energy throughout the U.V. region, such as sulisobenzone, oxybenzone, and dioxybenzone, may be the most successful for this use if they are used in adequate amounts. Table 3 lists some sunscreen agents and their tentative evaluations by the FDA OTC Panel on Topical Analgesic, Antirheumatic, Otic, Burn, Sunburn Treatment and Prevention Drugs.

Efficacy

Although the pharmacist cannot control the formulation of the various available sunscreen products, a knowledge of the specific active ingredients and their concentrations helps differentiate a good product from a mediocre one. For example, the sunscreen product that has a larger molar absorptivity and a higher concentration of the sunscreen is the better product. In addition, sunscreen agents that have a low or intermediate molar absorptivity can be made more effective by increasing the concentration of the active ingredient. For example, if the compound isoamyl *p-N,N*-dimethylaminobenzoate (molar absorptivity = 28,083) is used in a sunscreen product, its concentration should be at least 2.5 percent; if used in a suntan product, the concentration may be reduced to less than 2 percent, probably to 1.0 to 1.5 percent. In contrast, glyceryl *p*-aminobenzoate (molar absorptivity = 17,197) is about 59 percent

$$\left(\frac{17{,}197}{28{,}083} \times 100 = 59 \text{ percent}\right)$$

as efficient as isoamyl *p-N,N*-dimethylaminobenzoate and should be used at a higher concentration in sunscreen products and at a lower concentration (approximately one-half) in suntan products.

Factors which can influence the effectiveness of sunscreen products are:

□ Its pH. If the pH is raised or lowered, the fraction of the ionized and un-ionized sunscreen agent changes and changes the position of the peak absorbance, possibly shifting it away from the 290- to 320-nm U.V. light range.

□ Its solvent system. Various solvent systems, such as ethanol and the oil phase of an emulsion vehicle, can direct the position of the peak absorbance of the sunscreen. Shifts of the peak away from the 290- to 320-nm U.V. light range can compromise the sunscreen's effectiveness.

□ Its stability. The sunscreen must remain stable for the desired period of protection.

□ Thickness of the residual layer on the skin.

Suntan products

There are instances when the patient's needs are not therapeutic but cosmetic—the desire for a tan. For cosmetic needs, the patient may desire a suntanning product. In some cases, suntan products differ from sunscreen products only by having a lower concentration of the sunscreen agent. The concentration of the active ingredient is an important factor in judging the use and the effectiveness of a product. For example, SunDare Lotion, a suntan product, contains 1.75-percent cinoxate but Maxafil Cream, a sunscreen product, contains 4 percent—about twice as much as the suntan product—and 5-percent menthyl anthranilate, another sunscreen. Selection of a sunscreen can also be based on the amount of U.V. light it absorbs. For example, suntan products can contain a sunscreen agent that blocks wavelengths of less than 320 nm but allows wavelengths of more than 320 nm to penetrate, producing a light, transient tan. Others contain a weakly absorbent sunscreen agent, which allows a significant fraction of all the U.V. light to reach the skin.

Suntan products do not "promote" a tan. Some, including cocoa butter and mineral oil alone or with staining materials such as iodine or tannic acid, do not contain a sunscreen agent. None of these products provides protection from the sun. The products mainly stain and lubricate the skin and do not reverse the aging process caused by U.V. light. The FDA OTC Panel has stated that "Claims such as 'promotes tanning' for sunlight protective agents are unsubstantiated."[21]

Some suntan products contain dihydroxyacetone and a small amount of sunscreen. Dihydroxyacetone darkens the skin by interacting with keratin in the stratum corneum. The emphasis of these products is on the cosmetic tan produced and not on protection, although they may contain a small amount of sunscreen and do darken the skin.

Guidelines for product selection

Before recommending a sunscreen or suntan product, the pharmacist should know the identity of the active ingredient and its maximum absorption, molar absorptivity, and concentration (see Table 3). An *in vivo* evaluation is also useful in judging a product.[22] The physical characteristics (molar absorptivity and maximum absorption) are available in Table 2. The identity and concentration of the active ingredients can be supplied by the manufacturer but also should be on the label. Without this information, recommendations can be based only on intuition or personal experience. If the information is not supplied by the manufacturer, recommendations should be limited to products which indicate the identity and concentration of the active ingredients.

Studies that compare several sunscreen products in humans can serve as a basis for professional judgment. Cripps and Hegedus[22] evaluated 17 sunscreen products. They used a mean PF to evaluate each product. Table 4 shows that products that contain 5 percent aminobenzoic acid (PABA) are superior to those that contain PABA esters. However, PABA esters are generally used in a

Table 3. Tentative Evaluation of Sunscreen Agents[a]

Sunscreen agent	Dosage range	Category[b]	Safety	Effectiveness
Allantoin	—	II	—	Not effective
Aminobenzoic acid	5% hydroalcoholic 5-15% creams and ointments	I	Safe	Effective—absorbs U.V. light at 290-320 nm.
Cinoxate (2-ethoxyethyl *p*-methoxycinnamate)	1-3%	I	Safe	Effective—1% solution absorbs U.V. light at 280-320 nm; 10% concentration absorbs U.V. light at 270-328; maximum absorption at 310 nm.
Digalloyl trioleate (mix of several derivatives of tannic acid)	2-5%	I	Safe	Effective—absorbs U.V. light at 200-315 nm; maximum absorption at 297 nm.
Dihydroxyacetone with lawsone	—	I	—	—
2-Ethylhexyl p-methoxycinnamate	2.5-5%	I	No reported adverse reactions	Effective—1 mg% allowed 16% transmission at 310 nm.
Glyceryl *p*-aminobenzoate	2-3%	I	Safe—a few cases of contact dermatitis and photo contact dermatitis have been reported	—
Homosalate	4-15%	Not established	Safe	Prevents tanning at 15%; permits tanning at 8%.
Menthyl anthranilate	—	I as sunburn protective I as suntan preventive	—	Absorbs U.V. light at 300-360 nm; maximum absorption between 332 and 345 nm.
p-Methoxycinnamic acid diethanolamine	8-10%	III	No reported adverse reactions	Effective—maximum absorption at 290 nm; 4% transmission at 25 mg%.
3-(4-Methylbenzidine) camphor	1-2.5%	III	Safe when used as directed	Effective—1% transmission at 310 nm in concentration of 13.5%; absorbs U.V. light at 280-310 nm.
2-Mole propoxylate salt of *p*-aminoethylbenzoic acid	1-5%	III	No reported adverse reactions	1, 2.5, and 5% protected at 20, 40, and 60 MED, respectively.
Oxybenzone (2-hydroxy-4-methoxybenzophenone)	0.5-2 %	I	Safe when used as directed	Controls U.V. light at 320-400 nm and absorbs major portion of U.V. light at 280-320 nm.
Padimate A [pentyl *p*-(dimethylamino) benzoate]	1-3.6%	I	—	—
Padimate O [2-ethylhexyl *p*-(dimethylamino) benzoate]	1.4-4%	I	Does not appear to be a skin sensitizer or primary irritant	Effective.
2-Phenylbenzimidazole	1-4%	I	Safe	16% transmission at 290-310 nm
Titanium dioxide	1-15%	I	Safe	Scatters U.V. light at 290-700 nm.

[a]By the FDA OTC Panel on Topical Analgesics, Antirheumatic, Otic, Burn, Sunburn Treatment and Prevention Drugs. (This table is incomplete until the panel publishes its final report.) A common method for evaluating these agents is not yet available; thus, the most effective ingredient and/or product of those listed as safe and effective cannot be chosen from the information listed here. However, products containing agents listed as both safe and effective, if used in the appropriate concentrations, probably will be the more successful sunscreens. No data available (Category III) for 2-ethylhexyl-4-phenylbenzophenone-2-carboxylic acid or dihydroxyacetone with lawsone.

[b]Category I: safe and effective
Category II: not safe and/or effective
Category III: insufficient information

concentration of less than 5 percent. A study by Pathak *et al.*[23] showed that alcoholic preparations of 5 percent PABA and preparations that contain 2.5 percent isoamyl *p-N,N*-dimethylaminobenzoate were more effective than commercial products tested. Another product evaluation substantiates this finding in products that contain 5 percent PABA.[21] Several investigators [23 24] agree that aminobenzoic acid is more effective as a sunscreen than popular, proprietary products, but they disagree that PABA esters are less effective than the parent compound, aminobenzoic acid. Nevertheless, 5 percent PABA seems to yield the best results as a sunscreen product—the *Drugs of Choice, 1974-75* lists Pabanol, Solbar, and Sunstick as satisfactory.[25]

Table 4. Sunscreen Protection at 305 nm[a]

Sunscreen	Protection Factor (PF)[b]			Number of subjects
	Mean MED's	*Standard deviation*	*Range*	
Pabanol (5% aminobenzoic acid)	17.6	9.7	10–21	23
Presun (5% aminobenzoic acid)	17.6	9.7	10–21	23
Maxafil (4% cinoxate, 5% menthyl anthranilate)	9.6	5.7	6–14	23
Sea & Ski (glyceryl *p*-aminobenzoate)	8.3	4.6	5–11	13
RVPaque (red petrolatum, zinc oxide, cinoxate)	7.7	4.4	6–9	13
Solbar (3% oxybenzone, 3% dioxybenzone)	6.7	3.8	5–10	23
Sunswept (3.5% digalloyl trioleate)	6.6	3.3	5–9	23
Estee Lauder's U.V. Screening Lotion (padimate)	6.6	3.0	5–8	16
UVAL (10% sulisobenzone)	6.6	3.4	6–9	16
Afil Cream (5% titanium dioxide, 5% menthyl anthranilate)	6.3	3.5	6–8	16
Coppertone (homosalate)	6.0	2.6	4–7	17
Pan Ultra (diphenyl ketone)	6.0	2.5	4–7	17
Pabafilm (padimate)	5.9	3.4	4–9	23
Sungard (10% sulisobenzone)	5.9	3.2	3–8	17
SunDare (cinoxate)	5.9	2.4	5–7	17
Block Out (padimate)	5.5	3.1	4–7	17
RVP (red petrolatum)	3.2	2.1	2–4	18

[a] Adapted from D. J. Cripps and S. Hegedus, *Arch. Dermatol.*, **109**, 202(1974).

[b] Protection factor (MED's) of 17 sunscreens applied in concentrations of 30 μ l/cm^2, tested at 305-nm radiation (4-nm half-bandwidth).

Summary

Pathak *et al.*[23] suggest that a preventive program using an appropriate sunscreen may possibly prevent or minimize degenerative cutaneous changes, such as solar keratosis and skin cancer, which can result from repeated and long exposure to sunlight.

Although it is possible to discourage too much sunbathing, there is no escape from the sun. Protective habits which prevent the undesirable results of overexposure should be encouraged. They should be started at an early age because the aging process caused by the sun is insidious and cumulative. If a tan is desired, short exposures to the sun, which are gradually extended as the sunbathing season progresses, followed by generous applications of a good sunscreen can be recommended. The sunscreen should be reapplied after bathing, after excessive exercise or sweating, and at about 1- to 2-hour intervals. People on therapy that includes photosensitizing medication should be cautioned against exposure to the sun and advised to use physical protection, such as a hat, protective clothing, and concomitant use of an effective sunscreen. Although it is an often overlooked responsibility, evaluating or selecting the proper sunscreen or suntan product is an important health service for the pharmacist to fulfill.

References

1. F. Dyer, *New Sci.*, 228(July 31, 1969).
2. K. V. Sanderson, in "Comparative Physiology and Pathology of the Skin," A. J. Rook and G. S. Walton, Eds., Davis, Philadelphia, Pa., 1965, p. 637.
3. D. M. Pillsbury *et al.*, "Dermatology," Saunders, Philadelphia, Pa., 1956, p. 1145.
4. N. Tobias, "Essentials of Dermatology," 6th ed., Lippincott, Philadelphia, Pa., 1963, p. 328.
5. M. Segi, Monograph No. 10, 245, U.S. Nat. Cancer Inst., 1963.
6. Z. W. Zagula-Mally *et al.*, *Cancer*, **34**, 345(1974).
7. J. Belisario, "Cancer of the Skin," Butterworth, London, England, 1959, p. 15.
8. J. A. Elliott and D. G. Welton, *Arch. Dermatol. Syphilol.*, **53**, 307(1946).
9. V. A. Belinsky and L. N. Guslitzer, in "Tenth International Cancer Congress Abstracts, May 22-29," 1970, p. 109.
10. F. Urback *et al.*, in "Tenth International Cancer Congress Abstracts, May 22-29," 1970, p. 109.
11. H. Auerbach, *Publ. Health Rep.*, No. 76, Washington, D. C., 1961, p. 345.
12. G. J. McDonald and E. Bubendorf, in "Tumors of the Skin," Anderson Hospital and Tumor Institute, Houston, Texas, Year Book Medical, Chicago, Ill., 1964, p. 23.
13. M. Movshovitz and B. Modan, *J. Nat. Cancer Inst.*, **51**, 77(1973).
14. Editorial, *Br. Med. J.*, **3**, 72(1974).
15. F. Daniels and R. A. Alberty, "Physical Chemistry," 2d ed., Wiley, New York, N.Y., 1961, p. 654.
16. D. M. Pillsbury *et al.*, "Dermatology," Saunders, Philadelphia, Pa., 1956, p. 1241.
17. G. Goldman and E. Epstein, Jr., *Arch. Dermatol.*, **100**, 447(1969).
18. R. F. Dahlen *et al.*, *J. Invest. Dermatol.*, **55**, 165(1970).
19. Editorial, *Br. Med. J.*, **2**, 494(1970).
20. J. A. Johnson *et al.*, *Dermatologica*, **147**, 104(1973).
21. Summary Minutes of Meetings 1-16, OTC Panel on Topical Analgesic, Antirheumatic, Otic, Burn, Sunburn Treatment and Prevention Drugs, Division of OTC Drug Evaluation, Bureau of Drugs, Department of Health, Education, and Welfare, Rockville, Md., Mar. 1973-Jan. 1975.
22. D. J. Cripps and S. Hegedus, *Arch. Dermatol.*, **109**, 202(1974).
23. M. A. Pathak *et al.*, *N. Engl. J. Med.*, **280**, 1461(1969).
24. I. Willis and A. M. Kligman, *Arch. Dermatol.*, **102**, 405(1970).
25. V. H. Witten and R. J. Helfman, in "Drugs of Choice, 1974-1975," W. Modell, Ed., Mosby, St. Louis, Mo., 1974, p. 650.

Products 25 SUNSCREEN AND SUNTAN

Product (manufacturer)	Sunscreen agent	Other
A-Fil Cream (Texas Pharmacal)	menthyl anthranilate, 5%	titanium dioxide, 5%
Block Out (Sea & Ski)	padimate, 3.6%	alcohol, 70%; moisturizers; fragrance
Coppertone Nosekote (Plough)	homosalate, 7%	—
Coppertone Shade Lotion (Plough)	homosalate, 8% oxybenzone, 3%	—
Coppertone Suntan Foam, Lotion, Oil, and Spray (Plough)	homosalate, 8% (foam, lotion) 9% (oil, spray)	—
Coppertone Tanning Butter and Butter Spray (Plough)	homosalate, 6% (butter) 8% (spray)	cocoa butter, coconut oil
Dark Tanning Butter (Sea & Ski)	—	acetylated lanolin, cocoa butter, mineral oil, moisturizers, emollients
Dark Tanning Oil (Sea & Ski)	padimate, 1.1%	mineral oil, emollients, moisturizers
Eclipse (Herbert)	glyceryl *p*-aminobenzoate, 3% padimate O, 3%	alcohol, 5%; oleth-3 phosphate; petrolatum; synthetic spermaceti; glycerin; mineral oil; lanolin alcohol; cetyl stearyl glycol; lanolin oil; triethanolamine; carbomer 934P; benzyl alcohol, 0.5%; perfume
Florida Tan Tanning Oil and Dark Tanning Oil (Florida Tan)	aminobenzoic acid	cocoa butter, coconut oil, aloe, almond, lanolin, banana, fragrance
Golden Tan Lotion (Sea & Ski)	padimate, 1%	cocoa butter, mineral oil, lanolin, alcohol
Indoor/Outdoor Foam and Lotion (Sea & Ski)	padimate, 1.05%	dihydroxyacetone, 4%; lanolin; glycerin (foam only); mineral oil
Maxafil Cream (Texas Pharmacal)	menthyl anthranilate, 5% cinoxate, 4%	—
Mentholatum Stick (Mentholatum)	padimate A	petrolatum, menthol, camphor, essential oils
Natural Woman Suntan Lotion (LaMaur)	oxybenzone dioxybenzone	—
Pabafilm (Owen)	isoamyl *N,N*-dimethylaminobenzoate, 2.5%	alcohol, 70%
Pabagel (Owen)	aminobenzoic acid, 5%	alcohol, 57%
Pabanol (Elder)	aminobenzoic acid, 5%	alcohol, 70%
Paba Sun Lotion (Amer. Pharm.)	aminobenzoic acid	allantoin, cocoa butter, vitamins A, D, and E, sesame oil, avocado oil
Palmer's Cocoa Butter Formula (Browne)	—	cocoa butter; vitamin E, 0.1%; allantoin, 0.1%; mineral oil; microwax
Q. T. Quick Tanning Foam and Lotion (Plough)	homosalate, 8%	dihydroxyacetone
RVPaba Stick (Elder)	aminobenzoic acid	red petrolatum
RVPaque (Elder)	cinoxate	red petrolatum, zinc oxide
RVP Cream (Elder)	—	red petrolatum, hydrocarbon oil, ointment base
RVPlus (Elder)	—	red petrolatum, titanium-coated mica platelets
Sea & Ski Lotion (Sea & Ski)	glyceryl *p*-aminobenzoate, 2%	glycerin, mineral oil, lanolin, sesame oil
Snootie (Sea & Ski)	padimate, 2.5%	glycerin, stearic acid, dimethicone
Solar Cream (Doak)	aminobenzoic acid, 4%	titanium dioxide, 12%; water-repellent cream base, 84%
Solbar (Person & Covey)	dioxybenzone, 3% oxybenzone, 3%	—

roduct (manufacturer)	Sunscreen agent	Other
udden Tan Foam and Lotion by Coppertone (Plough)	homosalate, 6.25%	dihydroxyacetone
unDare Clear (Texas Pharmacal)	cinoxate, 1.75%	alcohol, 51.8%
unDare Creamy (Texas Pharmacal)	cinoxate, 2%	lanolin derivative
unswept (Texas Pharmacal)	digalloyl trioleate, 3.5%	—
uper Shade Lotion by Coppertone (Plough)	aminobenzoic acid, 5%	—
an Care by Coppertone (Plough)	—	glycerin, stearic acid, glyceryl monostearate, isopropyl myristate, polyethylene glycol 75, lanolin
ega-Tan Foam (Ortega)	glyceryl *p*-aminobenzoate	emulsifier, alcohol, aromatics
ropic Sun Oil and Butter (Sea & Ski)	padimate, 1.1% (oil only)	cocoa butter, coconut oil, almond oil, mineral oil, lanolin
val Sun'n Wind Stick (Dorsey)	padimate A, 3%	—
val Sunscreen Lotion (Dorsey)	sulisobenzone, 10%	—

External Analgesic Products

Paul Skierkowski
Nancy Burdock

Questions to ask the patient

Is the pain in a joint or in the muscle?

How long have you had the pain?

Is the pain a result of an accident or overwork?

(If the pain is in a joint) Is the joint red, swollen, or warm to the touch?

Have you experienced abdominal pain, nausea, or pain when urinating?

Does the pain radiate to other areas?

Do you have a fever or other "flu" symptoms?

What treatments have you tried? How well did they work?

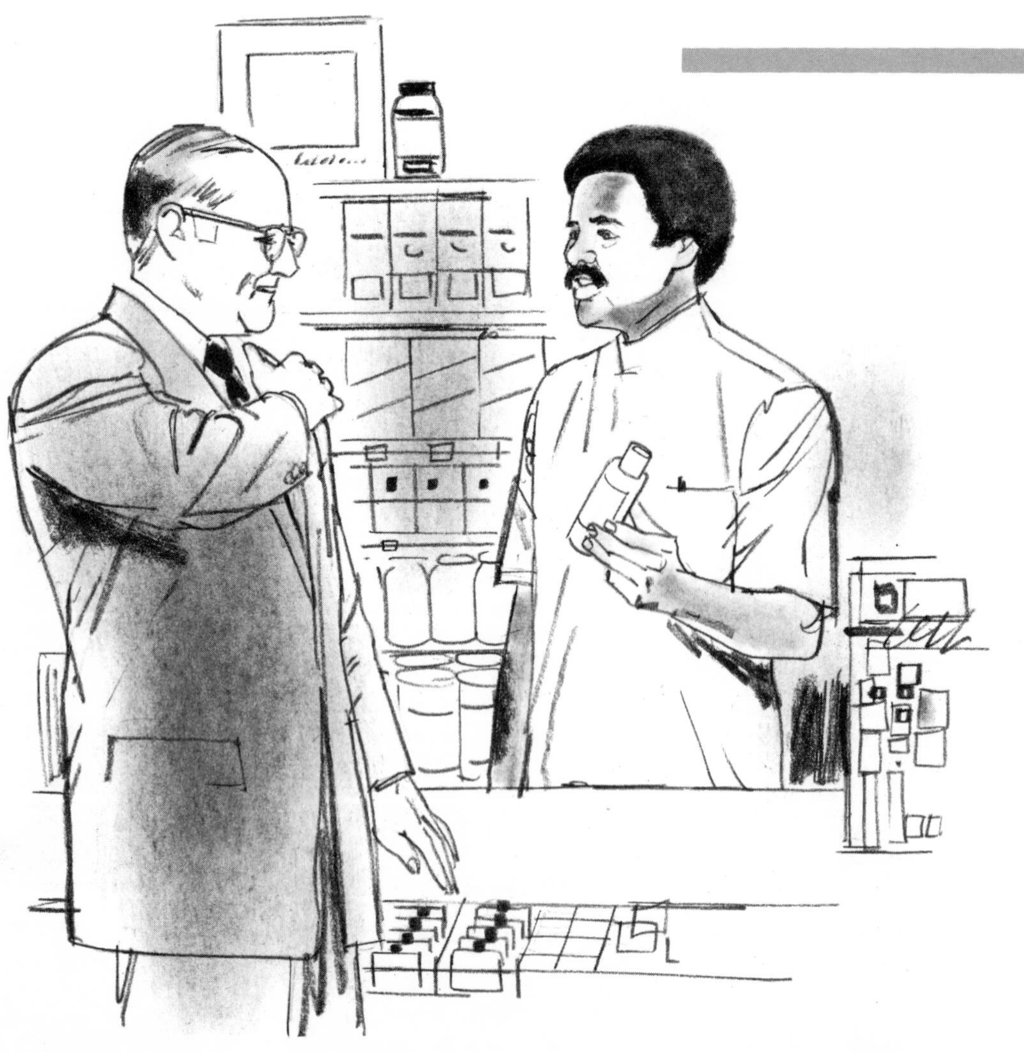

CHAPTER 26

The external use of analgesics and anesthetics is associated with conditions such as burn, sunburn, dental pain, hemorrhoids, muscular pain, etc. This chapter deals with the use of external analgesics for skeletal muscle pain. (For additional information, see Chapter on Internal Analgesic Products.)

Pain receptors are present in most areas of the body, including skeletal muscles. Stimuli activating these receptors cause sensory impulses which are translated into a pain perception. The threshold of response varies greatly among individuals.[1]

Etiology of muscular pain

Skeletal muscle pain is quite common, especially in an urban society where people are not accustomed to strenuous exertion. When people do strain themselves, their muscles become sore and painful to move. Muscle pain also can occur as a result of prolonged, fixed, and stressful positions such as bending over for long periods. Tension and anxiety may also induce prolonged tonic contraction of muscle, causing pain.[2]

The shoulder area, because of its location and structure, is subject to more stress and strain than any other articulation of the body. In addition to all its other activities, its pendulum structure makes it continuously subjected to the pull of gravity. A painful shoulder is more prevalent among older people but frequently occurs in athletes and with certain occupations, such as painting, where the arms are used vigorously and repetitively.[3]

Acute, temporary stiffness and muscle pain also can result from cold, dampness, temperature changes, and air currents. In some cases, internal stimuli such as tension, constipation, GI distention, and other minor disorders are reflected as shoulder pain. These are likely to be acute and self-limiting episodes, and elimination of the cause and symptomatic treatment provide relief. Poor posture is also a frequent cause of skeletal muscle pain.

Bursitis is an inflammation of the bursae of the body and is a common cause of pain in the shoulder. It may be acute, due to trauma, or chronic, in which case other causes such as infection should be suspect. Bursitis is characterized by localized pain, tenderness, and swelling. Limitation of motion of adjacent joints is common.[4]

Arthritic pain is caused by swelling of joints. When the joint is at rest, the pain is usually relieved; when in use, especially in a twisting motion, the pain is more persistent. Stiffness is also a constant symptom, most prominent upon first arising. Although arthritis is a chronic systemic disease, local treatment of painful joints can give temporary symptomatic relief.

When counseling patients about pains thought to be associated with skeletal muscles, the pharmacist should inquire into activities which may have brought on the condition. This information can eliminate other organic problems that may be misinterpreted as skeletal muscle pain. For example, a posteriorly perforating duodenal ulcer can cause pain radiating into the back, and spine disease may cause radial pain in the muscle of the thigh. However, if the pain developed after spending the day weeding a garden or painting a ceiling, it can generally be relieved by the use of external and/or internal analgesics.

Treatment: counterirritants

The topical OTC products for the symptomatic relief of pain due to sprains, strains, sore muscles and joints, neuralgia, rheumatism, arthritic pain, and similar disorders contain counterirritants in their formulation. Counterirritants are agents that are applied locally to produce an inflammatory reaction with the object of affecting another site, usually adjacent to or underlying the surface irritated. The intensity of response of the skin depends on not only the nature of the irritant employed, but also its concentration, the solvent in which it is dissolved, and the period of contact.[5]

The counterirritant drug is applied to the skin where pain is experienced. Pain is only as intense as it is perceived, and the perception of other sensations from application of the counterirritant, such as massage and warmth, of most drugs so used, crowd out perception of the pain. Several theories have been proposed to explain the mechanism of action of the irritant drugs, but there is no unanimity of opinion. The theories involve: [6]

- ☐ Stimulation of sensory nerve endings, producing vasodilation in a remote area because of reflexes acting through the cerebrospinal axis.
- ☐ Stimulation of sensory nerve endings, producing localized vasodilation of the skin owing to axon reflexes.
- ☐ A summation of painful stimuli due to the local inflammatory insult produced by counterirritants.

Reflexes mediated through the cerebrospinal axis, originating from sensory nerve fiber stimulation, produce efferent stimuli that elicit a vascular dilator response in the viscera. The afferent sensory nerve fibers from the skin synapse in the spinal cord with efferent vasomotor fibers to the viscera (Fig. 1). Stimulation of the skin by a counterirritant increases the number of afferent stimuli to a segment of the spinal cord from which arise many visceral efferent fibers.

The axon reflex hypothesis suggests that sensory nerves are directly connected with the nerve network of the arterioles. For example, stimulation of the sensory nerves of the skin by a counterirritant causes a stimulus to pass along the nerves and then to the branches of the arterioles. This produces an increase in the flow of blood to the muscles which, with concomitant waste disposal and other chemical changes, leads to recovery.[7]

Counterirritants may also produce a summation of pain stimuli. The classical signs of skin inflammation are heat sensations, redness, pain, and swelling. In producing these effects, the counterirritants may also relieve visceral pain by causing intense stimulation of the areas of pain interpretation of the brain, partly abating visceral pain stimuli. According to this theory of their action, stimuli originating in the viscera or muscles are transmitted over fibers in a common pathway along with sensations from the skin. Stimuli from the viscera or muscles are referred to the same area of the spinal cord as the stimuli from the skin. If the intensity of the stimulation from the skin is increased by the irritant action of the drug, the character of the visceral or muscle pain becomes modified. With intense skin stimulation, the visceral pain stimuli may be partly or completely obliterated insofar as the sensorium is concerned. The patient's attention is diverted from the diseased, visceral structure by the application of the counterirritant drug.[8]

Undoubtedly, the action of counterirritants in relieving pain has a strong psychological component. However, the therapeutic merits, based upon established empirical observation, are well recognized. Whatever their mechanism of action, the judicious use of the counterirritant drugs has a place in medical practice.

Ingredients in OTC products

Most of the products used as counterirritants are volatile substances. They include methyl salicylate, camphor, menthol, thymol, turpentine oil, allyl isothiocyanate, and oils of clove, cinnamon, wormwood, myristica, chenopodium, and eucalyptus. Some formulations may include aspirin, methacholine chloride, histamine dihydrochloride, or triethanolamine salicylate as additional active ingredients.

Methyl salicylate. Methyl salicylate, occurring naturally as wintergreen oil, is the most widely used counterirritant. When it is rubbed on the skin, it produces mild irritation and is absorbed to an appreciable extent.[9] There may be systemic analgesic effects due to the absorption of the salicylate component; however, there is no clinical evidence to support this hypothesis.

Concentrations of methyl salicylate in various products range from 10 to 50 percent. Unfortunately, the pleasant odor of methyl salicylate may be the cause of fatal poisonings from ingestion of the substance by children—1 tsp can be fatal.[10] Federal law requires that liquid preparations containing more than 5 percent of methyl salicylate be dispensed only in child-resistant containers with warnings to use only as directed for external use and to keep out of the reach of children.

Camphor. Camphor is used for its local action as a rubefacient when rubbed on the skin. When it is not vigorously applied, however, it may only produce a feeling of coolness. Camphor also has a mild local anesthetic action, and its application to the skin may be followed by numbness. The recommended concentration for external use is 1 to 3 percent, but it is used in various preparations in concentrations of as high as 9 percent.

Menthol. Menthol is a natural product from mint oils or is prepared synthetically. It is applied topically, in concentrations of as high as 16 percent, for its mild anesthetic and counterirritant properties. Menthol has the particularly outstanding property of producing a feeling of coolness. The sensation is quite noticeable in the respiratory tract when low concentrations of menthol are inhaled as in many medicinal inhalant preparations. This is caused by the selective stimulation of nerve endings which are sensitive to cold.[11]

Thymol. Thymol is a natural or synthetic phenol used in various liquid and ointment preparations also for its antifungal and antibacterial properties. It is used in concentrations of 0.1 to 2 percent.

Turpentine oil. Turpentine oil is used for its counterirritant properties either full strength or as a component of various liniments. Many accidental poisonings occur by ingestion of an excessive amount of this substance.[12]

Allyl isothiocyanate. Allyl isothiocyanate is the active component of volatile oil of mustard. It is a powerful local irritant and, if applied in excessive concentrations for extended periods, it may produce severe vesication and even perforation of the skin with danger of subsequent infection. It is most often found as a minor component of ointment preparations, but is also available as a plaster.

Clove oil. Clove oil contains eugenol as its main constituent. It is also an ingredient in various ointment preparations and is widely used as a component of toothache preparations. It has strong counterirritant action.

Capsicum oleoresin. Capsicum oleoresin is an irritant product of cayenne pepper. Although not a volatile oil, it produces a feeling of warmth without vesicant action when it is applied to intact skin. It is usually used in concentrations of less than 1 percent.

Chloroform. Chloroform was widely used in liniment formulations for its quick-acting rubefacient and counterirritant properties. The FDA has now banned the use of chloroform in products intended for human use.

Other ingredients. Methacholine chloride in a concentration of 0.025 percent and histamine dihydrochloride and methyl nicotinate in concentrations of 0.1 to 1 percent are used for their local vasodilator properties. These agents produce sensitivity reactions in certain individuals.

Triethanolamine salicylate in a concentration of 10 percent acts as an analgesic without counterirritant properties. It is also readily absorbed to produce a systemic effect.[13]

Dosage forms

The OTC external analgesics usually are available as liniments, gels, lotions, and ointments.

Liniments. Solutions or mixtures of various substances in oil, alcoholic solutions of soap, or emulsions are called liniments. They are intended for external application and should be so labeled. They are applied to the affected area with friction and rubbing of the skin, the oil or soap base providing ease of application and massage. Liniments with an alcoholic or hydroalcoholic vehicle are useful in instances in which rubefacient, counterirritant, or penetrating action is desired; oleaginous liniments are used primarily when massage is desired. By their nature, oleaginous liniments are less irritating to the skin than alcoholic liniments.

Liniments generally are not applied to skin areas that are broken or bruised because excessive irritation or infection might result. The vehicle for a liniment should, therefore, be selected on the basis of the kind of action desired (rubefacient, counterirritant, or massage) and on the solubility of the desired components in the various vehicles.[14]

Gels. Gels used for the delivery of topical analgesics are more appropriately called jellies because they are generally clear and are of a more uniform, semisolid consistency. It has been the experience of these authors that a greater sensation of warmth is experienced with the gel than with equal quantities of the same product in a different dosage form such as a lotion. Therefore, patients should be advised against using excessive amounts of the gel formulation as an unpleasant burning sensation may be experienced.

Lotions. These liquid preparations are used for external application to the skin for the protective or therapeutic value of their constituents. Depending on the ingredients, they may be alcoholic or aqueous in nature and are often emulsions. Their fluidity allows rapid and uniform application over a wide surface area. Lotions are intended to dry on the skin soon after application, leaving a thin coat of their active ingredients on the skin's surface.

Ointments. These dosage forms are particularly desirable for external analgesics because percutaneous absorption may occur. Balms are aromatic ointments often containing balsam.

Factors influencing percutaneous absorption

Percutaneous absorption is the absorption of substances from the surface of the skin to areas beneath the skin, including entrance into the bloodstream. It is not usually intended that the medication enter the general circulation. However, once the drug substance has penetrated the skin, it is close to blood capillaries that feed subcutaneous tissue, and absorption into the general circulation is possible. Fortunately, most of the substances for topical use as counterirritants are nontoxic in the amounts generally absorbed.

Selection of the vehicle is as important as selecting the drug. The choice depends on the solubility, stability, and ionization of the active ingredient.[15] Staining properties, tackiness, or consistency may influence the patient's choice of a product.

The choice of vehicle for the medicinal agents determines the rate and degree of penetration. The degree and rate vary with different drugs and vehicles. For example, methyl salicylate is more lipid soluble than salicylic acid, from which it is derived. When applied to the skin from vehicles composed of fatty substances such as petrolatum, the methyl salicylate has greater penetration than salicylic acid. The amount of methyl salicylate absorbed is proportional to its concentration. Plasma levels of methyl salicylate obtained from bases such as petrolatum are higher than those obtained from propylene glycol vehicles.[16]

Among the most widely used vehicles are petrolatum, mineral oil, lanolin, and anhydrous lanolin. Preparations with these vehicles are greasier than creams and contain little or no water. "Greaseless" vehicles are oil-in-water formulations and are usually preferred for daytime use.[17]

Petrolatum is a purified mixture of hydrocarbons obtained from petroleum. It has protective and emollient properties when applied to the skin. Anhydrous lanolin differs from lanolin in that it contains practically no water. Because both are obtained from the fatlike substance from the wool of sheep, many individuals are allergic to them.[18]

Humidity and temperature have a definite influence on the absorption of substances through the skin. A ten-fold increase in the skin penetration of aspirin occurs when the temperature is raised from 50° to 98.6° F (10° to 37° C). A similar increase occurs when these substances are applied to completely hydrated skin as compared to skin at humidity of 50 percent. Hydration of the skin can be achieved by covering or occluding the skin with plastic sheeting to prevent loss of moisture from the skin or by use of oleaginous vehicles such as petrolatum.[19]

The site of application, the amount of inunction performed, and the period of time that the medication is permitted to remain in contact with the skin also influence percutaneous absorption. Percutaneous absorption seems more effective when the drug is applied to skin with a thin epidermis. Absorption from sites such as the palms of the hands and soles of the feet which have thick layers of epidermis is comparatively slow.

The longer the period of inunction, the greater the absorption. The massaging action produced by inunction may also produce some increased circulation at the site of application. Most preparations instruct the patient to "gently massage" the preparation into the skin. Products containing counterirritants and local anesthetics, when applied with massage, enhance relief of skeletal muscle pain.[20] The anesthetic agent is absorbed and acts on nerve endings, potentiating the analgesic effect.[21]

The longer the medication remains in contact with the skin, the greater the amount of drug absorbed. The preparations may be applied as often as needed. There seems to be little agreement on how often the preparations should be applied for optimal results.

Untoward effects

Hypersensitivity. Hypersensitive reactions to either active volatile oil components or to the vehicle are not uncommon. Reactions may be manifested as a generalized eruption at the site of application. Some patients manifest idiosyncrasy to salicylates.[22]

Toxicity. Ingestion of substances such as camphor and turpentine has resulted in death. The mean lethal dose of turpentine in adults is probably between 120-180 ml; ingestion of 2 g of camphor generally produces dangerous effects in adults. The amount of these substances which may be absorbed percutaneously is assumed to be small enough that there is little danger of toxicity.[23]

Cautions

External analgesics are intended for use on intact skin and should not be applied to broken skin or raw surfaces.

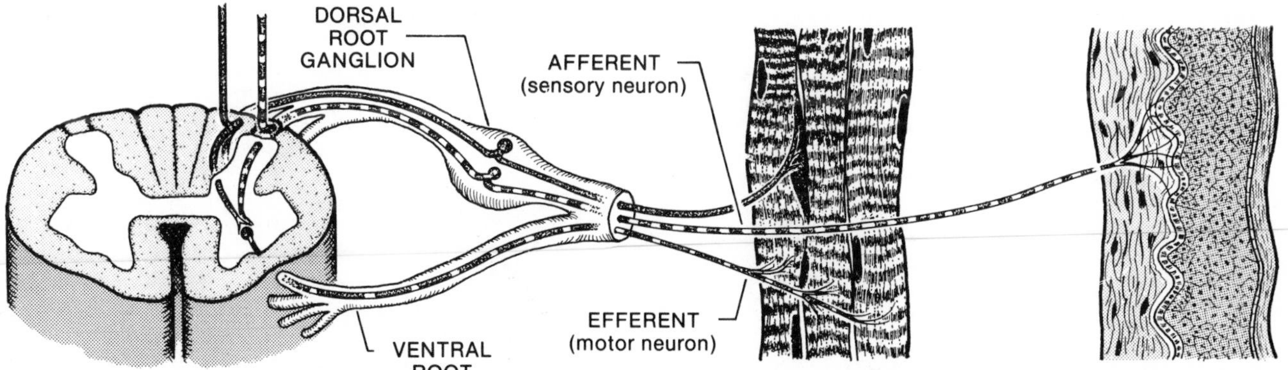

Figure 1. Reflex pathways showing the afferent (sensory) fibers, efferent (vasomotor) fibers, and their synapse in the spinal cord. Adapted from "The Ciba Collection of Medical Illustrations" by Frank H. Netter, M.D.

Their application to skin areas devoid of the normal barrier may lead to very rapid drug entrance into the bloodstream with consequent toxicity. These preparations should not be applied to sensitive mucous membranes, such as those inside the nose or mouth. They should not be used on children (unless the label on the preparation specifically states that the product is intended for this use) because percutaneous absorption is greater in children than in adults. Most package inserts available to the patient warn that, for conditions affecting young children, a physician should be consulted.

The following precautions and warnings apply to topical analgesic products: [24]

☐ Keep out of eyes and mucous membranes

☐ Do not apply to wounds or abraded skin

☐ Do not use on infants or small children

☐ For local application only: do not apply to large areas of the body

☐ Discontinue use if untoward reactions occur

☐ Frequency of application should be mediated by concentration, other ingredients, the vehicle, and directions for administration

☐ Contraindicated in individuals displaying an idiosyncrasy to salicylates.

Adjunctive measures

Although OTC preparations have merit of their own as therapeutic agents, they may be inferior to simple physical measures. Perhaps the most frequently used counterirritant is heat applied to the muscle with a hot-water bottle, a heating pad, a heat lamp, or a moist hotpack. However, these measures should not be used in conjunction with counterirritant drugs because severe burning or blistering of skin areas can occur. An advantage of external analgesic preparations over heat treatments is that they are less trouble to use and allow the patient freedom of movement while giving symptomatic relief.

Summary

If the use of an OTC external analgesic is indicated, the pharmacist should advise the patient about proper usage with appropriate advice concerning safety. The patient should also be advised that the preparation is intended only for temporary and symptomatic relief. As previously mentioned, a minor muscular pain may be caused by a more serious problem which cannot be ameliorated by an OTC preparation. If the condition persists, a physician should be consulted.

References

1. T. S. Szasz, *Arch. Neurol. Psychiatry*, **74**, 174(1955).
2. "Cecil-Loeb Textbook of Medicine," 13th ed., P. B. Beeson and W. McDermott, Eds., Saunders, Philadelphia, Pa., 1971, p. 153.
3. J. L. Hollander, "Arthritis and Allied Conditions," Lea and Febiger, Philadelphia, Pa., 1966, p. 1233.
4. "Handbook of Medical Treatment," M. J. Chatton *et al.*, Eds., Lange Medical Publications, Los Altos, Calif., 1970, p. 361.
5. D. M. Aviado, "Krantz and Carr's Pharmacologic Principles of Medical Practice," 8th ed., Williams and Wilkins, Baltimore, Md., 1972, p. 891.
6. "The Pharmacological Basis of Therapeutics," 5th ed., L. S. Goodman and A. Gilman, Eds., Macmillan, New York, N.Y., 1975, p. 951.
7. B. S. Post, *Arch. Phys. Med. Rehabil.*, **42**, 791(1961).
8. D. M. Aviado, "Krantz and Carr's Pharmacologic Principles of Medical Practice," 8th ed., Williams and Wilkins, Baltimore, Md., 1972, p. 892.
9. D. M. Aviado, "Krantz and Carr's Pharmacologic Principles of Medical Practice," 8th ed., Williams and Wilkins, Baltimore, Md., 1972, p. 893.
10. R. H. Dreisbach, "Handbook of Poisoning," Lange Medical Publications, Los Altos, Calif., 1971, p. 252.
11. "The Pharmacological Basis of Therapeutics," 5th ed., L. S. Goodman and A. Gilman, Eds., Macmillan, New York, N.Y., 1975, p. 951.
12. M. N. Gleason *et al.*, "Clinical Toxicology of Commercial Products," 3d ed., Williams and Wilkins, Baltimore, Md., 1969, p. 223.
13. "Facts and Comparisons," E. K. Kastrup, Ed., Facts and Comparisons, Inc., St. Louis, Mo., 1975, p. 503.
14. J. B. Sprowls and H. M. Beal, "American Pharmacy," Lippincott, Philadelphia, Pa., 1966, p. 268.
15. "Drugs of Choice, 1974-1975," W. Modell, Ed., Mosby, St. Louis, Mo., 1974, p. 611.
16. F. Reiss, *Am. J. Med. Sci.*, **252**, 588(1966).
17. "Drugs of Choice, 1974-1975," W. Modell, Ed., Mosby, St. Louis, Mo., 1974, p. 612.
18. "Remington's Pharmaceutical Sciences," 15th ed., J. E. Hoover *et al.*, Eds., Mack Publishing, Easton, Pa., 1975, p. 1532.
19. R. B. Stoughton, *Arch. Environ. Health*, **11**, 551(1965).
20. E. E. Gordon and A. Haas, *Ind. Med. Surg.*, **28(5)**, 217(1959).
21. "Report from Biological Sciences Laboratories," Foster D. Snell, Inc., Elizabeth, N.J., August 8, 1972.
22. K. L. Melmon and H. F. Morelli, "Clinical Pharmacology: Basic Principles in Therapeutics," Macmillan, New York, N.Y., 1972, p. 576.
23. M. N. Gleason *et al.*, "Clinical Toxicology of Commercial Products," Williams and Wilkins, Baltimore, Md., 1969, p. 223.
24. Minutes of the Fourth Meeting, OTC Panel on Topical Analgesics, Antirheumatic, Otic, Burn, Sunburn Treatment and Prevention Drugs, Food and Drug Administration, Rockville, Md., September 27 and 28, 1973.

Products 26 EXTERNAL ANALGESIC

roduct manufacturer)	Application form	Counterirritant	Other
bsorbent Rub (DeWitt)	lotion	camphor, 1.6%; menthol, 1.6%; methyl salicylate, 0.7%; wormwood oil, 0.6%; sassafras oil, 0.5%; capsicum, 0.03%	isopropyl alcohol, 69%; green soap, 11.6%; pine tar soap, 0.9%; *o*-phenylphenol, 0.5%; benzocaine, 0.5%
bsorbine Arthritic (W. F. Young)	lotion	methyl salicylate, menthol, methyl nicotinate	greaseless, stainless emulsion base
bsorbine Jr. (W. F. Young)	lotion	wormwood oil, thymol, menthol, chloroxylenol	acetone
ct-On Rub (Keystone)	lotion	methyl salicylate, menthol, camphor, eucalyptus oil, mustard oil	isopropyl myristate, balm base, lanolin
nalbalm (Central)	lotion	methyl salicylate, 5%; camphor, 2.5%; menthol, 0.5%	greaseless nonstaining emulsion base
nalgesic Balm (Lilly)	ointment	methyl salicylate, 15%; menthol, 15%	hydrocarbon waxes, lanolin, petrolatum, sorbitan sesquioleate, water-soluble base
nalgesic Balm (Parke-Davis)	ointment	methyl salicylate, 15 g/100 g; menthol, 15 g/100 g	—
ntiphlogistine (Roberts)	poultice	methyl salicylate, eucalyptus oil, salicylic acid	glycerin, kaolin, boric acid, peppermint oil
analg (Cole)	lotion	menthol, methyl salicylate, camphor, eucalyptus oil	greaseless base
aumodyne (North American)	gel	menthol	—
en-Gay (Leeming)	lotion	methyl salicylate, 15%; menthol, 7%	greaseless base
raska (Keystone)	lotion	methyl salicylate, menthol, camphor, monoglycol salicylate, methyl nicotinate, salicylamide	isopropyl alcohol
ounterpain Rub (Squibb)	ointment	methyl salicylate, 10.2%; menthol, 5.4%; eugenol, 1.4%	—
encorub (Roberts)	lotion	methyl salicylate, menthol, camphor, eucalyptus oil	—

Product (manufacturer)	Application form	Counterirritant	Other
Emul-O-Balm (Pennwalt)	lotion	menthol, 22.45 mg/ml; methyl salicylate, 22.45 mg/ml; camphor, 11.22 mg/ml	ribbon gum tragacanth, 8.37 mg/ml; methylparaben, 1.50 mg/ml; propylparaben, 0.30 mg/ml
End-Ake (Columbia Medical)	liniment	methyl salicylate, eucalyptus oil, menthol, camphor	—
Exocaine Plus (Kirk)	ointment	methyl salicylate, 30%; menthol crystals, 2%; clove oil, 1%	benzocaine, 5%
Exocaine Tube (Kirk)	ointment	methyl salicylate, 30%; clove oil, 1%	benzocaine, 5%
Heet (Whitehall)	lotion	methyl salicylate, capsicum, camphor	alcohol, 53%
Infra-Rub (Whitehall)	cream	methyl nicotinate, histamine dihydrochloride, capsicum oleoresin	glycol monosalicylate, lanolin
Lini Balm (Arnar-Stone)	aerosol foam	methyl salicylate, 15%; camphor, 2%; eucalyptus oil, 2%; menthol, 1%	polyoxyalkalene lanolin
Mentholatum (Mentholatum)	ointment	camphor, 9%; menthol, 1.35%	aromatic oils, petrolatum base
Mentholatum Deep Heating (Mentholatum)	ointment, lotion	methyl salicylate, 12.7% (ointment); 20% (lotion); menthol, 6%; eucalyptus oil (ointment); turpentine oil (ointment)	lanolin, greaseless base
Minit-Rub (Bristol-Myers)	ointment	methyl salicylate, 10%; menthol, 3.54%; camphor, 4.44%; eucalyptus oil, 1.77%	anhydrous lanolin, 4.44%
Mothers Friend Massage (S.S.S.)	lotion	—	cottonseed oil, glycerin, sorbitol, methylparaben, propylparaben, absorption base, fragrance
Musterole Deep Strength (Plough)	ointment	methyl salicylate, 30%; menthol, 3%; methyl nicotinate, 0.5%	—
Musterole Regular, Extra, and Children's Strength (Plough)	ointment	camphor, menthol, methyl salicylate, mustard oil, glycol monosalicylate	—
Neurabalm (S.S.S.)	lotion	methyl salicylate, menthol, eucalyptus oil, cajuput oil, camphor, chlorothymol	alcohol, 54%; acetone; benzocaine
Omega Oil (Block)	lotion	methyl salicylate, methyl nicotinate, capsicum oleoresin, histamine dihydrochloride	isopropyl alcohol, 44.4%
Panalgesic (Poythress)	lotion spray	methyl salicylate, 50%; camphor, 4%; menthol, 2%	emollient oils, 20%; alcohol, 18%; aspirin, 8%
Penetro Quick Acting Rub (Plough)	ointment	methyl salicylate, menthol, turpentine, camphor, thymol	pine oil
Sloan's (Warner-Lambert)	liniment	turpentine oil, 46.76%; pine oil, 6.74%; camphor, 3.35%; methyl salicylate, 2.66%; capsicum oleoresin, 0.62%	kerosene, 39.88%
Soltice Hi-Therm (Chattem)	cream	eucalyptus oil, 10 mg/g; methyl salicylate, 50 mg/g; menthol, 70 mg/g; camphor, 70 mg/g	greaseless base
Soltice Quick Rub (Chattem)	cream	eucalyptus oil, 10 mg/g; methyl salicylate, 50 mg/g; menthol, 50 mg/g; camphor, 50 mg/g	greaseless base
SPD (Amer. Pharm.)	cream, lotion	methyl salicylate, 10%; menthol; camphor; methyl nicotinate, 1%; capsicum oleoresin, 0.5% (cream)	washable greaseless base

Product (manufacturer)	Application form	Counterirritant	Other
Stimurub (Otis Clapp)	ointment	menthol, methyl salicylate, capsicum oleoresin	—
Surin (McKesson)	ointment	methyl salicylate, menthol, camphor	methacholine chloride, 0.25%; greaseless base
Vicks Vaporub (Vick)	external rub	camphor, menthol, turpentine spirits, eucalyptus oil, cedar leaf oil, myristica oil, thymol	—
Yager's Liniment (Yager)	liniment	turpentine oil, 8%; camphor, 1%	aqua ammonia, 1.4%; ammonium oleate
Zemo Liquid (Plough)	lotion	methyl salicylate, thymol, eucalyptol, menthol, phenol	sodium salicylate; sodium borate; benzoic acid; boric acid; alcohol, 35%
Zemo Liquid Extra Strength (Plough)	lotion	methyl salicylate, menthol, thymol, eucalyptol, phenol	sodium salicylate, sodium borate, benzoic acid, boric acid, alcohol, 40%

Topical Anti-Infective Products

Paul Zanowiak

Questions to ask the patient

What area of the skin is affected? How extensive is the area involved?

Is the skin broken?

How long have you had this condition? Have you had it before? Are other members of your family also affected?

Has the condition developed as the result of a previous rash or skin disorder?

Do you have a fever or other symptoms of the flu?

Do you have diabetes?

What treatments have you tried for this condition? Were they effective?

Are you presently using any medications?

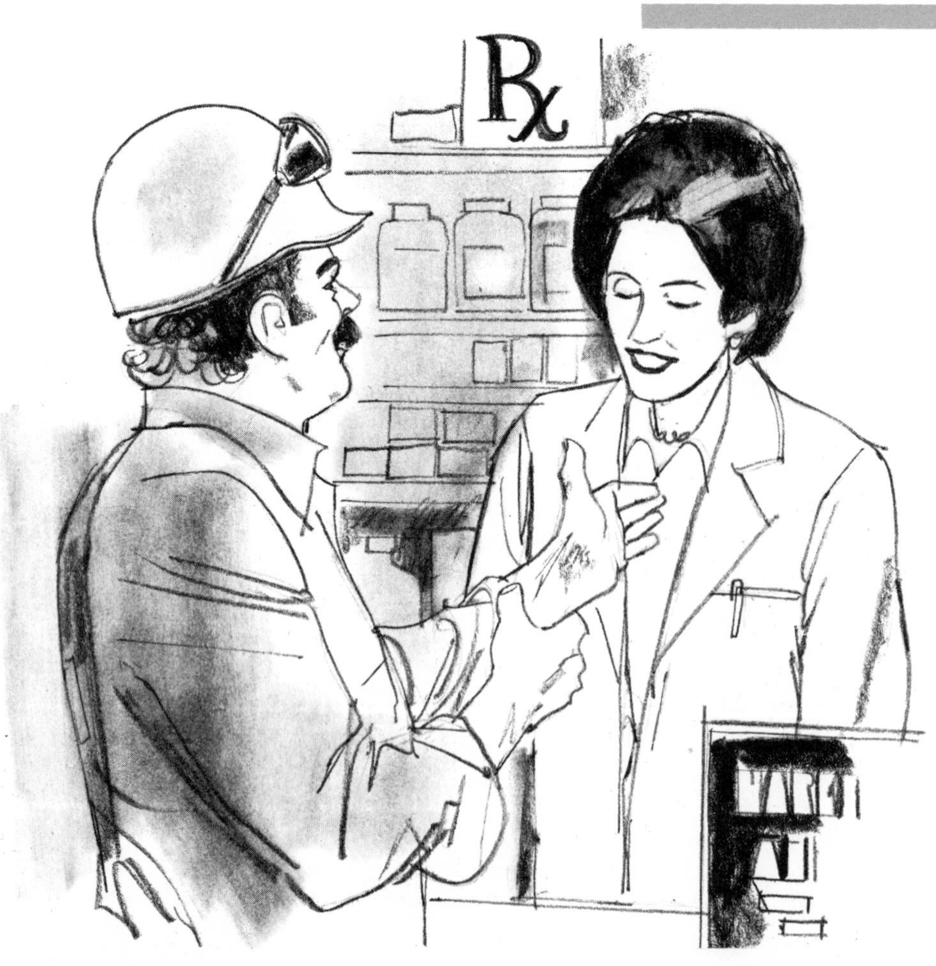

CHAPTER 27

By definition, this category of nonprescription drug products can include all products that are used to counteract infection (anti-infectives) on local tissue (topical). The active ingredients of these products are antimicrobial; most are antibacterial or antifungal. Because this product classification is so broad, discussion is limited to antimicrobial products for use in prevention and self-treatment of infections of the skin. (See individual chapters which deal with specific and localized conditions of the skin.)

Cutaneous infections

Bacterial

The normal flora of the skin contain various bacteria which are not invasive under normal conditions. However, when a breakdown in the defenses of the skin occurs or when a predisposing dermal problem exists, certain bacteria within the flora can invade dermal tissue to establish loci of infection and subsequent pus formation. Some of the factors that influence the incidence of all types of cutaneous infection are: change in the flora of the skin surface, the number of pathogens present, the water content of the skin, temperature, injury, pH, and scrubbing.

Bacterial infections of the skin can be classified as pyodermas (Fig. 1) because pus usually is present. They are caused primarily by β-hemolytic streptococci and hemolytic staphylococci.[1] The lesions result from external infection or reinfection, and they may be superficial or involve deeper dermal tissue. These pyodermic infections are primary (where no previous dermatoses existed) or secondary (where a predisposing dermal problem already exists). Organisms besides staphylococci or streptococci may be present in secondary pyodermas, including gram-negative bacteria (e.g., *Pseudomonas aeruginosa*) which are especially prevalent on warm, moist skin, such as the axillae, ear canals, and between the toes.

The primary pyodermic infections are impetigo, folliculitis, furuncles (boils), carbuncles, erysipelas, sweat gland infections, ecthyma, and pyonychia.[2,3]

Impetigo.[4] Impetigo vulgaris (caused by streptococci, staphylococci, or both) probably is the most superficial of the pyodermas, mainly involving surface areas. Direct contact with lesions or infected exudate generally is required for its transmission. Also, scrupulous hygiene is necessary to avoid reinoculation by spreading of the exudate. Thus, soiled dressings should not touch unaffected areas, and transport of exudate by clothing should be prevented. The patient's hands and nails should be kept clean, and scratching the lesions should be avoided.

Lesions initially are small red spots.[5] These evolve rapidly into characteristic vesicles (tiny sacs or blisters) filled with amber fluid. Exudation collects and forms yellow or brown crusts on the surface. Below the crust is a smooth, red, weeping surface. Direct spreading occurs rapidly when the exudation is not carefully removed. The eruptions can be circular with clear central areas and can occur in groups. The exposed parts of the body are most easily affected, but no area of the skin is immune if autogenous reinfection is not controlled. Impetigo is most common in children, where it is highly contagious.

Furfuraceous impetigo (pityriasis simplex faciei) is a superficial streptococcic infection, found almost exclusively in children. Lesions occur most often on the face; they are scaly, red, round patches of varying sizes. This impetigo seems to occur more often in cold weather, and depigmentation of the patchy areas may occur in previously affected areas.

The various forms of impetigo can occur as primary or secondary pyodermas. In the former, the responsible bacteria cause the infection directly (e.g., impetigo vulgaris). Some forms, however, can occur secondarily to the presence of other infections, injury, or general breakdown in skin defenses. Thus, impetigo Bockhart usually occurs as a secondary infection to another condition (furuncles, discharging ears, or wounds). Lesions characteristically are tiny, follicular pustules around hair shafts and may be encircled by narrow, red rings (areolae).

Folliculitis.[4] Follicular pustules are superficial or deep, depending on the pathogen and on the site involved. They involve only the hair shafts; surrounding tissue is not affected. Usually, the superficial forms are very similar to impetigo Bockhart, and they may be secondary infections. Areas of the skin which are regularly exposed to water, grease, oils, tars, etc. seem most easily affected.

Furuncles and carbuncles.[4] These pyodermas are generally staphylococcic infections with localization in or around hair follicles. The lesion may start as a superficial folliculitis but develops into a deep nodule. The fully established furuncle has elevated swelling, is erythematous, and is very painful. Furuncles are most common in males. Hairy areas and areas that are subject to maceration (skin softening due to moisture accumulation) and friction (collar, waist, buttocks, and thighs) seem most vulnerable. The initial erythema and swelling stage is followed by thinning of the skin around the primary follicle, centralized pustulation, destruction of the pilosebaceous structure, discharging of the core (plug), and central ulceration. Scarring often occurs. Chronic furunculosis is common, with new lesions appearing intermittently for months or years.

Furuncles can be secondary infections to other dermatoses or diseases. Diabetes mellitus and agammaglobulinemia may predispose a person to furuncles or carbuncles. Chronic cases of these pyodermas should be referred for urinalysis and blood sugar and sugar tolerance tests.

Carbuncles involve clusters of follicles with deeper and broader penetration over a larger area than furuncles. Furuncles may develop into carbuncles by infiltration or infection of adjacent follicles.

Sweat gland infections.[4] These staph infections originate in sweat and related apocrine glands; they may look like furuncles. Axillary apocrine sweat glands are the most common site, but other apocrine glands are also vulnerable (perianal, perimammillary, genital). Sweat gland infections may result as a secondary infection to an irritant; deodorant/antiperspirant products may produce

IMPETIGO VULGARIS

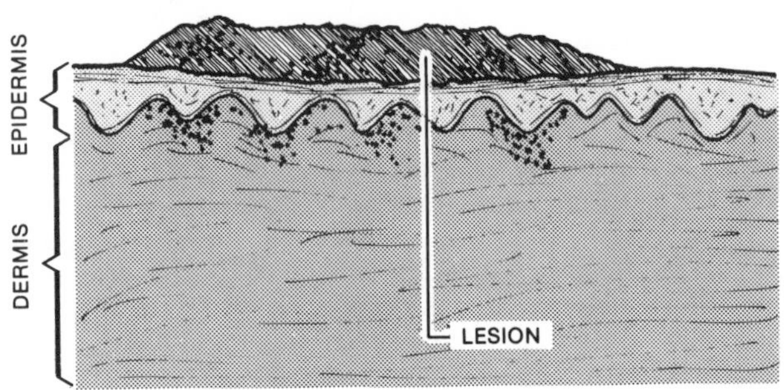

IMPETIGO BOCKHART

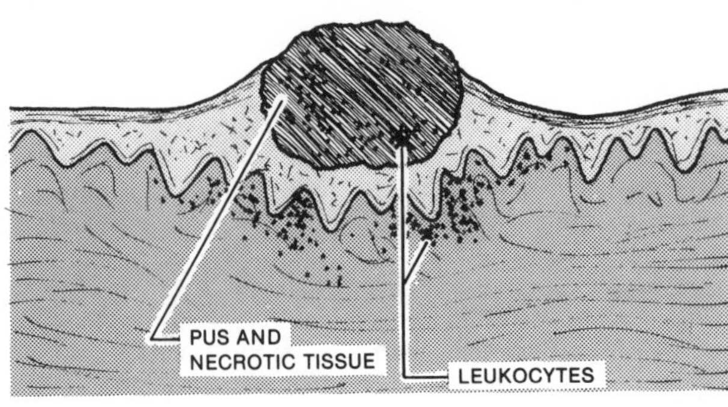

FOLLICULITIS-SUPERFICIAL

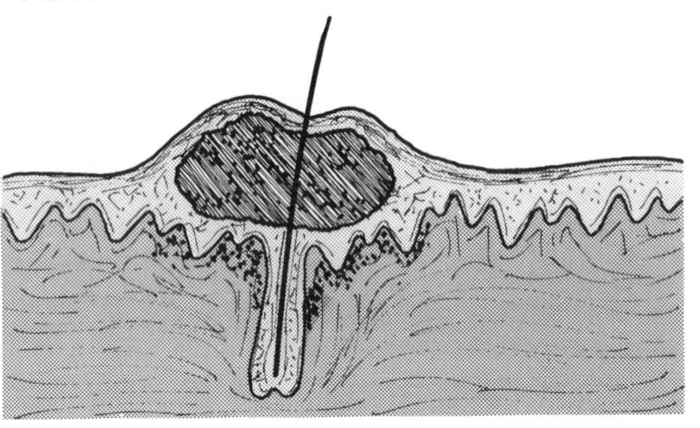

FOLLICULITIS-DEEP

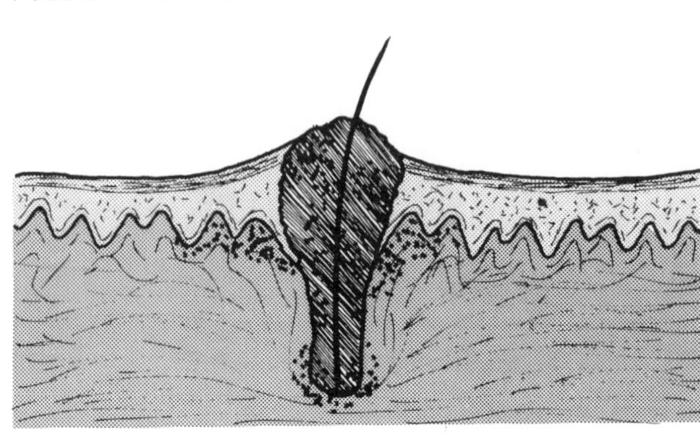

FURUNCLE

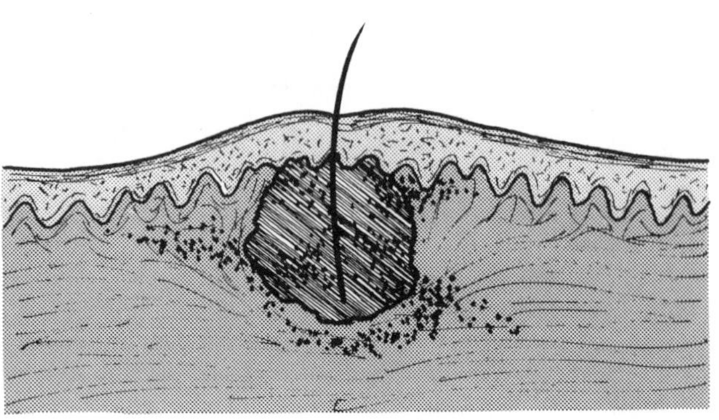

CARBUNCLE

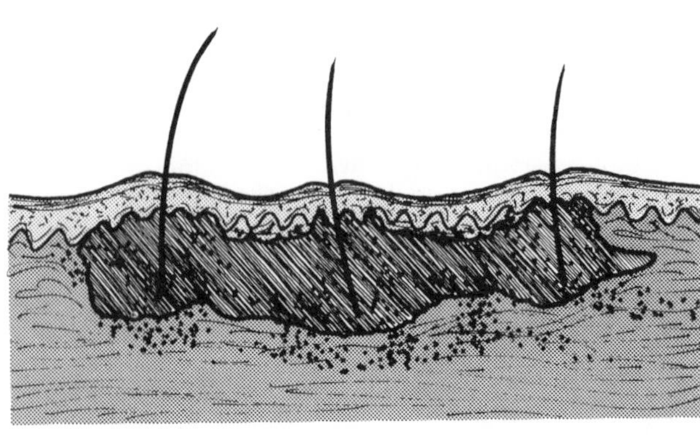

SWEAT-GLAND INFECTION

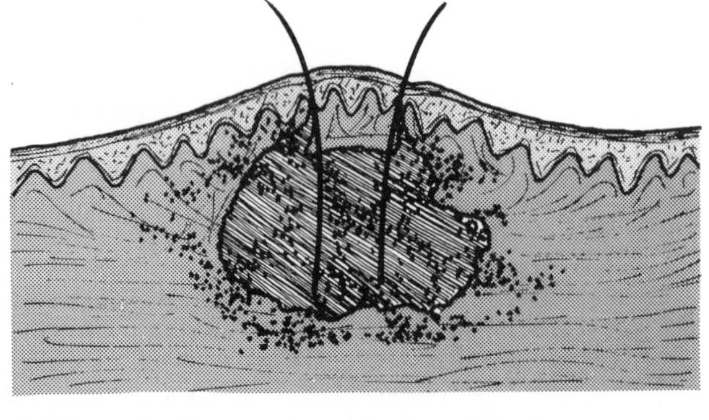

ECTHYMA

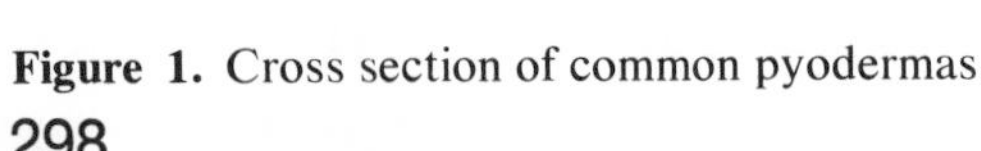

Figure 1. Cross section of common pyodermas.

an initial dermatitis. People with chronic skin conditions (acne, folliculitis) may be predisposed to sweat gland infections.[6]

Infants are subject to superficial infections (periporitis) and deeper and multiple abscesses of these glands. Generally, infants in poor health are more prone to such infections, which occur mainly as secondary infections to other skin disorders. Sweat gland abscesses in the axillae (hidradenitis axillaris) occur in adolescents and adults with an endocrine disorder.

Sweat gland infections begin as small, superficial, very tender pustules. They rapidly develop into hard, tender, bluish-red, elevated swellings. There can be many such abscesses. Within several days, softening usually occurs, and the abscess ruptures, exuding pus, blood, and serous fluid.

Ecthyma.[4] Ecthyma is a pyoderma that is very similar to impetigo, but it is deeper. Lesions begin as pustules and form deep crusts with red margins. Removal of the crusts results in pus-exuding, ulcerous wounds. This condition often occurs as a secondary infection to minor traumas (scratches). People with poor circulation seem predisposed to ecthyma, because the lower part of the legs is a common site.

Erysipelas.[6] This infection is caused by a β-hemolytic streptococcus. It is a cellulitis characterized by a rapidly spreading, red, and edematous plaque. Erysipelas is superficial and has sharply established borders and a glistening surface.[5] It occurs most often on the scalp and face and is usually accompanied by elevated temperature, chills, and malaise.

Pyonychia.[6] Pyonychia is a pyogenic infection of the nails with swelling and tenderness of surrounding tissue. Moderate pressure can force a pus exudate, and the nail may develop with irregularities. It is important that accurate recognition be made to avoid confusion with candidal or other fungal infections which can also affect nails.

Secondary pyodermic infections can occur where there is a break in the skin—after mechanical, burn, or chemical injury, or other dermatoses, scratching, etc.

Infectious eczematoid dermatitis.[6] This name refers to any chronic eczematous condition of the skin with an infectious component. Originally it was used to generally describe a secondary infection arising on the skin adjacent to an area of primary infection. In some cases of contact dermatitis caused by topical agents, this name also has been applied. Thus, this term is too general and confusing and probably should be avoided.

Otitis externa.[6] This inflammation involves the external ear and can be a secondary infection involving bacteria and fungi. It is essentially an inflammation, but microbial pathogens can be found in its exudate. It can occur secondarily, for example, to seborrheic scaling of the scalp. Lesions are characterized by redness, edema, crusts, and oozing. Real pus is rare, unless a true infection is also present in the ear canal. The anatomy of the ear makes cleanliness difficult. Because of the ear's warmth, darkness, and moisture, micro-organisms can flourish as secondary contributors to the original dermatitis. (See Chapter 19 for a complete discussion of otitis externa.)

Fungal infections

Fungal infections of the skin are often called dermatomycoses and are among the most common cutaneous disorders.[7, 8] Characteristically, they exhibit single or multiple lesions that may have mild scaling or deep granulomas (inflamed nodules). Superficial infections are called tinea, ringworm, and dermatophytosis. They affect hair, nails, and skin, and their general pathologic manifestations are caused mainly by three genera of fungi: *Trichophyton, Microsporum,* and *Epidermophyton. Candida* can also be involved.[6] Fungal infections of hairless skin generally are superficial, and the organisms are in or on the uppermost layers of the skin. In fungal infections of areas covered with heavy hair, the organisms are much deeper due to the penetration of hair follicles.

Tinea pedis (ringworm of the feet; athlete's foot).[7] This infection is caused by the several species of fungi already mentioned and may include *Candida albicans.* Its severity depends on the degree of resistance of the host and the specific, causative organism. Depending on the organism, the lesions are characterized by an erythematous and scaly dermatitis *(Epidermophyton floccosum)*; exudation and maceration with defined borders which are ringed with tiny vesicles *(C. albicans)*; acute vesicular formation between toes and on the soles of the feet with maceration and fissures *(Trichophyton mentagrophytes)*; and hyperkeratolytic thickening of the skin with few or no vesicles and inflammation *(T. rubrum).* (See Chapter 32 for a complete discussion of athlete's foot.)

Tinea capitis.[7] This infection is transmitted ,by direct contact with infected people or animals. It is caused by *Microsporum* and *Trichophyton.* The lesions are small papules infiltrated by broken hairs. The papules enlarge and form scaly, red patches. Inflammation, varying degrees of alopecia, and soft and wet, deeper lesions may occur.

Tinea cruris.[7] This infection is caused by *E. floccosum, C. albicans,* and species of *Trichophyton.* It occurs on the medial and upper parts of the thighs, with possible involvement of the pubic area (jock itch). The lesions have specific margins which are slightly elevated and more inflamed than the central parts; small vesicles can be found at the margins. Acute lesions are bright red and turn brownish in chronic cases, and they can scale. This condition is generally bilateral with severe pruritus.

Tinea corporis.[7] Species of *Trichophyton* and *Microsporum* are the causative organisms of this condition. The lesions involve glabrous (devoid of hair) skin and begin as small, circular, erythematous, scaly areas. They spread peripherally, and the borders may contain vesicles or pustules. Tinea corporis can easily be mistaken for an "eczema," because lesions can resemble eczematoid conditions.

Other fungal infections. Moniliasis, caused mainly by *C. albicans,* usually occurs in intertriginous (where two surfaces rub together) areas, such as the groin, axillae, interdigital areas, under breasts, and at the corners of the mouth; moisture and friction accelerate the condition.[7] Involvement of the mucous membrane appears as "thrush," vaginal candidiasis, and pruritus ani. Candidal paronychia involves the nails and is most common in people whose activities involve routine immersion of the hands in water. Systemic diseases such as diabetes, infection, or malignancy may lower general resistance and allow *C. albicans* infections to flourish. Certain drugs, e.g., antibiotics used locally in the GI tract, can do the same. Pregnancy is a predisposing cause of vaginal candidiasis.

Other fungal infections of the skin include tinea barbae (barber's itch or ringworm of the beard); tinea manum (hands); tinea versicolor (body trunk; brown in color); tinea circinata, which is generally ringed, red lesions that can agglomerate into polycyclic configurations;

tinea unguium (onychomycosis), a fungal infection of the nails, where the nail can become hypertrophic and can discolor and scale; and erythrasma (in axillary or pubic areas).[4,6]

Viral infections

Viruses are responsible for dermal diseases such as herpes simplex, herpes zoster, and verrucae (warts).

Herpes simplex.[4,9] Herpes simplex is a viral infection of the skin and mucous membrane. The caustive agent is a fairly large virus: herpesvirus hominis (HVH).[10] It has two strains—Type 1, which is common to herpes labialis; and Type 2, which is generally involved in genital herpes lesions and is transmitted venereally.

Herpes simplex (Type 1) develops as groups (few to many) of tiny vesicles filled with straw-colored fluid after an incubation period of 5 days.[5] The vesicles develop into blisters and plaques. The area may be reddened, slightly edematous, and uncomfortable—malaise, headache, and initial itching, stinging, and burning can accompany the lesions. Most occurrences heal spontaneously in about 10 days; however, there is a marked tendency for lesions to recur.[5] Tenderness of the lymph nodes of the area may occur. The lesions usually appear on the lips and nose (fever blisters, cold sores), fingers, and genital areas.[11]

Herpes zoster (shingles).[4,9] This viral infection is neurotropic in humans and is caused by a virus similar to that which causes chickenpox.[12,13] Lesions appear along the course of a nerve or group of nerves on one side of the body; the spinal ganglia seem to be the primary site. They appear suddenly and acutely as reddened, swollen, round plaques, ranging in size from about 0.5 cm to areas larger than a hand. They may be painful after formation of the lesions. It is possible for them to appear as successive "showers" or "crops" over several days.[11] The plaques develop into fairly large blisters, which become crusty in 2 to 14 days as they dry. The regional lymph nodes generally are tender. An episode is followed by a lasting immunity; recurrent cases are extremely uncommon.

Warts. Warts are benign, epithelial tumors of viral etiology. (See Chapter 32 for a complete discussion of warts and their treatment.)

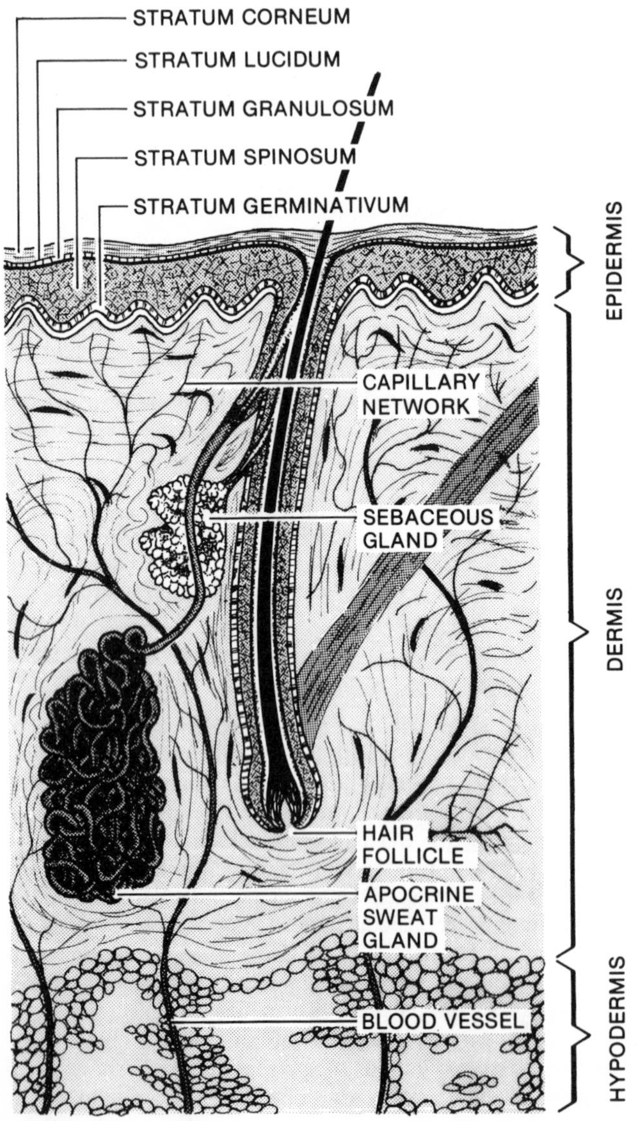

Figure 2. Cross section of human skin.

Anatomy and physiology of the skin

An understanding of the normal physiology and anatomy of the skin (Fig. 2) is basic to a thorough knowledge of adverse cutaneous reactions, including microbial infections.[14–18]

Normal skin ranges from 3 to 5 mm in thickness. The thickest skin is on the palms and soles; the thinnest is on the eyelids and parts of the genitals. The skin is divided into three main layers. The outermost layer (epidermis) is quite compact and nonvascular and consists of stratified, squamous epithelial cells. The next layer (dermis, corium) is vascular and is a connective tissue. These two layers are not similar in composition but adhere firmly to each other. The hypodermis is the innermost layer.

The epidermis is composed of several distinct layers. The innermost, in close association with the dermis, is the stratum germinativum. It consists of columnar/cuboidal epithelial cells. Above this is the prickle cell layer (stratum spinosum) which is composed of layers of polygonal epithelial cells. This layer is thicker in the palms than in hairy skin.

These two layers are involved in mitotic processes toward epidermal regeneration and repair. The prickle cells contain keratinocytes which are produced by cellular division in these layers of the epidermis. As the keratinocytes migrate to the skin's surface, they change from living cells to dead, thick-walled, flat, nonnucleated cells that contain keratin, a fibrous protein.

Above the prickle cell layer is the granular layer (stratum granulosum), which is several layers of flattened, polygonal cells. These cells contain granules of keratohyaline which are changed to keratin in the outermost layer of the skin (stratum corneum, or horny outer layer). The stratum lucidum is present only in areas of thick skin; it is between the granular layer and the stratum corneum. It is a narrow band of flattened, closely packed cells. These cells are believed to contain eleidin, a possible derivative of keratohyaline. The stratum corneum is composed of flat, scaly, dead tissue (keratinized). The outermost cells of this layer are flat or squamous plates. These plates are constantly desquamated or shed.

Throughout the basal layers of the dermis, dendritic processes exist between adjacent keratinocytes. Keratinocytes are the pigment-forming melanocytes that contain melanin precursors and melanin granules. The dead cells lost from the outer surface of the epidermis are replaced by new cells generated by the mitotic processes of the stratum spinosum and stratum germinativum. The newer cells push older ones closer to the surface. In the process, they become flattened, lose their water content, fill with keratin, and gradually die, taking their place on the surface of the skin.

The dermis supports the epidermis and separates it from the lower fatty layer. It consists mainly of collagen and elastin embedded in a mucopolysaccharide substance. Fibroblasts and mast cells are found throughout. The dermis also contains a network of nerves that are the neurovascular supply to the appendages in the dermis, i.e., hair follicles, sebaceous glands, and sweat glands. The main sublayers of the dermis are the papillary and reticular layers. The papillary layer is adjacent to the epidermis. It is very rich in blood vessels and the papillae probably act as conduits to bring blood nutrients near the avascular epidermis. The reticular layer, below the papillary layer, contains coarser tissue which connects the dermis with the hypodermis.

The hypodermis is made up of relatively loose connective tissue of varying thickness. It provides necessary pliability for the skin. In most areas this layer also includes a layer of fat (panniculus adiposus) which is involved in thermal control, food reserve, and as cushioning or padding.

Appendages of the skin

Hair follicle. A hair shaft is generated by a hair germ at the base of a hair follicle. The follicle basically is an inward tubular folding of the epidermis into the dermis. The hair within the follicle is a fiber of keratinized epithelial cells that grow as a result of multiplication of cells in the hair germ.

Sebaceous glands. Most sebaceous glands are located in the same areas as hair. They are appendages of the hair follicles. The ducts of these glands are lined with epithelial cells which are continuous with those of the basal layers of the epidermis. These glands produce sebum; they are holocrine, because the gland cells from which sebum is derived are destroyed in its production. Not all sebaceous glands are associated with hair follicles. They also are found in genital areas, around the nipples of the breast, and on the edges of the lips.

Sweat glands. Sweat glands develop from epithelial cells that proceed downward from the epidermis, and they are independent of hair follicles. They are long, hollow tubes that reach into dermal and hypodermal areas. Their secretory parts are in the hypodermis. The excretory ducts proceed upward through the epidermis as wavy or curved channels. Sweat is an eccrine secretion, and no part of the gland cell is destroyed. Sweat glands are found over much of the body.

Eccrine sweat glands. These glands are cholinergically innervated, although the nerve fibers are sympathetic. The heat regulation centers of the hypothalamus control overall secretion of the sweat glands. Emotional stress as well as heat can produce sweating. Sweat is basically a saline solution with some electrolytes, but it is devoid of carbohydrates, fats, or proteins. Much more sweat is produced by the true sweat glands (several liters per day) than by the apocrine glands.

Apocrine glands. These glands are located in the axillae, areolae of the nipples, and perianal and genital areas. They produce a milky secretion that appears in very small amounts on the skin and has a characteristic odor. They are erroneously called "sweat" glands. Apocrine glands are larger and deeper in the skin than true sweat glands.

The apocrines generally are attached to a hair follicle by a duct leading down into the coiled, secretory tubules of the gland. The tubules are covered by myoepithelium. This covering allows contraction to adrenergic stimulation. Thus, stimulation, as in stress, releases the secretion, which is odorless, until the bacteria of the skin utilize the fats present. This results in the characteristic pungent odor of apocrine "sweat." In the absence of apocrine secretions, such as in prepuberty, sweat is odorless.

Nails. The nails (onycho-) are modifications of the keratinized layer of the epidermis. The nail bed on which the nail plate lies derives from the basal epidermal layers. The body of the plate, at its periphery, is surrounded by the nail root. The root is derived from the nail groove, which is a process of the basal epidermal unit. The white area at the base is called the lunula, and the part of the nail groove that enfolds the plate at its margin is the eponychium. The hyponychium is a thick layer of stratum corneum immediately beneath the plate of the distal tip of the nail.

Normal function of the skin [15, 17]

The skin acts as a barrier between the environment and the body and protects the body against harmful external agents, e.g., pathogenic organisms and chemicals. The skin also contributes to sensory experiences. It is involved in temperature control, development of pigment, and synthesis of some vitamins. It is important in hydroregulation because it controls loss of moisture from the body and penetration of moisture into the body.

The skin, except for the stratum corneum, is living tissue and requires nutrition, including oxygen. The cells of all the layers use nutrients and excrete water and carbon dioxide. Most oxygen is supplied from the blood; a small amount is supplied from the air. Similarly, carbon dioxide is taken away from the tissues mainly by the blood, but some is "exhaled" directly to the atmosphere.

Dermal hydration

The water content of the skin is important to its normal health. Topical, nonmedicated preparations are available mainly for the physical control of moisture in the skin. The kind and degree of percutaneous absorption of various drugs, including anti-infective agents, are affected by the amount of water present in the various layers of the skin. Thus, the degree of skin hydration could promote percutaneous absorption to areas beyond those desired for the therapeutic activity of a drug. It also could restrict the degree of penetration. In either case, poor therapy would result. Also, promotion of absorption to the degree that the drug reaches the systemic circulation can be dangerous.

The loss of moisture from the skin and its penetration into the skin were thought to be controlled by a "barrier zone" which was believed to exist between the stratum corneum and stratum lucidum.[19] To date, the existence of the zone has not been proved conclusively. The postulation of its existence was based on the moisture content of the tissue which surrounds this area. The tissue below this area has regular blood flow and has about 70 percent moisture content. The corneous layers above the proposed zone have a lower moisture content, about 10 percent.[15] It is better to view the entire stratum corneum as a barrier, or water seal, because no definitive evidence exists for a "barrier zone" within the horny layer.

If the corneous layer "dries out" significantly, its elasticity is affected negatively. Returning water to the skin is the only means by which induced brittleness can be reversed. Hydration of the stratum corneum occurs by transfer of water from lower layers or by the accumulation of water (perspiration) caused by occlusive coverings at the surface (bandages, various vehicles). The accumulation of moisture by occlusive coverings seems to "open" the compactness of the stratum corneum, making penetration of this area by drug molecules easier.[20]

Sebum

The surface of the skin is covered with a mixture of fatty substances called sebum. The constituents include free fatty acids (mainly palmitic and oleic), triglycerides, waxes, cholesterol, squalene, and other hydrocarbons and traces of fat-soluble vitamins.[21] Sebum is a product of the sebaceous glands. It lubricates the skin surface to ensure suppleness and acts as a surface barrier to the loss of moisture from the deeper layers of the skin because of its fatty nature. Chemically, it prevents penetration of the skin by other substances, and it has some antiseptic and antifungal properties. The sebum is an emulsion of sweat and surface waste products of cutaneous cells.[19]

pH of the skin surface

The secretions that accumulate at the skin's surface are weakly acidic (pH of 4.5 to 5.5).[22] The pH varies slightly among individuals and among different areas of the body; it is somewhat higher in areas where perspiration evaporates slowly.[15] The acidic nature of the skin's surface is called the "acid mantle."

Jellinek [23] reported that the acid mantle is thought to be a protective mechanism because microbes tend to grow better at pH 6 to 7.5 and infected areas have comparably higher pH values than normal skin.

Peck and Russ [24] found that several fatty acids found in sweat inhibit microbial and fungal growth (propionic, caproic, and caprylic). The conclusion was that the importance of the "acid mantle" concept was not in the inherent pH, but in the specific compounds responsible for the acidity. It was also found that the ingredients of sebum have fungicidal and bactericidal properties.[25,26]

The buffer capacity of the secretions of the skin surface is another protective mechanism—when the pH is raised or lowered, the skin can readjust to its normal pH effectively.[15] The skin of some people takes longer to revert to a normal value. It was suggested that these people are prone to skin diseases.[27]

The skin's flora

A wide variety of micro-organisms lives on the surface of healthy, intact skin.[28] The individual species which make up the flora exist in a normal ecologic balance. The flora act as a defense mechanism to control the presence of potential pathogenic organisms and their possible invasion of the skin and body.

The emergence of infection by pathogenic organisms is related directly to the breakdown of the skin's "disinfecting," protective mechanism or to the development of an abundance of colonies of pathogenic organisms.[22] A breakdown in the normal ecologic balance may be potentiated by alterations in other defense mechanisms of the skin.

Normally, the stratum corneum has only about 10 percent water content, which ensures elasticity but which is generally below that needed to support luxuriant microbial growth.[22] An increase in moisture content can cause an imbalance in microbial growth, and superficial organisms can multiply freely, leading to infection. An imbalance of organisms in the acidic secretions of the sweat and sebaceous glands can foster infection. A break in the intact surface has a deleterious effect on the skin's defensive properties, especially when large numbers of pathogenic organisms are introduced to the inner layers.

Infection can be caused by excessive scrubbing of the skin (especially with strong detergents), excessive exposure to water, occlusion, increasing the skin's temperature, excessive sweating, excessive bathing, and injury.[22,29-31] Thus, the presence and extent of a microbial infection of the skin generally depend on the extent of breakdown of the skin and its defense mechanisms, the number of pathogenic organisms which are present, and the supportive nutrient environment for such organisms.[22]

Price [32] has distinguished between "resident" and "transient" skin flora. Certain organisms (resident) are normally found on the outer layers of the stratum corneum. Others (transient) change regularly as a result of a person's contact with inanimate objects, other people, etc.

The flora of various skin areas are diverse, including aerobic and anaerobic, staphylococci and corynebacteria, sarcinae, and occasional gram-negative rods.[33] The number of organisms in the various areas of the skin differs. Changes in kind and number of organisms occur in these constituent populations during different periods of life and during different seasons of the year.[22] Flora population varies between individuals; some have a constantly high microbial population.[33]

Treatment with topical products

When the pharmacist is asked for information about topical products for self-medication of adverse cutaneous conditions, the type of condition that exists should be ascertained first. Likewise, the pharmacist should be aware of the clinical manifestations and therapy of skin disorders other than infection (e.g., contact dermatitis, psoriasis) as well as eruptions caused by drugs.[34] Antimicrobial products should be considered only in cases of true infection.

The pharmacist can prevent erroneous self-medication by advising medical attention if the condition calls for it or suggesting a more appropriate OTC product. Incorrect self-medication can cause a delay in healing, possible deleterious progression of the disease, toxicity, obvious discomfort, and unnecessary cost.

MEDICAL ATTENTION IS WARRANTED IF:

☐ The condition has lasted for more than a few days.

☐ Appropriate treatments have not been successful, and the condition is getting worse.

☐ Applications of drug products have been used for several days over large areas, especially on denuded skin (checking for systemic toxicities); drainage is excessive and has occurred for several days; and improper cleaning of infectious exudate has led to widespread infection.

- ☐ There is predisposing illness, such as diabetes or systemic infection, or symptoms of such illness.
- ☐ Fever or malaise occurs.
- ☐ An unrecognized primary dermatitis (e.g., allergic dermatitis or primary irritation due to soap, chemicals, etc.) exists and has caused a secondary infection. (Such infections are generally difficult to treat with nonprescription drugs.)
- ☐ Lesions are "deep" and extensive.
- ☐ Lancing to aid drainage is necessary (because this often is not preferred therapy, it must not be done by the patient).
- ☐ There is doubt as to the causative organisms (bacteria or fungi, for example).

Probably the best approach to follow is to limit the use of OTC topical antimicrobial products to superficial conditions that involve minimal areas, when no predisposing or actual illness exists. Thus, self-administered, topical products should be viewed as extensions of supportive treatment (proper cleaning, proper hygiene, clean bandaging, etc.), not as "miracle" treatments. An anti-infective drug, in an appropriately designed (e.g., with a good rate of release of drug) vehicle or base, should be used to ensure bioavailability and appropriate penetration of the skin. Proper use of the drug with a regimen of cleanliness should then achieve therapeutic success and keep the infection from spreading while normal anti-infective defenses "take over" the infecting organisms. The tissue can then regenerate normally.

Medical attention should be sought in all but the most superficial, uncomplicated skin infections, especially if it appears that systemic medication is needed. Deep-seated and complicated secondary infections must have medical attention. Improper lancing as self-treatment can cause scarring and spreading of the condition by infected exudate; secondary infections can further complicate the situation. Scars subsequent to chronic carbuncles in children are a result of improper self-treatment.

The pharmacist should advise on the proper use of bandaging. Bandages are occlusive; they foster hydration of the epidermis, and therefore, increase penetration of drugs. Different types of bandages can produce different degrees of occlusiveness. Plastic wrappings are the most effective in this regard. Processes which can cause maceration (occlusive wet dressings and adhesive bandages) must be avoided except to promote "pointing" or "coming to a head" for drainage of pus, as with carbuncles.[3] Hot compresses, applied without injury, can promote "pointing."

In addition to treating dermal infections, certain topical antimicrobial agents are used to prevent infection of the skin. Deodorant soaps with these agents are popular, although their efficacy has not been proved. Skin antiseptic products also are available for general prophylactic use.

Supportive procedures common to the treatment of all skin infections also have been documented.[3] Because skin infections are triggered by external infection and reinfection, precautions should be taken to prevent their continuation or extension through self-reinoculation. Soiled bandages or clothing should not touch unaffected areas (infected clothes should be washed separately); such areas should be cleaned regularly or protected by suitable antiseptic products. The hands should be kept very clean. Direct contact with others should be avoided. In children, a special effort must be made to prevent manipulation of the lesions. Irritation from drug products, tight clothing, bandaging, etc., make the skin vulnerable to further spread of the infection; drying or lubricating powders may be used in these areas to minimize chafing.

Scrubbing or prolonged soaking of the lesions should be avoided to prevent extension of the pathogens by maceration of the area. General cleaning with water and nonirritating soap is adequate. Mild, antiseptic soaps may be helpful in the prevention of pyodermas but are not very effective in treatment.[35] They can be used prophylactically to control skin bacteria, but they are not effective against bacteria deep in the epidermis. However, certain halogenated salicylanilides incorporated into these soaps have been shown to cause contact dermatitis or photodermatitis.[22]

In secondary infections, treatment should be aimed at the primary disease condition which will minimize the secondary infection. Thus, systematic treatment of the secondary infection becomes less complicated. Development of a predisposing illness, e.g., diabetes mellitus, in patients with recurring carbuncles, must be watched for, diagnosed medically, and treated appropriately.

Many of the drugs used topically for cutaneous infections are prescription only, and there are strong indications by some medical writers for their exclusive use in such conditions. This signals a significant questioning of the therapeutic efficacy of nonprescription drugs for other than the most superficial cutaneous infections.

Treatment of bacterial infections

Impetigo vulgaris. Several general factors important in the effectiveness of topical agents in treatment of impetigo and other skin infections are the specific antimicrobial spectrum of the drug, supportive hygienic measures, the extent of lesions, and the manner of using the topical product.[22]

It is impossible for the pharmacist to know the exact pathogen involved in a particular infection; therefore, the pharmacist should know which general antibiotics are useful for impetigo. Local treatment with bacitracin and neomycin ointments generally is effective.[5] These antibiotics are available as nonprescription products and have minimal systemic use. Bacitracin is less sensitizing than neomycin. Sulzberger *et al.*[3] point out that the anti-infective drug should be applied at the base of the lesion after careful removal of the crust to promote better penetration into the lesion by the drug. This is done by soaking the crust in a hydrogen peroxide solution and (with medical assistance) gently removing the crust with forceps. Heller[36] suggests gently swabbing away the crusts with soap and water, followed by frequent applications of antibiotic ointments that have useful antimicrobial spectra, such as neomycin, bacitracin, and polymyxin B sulfate, in combination. Oozing after removal of the crust can be controlled by minimal applications of aqueous silver nitrate (2 to 10 percent).[3] This procedure should be performed by a physician.

Ammoniated mercury ointment (5 to 10 percent) has some effectiveness.[3] Other possible agents include iodochlorhydroxyquin ointment and cream, precipitated sulfur, salicylic acid, and ichthammol in petroleum, as compounded prescriptions. These have been used, probably with varying degrees of success, and are not recommended.

Proper use of topical antibiotics should cure the infection in 14 to 21 days.[37] Ointments should be applied at least three times a day to ensure continuous medication; intermittent applications can prolong the infection. Infected areas should be cleaned and patted dry after cleaning unaffected areas.[3] If lesions recur after topical management is stopped, a physician should be consulted for systemic antibiotic therapy. However, some physicians claim that systemic antibiotics are the only therapy for impetigo and feel that their topical use should be discouraged.[38] For example, Duncan[39] recommends that topical antibiotics be discouraged in treatment of impetigo because these products are ineffective, they trigger dermatoses, and they render systemic drugs ineffective. The last criticism seems unduly restrictive. The pharmacist can recommend topical antibiotic preparations for localized, uncomplicated impetigo.

Impetigo Bockhart. During the acute stage, these lesions probably are best treated by a physician. A suggested procedure is surgical opening of the pustules followed by direct application of antimicrobial agents.[3] Then, the lesions can be treated with topical remedies, such as bacitracin and neomycin.

Folliculitis. Sulzberger *et al.*[3] suggest that superficial folliculitis be treated the same as superficial impetigo, i.e., with OTC preparations. Antibacterial cleansers and combinations of polymyxin B sulfate-neomycin-gramicidin in nongreasy (nonocclusive) bases can be used.[39] However, widespread or recurrent cases should be referred to a physician because they may call for systemic antibiotics, selected on the basis of culture and sensitivity tests. Deeper lesions can be treated the same as furuncles and require medical attention.

Furuncles and carbuncles. Topical antibiotics generally cannot reach the seat of these infections because the pathogens are deep in the follicles. However, they may help prevent spreading of lesions across the surface of the skin. Dressings should be avoided because pustules can form beneath them.[39] Warm compresses help in "pointing."

Furuncles and carbuncles should not be squeezed or roughly manipulated. Immobilization of the affected area generally is helpful.[3] When the lesion points, aseptic and careful lancing helps drainage. However, deep incisions are contraindicated because they can destroy the "walling," and cause spreading of the lesion and scarring.

Cleanliness and preventive measures against self-reinfection are important in management of furuncles and carbuncles. Diabetics with furuncles and carbuncles should be referred to a physician. Irritating agents and maceration should be avoided.[3] If the lesions are extensive and multiple or on the face, systemic antibiotics (e.g., erythromycin) should be used.

Sweat gland infections. Superficial sweat gland abscesses are treated effectively with a therapeutic regimen similar to that for impetigo.[3] For deeper abscesses, therapeutic management similar to that for furuncles is suggested. Where necessary, hair should be shaved before topical medication is applied.

Ecthyma. Treatment of ecthyma is similar to that of impetigo. Local antibiotics (neomycin, polymyxin B sulfate, bacitracin) can be used with appropriate cleaning agents. However, topical therapy takes longer and should be used only where very few lesions are involved. Duncan[39] suggests treatment with systemic antibiotics for 10 days.

Erysipelas. This cutaneous infection needs systemic antibiotics for effective treatment.[3 6 39 40] Parenteral penicillin usually is the agent of choice. Improvement occurs within 48 hours, and antibiotic therapy (oral) should be continued for at least 1 week thereafter.[39]

Pyonychia. The pharmacist should refer patients with pyonychia to a physician because OTC therapy generally is ineffective. Suggested treatment of bacterial infection of the nails consists of hot, wet dressings with a mild antiseptic solution, including potassium permanganate (1:4,000 or less) and silver nitrate (0.1 to 0.5 percent).[3] Between applications, antiseptic ointments with bandaging can be used. If these procedures are ineffective, administration of systemic antibiotics is necessary.

Treatment of fungal infections

Fungal infections are called dermatomycosis, dermatophytosis, ringworm, and tinea. The dermatomycoses include all the infectious alterations of the skin and its appendages produced by fungi and their byproducts. The key to successful treatment is accurate diagnosis of the causative fungus. Treatment varies depending on the degree of inflammation, the organism involved, and the site of infection. For example superficial tineas due to *Trichophyton, Microsporum,* or *Epidermophyton* are treatable with topical OTC preparations; *Candida* infections are not. However, tinea infections involving the scalp or bearded areas may penetrate the hair shaft and be difficult to reach with topical antifungal agents. Similarly, fungal infections involving the nail areas of the hands or feet cannot be treated effectively with these agents. Another problem is differential self-diagnosis between tinea infections and *Candida* or nonfungal dermatoses (e.g., psoriasis, contact dermatitis, seborrhea) in their acute or chronic stages.

The pharmacist must exercise care in cases presented for recommendation of OTC medication. In general, if the problem is a mild flareup of a suspected tinea infection of the foot or groin, conservative self-medication should provide relief of symptoms in a few days. Suspected tinea infection of other body areas should be diagnosed by a physician.

Griseofulvin, orally administered, probably is the most effective antifungal medication. However, this is not an OTC drug. In various superficial tinea infections (cruris, pedis, capitis), griseofulvin elicits rapid results, but is not effective against infections caused by *C. albicans* or against tinea versicolor.[41] Tinea cruris responds to iodochlorhydroxyquin (3-percent cream or suspension).[42] Preparations containing undecylenates have some use in superficial dermatomycoses (e.g., athlete's foot).[43] They are weakly effective for more extensive use. Tolnaftate is effective topically against the organisms which cause tinea and ringworm but ineffective against candidal organisms.[43] It is used topically in conjunction with oral griseofulvin to provide effective therapy for chronic lesions.

Peeling (exfoliation) the stratum corneum helps ameliorate some fungal infections. Sulfur and salicylic acid ointments, dilute iodine solutions, carbol-fuchsin solution (Castellani's paint), and benzoic and salicylic acids ointment help soften the skin for peeling.[5 42] Triacetin (spray, powder, cream) has been used to treat superficial fungal infections. Sodium propionate and undecylenic acid in combination with zinc salts of triacetin have achieved some popularity as fungistatic agents.[37]

Cutaneous candidiasis is usually found in areas of chafing. Greasy products should be avoided; creams, powders, and lotions are preferred. Iodochlorhydroxyquin (3-percent cream or lotion) and nystatin are suggested for these infections.[42]

Onychomycosis is a fungal infection of the nails. Hasegawa[44] has suggested treatment with griseofulvin for *Trichophyton* or *Epidermophyton* infections. For monilial infections, nystatin cream is effective. If the invading organism is *C. albicans,* exposure to water must be avoided; 2 to 4 percent thymol in chloroform (nail paint) has been reported as beneficial.[45]

Desiccation and exposure to light and cooler temperatures are supportive procedures for cutaneous fungal infections. In general, a regimen of oral griseofulvin (prescription-only item) and topical tolnaftate is most effective for dermal, fungal infections. Therefore, referral to a physician in such cases is advisable. The other agents listed above are not as effective; they are more useful in superficial infections. Thus, it is important that these conditions be accurately diagnosed and proved by laboratory confirmation before therapy is recommended. Primary cases of cutaneous viral infections usually are self-limiting and should not be exposed to therapeutic risk or morbidity.[46] The selection and use of any antiviral drug should be carefully weighed against allowing the condition to "run its course."

Treatment of viral infections

Herpes simplex is self-limiting, generally clearing up in about 10 days; therefore, a "therapeutic nihilism" approach to medication for herpes simplex has been suggested.[4] This means that no specific drug is widely effective or needed and that palliative treatment to counter discomfort is sufficient.

Topical use of lidocaine [2.5-percent (OTC) ointment] is sufficient to ameliorate the discomfort of herpes simplex; emollients (petrolatum) can be used for the cracking and crusting.[41] Thymol iodide powder, a 2- to 5-percent tannic acid solution, or zinc oxide paste also can be used to ease discomfort. For itching, mentholated petrolatum or camphor spirit have been used with varying degrees of success. Secondary bacterial infection should be treated with systemic antibiotics. Products that contain sunscreens could be useful for cases triggered by sunlight, but such infections, if close to the eyes, need ophthalmologic consideration.[47]

For herpes zoster, only symptomatic treatment is possible with OTC medication (e.g., simple dusting powders, drying and cooling lotions, cool oatmeal baths, and anesthetic ointments).[4, 48] For severe pain that may accompany this condition, opiates often are necessary. Oral steroids, which improve the condition, also are helpful. Medical attention is often required for herpes zoster.

Percutaneous absorption

The therapeutic efficacy of topically applied anti-infective drug products depends on the ability of the active ingredients to transfer from the vehicle, or base, to the skin and to reach and remain at the appropriate dermal level for which therapy is intended. They should not penetrate to deeper tissue. If they are absorbed into the general circulation, toxicities can result. Topical drug products must be designed and evaluated carefully for maximum therapeutic effect and safety. Thus, bioavailability, absorption, and the relationship of the active ingredients to the nontherapeutic base are important.

The base in which an active ingredient is incorporated for topical use in anti-infective and other topical products significantly affects the absorption and therapeutic effect of the drug. Once it is released from the base, the drug must penetrate the various layers of the skin to reach the appropriate zones of activity. Even in cases where the drug is to treat only the surface of the skin, absorption must be considered because toxicities can result from improper base or vehicle selection.

Absorption of drugs through wounds, burns, chafed areas, and various dermatoses, where the integrity of the stratum corneum has been altered, is uncontrolled.[49] These conditions result in "artificial shunts" of the absorptive processes, causing excessive absorption.[50]

Molecules that are absorbed must pass through the sebum, the stratum corneum, the lower layers of the epidermis, the papillary dermis, and the capillary walls; then, they enter the blood stream or lymphatic circulation.[50] This movement is against varying degrees of resistance at each level.

The stratum corneum has the general characteristics of a semipermeable membrane and is usually the rate-limiting barrier to absorption. Passage of molecules through it is completely passive.[51] After a molecule has crossed the stratum corneum, generally, there is little resistance to its transfer across the rest of the epidermal layers into the dermis.[51] Passage of molecules through the horny cells (transcellular) of the stratum corneum (bulk diffusion) is probably the main means of transport of molecules into and through the skin.[51] Lipid-soluble molecules in this process enter the lipid-containing cellular membranes and pass through the nonpolar and lipoidal cellular matrices. Water-soluble molecules (small and polar) enter the protein part of the membrane and cross the lipid cellular parts probably through the small pores that exist between the protein units. These pores, or channels, are filled with water. When the corneum is hydrated beyond normal, they enlarge, and diffusion is accelerated.[51] Thus, occlusion of the surface, which increases hydration of the corneum, can lead to increased absorption of certain drugs.

Another route of transport of molecules through the skin has been attributed to diffusion through the sebaceous and sweat glands (shunt diffusion).[51] The stratum corneum usually does not involve these glands, and the transport by this mechanism is not hindered by this layer. However, the openings of these units on the surface of the skin constitute a very small part (1/1000) of the total dermal area; even if the transport of molecules by this route were rapid, only a small amount of drug could be absorbed in this manner.[51]

A third route of percutaneous absorption is diffusion between cells (intercellular) of the stratum corneum.[51] This pathway is probably most involved with transport of electrolytes, which have low lipid permeability. Thus, the intercellular route does not seem to have a role other than electrolyte transport in percutaneous absorption.

The passive transport of molecules through the stratum corneum involves a delay period after application of the drug product, which "charges" the surface membranes with the drug, and a steady rate of transfer after the delay period.[50] The transfer lasts as long as the chemical molecules exist in sufficient quantity at the site of application and are removed from deeper areas.

Blaug,[52] Brisson,[51] and Idson[50] have reviewed the factors that influence penetration of the skin. They are:

- ☐ The condition of the skin—intact or injured. Intact skin makes it difficult for chemicals to penetrate; damage to the stratum corneum (by injury, burns, scratching, disease) results in marked penetration by drugs. Similarly, treatment of the skin with organic solvents or keratolytics leads to increased permeability.[52]
- ☐ Age of the skin. There are indications that the skin of infants is more permeable than adult skin and that dermal changes in the elderly result in changed absorption characteristics.[53, 54]

☐ Increased rate of blood flow to the skin.[55] The influence of blood rate on penetration through the corneous layers has not been clearly demonstrated. However, it is probable that an increase would lead to higher permeability rates through the corneum because of the rapid removal of molecules from the lower tissue.[50]

☐ Hydration of the stratum corneum.

☐ Occlusion. Occlusive bandaging leads to increased hydration of the corneum and temperature which can elicit increased rates of permeability.[56-58]

☐ Dehydration (dry skin). Dehydration causes brittleness which results in cracking of the skin and increases permeability.[51]

☐ Thickness of the epidermal layers.[50 51]

☐ The solubility characteristics of the penetrating molecule.

☐ The concentration, the duration of exposure to the drug, and the size of the absorption site.[50]

☐ The nature and design of the vehicle or base in which a drug is incorporated.

Ingredients in OTC products

Various drugs are used for topical application to prevent or treat infection.[2 5 33 41 48 59-62] The major classes of drugs used are antiseptics, antifungal agents, and antibiotics.

Antiseptics

Hexachlorophene. Hexachlorophene previously had wide success as a topical antiseptic; it is now a prescription-only drug. Emulsions that contain 3 percent hexachlorophene are effective antiseptic/cleansing products used for handwashing of hospital personnel, surgical hand scrubs, and preoperative skin preparations.[62] Repeated use leaves an antimicrobial residual film on the skin, because hexachlorophene has a substantive (binding) property.

Halogenated salicylanilides and related compounds. Tribromsalan (TBS), dibromsalan (DBS), fluorosalan, triclocarban (TCC), and cloflucarban are antimicrobial agents used in soaps. Although bithionol is no longer approved for use in drug and cosmetic products, bithionol-containing products may still be on the shelves of pharmacies.[63]

The Food and Drug Administration (FDA) has indicated its intent to curtail the use of several halogenated salicylanilides, including TBS and DBS, because of their potential as photosensitizers.[64] Safer alternative agents exist, and the FDA feels that the risk-to-benefit ratio is improper for continued use of these chemicals in soaps. People who are sensitized to antimicrobial soaps should be cautious about using soaps that are not carefully labeled.[63]

There is concern that the widespread use of antimicrobial soaps can lead to disruption of the skin's normal flora. In general, the agents in the soap kill gram-positive flora, and effective and long-term reduction of the microbes can cause proliferation of the pathogenic gram-negative species.[65-67] Extensive use of anti-gram-positive agents in hospitals and nursing homes may produce a large increase in gram-negative infections among the "captive" populations in these institutions.[68] However, absolute proof of antimicrobial agents in soaps as the causative agent for gram-negative cutaneous infections has not been shown.

Alcohols. Ethanol (70 percent) and isopropyl alcohol are included in topical anti-infective products for their bactericidal effects.[47 60]

Ethanol. Seventy-percent aqueous solution of ethanol has good bactericidal activity, acts relatively quickly, but has little residual effect. It rapidly denatures cellular protein of micro-organisms, lowers the surface tension of bacteria to help in their removal, and has a solvent effect on sebum. However, it is neither an effective antiviral agent, nor does it kill spores. It is not a desirable wound antiseptic because it irritates (stings) already damaged tissue. The coagulum formed may, in fact, protect the bacteria.

Ethanol (70 percent) solution is called "rubbing alcohol" and may contain denaturants. It is not a recognized skin sensitizer. However, excessive exposure in high concentrations can dehydrate the corneum. Systemic ingestion produces usual alcoholic intoxication and severe GI distress. Denaturants worsen the GI symptoms.

Isopropyl. Isopropyl alcohol has somewhat stronger bactericidal activity and lower surface tension than ethanol. In general, it is used like ethanol solutions for cleaning and for its antiseptic effect on the skin. It can be used undiluted or as 70-percent aqueous solutions. Denaturants are not added because isopropyl alcohol itself is not potable. Isopropyl alcohol has a greater potential for "drying" the skin because its lipid solvent effects are stronger than those of ethanol. It may be gently swabbed over the ear to prevent otitis externa, when conditions may precipitate it, e.g., after swimming.

Halogen compounds. These antiseptics include sodium hypochlorite and iodine-containing compounds.[47 60]

Sodium hypochlorite. The antimicrobial effect of sodium hypochlorite results from liberation of elemental chlorine. Concentrated solutions (5 percent) are very irritating to tissue and are used as disinfectants (for utensils, swimming pools). Dilute solutions (0.5 percent or less) (Modified Dakin's) have been used as topical antiseptics with varying degrees of success.

Iodine. Solutions of elemental iodine or those that release iodine from chemical complexes are used as skin antiseptics prior to surgery and as wound antiseptics. Their antimicrobial effect is attributed to their ability to oxidize microbial protoplasm. Caution must be taken that strong iodine solution (Lugol's) not be used as an antiseptic. Iodine solution (2 percent I, 2.5 percent NaI) is used as an antiseptic for superficial wounds. Iodine tincture (2 percent I, 2.5 percent NaI, about 50 per cent alcohol) is less preferable than the aqueous solution (2 percent) because it is irritating to tissue. However, it has the advantage of not freezing at low temperatures.

In general, bandaging should be discouraged after iodine applications to avoid tissue irritation. Iodine solutions stain skin, are irritating to tissue, and can cause sensitization in some people.

Iodoform. Iodoform has minimal antibacterial activity in itself. However, the slow liberation of free iodine, when it is exposed to body secretions, exerts an antiseptic effect. It has been used on gauze for use in abscessed cavities. However, this use has questionable therapeutic efficacy and should be discouraged.

Povidone-iodine. Povidone-iodine is an organic complex used in topical nonprescription antiseptics to treat minor infections of the mucous membranes and cutaneous tissue and as a preoperative antiseptic. Percentage of the active ingredient varies according to product type, i.e., 1 percent in ointments, 0.75 percent in shampoos and skin antiseptics. As an antiseptic, it is less effective than iodine solutions but effectively controls minor infections. Organic iodine compounds usually are less irritating, less toxic, and less sensitizing than inorganic sources, but they are somewhat less effective as antiseptics. Therefore, the organic iodine complexes (e.g., povidone-iodine) generally have better patient acceptance (they are nonstinging and nonstaining) than solutions of elemental iodine. Their efficacy in combating cutaneous infection, although less than that of elemental iodine solutions, is recognized.

Mercurial compounds. Several mercurial compounds have antiseptic/disinfectant properties.[47 60] In general, however, they are considered poor antiseptics for wounded skin because serum and tissue proteins reduce their antimicrobial potency. If these compounds are used extensively or on large areas of abraded skin, mercury can be absorbed and can become a systemic poison; therefore, their use should be discouraged.

Inorganic salts of mercury are tissue irritants. The toxic properties are reduced when the mercury is incorporated into an organic compound. However, some investigators believe that the alcoholic component of mercurial tinctures has greater antimicrobial effect than the mercurial component.[47]

Several organic mercurials (nitromersol, phenylmercuric salts, thimerosal, and merbromin) are incorporated into topical antimicrobial, nonprescription products. These compounds can cause rashes because they are contact sensitizers.

Nitromersol. Nitromersol is more effective as an antiseptic than soluble inorganic compounds of mercury, but less effective than alcohol. It is not a serious tissue irritant and is available as a tincture in 1:200 dilution.

Phenylmercuric salts. These salts inhibit growth of gram-positive and gram-negative bacteria and topical fungi. They are not as effective as ethanol as skin antiseptics. However, their activity is not reduced, as is that of ethanol, in the presence of serum proteins or soaps, which may cause deactivation of some antiseptics by coagulation or precipitation.

Thimerosal. Thimerosal has antibacterial and antifungal properties, but it is less effective than ethanol. It is found in several types of topical products, including aqueous solutions, tinctures, ointments, creams, and aerosols. Systemic toxicity occurs less frequently with thimerosal than with the mercurials because the mercury in thimerosal is tightly bound to the organic configuration. The usual concentration is 0.1 percent.

Merbromin. Merbromin is less effective as a skin antiseptic than the other organic mercurials. However, it is used as a preoperative germicide (2 percent, aqueous). Serous fluids reduce its antimicrobial potency.

Silver compounds. The silver ion has an antiseptic effect because of its ability to precipitate the protein of cellular components of micro-organisms.[47 60] Soluble inorganic silver salts and organic silver compounds have been used as topical antiseptics; except for silver nitrate, most silver compounds are used less and less with the advent of more effective antiseptic agents. In general, silver salts are precipitated relatively quickly by chloride in cell components. The organic silver compounds are less irritating to tissue than the inorganic salts but are less effective as antimicrobial agents.

Silver nitrate. Silver nitrate is a fairly potent bactericide at a concentration of 1:1,000; at 1:10,000 it is bacteriostatic. Aqueous solutions (0.5 percent) are used on dressings for second- and third-degree burns to prevent infection. Extensive use, however, can deplete chloride ions and cause electrolyte imbalance.

Toughened silver nitrate. Toughened silver nitrate pencils can be used to cauterize minor wounds (shaving) and to treat warts. Mild silver protein and colloidal silver iodide are nonprescription forms of silver. However, they have minimal antiseptic efficacy.

Surface-active agents. Soaps and quaternary ammonium compounds are included in topical anti-infective products. In addition to their antiseptic properties, the agents are used for their cleansing properties.[47 60]

Soaps. Soaps are anionic surfactants. They are used as supportive treatment (cleansing) for the prevention of skin infections. Their actual antiseptic properties are minimal.

Quaternary ammonium compounds. These compounds are cationic surfactants that have antimicrobial activity upon gram-positive and gram-negative bacteria, but not upon spores. Gram-negative bacteria are more resistant than gram-positive ones; thus, they need a longer period of exposure. The "quats" emulsify sebum and have a detergent effect to remove dirt, bacteria, and desquamated epithelial cells. Their antimicrobial activity is caused by disrupting membranes and denaturing lipoproteins. These compounds are inactivated by anionic ones (soaps, base/vehicle ingredients, such as viscosity builders).

Nonprescription quat products include benzalkonium chloride, benzethonium chloride, and methylbenzethonium chloride. These compounds are formulated as creams, dusting powders, and aqueous or alcoholic solutions. Concentrates are available for dilution to proper concentration for topical use. If mistakenly used undiluted, these concentrates can cause serious irritation. Quat compounds are irritating to the eyes, and caution must be used in this regard. For use on broken or diseased skin, concentrations of 1:5,000 to 1:20,000 should be used; on intact skin and minor abrasions, a concentration of 1:750 is useful.

Methylbenzethonium chloride is effective against micro-organisms that split urea to form ammonia. It is used as a diaper rinse and for application to areas that are subject to irritation from ammonia formation: groin, thighs, and buttocks.

Oxidizing agents. The oxidizing agents used as antiseptics in topical preparations include hydrogen peroxide, potassium permanganate, and potassium chlorate.[47 60]

Hydrogen peroxide. Hydrogen peroxide (3-percent solution) is the most widely used of these compounds; sodium and zinc peroxides are also used. Enzymatic release of oxygen from hydrogen peroxide occurs when it comes into contact with blood and tissue fluids. The mechanical (fizzing) effect of the release of oxygen has a cleansing effect on a wound, but organic matter reduces its effectiveness. The duration of action is only as long as the period of active oxygen release. Using hydrogen peroxide on the intact skin is of doubtful value, because release of the nascent oxygen is too slow. This compound must be used only where the released gas can escape; therefore, it should never be used in abscesses nor should bandages be applied too soon after its use.

Potassium permanganate. Potassium permanganate is a strong oxidizing agent, but it rapidly decomposes in the presence of organic material. Its use as an antiseptic is questionable.

Potassium chlorate. Potassium chlorate solutions have been used for treatment of mucous membranes of the mouth. However, its potential toxicity overshadows its usefulness.

Acids. Acids are used in topical preparations because they kill or inhibit the growth of bacteria.[47 60]

Boric acid. This weak acid has been used as a topical antiseptic and eyewash. The aqueous solution (2.5 percent) inhibits growth of bacteria; it does not kill many forms of bacteria. Boric acid is an extremely dangerous systemic poison. Boric acid powder or solutions used on abraded skin can be absorbed readily to cause severe systemic poisoning: nausea, vomiting, diarrhea, exfoliative dermatitis, kidney damage, and acute circulatory failure. The minor therapeutic value of this compound, when compared to its potential as a poison, has led to the general recommendation that it no longer be used as a therapeutic agent.

Acetic acid (5 percent). This acid has been used as a bactericide. *Pseudomonas* appears particularly vulnerable to it, and it has been used for surgical dressings. Acetic acid is also used for otitis externa and "swimmer's ear."

Phenolic compounds. In very dilute solutions, phenol is an antiseptic and disinfectant.[47 60] It is bacteriostatic at a 1:500 concentration, bactericidal and fungicidal at 1:50 concentration, but it is ineffective against spores. Phenols and substituted phenols precipitate and denature cellular proteins. Their antimicrobial activity continues in the presence of organic matter.

Phenol. Phenol has local anesthetic activity and is claimed to be an antipruritic in concentrations of 1:100 to 1:200, as in phenolated calamine lotion. In aqueous solution of more than 1 percent, it is a tissue irritant and should not be used on skin.

Mixtures of phenol and camphor in oily solutions are "old favorites" as nonprescription antiseptics for use on minor cuts and burns, insect bites, athlete's foot, fever blisters, and cold sores. However, if they are applied to moist areas, lesions can occur because these products contain relatively high amounts of phenol, e.g., 4 percent. These products should be used with caution.

Liquefied phenol. A solution of phenol crystals dissolved in 10 percent water is used locally. It is used like trichloroacetic acid to "peel down" lesions. Liquefied phenol is too caustic for unaffected, intact skin, and it should be applied very carefully to the lesion, e.g., with a protective coating of petrolatum around the lesion.

Substituted phenols. Substituted phenols, including the halogenated phenols (e.g., hexachlorophene) and the alkyl substituted phenols have more bactericidal effects than phenol. Halogenation of a phenolic compound increases the antiseptic properties. Di- and trihalogenated forms have greater potency but are less water soluble than monohalogenated phenols.

Cresols are alkyl derivatives of phenol. Three isomers, the *ortho, meta,* and *para* forms all have similar disinfectant properties. They are used mainly as disinfectants of inanimate surfaces and objects. Cresol is more potent than phenol but does not have a greater potential for toxicity.

Resorcinol is somewhat antibacterial and antifungal but is much less potent than phenol; its systemic effects are the same as those of phenol. As an ointment (2 percent or more), it has been used in treating ringworm and several dermatoses. However, other topical agents (e.g., tolnaftate) are more effective in the treatment of ringworm. Resorcinol monoacetate exerts even milder but longer action because it releases resorcinol slowly. Both resorcinol and the monoacetate are used in acne preparations mainly for their keratolytic effect; their antiseptic effects are best described as mild or minor.

Hexylresorcinol (0.1-percent dilution) is a general antiseptic, but it is irritating and may produce sensitivity. Thymol and chlorothymol are also alkyl derivatives of phenol with minor antibacterial and antifungal properties.

Dyes. The coal-tar dyes are synthetic organic compounds, some of which have antiseptic properties.[60] Several have wound-healing properties, and others are used in various diagnostic procedures.

Scarlet red. This is an azo dye that is used more for its positive healing effect on wounds than as an antiseptic. It stimulates cellular proliferation and is used to treat burns and other dermal lesions. The azo dyes (5 percent, ointment) are not recommended as topical antimicrobials.

Acridine dyes. The acridine dyes are yellow and are flavines. Proflavine and acriflavine are used therapeutically as topical antimicrobial agents. Their strongest antibacterial action occurs in alkaline media on gram-positive organisms at dilutions of 1:1,000 to 1:10,000. These agents have not become popular for topical use.

Gentian violet. This is a methylrosaniline dye that kills gram-positive organisms and many fungi. It is used in concentrations of 1:1,000 to 1:5,000.

Methylene blue. This dye is a bacteriostatic agent. It is used as a urinary antiseptic, but rarely, if ever, as a topical agent.

Sulfur. Sulfur alone is not antiseptic. It has been speculated that its mild germicidal effect is caused by the formation (by micro-organisms or cutaneous tissue) of hydrogen sulfide and pentathionic acid. It is used in topical medications more for its keratolytic (peeling) properties, which are useful for treatment of various dermatoses.[60] However, when used topically, sulfur can promote comedo formation.

Ichthammol. Ichthammol (ammonium ichthosulfonate) is a sulfonated and neutralized (ammonia) derivative of the distillate of bituminous rock or shists.[60] It has little value as a topical antiseptic but has been used as a "drawing salve" for boils. It is a viscous, brownish-black semiliquid that has a characteristic, bituminous odor and an emollient effect. It is less common now than in the past.

Iodochlorhydroxyquin. This compound is an antibacterial and antifungal agent and is available in nonprescription products as a cream or ointment (3 percent) and vaginal inserts and powders.[60] It is considered an effective compound.

Antifungal agents

Fatty acids. Sweat has antifungal properties probably caused by its fatty acid content.[47 60] Sodium propionate is a fatty acid derivative which is used as a topical antiseptic; it has mild fungistatic activity. It has been used in topical products in concentrations of as much as 10 percent and with undecylenic acid. Undecylenic acid has the greatest antifungal activity of the fatty acids. It may cause irritation and sensitization and should be discontinued if these occur. It is basically fungistatic and needs long exposure at high concentrations to achieve a fungicidal effect. It is used in combination with its zinc salt in ointment, cream, powder, and aerosol forms (5-percent acid, 20-percent salt) for an additive antifungal effect.

Tolnaftate. Tolnaftate is a topical, nonprescription antifungal agent that is effective against all species of fungi, except *C. albicans,* that cause cutaneous infections, including tinea (ringworm).[47 60] However, complete clearing of cutaneous lesions may take several months. Nevertheless, tolnaftate is probably the most effective topical antifungal, OTC drug available. Fungal infections of the nails, palms of the hands, and soles of the feet are not very responsive to tolnaftate or any topical treatment. Combination therapy in such cases is appropriate, i.e., oral therapy (griseofulvin) with tolnaftate.[43]

Salicylanilide. Salicylanilide is a fungistatic agent that is used mainly for tinea capitis (5 percent, ointment).[47 60] Its derivatives are used in antiseptic soaps.

Selenium sulfide. Selenium sulfide is effective in the treatment of tinea versicolor and seborrheic dermatitis of the scalp.[47 60] It is also used in OTC topical products to control dandruff, usually as a detergent-suspension. Contact with the eyes and sensitive skin areas should be avoided because of its potential as an irritant. Although not absorbed to a significant degree through the skin, it is hazardous if swallowed, producing CNS effects and respiratory and vasomotor depression.

Triacetin. Triacetin is used in the treatment of superficial fungal infections.[47 60] Its activity is caused by the slow release of acetic acid due to action upon it by enzymes of fungi and skin. It is a nonprescription drug, available in aerosol (15 percent), cream (25 percent), and powder (33 percent). Because its activity depends on the slow release of acetic acid, triacetin probably is best viewed as effective only in the most superficial of fungal infections of the skin.

Benzoic acid and salicylic acid ointment. This ointment (Whitfield's Ointment) is used in the treatment of cutaneous fungal infections because of its keratolytic effect.[47 60] It peels the skin and removes the debris upon which organisms can grow, making deeper infections accessible to specific, topical antifungal compounds.

Dyes. Gentian violet and carbol-fuchsin solutions have been used for superficial fungal skin infections.[47 60] However, they are not significant antifungal agents and have the distinct disadvantage of staining. More effective antifungal agents, e.g., tolnaftate, have replaced these dyes in treatment of topical fungal infections.

Antibiotics

The major nonprescription, topical antibiotics are bacitracin, gramicidin, neomycin, and polymyxin B sulfate, alone or in combination.[5 47 59] The rationale for their use in combination is to ensure a broad spectrum of antibacterial activity through additive spectra of the individual component antibiotics.

Bacitracin. Bacitracin is a polypeptide antibiotic that prevents the completion of synthesis of bacterial cell membranes. Its main action is against gram-positive and gram-negative pathogens. It can be used topically (for bacterial infections) and parenterally because it is not absorbed through GI mucosa. Because it is nephrotoxic, excessive topical use, especially in vehicle bases that promote percutaneous absorption, should be avoided. Resistance to it is rather uncommon, and hypersensitivity is rare. It is unstable in aqueous solution and when it is exposed to light.

Gramicidin. Gramicidin is a polypeptide antibiotic that is effective against gram-positive bacteria. It cannot be absorbed after oral administration and has significant systemic toxicity (hemolysis and kidney and liver damage) that precludes parenteral use.

Neomycin. This aminoglycoside antibiotic is effective against gram-positive bacteria by its intervention in protein synthesis. Of the topical antibiotics, it is the one most likely to sensitize. Neomycin is used orally for GI tract infections and to "sanitize" the bowel before intestinal surgery. As such, it is minimally absorbed. However, if sufficient levels are reached in the blood, kidney damage and ototoxicity can result. Therefore, its major use is in topical treatment of cutaneous infections, where the chance for such toxicity is rare.

For topical use, neomycin is available in cream and ointment forms. Staphylococci and coliform bacilli can develop resistance to neomycin. To avoid this, neomycin generally is used in combination with polymyxin or bacitracin.

Polymyxin B sulfate. Polymyxin B sulfate is effective against gram-negative bacteria but not against gram-positive bacteria or fungi. It alters membrane permeability of bacteria and is not absorbed from the GI tract. Polymyxins do not readily develop resistant strains of bacteria but may cause renal damage and paresthesia if sufficient concentrations reach the blood. In topical use, such toxicity is rare.

Therapeutic efficacy and safety

Therapeutic efficacy and safety must be the primary concerns in the development and manufacture of topical anti-infective products and all drug products. Once a dosage form is marketed, it must be checked continually to ensure that it is, in fact, safe and effective. In the *Federal Register* of January 5, 1972, the FDA first indicated its intent to establish regulations to maintain efficacy and safety for nonprescription drug products.[69] Panels of experts were established to conduct evaluations toward recommendations for regulations to be used by the FDA to maintain desired levels of safety and therapeutic efficacy for OTC products. The OTC Panel on Topical Antimicrobials I made its recommendations in September, 1974.[70] Currently, a second Panel considering the remaining topical antimicrobials is compiling its recommendations.[71] The Antimicrobial I Panel offers guidelines for determining the efficacy and safety of nonprescription, antimicrobial drug products. These guidelines should be weighed against the opinions of other published authorities.

Tables 1, 2, and 3 outline the recommendations of the Panel concerning the degree of safety and effectiveness of the various topical antimicrobial agents it evaluated.

Table 1. Compounds Recommended as Safe and Effective (Category I)[a]

Use	Compounds[b]
Antimicrobial soap	None
Health care personnel handwash.	None
Patient preoperative skin preparation.	Tincture of iodine
Skin antiseptics	None
Skin wound cleanser	Benzalkonium chloride Benzethonium chloride Hexylresorcinol Methylbenzethonium chloride
Skin wound protectant	None
Surgical hand scrub	None

[a] By the OTC Panel on Topical Antimicrobials I (FDA), from *Fed. Regist.*, **39**, 33103(1974).

[b] Of those considered by the Panel.

Table 2. Compounds Generally Not Recognized as Safe and Effective (Category II)[a]

Use	Compounds[b]
Antimicrobial soaps	Fluorosalan Hexachlorophene Phenol (more than 1.5% aqueous/alcoholic) Tribromsalan
Health care personnel handwash	Fluorosalan Hexachlorophene Phenol (more than 1.5% aqueous/alcoholic) Tincture of iodine Tribromsalan Triclosan
Patient preoperative skin preparation	Cloflucarban Fluorosalan Hexachlorophene Phenol (more than 1.5% aqueous/alcoholic) Tribromsalan Triclocarban Triclosan
Skin antiseptic	Cloflucarban Fluorosalan Hexachlorophene Phenol (more than 1.5% aqueous/alcoholic) Tincture of iodine Tribromsalan Triclocarban
Skin wound cleanser	Cloflucarban (as formulated in products other than bar soaps) Fluorosalan Hexachlorophene Phenol (more than 1.5% aqueous/alcoholic) Tincture of iodine Tribromsalan Triclocarban (as formulated in products other than bar soaps)
Skin wound protectant	Cloflucarban Fluorosalan Hexachlorophene Phenol (more than 1.5% aqueous/alcoholic) Tincture of iodine Tribromsalan Triclocarban
Surgical hand scrub	Cloflucarban Fluorosalan Hexachlorophene Phenol (more than 1.5% aqueous/alcoholic) Tincture of iodine Tribromsalan Triclocarban Triclosan

[a]By the OTC Panel on Topical Antimicrobials I (FDA), from *Fed. Regist.*, **39**, 33103 (1974).

[b]Of those considered by the Panel.

The Panel used three categories to classify the degree of safety and efficacy for the various topical antimicrobial agents it reviewed:

Category I: The ingredients that have been evaluated (by the Panel) as safe and effective for OTC topical use within the "use" groups or categories established by the Panel.

Category II: The ingredients that the Panel found to be ineffective and/or unsafe for OTC topical use, within the "use" categories established by the Panel.

Category III: The ingredients for which the Panel found insufficient data to permit a classification under Category I or II. For these ingredients, the Panel recommended that time be allowed for further development and submission of data toward further review. This would result in placing Category III items into Category I or II.

The Panel concerned itself mainly with antimicrobial soaps. It expressed concern that some soap/detergent bars with antimicrobial ingredients might be treated as cosmetics and not drug products under the law, allowing possible lesser regulation at this time. It recommended that these products have effective regulations, whether they were classed officially as cosmetics or drugs.

The above concern centers around the opinion of some dermatologists that widespread use of these soaps can lead to infection by pathogenic "residents" of the skin by upsetting normal flora balance and that several agents that are used in antimicrobial soap bars can have photosensitivity potential. The Panel acknowledged that current data cannot substantiate a definite conclusion as to the possible deleterious effect that vast changes in the skin's normal flora can cause. Additional data on the relationships of concentration, contact time of antimicrobial agents with the skin, number of exposures, and the total microbial population of the flora are needed. Thus, the risk-to-benefit factor is not yet definite.

Under these circumstances, the Panel feels caution is necessary with the use of these compounds/products. It recommended that the antimicrobial content of soap be adjusted to concentrations that reduce the flora only enough to produce a deodorant effect. The Panel's report noted that experts have estimated that a 70 percent "kill" of normal flora yields a deodorant effect.[70] Some antimicrobial soap bars can reduce 90 percent or more of gram-positive organisms; so large an activity might be harmful.

A comparison of the antimicrobial ingredients reviewed by this Panel shows that not all of the compounds discussed in earlier sections of this chapter were included. Some topical antimicrobials were referred to the Antimicrobial II Panel for formal recommendations to FDA and publication in the *Federal Register*. Also, compounds mentioned in earlier sections are being evaluated by other OTC Panels (e.g., camphor and menthol by the OTC Panel on Topical Analgesics). A review of the work and recommendations of the OTC Panel on Topical Antimicrobials I gives significant insight into the opinions of experts as to safety and efficacy of topical antimicrobials.

The OTC Panel on Topical Antimicrobials II has not completed its evaluations and recommendations as of this writing; only the minutes of this Panel's meetings are available.[71] This Panel is reviewing and evaluating the safety and therapeutic efficacy of antibiotic ingredients in topical, nonprescription drug products and topical antimicrobials referred to it by other OTC Panels. It deals with antibiotic ointments, creams, and powders that are used to prevent cutaneous infections and that help to heal superficial or minor cuts, abrasions, and burns of the skin.

Table 3. Compounds for Which Available Data Are Insufficient to Permit Final Classification (Category III) [a]

Use	Compounds [b]
Antimicrobial soaps	Cloflucarban Chloroxylenol Phenol (1.5% or less aqueous/alcoholic) Triclocarban Triclosan
Health care personnel handwash	Benzalkonium chloride Benzethonium chloride Cloflucarban Hexylresorcinol Iodine complexed with phosphate ester of alkylaryloxypolyethylene glycol Methylbenzethonium chloride Nonoxynol-iodine Chloroxylenol Phenol (1.5% or less aqueous/alcoholic) Poloxamer-iodine Povidone-iodine Triclocarban Undecoylium chloride-iodine
Patient preoperative skin preparation	Benzalkonium chloride Benzethonium chloride Hexylresorcinol Iodine complexed with phosphate ester of alkylaryloxypolyethylene glycol Methylbenzethonium chloride Nonoxynol-iodine Chloroxylenol Phenol (1.5% or less aqueous/alcoholic) Poloxamer-iodine Povidone-iodine Undecoylium chloride-iodine
Skin antiseptic	Benzalkonium chloride Benzethonium chloride Hexylresorcinol Iodine complexed with phosphate ester of alkylaryloxypolyethylene glycol Methylbenzethonium chloride Nonoxynol-iodine Chloroxylenol Phenol (1.5% or less aqueous/alcoholic) Poloxamer-iodine Povidone-iodine Triclosan Triple dye Undecoylium chloride-idodine
Skin wound cleanser	Nonoxynol-iodine Iodine complexed with phosphate ester of alkylaryloxypolyethylene glycol Chloroxylenol Phenol (1.5% or less aqueous/alcoholic) Poloxamer-iodine Povidone-iodine Triclosan Undecoylium chloride-iodine
Skin wound protectant	Benzalkonium chloride Benzethonium chloride Hexylresorcinol Iodine complexed with phosphate ester of alkylaryloxypolyethylene glycol Methylbenzethonium chloride Nonoxynol-iodine Chloroxylenol Phenol (1.5% or less aqueous/alcoholic) Poloxamer-iodine Povidone-iodine Triclosan Undecoylium chloride-iodine
Surgical hand scrub	Benzalkonium chloride Benzethonium chloride Hexylresorcinol Iodine complexed with phosphate ester of alkylaryloxypolyethylene glycol Methylbenzethonium chloride Nonoxynol-iodine Chloroxylenol Phenol (1.5% or less aqueous/alcoholic) Poloxamer-iodine Povidone-iodine Undecoylium chloride-iodine

[a] By the OTC Panel on Antimicrobials I (FDA), from *Fed. Regist.*, **39**, 33103(1974).

[b] Of those considered by the Panel.

It would not be proper to speculate on expected recommendations of the Panel concerning topical antibiotics, etc., at this time. Again, this Panel's activities should be followed closely and its recommendations and regulations that will issue from them studied carefully. They should be weighed against other published information concerning topical antimicrobial products for self-medication in making decisions about the therapeutic value of available products.

Guidelines for product selection

A person's medication profile provides information to assist in product selection—known allergens can be avoided, judicious estimates as to possible cross-sensitization made, the general sensitivity of the skin to irritation can be ascertained, the possibility of drug interactions can be avoided, and possible predisposing illnesses or conditions can be uncovered.

The quality of hygienic procedures being practiced is useful information to determine in uncovering the basic reason for a long-lasting infection (continual reinfection). Bandaging practices can point to reasons for irritation, maceration, and spreading of lesions. Thus, selection of the best topical antimicrobial agent for use as a general prophylactic skin antiseptic can be narrowed down by reviewing the medical profile and history and conducting an interview with the patient. Such information also assists in prevention of allergic manifestations by the antiseptic and avoidance of possible cross-sensitivities and potential irritants.

With the necessary information, the pharmacist can make a more rational choice of an appropriate agent for self-medication of a cutaneous infection. In some cases, medical diagnosis supported by lab tests and referral for medical attention are necessary. Otherwise, the generally accepted principles of therapy for skin infections apply: self-medication is best reserved for superficial, uncomplicated skin infections; self-medication needs appropriate supportive procedures (i.e., proper hygiene); and the more serious cutaneous infections should be treated with systemic medications by a physician. Thus, if the pharmacist determines that a prescription drug is vastly superior in therapeutic efficacy to a nonprescription item, a physician should be consulted.

Once the therapeutic agent is selected, the proper drug product type must be chosen—powder, solution/tincture, ointment, cream, aerosol. Powders can be used for chafed, moist areas of superficial infections but not on open lesions; occlusive ointments for hydration of the skin to help penetration of the epidermis; and water-washable creams for hairy areas or when occlusion is not appropriate.

The pharmacist should be aware of possible allergens in the base formula of the product. Hypoallergenic cosmetics can be a useful parameter in this regard; perfumed products and those that contain ingredients that have been recognized as sensitizers [lanolin derivatives and some preservatives (e.g., parabens) and emulsifying agents] should be avoided. If a quaternary ammonium antiseptic is used, the pharmacist should caution against using products which could render the quat ineffective, such as an anionic agent used with the quat (soaps or cleaning agents that have anionic emulsifiers).

The pharmacist also should advise on the proper use of the suggested product. The advantages and disadvantages of creams and ointments must be weighed for each case. Similarly, the use of lotions or suspensions rather than semisolid dosage forms must be determined. For infections, intermittent applications are considered poor therapy; regular applications are preferable. Overmedication, however, can lead to irritation and possible systemic absorption and toxicity. An appropriate "thickness" of application should be suggested to avoid overmedication and to ensure therapeutic concentrations at the lesions. The need for cleanliness and avoidance of all situations that could cause reinfection must be stressed to the patient. Also, bandaging and its effects on the infection should be explained.

The progress of the condition should be monitored. If other eruptions or dermatitis, indications of irritation or maceration, spreading or "deepening" of the lesions, or denuding of the skin by the product occurs, self-medication should be stopped and medical attention sought. If the condition does not respond positively in a reasonable period, a physician should be consulted.

Summary

Topical antimicrobials are used to treat and prevent cutaneous infections caused by bacteria, fungi, and viruses. Proper design and formulation of topical antimicrobial products are important to the selection of appropriate therapeutic agents and products. The patient interview is essential in ascertaining whether self-medication or professional medical attention is appropriate. If OTC products are used, the pharmacist should instruct the patient on their use and on supportive procedures.

A review of the viewpoints of the FDA OTC Panels concerning topical antimicrobial and antibiotic products emphasizes the need for constant evaluation of therapeutic efficacy and safety of nonprescription drug products. The pharmacist should keep current with the regulations that will result from the OTC Panels' recommendations.

The pharmacist should be available to answer inquiries concerning cutaneous disorders, to assist in judicious product selection for self-medication, and to indicate the need for medical attention as a wiser alternative to self-medication, should the conditions warrant it.

References

1. E. L. Laden, in "Modern Dermatologic Therapy," T. H. Sternberg and V. D. Newcomer, Eds., McGraw-Hill, New York, N.Y., 1959, pp. 374-377.
2. E. L. Laden, in "Modern Dermatologic Therapy," T. H. Sternberg and V. D. Newcomer, Eds., McGraw-Hill, New York, N.Y., 1959, pp. 386-403.
3. M. B. Sulzberger *et al.*, "Dermatology: Diagnosis and Treatment," 2d ed., Year Book Medical, Chicago, Ill., 1961, pp. 277-305.
4. M. B. Sulzberger *et al.*, "Dermatology: Diagnosis and Treatment," 2d ed., Year Book Medical, Chicago, Ill., 1961, pp. 417-427.
5. B. M. Barker and F. Prescott, "Antimicrobial Agents in Medicine," Blackwell Scientific Publications, London, England, 1973, pp. 18-149.
6. E. L. Laden, in "Modern Dermatologic Therapy," T. H. Sternberg and V. D. Newcomer, Eds., McGraw-Hill, New York, N.Y., 1959, pp. 374-403.
7. E. T. Wright, in "Modern Dermatologic Therapy," T. H. Sternberg and V. D. Newcomer, Eds., McGraw-Hill, New York, N.Y., 1959, pp. 404-420.
8. M. B. Sulzberger *et al.*, "Dermatology: Diagnosis and Treatment," 2d ed., Year Book Medical, Chicago, Ill., 1961, pp. 306-356.
9. G. D. Baldridge, in "Modern Dermatologic Therapy," T. H. Sternberg and V. D. Newcomer, Eds., McGraw-Hill, New York, N.Y., 1959, pp. 439-453.

10. "The Merck Manual," 12th ed., D. N. Holvey, Ed., Merck, Rahway, N.J., 1972, pp. 33-37.
11. M. B. Sulzberger *et al.*, "Dermatology: Diagnosis and Treatment," 2d ed., Year Book Medical, Chicago, Ill., 1961, pp. 417-421.
12. M. B. Sulzberger *et al.*, "Dermatology: Diagnosis and Treatment," 2d ed., Year Book Medical, Chicago, Ill., 1961, pp. 421-427.
13. H. Blank and G. Rake, "Viral and Rickettsial Diseases," Little, Brown, Boston, Mass., 1955, pp. 71-96.
14. F. J. Ebling, in "Handbook of Cosmetic Science," H. W. Hibbott, Ed., Pergamon Press, Oxford, England, 1963, pp. 1-22.
15. J. S. Jellinek, "Formulation and Function of Cosmetics," 2d ed., Wiley, New York, N.Y., 1970, pp. 4-14.
16. E. Voss, *Fla. Pharm. J.*, **4-6,** 25-30(1971).
17. J. A. A. Hunter, *Br. Med. J.*, **4,** 340-342, 411-413(1973).
18. D. M. Pillsbury, "A Manual of Dermatology," Saunders, Philadelphia, Pa., 1971, pp. 1-53.
19. S. M. Blaug, in "Prescription Pharmacy," 2d ed., J. B. Sprowls, Jr., Ed., Lippincott, Philadelphia, Pa., 1970, pp. 230-231.
20. B. Idson, *J. Pharm. Sci.*, **64,** 910(1975).
21. A. M. Kligman, "The Epidermis," Academic Press, New York, N.Y., 1964, p. 387.
22. F. G. Weissman, *Drug Intell. Clin. Pharm.*, **8,** 535(1974).
23. J. S. Jellinek, "Formulation and Function of Cosmetics," 2d ed., Wiley, New York, N.Y., 1970, p. 13.
24. S. M. Peck and W. R. Russ, *Arch. Dermatol. Syphilol.*, **56,** 601(1947).
25. S. Rothman *et al.*, *J. Invest. Dermatol.*, **8,** 81(1947).
26. J. M. L. Burtenshaw, *J. Hyg.*, **42,** 184(1942).
27. V. W. Burckhardt and W. Baumle, *Dermatologica*, **102,** 294(1951).
28. A. M. Kligman, in "Skin Bacteria and Their Role in Infection," H. I. Maibach and G. Hildrick-Smith, Eds., McGraw-Hill, New York, N.Y., 1965, pp. 13-31.
29. M. T. Hojya-Tomoka *et al.*, *Arch. Dermatol.*, **107,** 723(1973).
30. L. F. Montes and W. H. Wilborn, *Br. J. Dermatol.*, **81,** 23(1969).
31. R. R. Marples, in "Skin Bacteria and Their Role in Infection," H. I. Maibach and G. Hildrick-Smith, Eds., McGraw-Hill, New York, N.Y., 1965, pp. 33-42.
32. P. B. Price, *J. Infect. Dis.*, **63,** 301(1938).
33. P. Dineen, in "Drugs of Choice, 1974-75," W. Modell, Ed., Mosby, St. Louis, Mo., 1974, pp. 113-117.
34. W. Bruinsma, "A Guide to Drug Eruptions," Excerpta Medica, Amsterdam, The Netherlands, 1973, pp. 45-48, 87-103.
35. R. R. Leonard, *Arch. Dermatol.*, **95,** 520(1967).
36. G. Heller, *J. Am. Med. Assoc.*, **215,** 1669(1971).
37. H. C. W. Stringer, *Drugs*, **6,** 413-416(1973).
38. W. C. Duncan, *Postgrad. Med.*, **52,** 98-99(1972).
39. W. C. Duncan, *Postgrad. Med.*, **52,** 96-101(1972).
40. "The Merck Manual," 12th ed., D. N. Holvey, Ed., Merck, Rahway, N.J., 1972, pp. 1446-1447.
41. R. C. V. Robinson, in "Pharmaceutical Therapeutics in Dermatology," M. Waisman, Ed., Charles C Thomas, Springfield, Ill., 1968, pp. 49-64.
42. E. T. Wright, in "Modern Dermatologic Therapy," T. H. Sternberg and V. D. Newcomer, Eds., McGraw-Hill, New York, N.Y., 1959, pp. 404-420.
43. "AMA Drug Evaluations," 2d ed., Publishing Sciences Group, Acton, Mass., 1973, pp. 595-605.
44. J. M. Hasegawa, *Postgrad. Med.*, **47,** 239-241(1970).
45. J. W. Wilson, *Arch. Dermatol.*, **92,** 726(1965).
46. C. M. Davis, *Postgrad. Med.*, **52,** 109-114(1972).
47. F. Pascher, in "Drugs of Choice, 1974-75," W. Modell, Ed., Mosby, St. Louis, Mo., 1974, pp. 609-628.
48. F. H. Meyers *et al.*, "Review of Medical Pharmacology," Lange Medical Publications, Los Altos, Calif., 1970, pp. 512-515.
49. I. H. Blank *et al.*, *J. Invest. Dermatol.*, **30,** 187(1958).
50. B. Idson, *J. Pharm. Sci.*, **64,** 901-924(1975).
51. P. Brisson, *Can. Med. Assoc. J.*, **110,** 1182(1974).
52. S. M. Blaug, in "Prescription Pharmacy," 2d ed., J. B. Sprowls, Jr., Ed., Lippincott, Philadelphia, Pa., 1970, pp. 231-239.
53. R. J. Feldman and H. Maibach, *J. Invest. Dermatol.*, **54,** 399(1970).
54. C. F. H. Vickers, in "Modern Trends in Dermatology," 3d ed., R. M. B. McKenna, Ed., Butterworth, London, England, 1966, pp. 84-109.
55. R. K. Winkelmann, *Br. J. Dermatol., Suppl. 4*, **81,** 11(1969).
56. R. B. Stoughton and W. Fritsch, *Arch. Dermatol.*, **90,** 512(1964).
57. A. W. McKenzie and R. B. Stoughton, *Arch. Dermatol.*, **86,** 608(1962).
58. M. B. Sulzberger and V. A. Witten, *Arch. Dermatol.*, **84,** 1027(1961).
59. "AMA Drug Evaluations," 2d ed., Publishing Sciences Group, Acton, Mass., 1973, pp. 569-578.
60. D. W. Esplin, in "The Pharmacological Basis of Therapeutics," 4th ed., L. S. Goodman and A. Gilman, Eds., Macmillan, New York, N.Y., 1970, pp. 1032-1066.
61. P. S. Herman and W. M. Sams, Jr., "Soap Photodermatitis," Charles C Thomas, Springfield, Ill., 1972, pp. 17-61.
62. "AMA Drug Evaluations," 2d ed., Publishing Sciences Group, Acton, Mass., 1973, pp. 645-655.
63. A. A. Fisher, "Contact Dermatitis," 2d ed., Lea and Febiger, Philadelphia, Pa., 1973, pp. 197-216.
64. *Fed. Regist.*, **39,** 33102(1974).
65. W. R. Markland, *Nord. Briefs*, **465,** 3(1975).
66. N. J. Ehrenkranz *et al.*, in "Antimicrobial Agents and Chemotherapy, 1966," American Society for Microbiology, Ann Arbor, Mich., 1966, pp. 255-264.
67. R. A. Amonette and E. W. Rosenberg, *Arch. Dermatol.*, **107,** 71-73(1973).
68. J. N. Braun and C. O. Solberg, *Br. Med. J.*, **2,** 580(1973).
69. *Fed. Regist.*, **37,** 85(1972).
70. *Fed. Regist.*, **39,** 33103(1974).
71. Summary Minutes of Meetings, OTC Panel on Antimicrobials II, Division of OTC Drug Evaluation, Bureau of Drugs, Department of Health, Education, and Welfare, Rockville, Md., 1974-1975.

Products 27 TOPICAL ANTI-INFECTIVE

Product (manufacturer)	Antiseptic	Antifungal agent	Antibiotic	Other
Achromycin Ointment (Lederle)	—	—	tetracycline hydrochloride, 3%	—
Aftate Antifungal Spray Liquid, Spray Powder, Powder, and Gel (Plough)	—	tolnaftate, 1%	—	—
Argyrol Stabilized Solution (Smith, Miller & Patch)	silver protein, 10 and 20%	—	—	edetate calcium disodium, 1.1%
Aureomycin Ointment (Lederle)	—	—	chlortetracycline, 3%	—
Baciguent Ointment (Upjohn)	—	—	bacitracin, 500 units/g	—
Bactine Aerosol (Miles)	methylbenzethonium chloride chlorothymol	—	—	isopropyl alcohol, 3.7% octoxynol

Product (manufacturer)	Antiseptic	Antifungal agent	Antibiotic	Other
Baximin Ointment (Columbia Medical)	—	—	polymyxin B sulfate, 5,000 units/g bacitracin, 400 units/g neomycin sulfate, 5 mg/g	—
Betadine Solution, Microbicidal Applicator, Swab Aid, Swab Sticks, Gauze Pads and Whirlpool Concentrate (Purdue Frederick)	povidone-iodine, 10%	—	—	—
Betadine Surgical Scrub, Surgi-Prep Sponge Brush, and Shampoo (Purdue Frederick)	povidone-iodine, 7.5%	—	—	detergents
B.F.I. Powder (Calgon)	boric acid menthol 4-pentyloxyphenol	thymol	—	bismuth formic iodide zinc phenolsulfonate bismuth subgallate aluminum potassium sulfate eucalyptol
Clorpactin WCS 90 Powder (Guardian)	available chlorine, 3–4%	—	—	—
Clorpactin XCB (Guardian)	available chlorine, 4–4.9%	—	—	—
Drest (Dermik)	alkylisoquinolinium bromide, 0.15% benzalkonium chloride, 0.125% povidone	—	—	alcohol, 14.1% protein greaseless gel
Epi-Clear Antiseptic Lotion (Squibb)	benzoyl peroxide, 5 and 10%	—	—	—
Isodine Antiseptic Skin Cleanser (Blair)	povidone-iodine, 7.5%	—	—	—
Isodine Antiseptic Solution and Ointment (Blair)	povidone-iodine, 10%	—	—	—
Lubraseptic Jelly (Guardian)	*o*-phenylphenol, 0.1% *p-tert*-pentylphenol, 0.02% phenylmercuric nitrate, 0.007%	—	—	—
Mercurochrome (Hynson, Westcott & Dunning)	merbromin, 100%	—	—	—
Merlenate Ointment (North American)	phenylmercuric nitrate, 1.15%	undecylenic acid, 5%	—	—
Myciguent Cream and Ointment (Upjohn)	—	—	neomycin sulfate, 5 mg/g	—
Mycitracin (Upjohn)	—	—	polymyxin B sulfate, 5,000 units/g bacitracin, 500 units/g neomycin sulfate, 5 mg/g	—
Neo-Polycin Ointment (Dow)	—	—	polymyxin B sulfate, 400 units/g bacitracin zinc, 400 units/g neomyxin (as sulfate), 3 mg	fuzene base polyethylene glycol dilaurate polyethylene glycol distearate light liquid petrolatum synthetic glyceride wax white petrolatum

Product (manufacturer)	Antiseptic	Antifungal agent	Antibiotic	Other
Neosporin Ointment (Burroughs Wellcome)	—	—	polymyxin B sulfate, 5,000 units/g bacitracin zinc, 400 units/g neomycin sulfate, 5 mg/g	white petrolatum
Obtundia First Aid Spray (Otis Clapp)	cresol–camphor complex	—	—	—
Ova Nite (Milroy)	benzalkonium chloride, 0.02%	—	—	nonionic surfactant edetate disodium, 0.25%
Polycin (Dow)	—	—	polymyxin B sulfate, 8,000 units/g bacitracin zinc, 400 units/g	polyethylene glycol dilaurate polyethylene glycol distearate light liquid petrolatum white petrolatum synthetic glyceride wax
Polysporin Ointment (Burroughs Wellcome)	—	—	polymyxin B sulfate, 10,000 units/g bacitracin zinc, 500 units/g	white petrolatum
Prophyllin Solution and Ointment (Rystan)	—	sodium propionate, 1% (solution) 5% (ointment)	—	chlorophyll, 0.0025% (solution) 0.0125% (ointment)
Quinalor Compound Ointment (Squibb)	halquinols, 0.5% benzoyl peroxide, 10% menthol	—	—	methyl salicylate polyethylene glycol mineral oil
Sea Breeze (Sea Breeze)	eugenol boric acid camphor	benzoic acid	—	alcohol, 43% peppermint oil clove oil eucalyptus oil
Spectrocin Ointment (Squibb)	—	—	neomycin, 2.5 mg/g gramicidin, 0.25 mg/g	—
Sperti Ointment (Whitehall)	phenylmercuric nitrate, 1:10,000	—	—	shark liver oil, 3% yeast cell derivative, 2,000 units skin respiratory factor/30 g
Terramycin Ointment with Polymyxin B Sulfate (Pfipharmecs)	—	—	oxytetracycline hydrochloride, 30 mg/g polymyxin B sulfate, 10,000 units/g	—
Triple Antibiotic Ointment (North American)	—	—	polymyxin B sulfate, 5,000 units/g bacitracin, 400 units/g neomycin sulfate, 5 mg/g	—
Vioform Ointment and Cream (Ciba)	iodochlorhydroxyquin, 3%	—	—	petrolatum base (ointment) water-washable base (cream)
Zea Sorb Powder (Stiefel)	chloroxylenol, 0.5%	—	—	microporous cellulose, 45% aluminum dihydroxy-allantoinate, 0.2%
Zemo Soap (Plough)	triclocarban	—	—	—
Zephiran Chloride Solution and Spray (Winthrop)	benzalkonium chloride, 0.13%	—	—	—
Zephiran Towelettes (Winthrop)	benzalkonium chloride chlorothymol	—	—	alcohol, 20% perfume

Acne Products

Raymond E. Hopponen

Questions to ask the patient

What types of medication are you currently using?

What treatments have you used? How effective were they?

What types of cosmetics and/or hair preparations do you use?

Are the blemishes only whiteheads and blackheads or are there also closed cysts under the skin?

Are the blemishes hot, red, swollen, or painful?

How old are you?

How long have you had acne?

Are you now or have you been under a physician's care for this condition?

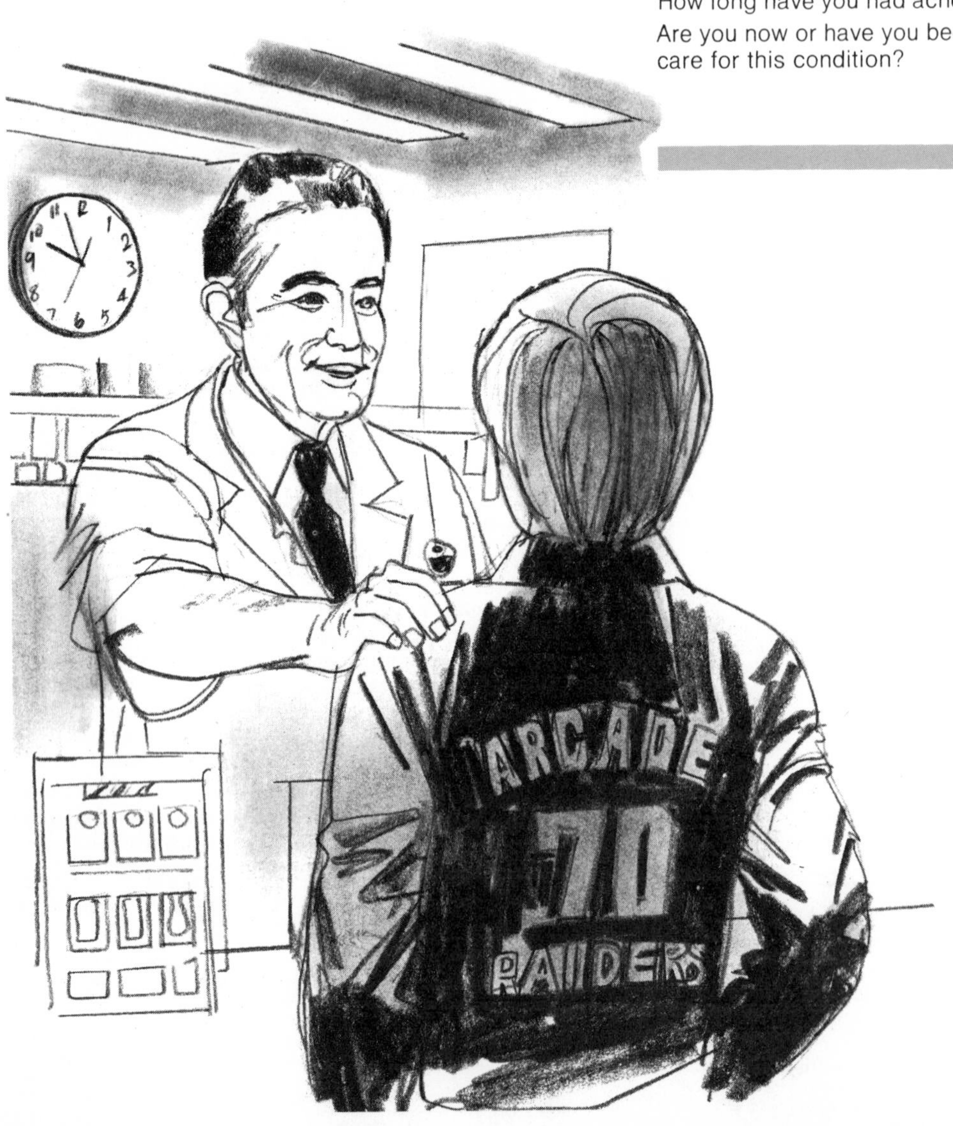

CHAPTER 28

Acne vulgaris is a chronic skin condition characterized mainly by comedones. It is most common on the face, chest, and back. In more severe cases, inflammation, pustules, cysts, and scarring may occur. Although acne does not pose a severe physical threat, it should not be ignored. It can be the cause of a great amount of emotional stress and anguish. Acne occurs most often in adolescence, a period during which many social and psychological adjustments are made and personal appearance and peer acceptance are important. It can also occur after adolescence.

Incidence

Studies concerning the incidence of acne in teenagers indicate that it is nearly universal in this group. Burton *et al.*,[1] in a study of 1,555 children from 8 to 18 years, reported 100 percent recognizable acne at ages of maximum incidence—14 years for girls and 16 for boys. They also found that 50 percent of the girls and 78 percent of the boys had acne severe enough to be termed clinical. Subclinical lesions were detected in about one-third of the 8- to 9-year group. Schacter *et al.*[2] found that only 10 to 11 percent of the high school students who were studied had sought medical help for acne, but about 60 percent were self-medicating.

Effect of Diet

The frequency of acne in adolescence, its remissions and recurrences, and its variability in response to treatment have prompted various theories implicating habit, diet, personality, and physiology as factors that affect it. Most of the theories have been disproved; diet, however, remains controversial.[3] Although several studies have demonstrated that chocolate does not affect the course of acne, some clinicians remain unconvinced and suggest it be removed from the diet.[4] No convincing evidence has been presented to implicate other dietary factors such as nuts, fats, colas, or carbohydrates, and many clinicians now feel that dietary restrictions for individuals with acne are an unwarranted imposition. Iodides and bromides which are secreted in the sweat do cause acneiform eruptions when they are ingested in substantial amounts as in therapeutic agents containing these ions. The amount of iodine in seafood or iodized salt is not significant.

Etiology/signs and symptoms

Acne vulgaris commences in the pilosebaceous units in the dermis (Fig. 1). These units consist of a hair follicle and the associated sebaceous glands. They are connected to the surface of the skin by a duct (infundibulum) through which the hair shaft passes. On the smooth skin of the body, the hair is very fine or absent. The sebaceous glands are most common on the face, chest, and back. They produce sebum, a mixture of fats and waxes, which maintains proper hydration in skin and hair. The sebum moves to the surface of the skin along the hair follicle and spreads over the surface to retard water loss.

Noninflammatory acne. The cause of acne is an increase in the activity of the sebaceous glands and of the epithelial tissue lining the infundibulum. This increase is induced by the increased production of hormones, especially androgenic hormones, as a person approaches puberty. The glands produce more sebum causing increased oiliness of the skin. The epithelial tissue, which is continuous with the epidermis, becomes thinner as it extends down into the follicle. Normally, it continually sloughs off and moves to the surface of the skin with the sebum. In the acne condition, the epithelial cells become more distinct and durable and stick together to form a coherent, horny layer which blocks the follicular channel.[5] This impaction plugs and distends the follicle to form a microcomedo. As more cells and sebum are added, the comedo becomes visible (whitehead) and is called a "closed" comedo, i.e., its contents do not reach the surface of the skin (Fig. 2). It is not easily expressed with a comedo extractor and may need to be lanced with a surgical blade before the plug can be extruded. If the plug enlarges and protrudes from the orifice of the follicular canal, it is called an "open" comedo, i.e., its contents open to the surface. The tip may darken (blackhead) because of the accumulation of melanin that is produced by the epithelial cells of the follicular lining.[6] Open comedones can be expressed easily with a comedo extractor. Although sebum is still produced, the sebaceous glands shrink during comedo formation. Acne that is characterized by closed and open comedones is called "noninflammatory acne."

The hair in the follicles is important in the development of comedones. If it is thin and small or in a rudimentary stage, it does not maintain an open channel and becomes entrapped in the plug. The heavier hair of the scalp and beard can push the developing plug to the surface and prevent comedo formation.

Inflammatory acne. "Inflammatory" acne is characterized by inflammation (surrounding the comedones), papules, pustules, and nodulocystic lesions. It is more likely to cause permanent scarring than noninflammatory acne. Inflammatory acne begins in closed comedones, rarely in open ones. As the microcomedo develops, it distends the follicle, which causes a thinning of the walls. Primary inflammation of the follicle wall develops with the disruption of the epithelium and the infiltration of lymphocytes into the adjacent areas of the dermis.[7] The process may stop at this point or proceed to a more severe inflammatory reaction in which the follicle wall ruptures and the contents of the follicle leak into the surrounding tissue. The inflamed follicles or pustules either heal in about a week or develop into cysts or sterile abscesses, which can lead to scarring and permanent disfigurement. Fingering or picking facial blemishes or attempting to express closed comedones can cause the development of inflammatory lesions by rupturing the follicles.

The sebaceous follicle contains epithelial cells, micro-organisms, and sebum. The epithelial cells are not involved in the initial inflammation of the follicular wall, but they can contribute to the inflammatory process if the follicle ruptures and they enter the surrounding tissue. The main micro-organisms which contribute to the inflammatory process are *Corynebacterium acnes* and one or two species of cocci. They are the predominant flora of normal skin and are not considered pathogens. These flora are not found in the damaged follicle walls nor in the inflammatory infiltrate of the primary phase of the inflammatory reaction. They rapidly die off when the follicle wall ruptures but may play a role as foreign substances in the inflammatory process of the invaded tissue.[5]

Sebum seems to be important in initiating follicular inflammation and contributing to inflammation of the surrounding tissue. Normal sebum does not contain free fatty acids and is nonirritating. However, in the presence of lipolytic enzymes, triglycerides of the sebum are split and release fatty acids which are irritating to tissue. The normal bacterial flora (especially *C. acnes*) of the sebaceous duct are the source of the enzymes responsible for the splitting of the glycerides.[8] Oral tetracycline can control inflammatory acne because it reduces the bacterial population and the concentration of free fatty acids in the sebaceous follicle.[3, 8]

The presence of pustules or cysts indicates inflammatory acne, a type that should be treated by a physician. Treatment requires prescribed medication and possible excision and drainage of lesions. Because of the danger of permanent scarring, medical help should be sought.

Aggravating factors

Many women with acne experience a flareup of symptoms during the premenstrual part of their cycle. The flareup cannot be explained on the basis of hormone levels alone, although the change in the level of progesterone has been implicated. Changes in sebaceous activity have also been claimed to be responsible. Cunliffe and Williams [9] have suggested that the premenstrual flareup, which occurred in 60 to 70 percent of women with acne, is caused by a reduction in the size of the orifice of the pilosebaceous duct. Measurements of the diameter of orifices during the complete cycle have shown that the size was markedly reduced during the premenstrual phase.

Hydration also decreases the size of the pilosebaceous duct orifice, a change which is reversible.[10] This explains the exacerbation of acne in high humidity or conditions where frequent and prolonged sweating occur.

Local irritation or friction can increase the incidence of acne symptoms. Rough or occlusive clothing, headgear straps, and pieces of equipment used in athletics often aggravate acne conditions. Resting the chin or cheek on the hand frequently or for long periods creates localized conditions conducive to pustule formation in individuals who are prone to acne.

Kligman and Mills [11] described "acne cosmetica," a condition resembling noninflammatory acne vulgaris, which was found in about one-third of adult women who were examined, but not in adult men. The lesions of acne cosmetica are typical, closed, noninflammatory comedones and cannot be distinguished from similar lesions of acne vulgaris. The condition was attributed to cosmetics because a comparable condition was not noted in men. Additionally, one-half of the bases of cosmetic creams used by these women were comedogenic in rabbit ear tests and on the skin of human volunteers. The condition responded readily to treatment with tretinoin.

Acne cannot be cured. In most cases, however, with currently available therapeutic regimens, symptoms can be reduced and permanent scarring can be minimized. Because acne persists for long periods, frequently from adolescence to the early twenties, treatment must also be long term. Periods of remission or reduction in severity of lesions may occur, especially in summer, but treatment should be resumed when necessary.

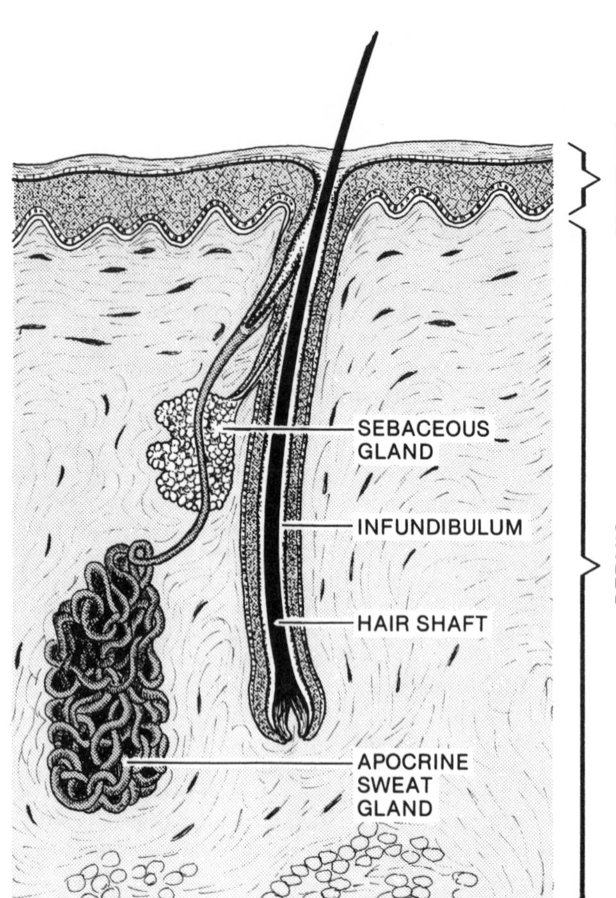

Figure 1. Normal pilosebaceous unit.

Treatment

Treatment of acne with OTC products involves removing excess sebum from the skin, preventing closure of the pilosebaceous orifice, minimizing conditions which are conducive to acne (e.g., covering lesions with cosmetics). Controlling inflammation and infection, suppressing or altering hormonal activity, and correcting destructive effects should be left to a physician.[12]

Removal of excess sebum. The best method for removal of excess sebum from the skin is a conscientious

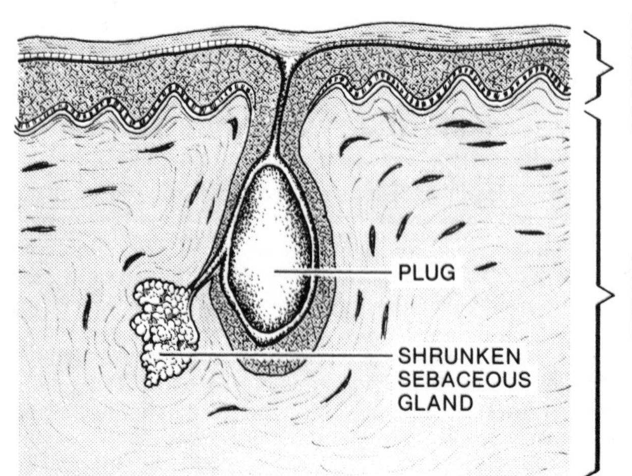

Figure 2. Closed comedo.

program of daily washing. The affected areas should be washed thoroughly three times a day with warm water, soap, and a soft washcloth. Scrubbing should be gentle to avoid damage and should last several minutes to take advantage of the keratin-softening effect of soap. Washing time is insufficient to hydrate the skin enough to decrease the size of the pilosebaceous duct orifice. The purpose of washing is to produce a mild drying of the skin and, perhaps, mild erythema.[3] Washing causes barely visible peeling which can loosen comedones. If washing produces a feeling of tautness, intensity of the washing should be reduced.

Toilet soaps usually produce satisfactory results. Although soap that contains antibacterial agents has been suggested for use in the control of acne, no conclusive evidence has been presented to show its value over nonmedicated soap. There also seems to be little rationale for the use of soaps that contain sulfur, salicylic acid, or resorcinol. If the affected area is properly rinsed, these added medications are washed away. Soap substitutes that contain surface active agents (ionic or nonionic) have been suggested for use in acne because they are less drying to the skin. However, because a mild degree of drying is desirable, an ordinary facial soap should be tried first. If it is inconvenient to wash the skin during the day, a cleansing pad that contains alcohol, acetone, and a surface active agent can be used. Some cleansing preparations contain pumice, polyethylene, or aluminum oxide particles to add abrasive action to the cleansing effect. However, these products are more expensive than soap, and it is doubtful whether they are more advantageous than using soap and a soft washcloth.

Because the treatment of acne is aimed at removing excess sebum from the skin, other topically applied fats and oils should be eliminated, e.g., cosmetics that contain fats. Hair dressings should contain a minimum of oil and should not be used in excessive amounts. "Pomade acne" has been reported to be caused directly by the long-term use of hair dressings that contain petrolatum or liquid petrolatum.[13] It appears as comedones on the forehead and temples. Frequent shampooing of the hair should be encouraged because acne is usually accompanied by an oily scalp.

Prevention of pilosebaceous orifice closure. Topical agents that cause mild irritation and desquamation are used to prevent closure of the pilosebaceous orifice. The irritant effect of these peeling agents causes an increased rate of turnover of the epithelial cells lining the follicular duct.[3] Peeling agents also cause keratolysis, which reduces the cohesiveness of the follicular lining. The net effect of this therapy reduces the tendency to form new comedones and loosens the structure of formed comedones to help their extrusion.

Ingredients in OTC products

The mildest agents—the ones which usually are tried first—are sulfur, resorcinol, and salicylic acid.

Sulfur. Sulfur is usually used in the precipitated or colloidal form at concentrations of 2 to 10 percent. The higher concentrations produce a more intense effect. Other forms, such as zinc sulfide and sodium thiosulfate, are milder. Sulfur presents a paradox in that it helps resolve formed comedones but may promote the formation of new ones. Mills and Kligman[14] showed that sulfur (but not thiosulfates or sulfides) is comedogenic in rabbit ear tests and on human volunteers. They suggest the use of the more effective agents, benzoyl peroxide and tretinoin, instead of sulfur. The comedogenic effect of sulfur suggests that, for mild effects, resorcinol or salicylic acid is better. However, habit and established practices are slow to change, and sulfur will probably continue to be used for some time.

Resorcinol and salicylic acid. Resorcinol is usually used in concentrations of 1 to 4 percent; resorcinol monoacetate is milder and can be used at higher concentrations. Resorcinol can produce a dark-brown scale on some black-skinned people, and they should be forewarned.[15] The reaction is reversible when the medication is discontinued. Salicylic acid is used in concentrations of 0.5 to 2 percent. The combination of resorcinol and salicylic acid in an alcohol solution is advantageous because it dries quickly and does not leave a visible film. Resorcinol and salicylic acid are often added to preparations that contain sulfur to increase the total activity.

Benzoyl peroxide. Benzoyl peroxide is a primary irritant which increases the growth rate of epithelial cells, causing an increased rate of sloughing and promoting resolution of comedones.[16] It is used in concentrations of 5 to 10 percent (the lower concentration is suggested at the beginning of treatment). Benzoyl peroxide is applied at night after washing the affected area with soap and water. Fair-skinned individuals may find it better to leave it on for only 2 hours at a time until the skin becomes conditioned. Benzoyl peroxide produces a feeling of warmth, slight stinging, and reddening of the skin. If the stinging or burning is excessive after an application, the preparation should be removed with soap and water and not reapplied until the next day. Because benzoyl peroxide is highly irritating, it should not be used on the eyelids, lips, or neck. Other sources of irritation, such as sunlamps, should be discontinued, and it may be necessary to reduce the vigor and frequency of washing. Because benzoyl peroxide is an oxidizing agent, it may bleach colored fabrics. Its potential explosiveness has been eliminated in commercial preparations by combining it in a 35:65 ratio with dicalcium phosphate.

Other treatment

Although the oral use of tetracycline is successful in the treatment of inflammatory acne, the value of topical applications of antibacterial agents has not been proved. Because acne is not an infection, topical antibacterial agents generally are ineffective. These agents cannot reach the anaerobic *C. acnes* because the organisms are found in the deeper areas of the follicle. However, Fulton[17] found that topical solutions of erythromycin decrease the number of inflammatory lesions. A 2-percent solution of erythromycin compounds in a 2:2:1 mixture of ethanol, ethylene glycol monomethyl ether, and propylene glycol reduced the level of free fatty acids of the follicles to the level reached by oral tetracycline. The hypothesis is that the lipid-soluble antibiotic can penetrate the sebaceous follicle to suppress *Corynebacterium.* It would seem, however, that the proven effectiveness and convenience of oral tetracycline is preferable to the potential variability of effectiveness of topical antibacterial solutions. Erythromycin and oral tetracycline are available by prescription only.

Tretinoin (retinoic acid), the acid form of vitamin A, is the most effective available topical agent for the treatment of acne. It is a strong primary irritant, similar to benzoyl peroxide but more effective, that prevents closure of the pilosebaceous orifice.[18] Tretinoin is available (prescription only) as a 0.05-percent solution in a mixture of equal parts of 95 percent ethanol and polyethylene glycol; as pads saturated with the solution; and as a vanishing cream containing 0.1 percent tretinoin. The products are applied at night. They cause a feeling of warmth or slight stinging.[19] The acne may seem to worsen during the first few weeks of therapy; optimum results occur in 3 to 4 months. Care should be taken to avoid touching the eyes, nose, and mouth with tretinoin. Other topical agents should be discontinued before using tretinoin. The face should be washed only twice a day to avoid excessive irritation; tretinoin should not be applied to wet skin because it causes excessive stinging. Exposure to sun lamps and strong sunlight also should be avoided because of the increased sensitivity of the skin.

Treatments that have been abandoned or have not been proved effective include oral vitamin A, laxatives, bacterial vaccines, and digestive aids, such as pancreatin, pepsin, bile salts, and acidophilus bacterial cultures.

Exposure to sunlight is often beneficial in acne conditions. Because of this, improvement is often noted during the summer months. The improvement is believed to result from the irritant properties of the ultraviolet wavelength of sunlight which stimulates increased proliferation of the epithelium. Ultraviolet lamps produce the same effect, but they are not generally recommended for self-medication because of the difficulty of determining and regulating the amount of exposure necessary to produce mild erythema. The danger of falling asleep under the lamp can be avoided by having someone else time the exposure. If a sunlamp is used, care must be taken to adequately protect the eyes from the damaging effect of the light.

Secondary formulation factors

Suspensions, lotions, creams, and gels are generally used as the vehicles to carry anti-acne medication to the skin. Lotions and creams should have a low fat content so that they do not counteract drying and peeling. Ethyl or isopropyl alcohol added to liquid preparations and gels hastens their drying to a film. Nonfatty gels, in particular, are slow drying if they are formulated in a completely aqueous base.

Thickening agents in all preparations should not dry to a sticky film. The solids of most preparations leave a film which is not visible and does not need coloring to blend with the skin. Some products, however, are intended to hide blemishes by depositing an opaque film of insoluble masking agents, such as zinc oxide, on the skin. These products need tinting to improve their cosmetic effect.

Guidelines for product selection

Only noninflammatory acne should be self-medicated. Individuals exhibiting characteristics of inflammatory acne should be referred to a physician. A medication history should be taken and should include previous measures taken to control the acne and which medications were used, when, and for how long. The history should also include the degree of success and personal acceptance of the preparation that was tried. Subjective data on a person's attitude toward treatment and willingness to actively participate in a program of skin care should be determined.

The success of a program to control acne depends on patient willingness to devote the time and effort required to carry out a continued, daily regimen of washing the affected areas and applying medication. A clear explanation of the acne process should be given and misconceptions corrected. The pharmacist should advise on scalp and hair care, the use of cosmetics, and, above all, the need for long-term, conscientious care.

Claims made for OTC products for acne relief must be studied carefully for their accuracy. A variety of creams, lotions, antiseptics, and skin peels is available, and formulas should be carefully examined before a value judgment is made.

If a medication has not previously been used consistently, one of the milder peeling agents should be recommended. Resorcinol or salicylic acid preparations might be suggested before those which contain sulfur, which is potentially comedogenic. These preparations along with conscientious washing with soap, water, and a washcloth may control the acne in many cases. If a milder agent was tried conscientiously without success, benzoyl peroxide should be tried. However, the cautions on its very irritating properties should be observed. Cases of acne that continue to be resistant to control should be referred to a physician.

Summary

Acne vulgaris occurs almost universally in young adults from early teens to mid-twenties and occasionally appears in older people. Acne is generally not amenable to a cure, but it can be controlled to improve appearance and to prevent the development of severe acne and its resultant scarring. With understanding and reassurance, acne sufferers may be made to understand that care must be given to the affected areas for a long time.

References

1. J. L. Burton *et al., Br. J. Dermatol.*, **85**, 119(1971).
2. R. J. Schacter *et al., N. Y. State J. Med.*, **71**, 2886(1971).
3. R. M. Reisner, *Pediatr. Clin. North Am.*, **20**, 851(1973).
4. J. E. Fulton *et al., J. Am. Med. Assoc.*, **210**, 2071(1969).
5. A. M. Kligman, *J. Invest. Dermatol.*, **62**, 268(1974).
6. D. Blair and C. A. Lewis, *Br. J. Dermatol.*, **82**, 572(1970).
7. R. K. Freinkel, *N. Engl. J. Med.*, **280**, 1161(1969).
8. R. K. Freinkel *et al., N. Engl. J. Med.*, **273**, 850(1965).
9. W. J. Cunliffe and M. Williams, *Lancet*, **2**, 1055(1973).
10. M. Williams *et al., Br. J. Dermatol.*, **90**, 631(1974).
11. A. M. Kligman and O. H. Mills, *Arch. Dermatol.*, **106**, 843(1972).
12. S. B. Frank, "Acne Vulgaris," Charles C Thomas, Springfield, Ill., 1971, p. 175.
13. G. Plewig *et al., Arch. Dermatol.*, **101**, 580(1970).
14. O. H. Mills and A. M. Kligman, *Br. J. Dermatol.*, **86**, 620(1972).
15. S. B. Frank, "Acne Vulgaris," Charles C Thomas, Springfield, Ill., 1971, p. 184.
16. P. Vasarenish, *Arch. Dermatol.*, **98**, 183(1968).
17. J. E. Fulton, *Arch. Dermatol.*, **110**, 83(1974).
18. A. M. Kligman *et al., Arch. Dermatol.*, **99**, 469(1969).
19. A. M. Kligman *et al., Postgrad. Med.*, **55**, 99(1974).

Products 28 ACNE

Product (manufacturer)	Application form	Sulfur	Resorcinol/ salicylic acid	Antibacterial	Other
Acnaveen (Cooper)	cream bar	2%	salicylic acid, 2%	—	soapless detergents
Acne Aid (Stiefel)	cream lotion	2.5% (cream) 10% (lotion)	resorcinol, 1.25% (cream)	chloroxylenol, 0.375% (cream)	alcohol, 10% (lotion)
Acne-Aid Detergent Soap (Stiefel)	cleanser	—	—	—	sulfated surfactants hydrocarbon hydrotropes, 6.3%

Product (manufacturer)	Application form	Sulfur	Resorcinol/ salicylic acid	Antibacterial	Other
Acnesarb (C&M)	solution	—	salicylic acid, 3%	methylbenzethonium chloride, 0.08%	isopropyl alcohol, 63% boric acid, 2%
Acnomel (Smith Kline & French)	cream cleanser	8% (cream) 4% (cleanser)	resorcinol, 2% (cream) 1% (cleanser)	—	—
Acnotex (C&M)	lotion	8%	salicylic acid, 2.25%	methylbenzethonium chloride, 0.08%	propylene glycol powder base acetone isopropyl alcohol, 22% perfume
Acnycin (Columbia Medical)	cream	5%	resorcinol, 2%	—	zinc oxide
Benoxyl (Stiefel)	lotion	—	—	—	benzoyl peroxide, 5 and 10%
Bensulfoid (Poythress)	lotion	colloidal, 2%	resorcinol, 2%	—	alcohol, 12% zinc oxide, 6% thymol, 0.5% hexachlorophene, 0.1% perfume
Betadine Skin Cleanser (Purdue Frederick)	cleanser	—	—	povidone-iodine, 7.5%	detergents
Brasivol (Stiefel)	cleanser	—	—	—	aluminum oxide neutral soap detergents (fine, medium, rough)
Cenac (Central)	lotion	colloidal, 8%	resorcinol, 2%	—	isopropyl alcohol, 30%
Clearasil Medicated Cleanser (Vick)	cleanser	—	salicylic acid, 0.25%	—	alcohol, 43% allantoin, 0.1%
Clearasil Regular, Tinted, and Stick (Vick)	cream stick	8%	resorcinol, 2% (cream) 1% (stick)	—	bentonite, 11.5% (cream) 4% (stick) alcohol, 10% (cream)
Clearasil Vanishing Formula (Vick)	cream	3%	resorcinol, 2%	—	bentonite, 10% alcohol, 10%
Contrablem (Texas Pharmacal)	gel	5%	resorcinol, 2%	—	alcohol, 9.5%
Cuticura (Purex)	ointment	precipitated	—	8-hydroxyquinoline	petrolatum mineral oil mineral wax isopropyl palmitate synthetic beeswax phenol pine oil rose geranium oil
Cuticura Acne Cream (Purex)	cream	—	—	—	benzoyl peroxide, 5% alcohol, 1%
Cuticura Medicated (Purex)	liquid	—	resorcinol salicylic acid	8-hydroxyquinoline sulfate phenol	alcohol, 28% boric acid chlorobutanol camphor glycerin
Epi-Clear (Squibb)	lotion	10%	—	—	alcohol, 10%
Epi-Clear Scrub Cleanser (Squibb)	cleanser	—	—	—	aluminum oxide, 38% (fine) 52% (medium) 65% (coarse)

Product (manufacturer)	Application form	Sulfur	Resorcinol/ salicylic acid	Antibacterial	Other
Epi-Clear Soap for Oily Skin (Squibb)	cleanser	—	—	—	sulfated surfactants, 6.3% hydrocarbon hydrotropes
Finac (C&M)	lotion	2%	—	methylbenzethonium chloride, 0.08%	powder base isopropyl alcohol, 8% perfume
Fomac Cream Cleanser (Dermik)	cleanser	colloidal, 2%	salicylic acid, 2%	—	soapless detergents
Fomac-HF (Dermik)	cleanser	—	—	chloroxylenol, 2%	—
Ionax Foam (Owen)	aerosol foam	—	—	benzalkonium chloride, 0.2%	polyoxyethylene ethers soapless surfactant
Ionax Scrub (Owen)	paste	—	—	benzalkonium chloride, 0.2%	granular polyethylene polyoxyethylene ethers alcohol, 10%
Klaron (Dermik)	lotion	colloidal, 5%	salicylic acid, 2%	—	alcohol, 13.1%
Komed (Barnes-Hind)	lotion	—	resorcinol, 2% salicylic acid, 2%	—	isopropyl alcohol, 22% sodium thiosulfate, 8% menthol camphor colloidal alumina
Komex (Barnes-Hind)	cleanser	—	—	—	sodium tetrahydrate decahydrate granules
Liquimat (Texas Pharmacal)	lotion	5%	—	—	alcohol, 22% tinted bases
Listerex Herbal Lotion (Warner-Lambert)	cleanser	—	salicylic acid, 2%	—	polyethylene granules surface-active cleansers
Listerex Regular Lotion (Warner-Lambert)	cleanser	—	—	—	thymol, 0.16% polyethylene granules surface-active cleansers menthol eucalyptol
Loroxide (Dermik)	lotion	—	—	chlorhydroxyquinoline, 0.25%	benzoyl peroxide, 5%
Lotio Alsulfa (Doak)	lotion	colloidal, 5%	—	—	colloidal clays, 95%
Lotioblanc (Arnar-Stone)	lotion	—	—	—	zinc sulfate sulfurated potash
Medicated Face Conditioner (MFC) (Mennen)	liquid	—	salicylic acid, 1%	—	alcohol, 55%
Microsyn (Syntex)	lotion	—	resorcinol, 2% salicylic acid, 2%	—	sodium thiosulfate, 8% colloidal alumina menthol camphor
Multiscrub (Bristol-Myers)	cream	2%	salicylic acid, 1.5%	—	soapless detergents polyethylene resin granules, 26%
Oxy-5 (Norcliff-Thayer)	lotion	—	—	—	benzoyl peroxide, 5%
Persadox (Texas Pharmacal)	lotion cream	—	—	—	benzoyl peroxide, 5%
Persadox HP (Texas Pharmacal)	cream lotion	—	—	—	benzoyl peroxide, 10%
pHisoAc (Winthrop)	cream	colloidal, 6%	resorcinol, 1.5%	—	alcohol, 10%
pHisoDerm (Winthrop)	cleanser	—	—	—	entsufon sodium petrolatum lanolin cholesterols

Product (manufacturer)	Application form	Sulfur	Resorcinol/ salicylic acid	Antibacterial	Other
piSec (Owen)	cream	3.14%	—	benzalkonium chloride, 0.2%	polyoxyethylene ether
Postacne (Dermik)	lotion	microsize, 2%	—	—	alcohol, 29%
Quinalor Compound (Squibb)	ointment	—	—	halquinols, 0.5%	benzoyl peroxide, 10% menthol methyl salicylate polyethylene glycol mineral oil
Resulin (Schieffelin)	lotion half-strength lotion	8%	resorcinol, 4%	—	alcohol, 32%
Rezamid (Dermik)	lotion cream	microsize, 5%	resorcinol, 2%	chloroxylenol, 0.5%	alcohol, 28.5%
Sastid Plain (Stiefel)	cleanser	1.6%	salicylic acid, 1.6%	—	soapless surfactants
Seale's Lotion (C&M)	lotion	6.4%	resorcinol, 3.2%	—	sodium borate zinc oxide acetone bentonite
Seba-Nil (Texas Pharmacal)	solution	—	—	—	alcohol, 49.7% acetone polysorbate 80
Seba-Nil Cleansing Mask (Texas Pharmacal)	cleanser	—	—	—	polyethylene granules
Spectro-Jel (Recsei)	gel	—	—	cetylpyridinium chloride, 0.1%	isopropyl alcohol, 15% methylcellulose, 1.5% glycol–polysiloxane, 1%
Stri-Dex Medicated Pads (Lehn & Fink)	medicated pads	—	salicylic acid, 0.5%	—	sulfonated alkylbenzenes citric acid alcohol
Sulforcin (Texas Pharmacal)	lotion	5%	resorcinol, 2%	—	alcohol, 11.65%
Sulfur Soap (Stiefel)	cleanser	precipitated, 10%	—	—	—
Teenac (Elder)	gel	1.5%	—	—	mercuric sulfide, 0.5% urea
Thera-Blem (Noxell)	cream	2%	resorcinol, 1.5%	phenol, 0.5%	menthol, 0.5% camphor, 0.5%
Therac (C&M)	lotion	colloidal, 4%	salicylic acid, 2.35%	—	bentonite perfume
Therapads (Fuller)	pads	—	salicylic acid, 1.5%	—	alcohol, 50%
Therapads Plus (Fuller)	individual wipes	—	salicylic acid, 1.5%	—	alcohol, 70% sodium alkyl aryl polyether sulfonate, 0.1%
Thylox Medicated Soap (Dent)	cleanser	magnetic, 8.8%	—	—	—
Tyrosum Packets (Summers)	cleanser	—	—	—	alcohol acetone polysorbate
Vanoxide (Dermik)	lotion	—	—	chlorhydroxyquinoline, 0.25%	benzoyl peroxide, 5%
Xerac (Person & Covey)	gel	4%	—	—	isopropyl alcohol, 44%

Dry Skin, Dandruff, Seborrhea, Psoriasis, and Eczema Products

Joseph R. Robinson

Questions to ask the patient

How long have you had this condition?

Which area of the skin is affected? Is the condition patchy or uniformly distributed?

Is the condition stable or does it fluctuate greatly? Can you relate the fluctuation to a cause?

Is your skin exposed to detergents or chemicals? What types of cosmetics do you use?

Is there a family history of skin disease, asthma, or hay fever?

Have you consulted a dermatologist? What was recommended?

What treatments have you used? How effective were they?

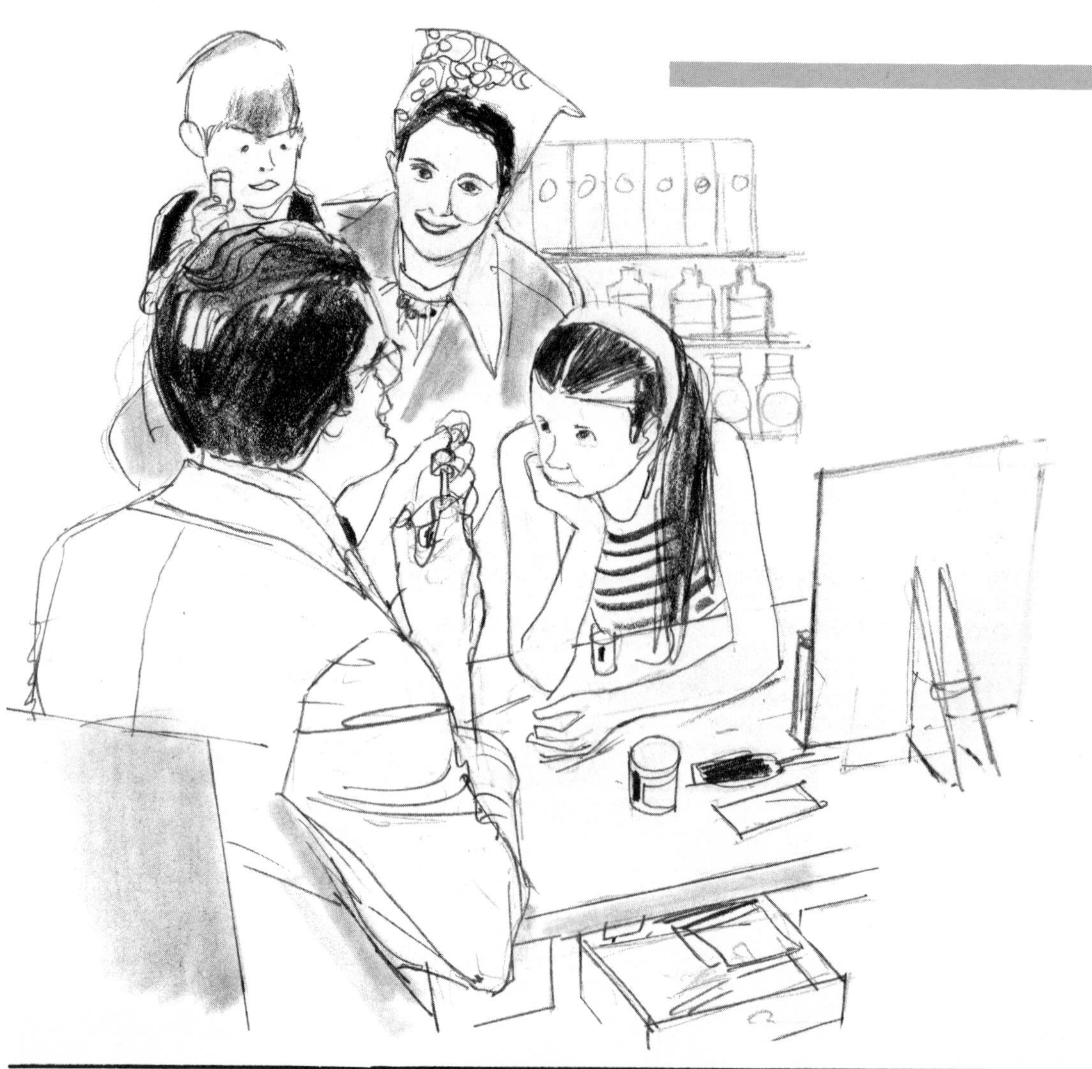

CHAPTER 29

Considering the extent of exposure of the skin to a wide variety of chemicals and environmental insults, it demonstrates remarkable resiliency and recuperative ability. (See Chapter 27 for a complete discussion of the anatomy and physiology of the skin.) Despite the fact that most people's skin is normal, advertising has created an image that few people have "normal" skin. Cosmetic and OTC drug advertisements have also been able to create the impression that many normal physiological processes are in fact abnormal or at least undesirable. There are, of course, metabolic, bacterial, fungal, viral, and other abnormalities of the skin that should be treated with drugs. Skin conditions such as dry skin, dandruff, seborrhea, psoriasis, and eczema must be considered from both the cosmetic and pathologic points of view so that the pharmacist can advise patients on the use of OTC products.

Dry skin

Everyone experiences dry or chapped skin. In some people it is seasonal or acute; in others it is chronic. Although dry skin is not life threatening, it is annoying and uncomfortable because of the attendant pruritus and, in some cases, pain and inflammation. In addition, dry skin is more prone to bacterial invasion than normal skin.

Dry skin can be characterized by one or more of the following signs and symptoms: roughness and flaking, loss of flexibility and elasticity, fissures, hyperkeratosis, and inflammation. The cardinal sign of a dry skin condition is a less than adequate moisture content in the stratum corneum of the epidermis. A lack of moisture may be caused by genetic or environmental conditions or pathologic states, or may occur as a normal consequence of the aging process. Thus, many conditions are classified either as dry skin or as chafed or chapped skin, atopic dermatitis, "winter dermatitis," senile pruritus, psoriasis, ichthyosis, soap dermatitis, miliaria, "bath itch," eczematoid dermatitis, and other associated dermatitides. Various OTC cosmetic products in an assortment of vehicles are available to correct a dry skin condition, or at least help alleviate some discomforting aspects. To evaluate the worth of these products in treating a dry skin condition, it is necessary to understand the condition and factors influencing the loss of moisture from the skin.

Maintenance of normal hydration

The mechanical properties of skin that are altered by dry skin conditions are related to the water content of the stratum corneum.[1] If the water content of the stratum corneum falls below about 10 percent, a dry skin condition will result. A great deal is now known regarding the mechanism and factors that influence the movement of water into and out of the skin.[2-6]

Water can be lost from the skin through perspiration via the sweat glands and through transepidermal diffusion. The volume of water lost through perspiration varies considerably with thermal and emotional conditions; as much as 2 liters/hour can be lost under extreme thermal stress. Diffusional loss is a relatively constant process. Its rate depends, in part, on humidity and skin surface temperature. Because human skin is such an effective barrier to diffusive loss of water, the daily loss from an adult skin surface (20,000 cm^2) is only about 120 ml.[7]

The entire stratum corneum acts as a barrier or water seal; there is not a distinct narrow "barrier zone" contained within the horny layer as had been proposed earlier.[1 5] Removal of this barrier results in an immediate 50-fold rise in the rate of water loss, roughly the same rate as from a free water surface.[2 3]

Perhaps the process of diffusion is better described as ". . . an equilibrium process, whereby as water leaves the skin surface more water is released from the lower skin. The barrier acts like a gate valve, opening and closing in response to concentration and temperature differences on the two sides of the skin membrane."[8]

Under normal circumstances, the water content of the skin is primarily a function of the:

☐ Diffusion rate of water from the lower epidermal and dermal layers to the epidermis;

☐ Ability of the stratum corneum to hold water; and

☐ Environmental conditions which increase or decrease the moisture level.

The rate of diffusion of moisture to the horny layer of skin is rapid. Blank[1] has shown that, by diffusion, water can be brought to the base of the epidermis from lower layers 50 to 100 times faster than it is lost from the surface of the epidermis to the environment. Thus, movement of moisture to the epidermal layer is not rate limiting. However, movement of moisture through the horny layer is relatively slow partly because of low water vapor permeability and pressure of the stratum corneum. Because of this slow movement of moisture, vasoconstriction or vasodilation has little influence on the water vapor pressure and content in the horny layer and no effect on diffusional water loss through it.

Perhaps the most critical factor to horny layer hydration is the ability of this layer to hold moisture. Blank[1] reported that a hydrophilic component of the stratum corneum was responsible for water retention. Research has been devoted to elucidating the composition and mechanism of action of this substance, called Natural Moisturizing Factor (NMF).[9-11]

Several components of NMF, e.g., lactate, polypeptides, hexosamines, pentoses, urea, pyrrolidine, carboxylic acid, inorganic ions, have been isolated and identified, but a quantitative formula for the specific organization of NMF in the skin and the specific mode of action of its components are unknown. One theory is that the components themselves bind water; another is that they keep the keratin layer organized to allow hydration of the keratin protein. A third theory postulates a combination of the first two because there is evidence for a "free" pool of water in the skin and another pool which is more tightly "bound" and hence, more difficult to remove.

Addition of hygroscopic materials of NMF to the skin surface results in only temporary hydration. Subsequent exposure to water or conditions conducive to dry skin causes a reversal of the hydrated state. Apparently, the components of NMF are not incorporated into the skin structure; they function only topically.

Environmental conditions influence the moisture content of the skin. Low humidity, high temperatures, and many other conditions cause moisture to leave the skin faster than it can be replaced, lowering the moisture level below the critical 10 percent that is required. Clearly, if low atmospheric moisture contributes to the dry skin condition, raising the relative humidity should improve the problem. Home and office humidifiers are valuable adjuncts in treating dry skin.

Factors influencing water loss from the skin

Temperature and humidity conditions. The horny layer becomes soft and pliable when moisture content is about 10 percent. This corresponds to a relative humidity of about 60 percent. Under normal indoor conditions, the water content of the stratum corneum is about 10 to 15 percent. At about 95 percent relative humidity, the water content of skin rises to approximately 65 percent; low relative humidity accelerates loss of moisture from the surface of the skin, leading to a dry skin condition.[12-16] Under the conditions of low temperature and humidity, the outer layer becomes colder or drier than the deeper layers. This results in lower flexibility of the corneum surface so that, when the skin is stretched or flexed, it cracks, causing an even faster rate of moisture loss from the skin surface. Of temperature and relative humidity, relative humidity seems to be the more important factor in skin dehydration. In addition to temperature and humidity, high wind velocity also causes more rapid evaporation of moisture from the skin surface.

Contact with nonaqueous solvents and surfactants. Middleton [4] theorizes that the water content of the corneum depends on the presence of hygroscopic substances. These substances are contained within the corneum cells by cell walls which are freely permeable to water but not to electrolytes and cannot be extracted unless the cell wall is damaged. The damage is achieved by physical disruption, by extracting the lipids from the cell with solvents, or by prolonged treatment with detergents.[17-20] The loss of hygroscopic substances resulting from this damage reduces the ability of the corneum to retain water, and a dry skin condition can result.

Physical damage. Removal of the stratum corneum generates an immediate dramatic rise in the rate of transepidermal water loss. However, within 1 or 2 days, there is about 50 percent return of the barrier function. The return is presumably caused by the formation of a temporary parakeratotic barrier and then slow return of the total barrier in 2 to 3 weeks.

Age of skin. As skin ages the entire epidermal layer thins, decreasing its capacity to retain moisture. The capacity of the stratum corneum to hold water is also decreased because of a decrease in the hygroscopic components. During the aging process there is a reduction in hormonal level with a subsequent lowering of sebum output. The lowered sebum output means less lubrication to the skin and less ability to retain horny layer moisture.[21] Finally, as skin ages it becomes hardened because of keratin cross-linking induced by a long-term exposure to ultraviolet radiation. The cross-linking is also associated with an increase in surface dryness and general pruritus.

Treatment of dry skin

The main objectives in treating a dry skin condition are to raise the level of moisture in the stratum corneum and to reestablish the integrity of this layer. Blank [1] has shown that water is the only true plasticizer for human corneum, but simply adding water to the skin, without the corneum being able to retain it, is not a useful approach. For example, hydration can be accomplished by soaking the dry skin, but unless the skin is immediately covered with an occlusive substance, such as petrolatum or plastic, it will quickly become dehydrated.

Several approaches to treating a dry skin condition are available.[22]

Moisturizing. In this approach the skin is hydrated, thereby thickening it several fold. If successful, it should eliminate most or all of the dry skin.

Chemically softening the keratinous epidermal layer. Chemically altering the keratin layer softens the skin and cosmetically improves its appearance. This approach does not need substantial addition of water, but all of the attendant dry skin symptoms may not be alleviated unless water is added to the keratin layer.

Lubricating the skin. This is more of a psychological approach—the skin feels smooth but is not necessarily hydrated or back to normal.

Most OTC and cosmetic products for dry skin attempt to treat the condition by one or more of these approaches.

An ideal moisturizer should fulfill certain conditions: [11]

- ☐ It should regulate and maintain the water level of the stratum corneum above the critical level (10 percent) but not to such a degree as to induce superhydration or maceration. Increasing hydration of the stratum corneum too much reduces its barrier efficiency, making it more susceptible to invasion by micro-organisms, irritants, and allergens.
- ☐ Its effectiveness should be independent of environmental changes.
- ☐ Continued application should not cause damage to the stratum corneum by the removal of or interference with its natural moisturizers.
- ☐ It should be nonirritating and nonsensitizing.
- ☐ It should be economical and readily available.
- ☐ It should be stable in cosmetic formulations.

Occlusives

Strianse [11] believes that an occlusive barrier alone that prevents evaporation of moisture from the skin does not fulfill these conditions. Additional moisture may not be retained by the skin—a hygroscopic moisturizer is needed with the occlusive agent. However, Anderson *et al.*[23] have shown that occluded dry skin (6 to 14 nights using a plastic film) showed an increased capacity to absorb water when hydrated at 95 percent relative humidity during the day for several days. It was their opinion that occlusion treatment of dry skin causes an enhanced metabolic rate in the epidermis which causes increased production of protein and low molecular weight, water-soluble materials that become part of the stratum corneum. Undoubtedly, from the point of view of time, it is preferable to add substances topically that would quickly return the damaged horny layer to its normal state than to occlude the site for a relatively long period.

Various occlusive agents for skin are available. The agents are called emollients presumably because they soften the skin and add lubricity. The influence of some substances on transepidermal water loss is shown in Table 1. Each of these substances attempts to provide an occlusive barrier and to add lubricity to the skin. In fact, all emollients are sold for their ability to reduce frictional forces.

Attempts have been made to formulate products that duplicate the normal oil mantle of the skin as a means of treating dry skin. However, sebum is not an effective barrier against moisture loss from the skin. It helps protect the horny layer from drying and helps reduce friction so that the skin remains flexible and smooth, aiding in the prevention of chapping. Squalene is a normal component of skin lipids and is a reasonably effective barrier. Glycerin represents a class of humectants that has been tried topically to promote a rehydration of skin. The *in vitro* data in Table 1 show that glycerin apparently promotes the loss of moisture from the skin which would lead to a worsening of the dry skin condition. However, *in vivo* studies with glycerin show that it indeed is beneficial in the dry skin condition. Petrolatum seems to be the most effective occlusive agent. Despite its success as an occlusive barrier, it is not well accepted by the consumer because of its oiliness and staining properties. Mineral oil is not as efficient a barrier as petrolatum, and silicones are even less efficient.[24 25]

Oils. Because sebum and skin surface lipids contain a relatively high concentration of fatty acid glycerides, vegetable and animal oils (peanut, safflower, cucumber, sesame, avocado, mink, turtle, etc.) have been used to treat dry skin. Their inclusion in dry skin products is presumably due to their unsaturated fatty acid content. These oils contribute to skin flexibility, but their occludent effect is less than that of petrolatum. Although there is a great psychological appeal to products containing these oils, their actual value in treating a dry skin condition is not documented.

Mineral oil products are adsorbed better than vegetable oil products, and oatmeal products are the least effective.[26] Adsorption onto and absorption into the skin increase with increases in temperature and concentration of the oil. Bath oils, which are applied at a high temperature but unfortunately at a low oil concentration, are moderately effective in improving a dry skin condition. Part of their effect is due to the slip or lubricity they impart to the skin which may be more important to the consumer than the occlusive properties.

Application of bath oils in the form of wet compresses has been shown to be quite effective in treating a variety of dry skin conditions.[27] However, with the exception of bath oils, there is a lack of consumer appeal for applied oil products; emulsion systems are preferred.

Emulsions. Oil-in-water (O/W) emulsions are preferred over water-in-oil (W/O) emulsions or pure oil products because they feel less greasy. O/W emulsions help alleviate the pruritus associated with dry skin by virtue of their cooling effect as the water evaporates from the skin surface. There is sufficient oil in most O/W emulsions to form a continuous film on the surface of the skin provided that waxes, gums, and other formulating agents provide an occlusive film after the water evaporates.[28] The thickness of the oil film on the skin from an O/W emulsion is less than that from a W/O emulsion because there is less oil. However, other ingredients in the product may contribute to correcting the dry skin condition. Rothman [29] believes that it makes very little difference whether a W/O or O/W emulsion is used. Mezei *et al.*[17] have indicated that the surfactants present in dispersion system products have the potential to further dry the skin.

Frequency of application of these products depends on severity of the dry skin condition as well as the hydration efficiency of the occlusive agent. Care must be exercised to avoid excessive hydration or maceration. In addition, although most commercial formulations generally are bland, contact with the eye or with broken abraded skin should be avoided because irritation from formulation ingredients is possible in these cases. This is especially true with emulsion systems because the surfactants in these systems can denature proteins.

Table 1. Effect of Applied Substances on Transepidermal Moisture Loss[a]

Substances	Effect on moisture loss
Glycerin	42% increase
Isopropyl palmitate	28% decrease
Lanolin, anhydrous	32% decrease
Petrolatum	48% decrease
Squalene	26% decrease

[a]Adapted from D. H. Powers and C. Fox, *Proc. Sci. Sect. Toilet Goods Assoc.*, **28**, 21(1957).

Ingredients in OTC products for dry skin

Urea and allantoin. Urea (10 to 30 percent), allantoin (0.3 percent), and allantoin complexes are claimed to soften keratin by disrupting its structure.[22] Urea is mildly keratolytic and increases water uptake in the corneum, giving it a high water binding capacity.[30 31] Urea accelerates digestion of fibrin at about 15-percent concentration and is proteolytic at 40 percent. It is considered harmless and has been recommended for crusted necrotic tissue. Ten-percent urea systems have been used on simple dry skin, and 20 to 30 percent systems have been used for difficult dry skin conditions, such as in podiatry. Animal or human urine has been used for centuries in the treatment of dry skin presumably due to the urea content. Allantoin is also considered a relatively safe compound but is apparently less effective than urea for softening keratin.

Glycerin. Many dry skin products use humectants in the formulation not only to prevent the product from drying out but also as active ingredients. Products containing 50-percent glycerin (e.g., glycerin and rose water) are used to treat a dry skin condition. The purpose of adding a humectant to a dry skin product is that it will be absorbed into the skin to help replace the missing hygroscopic substances, or, if that does not occur, the humectant on the surface of the skin will attract water from the atmosphere and serve as a reservoir to supply water to the stratum corneum. Unfortunately, glycerin does not penetrate into the skin, and high humidity is needed for it to attract water from the environment. (High relative humidity is precisely when the incidence of dry skin is the lowest.)

Glycerin increases the rate of transepidermal moisture loss, an effect that is apparently opposite to what is desired. A partial explanation for its mechanism of action is that it accelerates the diffusion of moisture from the dermal tissue to the surface and holds water in intimate contact with the skin. In this manner, it supplies moisture to the parched stratum corneum, but more importantly, it brings moisture from the dermal region into and through the horny layer. In addition, glycerin provides lubricity to the skin surface.

Hormones. Topical application of estrogenic creams improves the water holding capacity, proliferation of cells, plumpness, and overall appearance of the skin. However, the FDA limits the amount of hormone that can be contained in a cosmetic hormone cream, and these creams have no effect on the course of a dry skin condition. Although most of these products are in oleaginous or semi-oleaginous vehicles, it is difficult to separate the contribution of the base from that of the hormone. Hence, cosmetic hormone creams cause a plumping of the skin, perhaps a disappearance of the tiny crows feet lines, and can help alleviate the dry skin condition, but a good deal of this activity, if not all, is caused by the vehicle rather than the hormone.

Vitamin A. Topical application of vitamin A has little beneficial effect on a dry skin condition other than its occlusive properties. Vitamin A is extremely oil soluble and will penetrate human skin only at high concentrations. Vitamin A acid, or retinoic acid, is more water soluble than vitamin A and is an important topical agent in acne, psoriasis, and other conditions involving accelerated mitosis. Other oil-soluble vitamins such as E and D also have occlusive properties but no specific indication for the dry skin condition.

Dandruff

Dandruff is best defined as a chronic, noninflammatory condition of the scalp that is characterized by excessive scaling of scalp tissue.[32] It is not a disease but rather a normal physiological event much like growth of hair and nails, except that the end product can be seen on the scalp and is deemed socially unacceptable. The degree of scaling ranges from mild, involving only a few flakes on the scalp, to severe, where sections of the scalp or the entire scalp appear heavily laden with dandruff flakes. The condition is a trivial medical problem but has substantial cosmetic and social impact.

During 1974, sales for medicated shampoos were more than $100 million, representing 26 to 28 percent of the total shampoo market.[33,34] Advertisements have not only created *persona non grata* status for the dandruff sufferer, but they have also attempted to obliterate the difference between dandruff, a nonpathologic condition, and psoriasis and seborrhea, which are pathologic conditions.

Incidence

Dandruff appears at puberty, when many skin activities are altered. It reaches a peak in early adulthood, levels off in middle age, declines in advancing years, and disappears in old age. The process correlates very well with the proliferative activity of the epidermis; epidermal skin kinetics are intimately related to the dandruff condition. Excessive use of hair sprays and other cosmetics can also stimulate dandruff.

Everyone has epidermal scales in the scalp to a degree.[35] The difference between dandruff and the non-dandruff condition is the quantity of scales (see Table 2). Estimates of the prevalence of dandruff range from 2.5 to 70 percent of the population.[36,37] These divergent estimates are subjective. Based on visual estimation of the extent of dandruff scurf and an objective corneocyte count, about 18 percent of the population has moderately severe dandruff or worse, and 18 percent has mild dandruff.[35,38] The degree of dandruff serious enough to warrant medical treatment is a matter of individual criteria of acceptability insofar as the quantity of scales.

The scaling process

It is quite normal for epidermal cells on the scalp to slough off continually just as on other parts of the body. However, the rate of epidermal cell turnover in normal individuals is greater on the scalp than on other parts of the body.[39] The high rate of epidermal cell turnover on the scalp involves the infundibulum of the hair follicle.[40] Dandruff flakes often appear around a hair shaft due to the epithelial growth at the base of the hair. The hair restricts the elimination of sloughed keratin, creating a visible scale.

Table 2. Distinguishing Features of Dandruff, Seborrhea, and Psoriasis

Characteristic	Dandruff	Seborrhea	Psoriasis
Location	Scalp	Scalp and other areas of the body, e.g., axilla.	Scalp and other areas of the body, particularly those prone to stress (the folds of the elbows and knees, scalp, and face).
Influence of external factors	Generally a stable condition, does not fluctuate from week to week.	Influenced by many external factors, notably stress.	Influenced by irritation and other external stress.
Inflammation	Absent	Present	Present
Epidermal hyperplasia	Absent	Present	Present
Epidermal kinetics	Turnover rate is two times faster than normal.[a]	Turnover rate is about five to six times faster than normal.[a]	Turnover rate is about five to six times faster than normal.[a]
Percentage of parakeratotic cells	Rarely exceeds 5% of total corneocyte count.[b]	Commonly makes up 15–25% of corneocyte count.[b]	Commonly makes up 40–60% of corneocyte count.[a]

[a] Adapted from K. J. McGinley *et al.*, *J. Invest. Dermatol.*, **53**, 107(1969).
[b] Adapted from A. M. Kligman *et al.*, *J. Soc. Cosmet. Chem.*, **25**, 73(1974).

There seems to be only one major manifestation of dandruff—scaling. The visible scaling is a result of an increased rate of horny substance production on the scalp and the sloughing of large scales (squamae). Although epidermal turnover is normally greater on the scalp than on the rest of the body, in the dandruff patient it is even greater. Dandruff flakes appear white due to the presence of air in the clefts between the cellular fragments. This does not occur in the normal condition, because the horny substance breaks up in a much more uniform fashion.[32] The breakup pattern of the scalp horny layer is important to the visibility of the resulting flake. Scalp horny layer in normal individuals consists of 25 to 35 fully keratinized, closely coherent cells arranged in an orderly fashion. However, in dandruff, the intact horny layer usually has fewer than 10 cells, and nonkeratinized cells are common. With dandruff, crevices occur deep in the stratum corneum, resulting in cracking which generates large flakes. If the large clumps or flakes can be broken down to smaller units, the visibility of dandruff decreases. Thus, dandruff is characterized by accelerated epidermopoiesis, an irregular breakup pattern of the horny layer, and the shedding of cells in large flakes.

Dandruff vs. psoriasis and seborrhea capitis

The principal skin conditions that exhibit symptoms similar to dandruff are psoriasis and seborrhea capitis. All of these conditions involve an accelerated rate of keratin production, but psoriasis and seborrhea are distinctly different from dandruff. Many people consider dandruff an extension or mild form of seborrhea, but evidence shows this to be untrue.[35] Fortunately, an incorrect diagnosis between these conditions or no diagnostic distinction is not serious because the agents used to treat all of these conditions are similar, except in severe cases.

The rate of epidermal cell turnover in the dandruff patient is about twice that of normal individuals but is significantly less than that found in either psoriasis or seborrhea.[32] As the rate of keratin cell turnover increases, the number of incompletely keratinized cells (parakeratotic cells) increases. Parakeratosis is characterized by retention of nuclei in cells of the keratin layer. The number of these cells is a distinguishing factor between dandruff, psoriasis, and seborrhea. There are more in the dandruff condition than on normal scalps and even more in seborrhea and psoriasis. Parakeratotic cells in dandruff appear in clusters. This has been explained as a result of tiny foci of inflammation which are incited when capillaries squirt a load of inflammatory cells into the epidermis, resulting in accelerated growth of epidermis in a small area.[41] These microfoci are found in all scalps but are proportionately increased in dandruff.

The specific cause of this accelerated growth is unknown, but clearly, it is not as a result of micro-organisms. For many years, it was assumed that elevated levels of micro-organisms, particularly the yeast *Pityrosporon ovale*, on the scalp of dandruff patients were the cause.[37,42] The presence of these organisms does not lead to dandruff. The elimination of the organisms does not influence the dandruff; their accelerated growth occurs as a result of the dandruff condition which provides a favorable medium for growth.

Some observations or misconceptions regarding dandruff have recently been explained:[35]

- ☐ Dandruff is seasonal; it is mild in the summer months and most severe from October through December.
- ☐ Unlike seborrhea and psoriasis, dandruff is uniform and diffuse. Patchiness probably results from hair styles and brushing, which dislodge adherent flakes.
- ☐ Poor hygiene does not cause dandruff in a nondandruff patient, but it exacerbates existing symptoms.
- ☐ Dandruff is a very stable process and is not subject to sudden shifts in severity from week to week. It is less subject to outside stress than psoriasis and seborrhea.

Table 2 lists distinguishing features of dandruff, seborrhea, and psoriasis. In addition to these rather general differences, there are more elaborate cytologic differences.[43] For the pharmacist without access to extensive laboratory diagnostic aids, the site of the condition, the influence of external factors, and the overall severity of the condition are often useful in distinguishing the conditions.

Treatment of dandruff

There is no cure for dandruff, only control of the condition. Total removal of hair eliminates the dandruff condition. This is obviously a rather drastic approach to treatment and generally is unacceptable. Other approaches are available which decrease visible dandruff. At least four methods are used to reduce the visible flaking of dandruff:

- ☐ Using a keratolytic agent to dissolve dandruff flakes. Traditional keratolytic agents such as salicylic acid and sulfur are used in dandruff products to dissolve or lyse keratin and facilitate its removal from the scalp in smaller particles.
- ☐ Cleaning the hair and scalp frequently. Shampooing the hair and scalp at short intervals, perhaps daily, should control most forms of dandruff.
- ☐ Using cytostatic agents, e.g., selenium sulfide and zinc pyrithione, that reduce the rate of epidermal turnover.
- ☐ Dispersing the scales into smaller subunits so that they are less visible. Several agents such as detergents, chelating agents, and perhaps coal tar are used.

Some agents in OTC dandruff products possess antibacterial and antifungal activity. The antibacterial/antifungal approach to the control of dandruff is used because of the abnormally elevated flora in the dandruff patient. However, reduction of microbial count does not reduce dandruff unless these agents have a surface-active effect to disperse scales or reduce dandruff in another manner. The questionable statement "to prevent secondary infections" is not altogether acceptable as a rationale for inclusion of these agents.

Ingredients in OTC products for dandruff

Keratolytics. There are many types of keratolytic agents, many of which have distinctly different modes of action. For example, resorcinol is presumed to act as a keratolytic by its irritant effect which causes vesicle formation in the stratum corneum. Sulfur is believed to function by an inflammatory process, causing increased sloughing of cells. The keratolytic action of salicylic acid may be caused by lowering the pH of the skin, causing increased hydration of keratin, thus facilitating its loosening and removal.

Vehicle composition, time of contact, and concentration are important considerations to the success of a keratolytic. Strokosch[44-47] has shown that salicylic acid functions best as a keratolytic when used in an O/W emulsion base; sulfur shows its best activity in a non-emulsion base. Contact time is minimal in a shampoo; significant absorption/adsorption of the agent by the skin cannot occur during the brief period of contact while shampooing. Ointments which are applied a few times daily and left on are naturally much more effective. Salicylic acid at a concentration of 10 to 15 percent showed a keratolytic effect in 2 to 3 days, 3- to 5-percent concentrations in 3 days, and 1-percent concentrations took several days. "It is doubtful whether salicylic acid incorporated in the usual concentrations of 1-2% in pastes and ointments significantly impairs the normal barrier by its keratolytic action. It may, however, have a greater keratolytic effect on the abnormal parakeratotic stratum corneum."[48] Sulfur behaved in a similar manner. A 10- to 20-percent concentration is keratolytic after 1 or 2 days, 5 percent in 3 days, 3 percent in 7 days, and 1 percent in 10 days. Ointments and pastes are difficult to use on the hairy scalp and thus, aqueous and alcoholic preparations are preferable.

Keratolytic agents have a primary irritant effect, particularly on mucous membranes and the conjunctiva of the eye. They have the potential of acting on hair keratin as well as skin keratin, and hair appearance may suffer as a result. Toxic manifestations after application of resorcinol to abraded skin have been reported.[49,50]

Soaps and detergents. Vigorous washing of the scalp with a bland shampoo eliminates visible dandruff scale.[35] The frequency of shampooing to keep scurf under control is not fixed; the intervals become shorter as the severity of dandruff increases. Many bland shampoos leave a detergent residue on the scalp which perhaps interrupts the structure of the lipid-horny cell layer at the surface of the keratin layer. This causes subsequent sloughing of keratin to be in smaller, less visible subunits.

Cytostatic agents. Using cytostatic agents is the most direct approach to controlling dandruff. By increasing the time necessary for epidermal turnover, it is possible to bring about a dramatic decline in visible scurf. Selenium sulfide and zinc pyrithione at concentrations of 1 to 2 percent significantly reduce the rate of cell turnover. This cytostatic activity is not restricted to conditions where the rate of epidermal turnover is great but is also observed in normal skin, where application of these compounds proportionately lengthens turnover time. Kligman *et al.*[35,40] consider zinc pyrithione a slower acting agent than selenium sulfide, but the comparison involved 2.5 percent selenium sulfide, a concentration requiring a prescription, and 2 percent zinc pyrithione, an OTC product. Both products, at OTC concentrations, are effective in controlling dandruff.

The relative effectiveness of selenium sulfide and zinc pyrithione can be influenced by a number of factors. Okumura *et al.*[51] have shown that zinc pyrithione is strongly bound to both hair and skin and that the extent of binding correlates with clinical performance. Adsorption of this agent increases with increased contact time, increased temperature, increased concentration, and frequent application. Zinc pyrithione is bound to the external layers of skin and does not penetrate into the dermal region. The toxicity of these agents seems minimal, although burning of the skin, particularly under the fingernails, and some cases of conjunctivitis have been noted with selenium sulfide. Naturally, these agents should not be used on broken or abraded skin.

Dispersing agents. Dispersing the scales into smaller subunits decreases their visibility.[35] This can occur with detergents e.g., sodium lauryl sulfate. Kligman *et al.*[35] speculate that tars were ancient dandruff medications that depended on dispersion for their activity. Coal tars are traditional dermatologic agents, but they have undesirable side effects such as photosensitivity and retardation of wound healing. Coal tar products should probably not be recommended for dandruff unless the condition is refractory. The value of antiseptics such as quaternary ammonium compounds (QAC) in dandruff may be due more to dispersion of the flakes than to other activity. QAC's are known surface-active agents and can function in this capacity to reduce the size of the horny scale.

It seems that for mild forms of dandruff, simple washing with a bland shampoo at frequent intervals controls excess scaling. For more serious dandruff conditions, cytostatic agents such as selenium sulfide or zinc pyrithione can be used. The activity of medicated products increases with longer contact times; if shampoos are used, they should be left on the scalp for 5 to 10 minutes before rinsing. Because soaps and other components of medicated products can act as a "glue" to join together small flakes to make larger, more visible ones, it is important to rinse the hair thoroughly after shampooing.[35]

Seborrhea

Seborrheic dermatitis is a general term for a group of eruptions that occur predominantly in the area of greatest sebaceous gland activity. The most common form is seborrhea capitis which is characterized by greasy scales on the scalp, frequently extending to the middle one-third of the face with subsequent eye involvement. The distinctive characteristics of seborrhea are its common occurrence in the hairy skin, specifically the scalp, the appearance of the lesions which are well demarcated and are dull yellowish red, and the associated presence of greasy scales.[52]

Etiology

The cause of seborrhea is unknown. The characteristic accelerated cell turnover and enhanced sebaceous gland activity give rise to the prominent scale displayed in the condition, although there is not a quantitative relationship between the degree of sebaceous gland activity and susceptibility to seborrhea. Hence, predisposing factors are complex. It is almost universally accepted that seborrhea capitis is merely an extension of dandruff. Kligman *et al.*[35] dissent from this view offering evidence that seborrhea is a separate condition from simple dandruff. For example, they point out that the nucleocytes (parakeratotic cells) commonly make up 15 to 25 percent of the corneocyte count in seborrhea dermatitis but rarely exceed 5 percent in dandruff. This and other distinguishing features of the two conditions are shown in Table 2.

Differential diagnosis and treatment

Fortunately, misdiagnosis of the seborrhea condition as dandruff is not of great consequence because they both involve accelerated epidermal turnover with scaling as the principal manifestation. Hence, treatment is generally the same in both cases. However, some aspects of seborrhea capitis are worth noting. Dandruff is considered a relatively stable condition whereas seborrhea fluctuates in severity, often as a result of stress. Involvement of eyebrows and eyelashes with associated eyelid problems such as blepharitis is common in seborrhea but not in dandruff. Special precautions for eyelid involvement require control of the scalp condition as well as specific ophthalmic agents.

Psoriasis

Psoriasis accounts for approximately 5 percent of all visits to dermatologists in the U.S.[52] It is a chronic, sometimes acute, relapsing papulosquamous disease of the skin, characterized by well-defined, pink or dull red lesions covered with silvery scales.[52 53] The edge of the lesion is sharply delineated, and gentle scraping of the lesion will produce micalike scales. Psoriatic lesions have a marked predilection for certain areas of the body such as the scalp, the folds of the elbows and knees, and the genitoanal region. The condition is unpredictable in its course but has a tendency to be chronic.

Pathophysiology

It is generally accepted that there is a genetically determined predisposition to psoriasis because in more than one-fourth of the psoriatic patients, there is an associated family history. No age is exempt from the condition, and most cases develop between the ages of 10 and 50. It is rarely found in Negroes, Japanese, and American Indians. It is distributed almost equally between men and women.[54]

Skin in the psoriatic plaque is characterized by accelerated epidermopoiesis, proliferation of capillaries in the dermal region, extensive infolding of the epidermal-dermal junction, and invasion of the epidermis by polymorphonuclear leukocytes.[52] The greatly expanded surface area of the epidermal-dermal junction by infolding and the presence of two or three basal cell layers lead to a greatly exaggerated mitotic growth and epidermal thickness. Normal epidermal turnover is 25 to 30 days; in psoriatic plaque skin, it is 3 to 4 days or less.[54] At this rapid rate, the keratin produced has many parakeratotic cells, and the granular layer is absent in severe cases.

The specific biochemical event triggering formation of the psoriatic skin is unknown. It is possible that cyclic adenosine 3′,5′-monophosphate (cAMP) mediates the regulation of epidermal proliferation and that there may be a defect in the adenylcyclase-cAMP system in psoriatic skin.[55-57]

Psoriatic lesions frequently develop in sites of vaccination, scratch marks, surgical incisions, or in skin test sites and have been reported to be produced by shock and noise. In fact, the response to skin trauma is so predictable (Kobner's phenomenon) that it can be used in diagnosis. For example, when scaling is not evident, making diagnosis difficult, scales can be induced by light scratching. Endocrine factors have also been frequently implicated in psoriasis. The condition often improves or clears during pregnancy but may reappear after parturition.

Acute guttata psoriasis attacks often occur at puberty or following childbirth. This condition, which is characterized by many small lesions more or less distributed over the body, accounts for about 17 percent of psoriatic patients. A variety of systemic illnesses have precipitated psoriatic attacks. For example, the onset of psoriasis in children commonly follows a streptococcal tonsillitis. Hot weather and sunlight cause an improvement in the condition, and cold weather causes a considerable worsening.

Psoriasis in children is usually of the guttata variety. When these small lesions coalesce they form large characteristic plaques. "Pustular psoriasis," which may or may not be a form of psoriasis, is localized on the palms and soles. Pitting of the nails is a common characteristic of psoriasis and can frequently be used as a diagnostic aid.

The duration of psoriasis is variable. A lesion may last a lifetime or it could disappear quickly. The course of the disease is marked by spontaneous exacerbations and remissions. When the psoriatic condition is initiated by a guttata attack, the disease carries a better prognosis than that of a slower and more diffuse onset. When lesions disappear they may leave the skin hypo- or hyperpigmented.

A relationship exists between psoriasis and inflammatory polyarthritis (distinguished from rheumatoid arthritis by its onset), which is usually subacute and occurs in only one joint. Approximately 4 percent of all patients with polyarthritis also have psoriasis, with the skin manifestation of psoriasis preceeding the arthritis by many years. A more telling statistic is that psoriasis is found in the families of 40 percent of polyarthritis patients. The cause of this relationship is unknown, but there is a difference in the time course of psoriasis between patients with and without polyarthritis. For example, psoriasis of the nails occurs in 80 to 90 percent of patients with arthritis as compared to 30 to 40 percent in patients without arthritis.[52]

Differential diagnosis

Diagnosis usually is straightforward for simple psoriasis. Sites of involvement, the dry silvery appearance of the scale, and a small area of bleeding (Auspitz sign) after removal of the scales are characteristic. The bleeding puncta is the top of the capillary loop in the skin. Precipitating factors such as a recent vaccination, disease, pregnancy, trauma, etc., are useful factors in a preliminary diagnosis. However, other diseases can be confused with the psoriatic condition.

When the scalp or the flexural and intertriginous areas are involved, it is necessary to differentiate psoriasis from seborrhea and moniliasis. Psoriasis of the scalp generally produces dry, patchy adherent scales; seborrhea is usually a yellowish, oily scale (seborrhea oleosa) and tends to be more diffuse. If lesions are present in the groin, axilla, and inframammary region, diagnosis based on visual inspection can be difficult. Identification of the fungal organism from lesion scrapings proves the presence or absence of moniliasis. Distinguishing between seborrhea and psoriasis can sometimes be done on the basis of the scale color and appearance. In psoriasis, the plaque has a full, rich, red color with a particular depth of hue and opacity not normally seen in eczema and seborrhea. In dark-skinned races this color quality is lost. More elaborate histologic and pathologic techniques are available for a more precise diagnosis.[58-60]

Localized neurodermatitis, particularly in the genitoanal regions, may be confused with psoriatic lesions. In addition, circular or annular lesions of fungus conditions are easily confused with psoriatic lesions. In some individuals, psoriasis alternates with or is complicated by other diseases, such as seborrhea, making diagnosis much more difficult.

Treatment of psoriasis

Many patients are helped by very simple measures whereas others are refractory to the most formidable treatment. More potent agents to treat psoriasis should not be used until they are deemed necessary. A simple case of psoriasis may become worse and may lead to general exfoliative dermatitis, in which a general erythematous scale, covering the entire body, develops. For example, if the onset of a psoriatic condition is acute and the lesions are severely erythematous, local therapy should be soothing and nonirritating. A bland, nonmedicated cream should be used; as the acute process subsides and, in most patients, the usual thick-scaled plaques appear, more potent medication such as keratolytics can be used.

It is recommended that the plaque in psoriasis be removed or that an occlusive bandage be applied prior to application of a medicinal agent. The concern is that penetration of substances through the thick plaque is impeded unless the area is abraded or occluded. There is significant improvement in therapy when the plaque is removed prior to therapy or when occlusive covering of the drug is used. Psoriatic skin loses water 8 to 10 times faster than normal. In fact, when large areas of the body surface are involved, whole body skin water loss may be as much as 2 to 3 liters daily, in addition to normal perspiration loss. Evaporation of this volume of water requires over 1,000 cal, and thus, psoriatic patients may show increased metabolic rates and are prone to GI ulcer formation.

Psoriatic skin is more permeable to many substances than normal skin. It is expected that the barrier that normally prevents drug penetration through skin is disrupted in psoriasis, causing rapid drug entrance. There is a rapid response of this disorder to local treatment in the early stages and then a slowing of the rate of improvement as the skin barrier approaches normalcy.

The most direct approach to treating psoriasis is to reduce epidermal activity through the use of cytostatic agents such as topically applied corticosteroids and systemically administered methotrexate. These are prescription-only drugs. Systemically administered corticosteroids are usually contraindicated in all but the most severe forms of psoriasis. In addition to the normal side effects of corticosteroids, high doses cause an involution of the condition, but upon cessation of therapy, the disease is likely to be worse than it was initially.[53] The serious potential side effects and toxicity of methotrexate therapy are well known. Strict supervision of patients on methotrexate, including frequent blood analysis and regular liver biopsy, is essential.[61]

Ingredients in topical OTC products for psoriasis

Keratolytics. Salicylic acid (2 to 10 percent) is commonly used for psoriasis. Because it is an irritant, there is concern about worsening of the psoriatic condition. Salicylic acid in concentrations of 0.5 to 10 percent in a petroleum jelly base does not affect the rate of proliferation of psoriatic epidermal cells.[62] Keratolytics should be applied at low concentration initially, increasing the dose as the patient demonstrates a tolerance for the lower doses.

Tar products. As with many dermatologic diseases, there is a significant improvement in psoriatic skin conditions during the summer months, especially during periods without stress. In 1925, Goeckerman [63] introduced tar and U.V. light therapy for psoriasis. In order to enhance the beneficial effects of the light, crude coal tar was applied. For many years the therapeutic response with this form of therapy was believed to be caused by phototoxicity, but this theory has been challenged.[64, 65] U.V. light alone may be helpful for the condition, but the activity is significantly enhanced with coal tar. The combination is better than either agent alone. Some patients show a worsening of the condition when exposed to coal tar products.

Combinations of coal tar and keratolytics also are used. Many patients respond to salicylic acid (2 percent) and coal tar extract (10 percent) in cream or ointment form, applied several times daily. Similar therapy is the application of keratolytics during the day and coal tar at night. Bathing in coal tar or using a tar soap may be effective. The psychological component of therapy (attitude and belief in a particular agent) is important and should be considered.

Others. Ammoniated mercury with or without a keratolytic has been used. Its beneficial effect is doubtful, and its propensity toward causing sensitivity and potential systemic toxicity should seriously restrict its use.

Occlusion with a plastic film reduces the metabolic rate of skin and allows reformation of the granular layer in the psoriatic plaque.

Anthralin (dithranol) is an effective topical agent but has considerable burning and staining properties. A derivative of anthralin, triacetoxyanthracene, lacks the burning and staining effects of anthralin but is less effective.

Application of colchicine (1 percent) in hydrophilic ointment for several weeks has been tried. This is still an experimental approach, but the preliminary results are encouraging.[66]

Ingredients in internal OTC products for psoriasis

Antihistamines. The attendant pruritus of psoriasis may be alleviated with systemically administered antihistamines. The sedation properties of antihistamines also are useful where an associated emotional factor is involved. Because of this, some patients respond to tranquilizers in small doses or sedatives such as phenobarbital. Topical application of antihistamines is of questionable value.

Vitamin A. Vitamin A is believed to be involved in epidermal activity, but the consensus is that vitamin A is ineffective in the psoriatic condition. Preliminary results on topically applied tretinoin (vitamin A acid) are encouraging, but additional work is needed.

Other ingredients. Cyanocobalamin has been found to be generally ineffective. Vitamin D helps in cases complicated by hypocalcemia.

It has been customary for some physicians to recommend special diets for psoriatic patients, but this has not proved to be of benefit. The major point in diet control was to lower the cholesterol level, which is altered in many psoriatic patients. Other diet modifications included low protein and low tryptophan.

Summary

In summary, treatment of psoriasis, after proper diagnosis, should be initiated in a conservative manner, with the more potent agents reserved for situations where the condition does not respond. There is no cure for psoriasis, only a reduction in the severity of the condition. There is consensus that "guerrilla tactics are better than a frontal assault," with the more powerful agents held in reserve.[52] The following approach is suggested, keeping in mind that in eruptive or unstable forms of the disease, even mild sunlight may provoke a Kobner-type exacerbation:

- ☐ Discussion with the patient as to the nature of the condition so as to lead to a general acceptance of the disease. This may reduce stress or emotional instability.
- ☐ Rest, mild sedation, and simple local measures such as sunlight (U.V. light) and mild keratolytic products. The U.V. light should be used in suberythemal doses.

□ Tar products and weak topical corticosteroids in combination with U.V. light.

Corticosteroids, such as hydrocortisone, have a significant suppressive effect on psoriasis, but the danger of rebound limits their use. Other concerns with this form of therapy, in addition to systemic absorption of these potent steroids, are local atrophy which may result from prolonged use of these agents as well as reduction in tolerance to other agents. Relapse occurs more quickly after topical corticosteroids than after tar or anthralin therapy.

Eczema

The term "eczema" was formerly used for a large group of skin disorders of unknown etiology, many of which are now called by more specific names. When the cause of a particular skin condition was elucidated, the disease was given a different name, and the eczema nomenclature was dropped or modified.

"Eczema" is synonymous with dermatitis and eczematous dermatitis, and it may be considered a noninfectious, inflammatory dermatosis in which the affected skin is erythematous. It is a pattern of skin manifestations rather than a specific disease. The symptoms may include papules, vesicles, edema, and patches. Because pruritus generally accompanies the condition, excoriations, crusting, and secondary infections often occur as sequelae to the condition.[67] Eczema is, therefore, a symptom. At times, the eczematous condition resembles an inflammatory response. In fact, most dermatologists would accept the definition of eczema as "skin inflammation from whatever cause."

Eczema can be either acute or chronic. The clinical appearance of acute eczema is characterized by erythema, weeping, and vesicles; chronic symptoms are usually dry, thick, and very itchy skin. The main symptoms of eczema are pruritus and weeping of the skin. The itching may convert to pain over time, and the weeping may diminish, giving way to a scaly condition; at no time does the epidermal tissue appear normal. In the acute stages of eczema there is a uniform pattern of papular vesicles on an erythematous base. In the chronic form, the weeping is absent, but epidermal thickening and scaling are present.

Table 3. Abbreviated Classification of Eczema

Exogenous	Endogenous
Allergic dermatitis	Asteatotic eczema
Infective dermatitis	Atopic eczema
Irritant dermatitis	Hypostatic eczema
	Neurodermatitis
	Pityriasis alba
	Recurrent summer pompholyx
	Seborrheic eczema

Eczema is precipitated by external sources (exogenous) or by internal ones (endogenous) (Table 3).

Etiology of eczema

Exogenously induced eczema

The conditions of exogenously induced eczema are grouped under the general heading of contact dermatitis. The offending substance can irritate the skin upon first or multiple exposure or it can generate an allergic response. In either case, the result is an inflammatory response from the skin.

Irritant dermatitis. Application of a strong acid or base to the cutaneous surface of the skin causes irritation and a subsequent inflammatory reaction. However, there are many agents with a propensity to irritate. A primary irritant elicits a response in the majority of the population upon first exposure; secondary irritants cause an inflammatory response only if certain ancillary circumstances are met or if application of the agent is repeated.

The symptoms of irritant-induced contact dermatitis range from mild reddening, or erythema, accompanied by pruritus to actual necrosis and ulceration of the skin. Primary irritants cause pruritic erythema or perhaps ulceration; secondary irritants, which frequently generate a low-grade inflammation for a long period, tend to produce symptoms more closely related to chronic eczema (Table 4).

Table 4. Exogenously Induced Eczema

Characteristic	Weak or secondary irritant dermatitis[a]	Irritant dermatitis[b]	Allergic dermatitis[c]
Mechanism	Abrasion, desiccation, trauma, dryness, soreness, and fissuring precede eruption.	Direct insult to tissue. No preceding dryness or fissuring.	Immunological. Initial contact sensitizes, subsequent contact elicits a response. No preceding eruption.
Onset	Slow, over days, months, or years.	Sudden, response in 30 min to several days after exposure.	Sudden, response in 24–48 hours after exposure.
Symptoms	Hyperkeratosis, erythema, vesicles, and fissuring.	Erythema, vesicles, exudation, and sometimes necrosis.	Erythema, vesicles, edema, and necrosis.
Usual location	Hands	Hands	Hands and face
Patch test	Negative	Positive	Positive

[a]Cumulative insults are required.

[b]Single exposure to an offending agent.

[c]Multiple exposures are usually required.

In general, the factors influencing the development of skin irritation are the substance, climate, and the host.

The substance. Substances that can penetrate into and/or remain in the epidermis are irritating at a much lower concentration than those which cannot. The epidermis does not possess a vascular or lymphatic supply, and in order for a substance to be irritating to the skin, it would require penetration to the dermal area. The irritant property of camphor, menthol, coal tar, resorcinol, etc., is well known, but whether or not they function as primary or secondary irritants is a function of their concentration. With some substances, such as camphor, very high concentrations usually are needed to produce irritation to the intact skin, and there is no apparent buildup on the skin. Some of the coal tars, however, are very irritating at relatively low levels. Agents such as bithionol and hexachlorophene are bound to the epidermal layer, and repeated application can cause irritation. Thus, the degree of skin irritation from an applied substance is a function of the intrinsic irritation potential of the test material, its concentration, and its ability to remain bound to the skin.

Climate. The climate is important to the development of skin irritation. The microclimate depends on whether the skin is occluded or left open to the atmosphere. Occlusion causes the skin to become more hydrated and allows penetration of more of the irritating substance faster. The macroclimate refers to environmental conditions and their influence on the skin. Apparently, humidity conditions play a large role in the texture of the skin and its resistance to irritating substances.

The host. The biologic variability of human subjects to irritational insult is well known, but the cause of this is unknown. Aged skin is less prone to irritation than youthful skin, presumably because of the greater difficulty in drug penetration through aged skin. It has also been suggested that darker skinned races, in general, are less susceptible than the lighter skinned races to skin irritation, although the evidence for this is scant.

Concomitant administration of more than one substance plays a large role in skin irritation. A secondary irritant may not be irritating to the skin when applied alone but may show irritation when combined with an agent that promotes absorption, such as a surface-active agent. Damaged skin also encourages skin irritation.

Allergic dermatitis. An allergic reaction follows the combination of the tissues of antibodies or specifically primed cells (in the delayed type of reaction) with a specific antigen. Under normal circumstances, when an antigen or foreign substance enters the body, the body responds by producing a countersubstance, called an antibody. This antibody appears in the bloodstream to neutralize the antigen against which it was made.

In allergic individuals the antibody not only attaches itself to the antigen but also fixes itself to various tissues in the body such as the skin. The tissue to which a sensitizing antibody is attached becomes allergic, and subsequent exposure to the antigen causes an inflammatory response. With most allergens, only a small percentage of the population will become sensitized, even though a large population may have been exposed to the same allergen under the same conditions. This is suggestive of a kind of genetic predisposition or hereditary preparedness.

Some individuals react abnormally, with appropriate skin manifestations, to common substances such as mushrooms, strawberries, or shellfish, but the changes do not appear to be mediated by antibodies or delayed sensitivity, and they usually occur upon first exposure to the substance. Such changes are not allergic but are idiosyncrasies caused by an intrinsic factor or a defect in the tissues.

Allergic reactions are classified as immediate (anaphylactic), intermediate (Arthus), cytotoxic, and delayed (tuberculin) (Table 5).

Immediate (anaphylactic) reaction. In this case the antibody sensitizes the tissue cells passively. Administration of exogenous antigen reaches the sensitized cells, causing cell injury and release of pharmacologic agents. These agents cause further local changes, which usually include contraction of smooth muscle, increased vascular permeability, and edema. The cell injury from this type of reaction is transient, and most of the cells recover. Antihistamines suppress or modify the tissue changes in species of animals in which histamine is the most active pharmacologic agent. They do not prevent the reaction of antibody with the antigen but will prevent the release of histamine if given prophylactically.

Atopic dermatitis or eczema is sometimes associated incorrectly with anaphylactic allergy. Affected individuals show positive skin tests and develop allergic signs after exposure. However, normal treatment for allergy such as avoiding contact with allergen and administration of antihistaminic drugs seldom brings relief.

Intermediate (Arthus) reaction. In this reaction the antigen combines with the antibody in tissue spaces or in the circulation to produce a type of complex. The complex causes secondary changes to the tissue, depending on concentration and composition. The main change is massive infiltration of the extravascular tissues which usually occurs 2 to 4 hours after administration of the antigen. Administration of corticosteroids suppresses full development of the Arthus reaction.

Cytotoxic reaction. A cytotoxic reaction is one in which cells are damaged. In the allergic classification, it is restricted to cell damage caused by delayed sensitivity that is specific for the antigen in the susceptible target cell. The lysis of red cells by antibodies specified for the red cells is an example of reaction of an antibody to an antigen acquired by the cell. The cell that has adsorbed the antigen is usually damaged.

Delayed (tuberculin) reaction. This type of reaction takes a number of hours to reach a maximum response and occurs in the absence of demonstrable globulin antibody. The lesion produced is a diffuse reaction characterized by accumulation of fluid (edema). The allergic response may be inhibited by corticosteroids but is not altered by antihistamines.

The essential features of the delayed sensitivity reaction are its mediation by cells only and its passive transfer to normal subjects by cells only. No circulating antibodies can be detected. Allergic contact dermatitis can manifest different types of skin symptoms, some of which do not respond equally to the same drug therapy.

Infective dermatitis. Infective dermatitis is a skin condition caused by the presence of micro-organism toxins, not by the specific pathogenic activity of the organism. A satisfactory mechanism of action for this type of eczema has not been established, but it is known that inoculation of the skin of susceptible individuals with a bacterial culture or filtrate will produce an eczematous condition. It is presumed that bacterial toxins or antigens elicit the unfavorable response. The condition responds favorably to systemic antibiotics.

Endogenously induced eczema

Atopic eczema. This skin disease occurs primarily during childhood and early adulthood. It may begin shortly after birth and last many years or it may last only a year or two and disappear. The symptoms are erythema, scaling, and weeping, accompanied by severe pruritus. Unfortunately, secondary or associated infections are common, making diagnosis and treatment difficult. The etiology of the condition is unknown, but patients often have associated asthma or hay fever. Skin sensitivity to a wide range of agents is common; thus, skin tests are not very beneficial as diagnostic aids.

Asteatotic eczema. This eczema is characterized by dry and fissured skin and by scantiness or absence of the sebaceous secretions. It occurs mainly during the dry winter weather and in the aged.

Neurodermatitis. This is a chronic form of eczema found more often in women. It is often localized in the nape of the neck, legs, genitoanal region, and forearms. The areas of involvement are highly lichenified and become worse when continually rubbed or scratched. Emotional stress plays a role in this condition.[68]

Exogenous vs. endogenous eczema

Differentiation between endogenous and contact patterns of eczema are very important to initiate proper therapy. In most cases of contact dermatitis, an accurate diagnosis is readily made on the basis of the eczematous character, configuration, and location of the rash and itching. Eczema of the backs and sides of the fingers and hands, eyelids, genitoanal region, wrists, forearm, and feet is suggestive of the contact eczema. Occupational and leisure activities and family history are also useful diagnostic aids as well as recently used topical medicaments and cosmetics.[69–71]

In some cases of eczema (especially eruptions of the hands) there is a mixture of infectious eczematoid, atopic, and contact dermatitides. With contact dermatitis, once the skin reacts to one substance, it may be more vulnerable to other substances, making diagnosis and treatment more complicated. Allergic or primary irritant dermatitis may be a secondary eruption caused by an agent used in therapy, complicating one of the other forms of eczema.

The duration of the eruption can also be helpful. For example, atopic dermatitis lasts for months or years; contact dermatitis does not.

Treatment of eczema

Therapy for eczema must be approached cautiously in order to prevent exacerbation of the condition. In some forms of eczema the patient is sensitive to a wide variety of agents, and therapeutic entities may aggravate already inflamed skin. The time element of therapy should be considered. In contact eczema, drug therapy is needed for only a short time because withdrawal of the allergen or irritant ameliorates the condition. However, in atopic and other forms of dermatitis, therapy is needed for long periods. Useful modes of therapy for neurodermatitis are tranquilizers, sedatives, and especially, counseling.

For most forms of eczema it is worthwhile to protect the lesions from clothing and fingernails, especially in small children. A bland dressing often helps without resorting to additional drugs.

Particularly in acute eczema, the patient should be instructed to avoid soap and water (or use sparingly), friction from wool and rough clothing, heavy exercise, known irritants and allergens, and self-testing to identify the allergen (in the case of suspected allergen).[72 73]

Ingredients in OTC products for eczema

Protectants. To protect small areas of eczematous skin, zinc oxide paste (Lassar's), zinc oxide ointment, or paste-impregnated bandages can be used. Some of these topical products are astringents as well as protectants. For larger areas, soaking in aluminum acetate solution or water reduces the weeping. Covering the lesions or applying a drug with an occlusive barrier increases the degree of maceration of tissue and can also prevent heat loss. This may contribute to discomfort of the affected area.

Cooling agents. Cooling of the skin surface reduces the extent of pruritus. In the acute phase of eczema, soothing lotions applied as wet compresses are helpful, but aromatic substances such as menthol and camphor should be used cautiously in order not to exacerbate the condition. The cooling effect of a lotion or emulsion that is applied infrequently is only transitory. Orally administered antihistamines may be used for their sedative and antipruritic effects. Topically administered antihistamines

Table 5. Types of Allergic Reactions in the Skin[a]

	Anaphylaxis	Arthus reaction	Cytotoxic reaction	Delayed
Response mediated by:	Sensitizing antibody	Precipitating antibody	Antibody or cell	Cell
Skin test	Immediate wheal or flare	Arthus reaction with polymorph infiltration, appearing in 2–4 hours but may progress to necrosis for hours or days.	Immediate wheal and flare; granulomatous lesions with or without polymorphs, first appearing in 2–6 hours.	Delayed, tuberculin response.
Clinical manifestation	Erythema	Serum sickness	Eczema	Eczema
Skin or vascular changes	Urticaria; angioneurotic edema.	Allergic vasculitis; nodular vasculitis.	Purpura; homograft rejection.	Contact dermatitis; homograft rejection.

[a]Adapted from W. E. Parrish, "An Introduction to the Biology of the Skin," Blackwell Scientific Publications, Oxford, England, 1970.

should not be recommended or used because of their questionable efficacy and their significant tendency to become sensitizers. Antihistamines and corticosteroids act prophylactically to prevent further inflammation. They have no effect on existing inflammation and hence, improvement in the condition should be evaluated accordingly.

Astringents. Astringency is sometimes needed to reduce the extent of weeping. Baths or local compresses (15 to 30 minutes each) a few times daily help dry the weeping areas. More potent astringents should be reserved until the erythemal inflammation of the acute phase subsides in order not to further aggravate the eczema. Calamine lotion and other powder-based substances that dry a weeping condition through water adsorption or astringency should be avoided because of their tendency to crust. Removal of the crusts causes bleeding and potential infections.

Antiseptics. Antiseptics are necessary in infective dermatitis but should be used cautiously in the more general forms of eczema. Many of these agents have considerable sensitizing and irritating potential, particularly when they are used chronically. For example, neomycin should not be used for maintenance treatment of hypostatic eczema or genitoanal eczema.[71]

Keratolytics. Keratolytics are usually avoided in eczema unless extensive lichenification has occurred. These agents and those that reduce the mitotic activity of the epidermis, such as tars and anthralin, should be used cautiously.

Summary: psoriasis and eczema

The causative mechanisms of psoriasis and most types of eczema are unknown or at best, speculative. Even without a precise mechanistic understanding, sophisticated analytical techniques are available so that pathologic changes in the skin can be described in great detail. This allows for a more rational approach to therapy, even though it is, in many respects, empirical. It is very important that patients suffering from these dermatologic problems have proper diagnosis before attempting treatment with home remedies or OTC preparations. Overtreatment or improper treatment can often exacerbate the condition. For example, pruritus is a constant feature of eczema and a counterirritant might be indicated; application of a counterirritant for psoriasis might greatly aggravate the condition, particularly in its early stages. These conditions should not be lumped together and treated symptomatically but should be diagnosed correctly and then treated. The pharmacist can perform a very valuable service in this regard by serving in an informed triage role.

References

1. I. H. Blank, *J. Invest. Dermatol.*, **18,** 433(1952).
2. D. Spruit and K. W. Malton, *J. Invest. Dermatol.*, **45,** 6(1965).
3. S. Monash and I. H. Blank, *Arch. Dermatol.*, **78,** 710(1958).
4. J. D. Middleton, *Br. J. Dermatol.*, **80,** 437(1968).
5. R. H. Scheuplein, *J. Invest. Dermatol.*, **45,** 334(1965).
6. I. H. Blank, *J. Invest. Dermatol.*, **21,** 259(1953).
7. A. M. Kligman, in "The Epidermis," W. Montagna and W. C. Lobitz, Jr., Eds., Academic Press, New York, N.Y., 1964.
8. B. Idson, *Drug Cosmet. Ind.*, **28-29,** 108-110(August, 1972).
9. O. K. Jacobi, *Proc. Sci. Sect. Toilet Goods Assoc.*, **31,** 22(1959).
10. K. Laden, *Am. Perfum. Cosmet.*, **82,** 77(1967).
11. S. J. Strianse, *Cosmet. Perfum.*, **89,** 57(1974).
12. J. Hattingh, *Acta Dermatoverner (Stockholm)*, **52,** 438(1972).
13. F. A. J. Thiele and K. von Sinden, *J. Invest. Dermatol.*, **47,** 307(1967).
14. R. H. Wildnaur *et al.*, *J. Invest. Dermatol.*, **56,** 72(1971).
15. J. D. Middleton and B. M. Allen, *J. Soc. Cosmet. Chem.*, **24,** 239(1973).
16. K. A. Grice, *J. Invest. Dermatol.*, **57,** 108(1971).
17. M. Mezei *et al.*, *J. Pharm. Sci.*, **55,** 584(1966).
18. H. Baker, *J. Invest. Dermatol.*, **50,** 283(1968).
19. J. D. Middleton, *J. Soc. Cosmet. Chem.*, **20,** 399(1969).
20. I. H. Blank and E. B. Shapiro, *J. Invest. Dermatol.*, **25,** 391(1955).
21. R. M. Handjani-Vila *et al.*, *Cosmet. Perfum.*, **90,** 39(1975).
22. R. L. Goldenberg, *Skin Allerg. News*, **5,** 20(1974).
23. R. L. Anderson *et al.*, *J. Invest. Dermatol.*, **61,** 375(1974).
24. G. Barnett, in "Cosmetics: Science and Technology," 2d ed., M. S. Balsam and E. Sagarin, Eds., Wiley and Sons, New York, N.Y., 1972.
25. G. K. Steigleder and W. P. Raab, *J. Invest. Dermatol.*, **38,** 129(1962).
26. E. A. Taylor, *J. Invest. Dermatol.*, **37,** 69(1961).
27. I. I. Lubowe, *West. Med.*, **1,** 45(1960).
28. E. M. Seiner *et al.*, *J. Am. Podiatr. Assoc.*, **63,** 571(1973).
29. S. Rothman, "Physiology and Biochemistry of the Skin," The University of Chicago Press, Chicago, Ill., 1954, p. 26.
30. H. Ashton *et al.*, *Br. J. Dermatol.*, **84,** 194(1971).
31. D. P. Nash, *J. Am. Podiatr. Assoc.*, **61,** 382(1971).
32. A. B. Ackerman and A. M. Kligman, *J. Soc. Cosmet. Chem.*, **20,** 81(1969).
33. T. Gersten, *Cosmet. Perfum.*, **90,** 36(1975).
34. G. Barker, *Cosmet. Perfum.*, **90,** 71(1975).
35. A. M. Kligman *et al.*, *J. Soc. Cosmet. Chem.*, **25,** 73(1974).
36. S. Bourne and A. Jacobs, *Br. Med. J.*, **1,** 1268(1956).
37. F. C. Roia and R. W. Vanderwyk, *J. Soc. Cosmet. Chem.*, **20,** 113(1969).
38. K. J. McGinley *et al.*, *J. Invest. Dermatol.*, **53,** 107(1969).
39. H. Goldschmidt and A. M. Kligman, *Arch. Dermatol.*, **88,** 709(1963).
40. G. Plewig and A. M. Kligman, *J. Soc. Cosmet. Chem.*, **20,** 767(1969).
41. A. M. Kligman, *Cosmet. Perfum.*, **90,** 16(1975).
42. F. C. Roia and R. W. Vanderwyk, *J. Soc. Cosmet. Chem.*, **15,** 761(1964).
43. H. Goldschmidt and M. A. Thew, *Arch. Dermatol.*, **106,** 476(1972).
44. E. Strokosch, *Arch. Dermatol. Syphilol.*, **47,** 16(1943).
45. E. Strokosch, *Arch. Dermatol. Syphilol.*, **47,** 216(1943).
46. E. Strokosch, *Arch. Dermatol. Syphilol.*, **48,** 384(1943).
47. E. Strokosch, *Arch. Dermatol. Syphilol.*, **48,** 393(1943).
48. "Textbook of Dermatology," vol. 1, 2d ed., A. Rook *et al.*, Eds., Blackwell Scientific Publications, London, England, 1972, p. 253.
49. A. Osol *et al.*, "United States Dispensatory and Physicians' Pharmacology," 26th ed., Lippincott, New York, N.Y., 1967.
50. K. W. Chesterman, *J. Am. Pharm. Assoc.*, **NS 12,** 576(1972).
51. T. Okumura *et al.*, *Cosmet. Perfum.*, **90,** 101(1975).
52. "Textbook of Dermatology," vol. 2, 2d ed., A. Rook *et al.*, Eds., Blackwell Scientific Publications, London, England, 1972, pp. 1192-1234.
53. G. M. Lewis and C. E. Wheeler, "Practical Dermatology," 3d ed., Saunders, Philadelphia, Pa., 1967, pp. 207-218.
54. G. Weinstein, *Br. J. Dermatol.*, **92,** 229(1975).
55. J. J. Voorhees and E. A. Duell, *Arch. Dermatol.*, **104,** 352(1971).
56. R. K. Wright *et al.*, *Arch. Dermatol.*, **104,** 352(1971).
57. M. M. Mui *et al.*, *Br. J. Dermatol.*, **92,** 255(1975).
58. "Dermal Pathology," J. H. Graham *et al.*, Eds., Harper and Row, New York, N.Y., 1972, pp. 325-332.
59. M. Gordon *et al.*, *Arch. Dermatol.*, **95,** 402(1967).
60. E. J. Van Scott and T. M. Ekel, *Arch. Dermatol.*, **88,** 373(1963).
61. L. E. King, Jr., *Arch. Dermatol.*, **111,** 131(1975).
62. H. Pullman *et al.*, *Arch. Dermatol. Forsch.*, **251,** 271(1975).
63. W. H. Goeckerman, *Northwest Med.*, **24,** 299(1925).
64. L. Tanenbaum *et al.*, *Arch. Dermatol.*, **111,** 467(1975).
65. L. Tanenbaum *et al.*, *Arch. Dermatol.*, **111,** 395(1975).
66. K. H. Kaidbey *et al.*, *Arch. Dermatol.*, **111,** 33(1975).
67. "Textbook of Dermatology," vol. 2, 2d ed., A. Rook *et al.*, Eds., Blackwell Scientific Publications, London, England, 1972, pp. 256-294.
68. H. Baker, *Br. Med. J.*, **4,** 544(1973).
69. D. Munro-Ashman, *Br. J. Clin. Pract.*, **17,** 537(1963).
70. L. Fry, *Update Int.*, **1,** 113(1974).
71. D. G. C. Presbury, *Update Int.*, **1,** 334(1974).
72. R. B. Stoughton, *Arch. Dermatol.*, **92,** 281(1965).
73. I. Sarkany, *Nurs. Times*, 1211-1212(September 20, 1971).

Product (manufacturer)	Application form	Keratin softener	Humectant	Other
Aquacare (Herbert)	cream lotion	urea, 2%	glycerin	oleth-3 phosphate, petrolatum, triethanolamine, synthetic spermaceti, carbomer 934P, mineral oil, lanolin alcohol, cetyl stearyl glycol, lanolin oil, benzyl alcohol, perfume
Aquacare/HP (Herbert)	cream lotion	urea, 10%	glycerin	oleth-3 phosphate, cetyl stearyl glycol, petrolatum, triethanolamine, synthetic spermaceti, carbomer 934P, mineral oil, lanolin alcohol, lanolin oil, benzyl alcohol, perfume
Carmol (Ingram)	cream	urea, 20%	—	nonlipid base
Carmol Ten (Ingram)	cream	urea, 10%	—	nonlipid base
Clocream Ointment (Upjohn)	ointment	—	—	vitamins A and D, vanishing cream base
Corn Huskers Lotion (Warner-Lambert)	—	—	glycerin, 6.7%	alcohol, 5.7%; sodium alginate; galactomannan
Emulave (Cooper)	soap	—	glycerin	vegetable oils and dewaxed lanolin, 25%; colloidal oatmeal, 30%
Jergens Direct Aid (Jergens)	lotion	allantoin	—	deionized water, sorbitol, stearic acid, coceth-6, glyceryl dilaurate, glyceryl stearate, lard glyceride, stearamide, hydrogenated vegetable oil, isopropyl palmitate, polyethylene glycol 100 stearate, dimethicone, petrolatum, sodium carbomer 941, fragrance, methylparaben, quaternium-15, propylparaben, simethicone
Jergens for Extra Dry Skin (Jergens)	lotion	allantoin	glycerin	deionized water, coceth-6, glyceryl dilaurate, lard glyceride, mineral oil, isopropyl palmitate, stearic acid, dimethicone, methylparaben, sodium carbomer 941, fragrance, propylparaben, quaternium-15, simethicone
Jergens Hand Cream (Jergens)	cream	allantoin	glycerin	deionized water, stearic acid, alcohol, potassium stearate, propylene glycol dipelargonate, fragrance, lanolin oil, tetrasodium dicarboxyethylstearyl sulfosuccinamate, potassium carbomer 934, methylparaben, polysorbate 81, simethicone, salicylic acid, cellulose gum, propylparaben
Jeri-Bath (Dermik)	oil	—	—	dewaxed oil-soluble fraction of lanolin, mineral oil, nonionic emulsifier
Jeri-Lotion (Dermik)	lotion	—	—	dewaxed oil-soluble fraction of lanolin, mineral oil, nonionic emulsifier
Lubriderm (Texas Pharmacal)	cream	—	glycerin	lanolin derivatives, cetyl alcohol, petrolatum blend
Lubriderm (Texas Pharmacal)	lotion	—	—	lanolin derivatives, mineral oil, sorbitol, cetyl alcohol, triethanolamine stearate
Nivea (Beiersdorf)	cream	—	glycerin, 3%	water, 68%; mineral oil, 17%; petrolatum, 4%; waxes, 3.7%; wool wax alcohol, 2%; fatty alcohol, 1%; aluminum stearate, 0.4%; magnesium stearate, 0.01%; magnesium sulfate, 0.55%; fragrance, 0.29%; formaldehyde, 0.05%
Nutraderm (Owen)	lotion cream	—	—	mineral oil, aliphatic alcohols, balanced emulsifiers
Nutraplus (Owen)	cream lotion	urea, 10%	—	glyceryl stearate, acetylated lanolin, alcohol, isopropyl palmitate
Nutraspa (Owen)	liquid	—	—	dewaxed fraction of lanolin, mineral oil, soapless surfactant
Oilatum Soap (Stiefel)	soap	—	—	polyunsaturated vegetable oil, 7.5%
Saratoga Ointment (Blair)	ointment	—	—	zinc oxide, 14%; boric acid, 1.75%; eucalyptol, 1.1%; servum preparatum; white petrolatum
Sardo (Plough)	bath oil	—	—	mineral oil, isopropyl myristate, isopropyl palmitate
Sardoettes (Plough)	towelettes	—	—	mineral oil, isopropyl myristate, isopropyl palmitate
Sayman Salve (Carson)	ointment	—	propylene gycol	petrolatum, zinc oxide, camphor, lanolin

Products 29 DRY SKIN

Product (manufacturer)	Application form	Keratin softener	Humectant	Other
Shepard's (Dermik)	lotion	—	—	sesame oil
Siliderm (C&M)	lotion	—	glycerin	silicone, nonsensitizing lanolin, purified water, perfume, sorbic acid
Sofenol (C&M)	lotion	—	glycerin	peanut oil, lanolin, cetyl alcohol, stearyl alcohol, purified water, perfume, triethanolamine stearate, sorbic acid
Tega E (Ortega)	cream	—	—	vitamin E, 50 IU/g; cream base
Thilene 4-M (Quality Products)	lotion	allantoin, 0.25%	—	cleansers, wetting agents, emulsifiers, dispersants
Tridenol (Spirt)	liquid	—	—	olive oil, vegetable oils, nonionic surfactant
Wibi (Owen)	lotion	—	—	emulsifying wax, polyglycols, alcohol, menthol, glycerol
Woodbury for Extra Dry Skin (Jergens)	lotion	allantoin	glycerin	deionized water, alcohol, mineral oil, triethanolamine stearate, stearyl alcohol, lanolin, hydrogenated vegetable oil, cetyl alcohol, sodium carbomer 941, methylparaben, polyparaben, fragrance

Products 29 DANDRUFF/SEBORRHEA

Product (manufacturer)	Application form	Keratolytic	Cytostatic agent	Other
Anti-Dandruff Brylcreem (Beecham Products)	shampoo	—	zinc pyrithione, 0.1%	mineral oil, propylene glycol, paraffin wax, water, excipients
Breck One (Breck)	cream lotion shampoo	—	zinc pyrithione, 1.0%	anionic surfactants, 15.6%
Dalex (Herbert)	shampoo	—	zinc pyrithione, 1%	surfactants
Dandricide Rinse (King)	rinse	—	—	isopropyl alcohol, benzalkonium chloride, lauryl isoquinolinium bromide, polysorbate 80, sorbitol
Dandricide Shampoo (King)	shampoo	—	—	triethanolamine, lauryl sulfate, propylene glycol, lauramid diethanolamine, sodium undecylenic monoethanolamidosulfosuccinate, laneth-10 acetate, linoleamide diethanolamine, hydrolyzed animal protein, imidazolidinylurea, methylparaben, propylparaben
Danex (Herbert)	shampoo	—	zinc pyrithione, 1.0%	sodium methyl cocoyl taurate, magnesium aluminum silicate, sodium cocoyl isethionate, citric acid, fragrance
Diasporal (Doak)	cream	colloidal sulfur, 3% salicylic acid, 2%	—	isopropyl alcohol, 95%
Fomac Cream Cleanser (Dermik)	cleanser	colloidal sulfur, 2% salicylic acid, 2%	—	soapless detergents
Head & Shoulders Cream (Procter & Gamble)	shampoo	—	zinc pyrithione, 2%	anionic detergent
Head & Shoulders Lotion (Procter & Gamble)	shampoo	—	zinc pyrithione, 2%	lauryl sulfate, cocamide, ethanolamine, triethanolamine, magnesium aluminum silicate, hydroxypropyl methylcellulose
Ionil (Owen)	shampoo	salicylic acid, 2%	—	polyoxyethylene ethers (nonionic); benzalkonium chloride, 0.2%; alcohol, 12%

Product (manufacturer)	Application form	Keratolytic	Cytostatic agent	Other
Klaron (Dermik)	lotion	colloidal sulfur, 5% salicylic acid, 2%	—	greaseless, hydroalcoholic vehicle; alcohol, 13.1%
Long Aid Sulphur (Keystone)	ointment	salicylic acid, 0.89% sulfur, 0.39%	—	—
Meted (Texas Pharmacal)	shampoo	sulfur, 3% salicylic acid, 2%	—	highly concentrated detergents
Meted 2 (Texas Pharmacal)	shampoo	colloidal sulfur, 2.3% salicylic acid, 1%	—	mild detergent blend
Monique Dandruff Control (Quality Products)	shampoo rinse	—	—	benzalkonium chloride alkylisoquinolinium bromide
Neomark (C&M)	lotion	salicylic acid, 1.6%	—	coal tar solution, 2%; betanaphthol, 1%; resorcinol monoacetate, 1%; castor oil; isopropyl alcohol, 68%; purified water
Ogilvie (Tussy)	shampoo	—	—	sodium undecylenic sulfosuccinate
pHisoDan (Winthrop)	shampoo	precipitated sulfur, 5% sodium salicylate, 0.5%	—	entsufon sodium, lanolin cholesterols, petrolatum
Resorcitate (Schieffelin)	lotion	salicylic acid, 1.5%	—	resorcinol monoacetate, 1.5%; alcohol, 66%
Resorcitate with Oil (Schieffelin)	lotion	salicylic acid, 1.5%	—	resorcinol monoacetate, 1.5%; castor oil, 1.5%; alcohol, 81%
Rezamid Tinted (Dermik)	shampoo lotion	microsize sulfur, 2% (shampoo) 5% (lotion)	—	foaming cleanser; resorcinol, 2%; chloroxylenol, 0.5%; alcohol, 28.5%
Rinse Away (Alberto Culver)	liquid/gel	—	—	benzalkonium chloride, 0.12%; laurylisoquinolinium bromide, 0.12%
Sebaquin (Summers)	shampoo	—	—	diiodohydroxyquin, 3%
Sebaveen (Cooper)	shampoo	salicylic acid, 2% sulfur, 2%	—	colloidal oatmeal, 5%; emollients, 4%
Sebb (Max Factor)	shampoo	—	—	*N*-trichloromethylmercapto-4-cyclohexene-1,2-dicarboximide
Sebisol (C&M)	shampoo	salicylic acid, 2%	—	clorophene, 0.1%; betanaphthol, 1%; alkyl–aryl surfactant base (biodegradable); aliphatic alcoholamide conditioner; purified water
Selsun Blue (Abbott)	shampoo	—	selenium sulfide, 1%	surfactants
Soltex (C&M)	shampoo	—	—	clorophene, 0.1%; alkyl–aryl surfactant base (biodegradable); aliphatic alcoholamide conditioner; purified water
Sul-Blue (Columbia Medical)	shampoo	—	selenium sulfide, 1%	—
Sulfur-8 Hair and Scalp Conditioner (Plough)	ointment	sulfur, 2%	—	menthol, 1% triclosan, 0.1%
Sulfur-8 Shampoo (Plough)	shampoo	—	—	triclosan, 0.2%
Thylox PDC (Dent)	shampoo	—	—	zinc sulfide, salicylanilide
Vanseb (Herbert)	shampoo	sulfur, 2% salicylic acid, 1%	—	proteins, surfactants
Zincon (Lederle)	shampoo	—	zinc pyrithione, 1%	surfactants

Product (manufacturer)	Application form	Keratolytic/ Keratin softener	Tar product	Other
Alma Tar (Schieffelin)	bath	—	juniper tar, 35%	—
Alma Tar (Schieffelin)	shampoo	—	juniper tar, 4%	polyoxyethylene ether, edetate sodium, sulfonated castor oil, coconut oil, triethanolamine
Alphosyl (Reed & Carnrick)	lotion cream	allantoin, 2% (lotion, cream)	coal tar extract, 5%	hydrophilic base (lotion, cream)
DHS Tar (Person & Covey)	shampoo	—	coal tar, 0.5%	cleansing agents
Diasporal-Tar (Doak)	cream	colloidal sulfur, 3% salicylic acid, 2%	tar distillate, 5%	isopropyl alcohol, 90%
Epidol (Spirt)	liquid	salicylic acid, 3%	coal tar, 18%	—
Ionil T (Owen)	shampoo	salicylic acid, 2%	coal tar solution, 5% (equivalent)	polyoxyethylene ethers (nonionic); benzalkonium chloride, 0.2%; alcohol, 12%
Kay-San (Commerce)	cream	allantoin	coal tar	sodium salicylate, resorcinol, chloroxylenol
Lavatar (Doak)	bath oil	—	tar distillate, 25%	—
L.C.D. (Schieffelin)	cream solution	—	coal tar solution, 5.8% (cream) 100% (solution)	—
Mazon (Norcliff-Thayer)	cream	salicylic acid, 1%	coal tar, 0.87%	resorcinol, 1%; benzoic acid, 0.5%
Mazon (Norcliff-Thayer)	shampoo	sulfur, 1%	coal tar, 3%	—
Oxipor VHC (Whitehall)	lotion	salicylic acid	coal tar solution	benzocaine; alcohol, 81%
Packer's Pine Tar (Cooper)	soap	—	pine tar, 6%	soap chips, 93%
Pentrax (Texas Pharmacal)	shampoo	—	coal tar, 8.75%	highly concentrated detergents
Polytar (Stiefel)	soap bath oil shampoo	—	juniper, pine, and coal tars, 1% (soap, shampoo) 25% (bath oil)	surfactant base (soap, shampoo)
Poslam (Royd)	ointment	sulfur salicylic acid	tar distillate	phenol, 0.035%; zinc oxide; menthol; lanolin
Pragmatar (Smith Kline & French)	cream	salicylic acid, 3% colloidal sulfur, 3%	cetyl alcohol–coal tar, 4%; emulsion base	—
Psorelief (Columbia Medical)	cream	allantoin	coal tar solution	isopropyl myristate, psoralen
Psorex (Jeffrey Martin)	shampoo	allantoin, 0.2%	coal tar, 2%	surfactants
Psorex Medicated (Jeffrey Martin)	cream shampoo	allantoin, 0.25% (cream) 0.20% (shampoo)	coal tar, 0.50%	silicone base (cream) lanolin and protein base (shampoo) surfactants
Riasol (also known as Dermoil) (Blair)	lotion	—	—	phenol, 0.5%; mercury, 0.45% (as coconut oil soap); cresol, 0.75%
Supertah (Purdue Frederick)	ointment	—	coal tar fraction, 1.25%	zinc oxide, starch
Tarbonis (Reed & Carnrick)	cream	—	coal tar extract, 5%	hydrophilic base
Tar-Doak (Doak)	lotion	—	tar distillate	—

Product (manufacturer)	Application form	Keratolytic/ Keratin softener	Tar product	Other
Tarpaste (Doak)	paste	—	tar distillate, 5%	zinc oxide
Tarsum (Summers)	shampoo	salicylic acid, 5%	coal tar solution, 10%	—
Tegrin (Block)	cream lotion shampoo	allantoin, 0.2%	coal tar extract, 5%	—
Tersa-Tar (Doak)	shampoo	—	tar distillate, 3%	—
Vanseb-T (Herbert)	shampoo	sulfur, 2% salicylic acid, 1%	coal tar, 5%	sodium lauryl sulfate, sodium stearate, fatty alkylolamide condensate, hydrolyzed animal protein, polyethylene glycol 75, lanolin, silicone–glycol copolymer, imidazolidinylurea, perfume
Vanseb-T Tar (Herbert)	shampoo	sulfur, 2% salicylic acid, 1%	coal tar solution, 5%	proteins, surfactants
Zetar (Dermik)	lotion ointment	—	colloidal crude coal tar, 2%	zinc oxide talc
Zetar (Dermik)	shampoo	—	crude colloidal coal tar, 1%	chloroxylenol, 0.5%

Poison-Ivy and Poison-Oak Products

Henry Wormser

Questions to ask the patient

Have you been exposed to poisonous plants recently?
Have you had poison-ivy/oak/sumac rash before?
How long have you had the rash?
Where is it located? How extensive is it?
Are the lesions weeping?
What treatments have you tried? Were they effective?

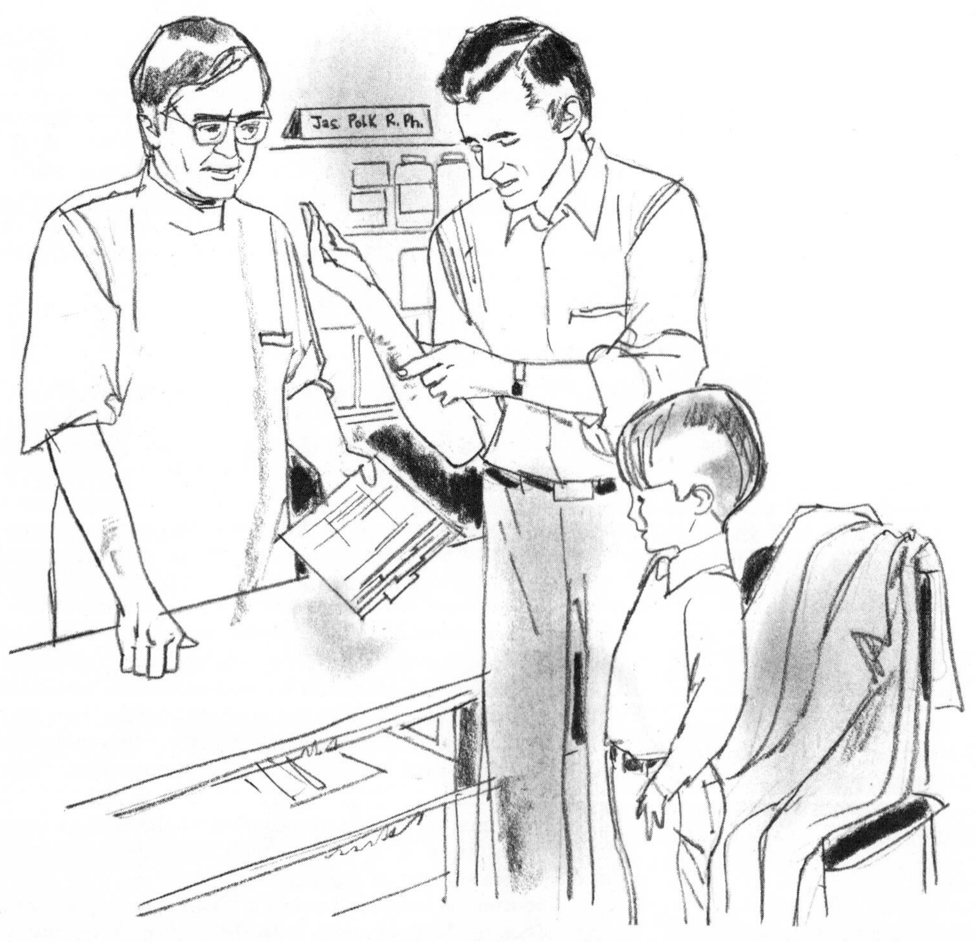

CHAPTER 30

Poison-ivy or poison-oak dermatitis is a common, seasonal, allergic contact dermatitis. It may be acute or chronic depending on the extent of exposure and the degree of sensitivity to the allergens. Symptoms range from transient redness to severe swelling and the formation of bullae; itching and vesiculation nearly always occur.

Causative plants

Many chemical substances and products (nickel and chromium salts, halogenated aromatic chemicals, epoxy resins, aniline derivatives) cause allergic contact dermatitis. Various plants and parts of plants—trees, grasses, flowers, vegetables, fruits, and weeds and airborne pollen—can also produce the allergy.[1] Among the 60 or more plants which can cause contact dermatitis, those which are most commonly encountered and which are responsible for the more severe lesions are poison-ivy (*Toxicodendron radicans*), western poison-oak (*T. diversilobum*), eastern poison-oak (*T. toxicarium*), and poison-sumac, or thunderwood, (*T. vernix*).[2] They belong to the Anacardiaceae family, members of which are both noxious and useful and are found in many parts of the world. Members include the Japanese lacquer-tree (*Rhus vernicifera*), which grows in Japan, China, and Indochina from which a rich furniture lacquer is obtained; the cashew nut tree (*Anacardium occidentale*), found in India, the East Indies, Africa, and Central and South America; and the mango tree (*Mangifera indica*), found in tropical areas. Cross-sensitivity can occur upon exposure to cashew nut shells, mango rinds, and furniture painted with natural lacquer.

Poison-ivy and poison-oak are the main causes of *Rhus* dermatitis in the U.S. Poison-ivy is particularly abundant in the eastern part of the U.S. and the southeastern part of Canada. It can be either a shrub or a vine and is readily identified by its characteristic leaves arranged in a cluster of three leaflets per stalk, by white berries produced in the fall, and by its climbing nature (Fig. 1). Western poison-oak is found along the Pacific coast area and in the southeastern U.S. It commonly grows as a bush without support, and the center leaf of the three-leaflet cluster resembles an oak leak. Poison-sumac, or poison-dogwood, is a coarse, woody shrub commonly found in swamps of the southern and eastern parts of the U.S. It differs from the other two plants by having 7 to 13 leaves per stalk.[3]

Dark-skinned people seem somewhat less susceptible to the dermatitis than others. Young people are more susceptible than the elderly, and newborns can readily be sensitized by applying the sap of the plant on the body.[4] It is estimated that at least 70 percent of the population of the U.S. would acquire the dermatitis if casually exposed to the plants. However, most estimates show about 40 percent incidence of the allergy.

Allergenic constituents

A phenolic oily resin, toxicodendrol, is present in all of the poisonous species and contains a complex active principle, urushiol. Urushiol is distributed widely in the roots, stems, leaves, and fruit of the plant, but not in the flower, pollen, or epidermis.[5] Therefore, contact with the intact epidermis of the plant is harmless—dermatitis occurs only if contact is made with a bruised or injured plant. The dermatitis cannot be contracted by emanation because neither toxicodendrol nor urushiol is volatile. However, smoke from burning plants carries a substantial amount of the resin and can cause serious reactions in susceptible individuals.

The identification and structure elucidation of the allergenic constituents of poison-ivy are credited mainly to the research of Dawson and co-workers[6-8] at Columbia University. They found four antigens, all possessing a 1,2-dihydroxybenzene or catechol nucleus with a 15-carbon atom side chain at position 3. The only difference among the antigens is the degree of unsaturation of the side chain. There is a saturated component (3-pentadecylcatechol, or 3-PDC), a mono-olefin (unsaturated at C-8), a diolefin (unsaturated at C-8 and C-11), and a triolefin (unsaturated at C-8, C-11, and C-14). Certain individuals who are hypersensitive to 3-PDC show cross-reactivity with other compounds such as resorcinol, hexylresorcinol, and the hydroquinones, but not with phenol itself.[9]

It has been reported that as little as 1 μg of crude urushiol causes dermatitis in sensitive individuals.[10] Direct contact with the plant is not necessary in a sensitive person; contact with the antigens can be made from an article that injured the plant or from particles of soot that contain antigenic material from the plant. Stroking a dog whose hair is contaminated is also a common source of the dermatitis. Contaminated clothing, a frequent source of antigens, is rendered harmless by machine laundering with an effective commercial detergent.

Two phases of contact dermatitis

The natural course of contact dermatitis is divided into two phases—a sensitization phase, during which a specific hypersensitivity to the allergen is acquired, and an elicitation phase, during which subsequent contact with the allergen elicits a visual dermatological response.[11] (See Chapter 27 for a discussion of the anatomy and physiology of the skin.) In the sensitization phase, urushiol components combine readily with epidermal proteins to form complete antigens on conjugated proteins. Each conjugate leaves the skin via the lymphatic system and is carried to the reticuloendothelial system where special globulins and antibodies are synthesized in response to the antigenic stimulus of the conjugate. In the elicitation phase, repeated contact with the allergen again produces the antigenic conjugate, this time causing a noticeable reaction. The reaction appears to be triggered by the association of specific immunologic elements carried to the skin in very low concentration by the blood with antigenic conjugates in the papillary layer of the dermis.

The interval between contact with the antigen and the appearance of the rash varies with the degree of sensitivity and the amount of antigen contacted. Reaction time, or the time between contact of sensitized skin with the allergen and the first sign of reaction, is usually not less than 12 hours.

Lesions vary from simple macules to vesicles and bullae. Contrary to popular belief, fluids in the vesicles and bullae are not antigenic, and patch tests with the fluids give negative reactions. Histologically, nonspecific inflammatory changes occur in the dermis and spongiosis followed by intraepidermal vesicles are seen in the epidermis in the acute stage of the disease. Bursting of the vesicles is a problem, because it may lead to secondary infection.

Signs and symptoms

Although the limbs, face, and neck are common sites of the dermatitis, all areas of the skin that come in contact with the sensitizing substance can be affected. Sometimes, distribution of the lesions is bizarre, especially if the antigenic agent is in the clothes or is transferred to various parts of the body by the fingers. Different parts of the body may not have the same sensitivity. Thus, the dermatitis may appear first in one area and later in another. The phenomenon is often called "spreading," but this description is inaccurate. Often, parts of the body that may sustain a heavy concentration of the allergen and exhibit more severe reactions will remain "hypersensitive" for several years.

The initial reaction following exposure to the antigen is erythema. The development of raised lesions (erythematous macules and papules) follows and finally, vesicles are formed caused by the accumulation of fluid in the epidermis. The initial lesions usually are marked by mild to intensive itching and burning. The affected area is often hot and swollen. It oozes and eventually dries and crusts.[12] Secondary bacterial infections may occur. Very rare complications include eosinophilia, kidney damage, urticaria, dyshidrosis, marked pigmentation, or leukoderma. The majority of cases of the dermatitis are self-limiting and will disappear in 14 to 20 days. Again, disappearance depends on the degree of sensitization and frequency of reexposure to the allergen.

The diagnosis of *Rhus* dermatitis can be made not only from the morphological appearance of the lesions but also from their distribution—linear streaking is common. A history of exposure facilitates the diagnosis. Toxicodendron plants are not photosensitizers. The dermatitis occurs on covered and uncovered parts of the body and does not require sunlight to develop.

Prophylaxis

Topical, or external, prophylactic measures for poison-ivy and poison-oak dermatitis that have been used include removal of the antigen by washing with soap and water or organic solvents, prior use of barrier creams, and/or use of detoxicants (oxidizing and complexing agents which chemically inactivate the antigen).[9] However, many investigators have shown that the benefits derived from these measures are questionable.[13-15] Removal of the antigen by washing has been largely ineffective probably because alkyl and alkenyl catechols of the sap, in contact with the skin, readily form a tightly bound complex with one or more specific proteins of the skin.

Kligman [9] tested 34 barrier preparations over a 2-year period on a group of highly sensitive people. The preparations were detoxicants that contained potassium permanganate, hydrogen peroxide, sodium perborate, iodine, iron and silver salts, etc. Kligman concluded that all the preparations were incapable of preventing the dermatitis. It is inferred by this conclusion that the antigen reacts rapidly and quite selectively with the skin and that irreversible damage occurs before preventive action can be taken. Enthusiastic claims have been made for zirconium oxide, a complexing agent which is used in many OTC products. Kligman [9] found it completely ineffective. In addition, several researchers have found extensive, sarcoid-like granulomas of glabrous skin that develop because of allergic hypersensitivity to insoluble zirconium oxide.[16-18]

Specific hyposensitization may be tried by administering repeated doses of *Rhus* antigens, but it is neither complete nor permanent; the original sensitivity returns in about 6 months after stopping the treatment.[19,20] Various forms of the plant antigens and several routes of administration have been used. Prophylaxis can be accomplished intramuscularly or orally. For equivalent effects, larger amounts of the oleoresin are required orally than parenterally. Sustained release is probably the major factor in the superior efficacy of the intramuscular route. Orally, there may be inactivation and imperfect absorption. Maximum hyposensitization is obtained with approximately 2 to 2.5 g IM and 2.5 to 3 g orally of the poison-ivy oleoresin antigen. If available, pure (less potent) pentadecylcatechol may be administered in doses of 2.5 to 3 g IM and 3.5 to 4 g orally.

Hyposensitization by administering crude extracts of oleoresins from plants has usually been ineffective because potency of the extracts varies and recommended dosages are usually far below those required. Three or four injections cannot provide clinical protection for moderately or extremely sensitive people. An alum-precipitated pyridine extract has been used with a weak to moderate degree of success. The outlook for successful hyposensitization has been improved by the availability of intramuscularly administered 3-PDC. Large amounts (1 to 3 g) may be needed in a course of 8 to 20 injections to provide clinical protection. The greater the sensitivity, the larger the amount needed. Administration of an antigenic substance to sensitive individuals involves a certain amount of risk. The exact course of treatment must be individualized and geared to the particular level of sensitivity and the person's capacity to tolerate the antigen without serious allergic reactions. If the dermatitis appears during prophylactic treatment, the treatment should be stopped for the duration of the eruption.

Hyposensitization is temporary, and maintenance doses of the antigen should be administered at predetermined intervals. Hyposensitization generally results in milder and shorter reactions and lessens the tendency of the reaction to "spread" to other parts of the body. It is important that the dermatitis be properly diagnosed by a qualified dermatologist prior to hyposensitization because prophylactic administration of Toxicodendron antigens has no effect on similar kinds of contact dermatitis. The only objective proof of successful hyposensitization is a negative or weakly positive patch-test reaction to the antigens at a previous, strongly positive reaction site.

The best prophylaxis for allergic contact dermatitis is complete avoidance of the allergen. People should be taught to recognize and avoid the poison-ivy and poison-oak group of plants and to carefully observe and search surrounding terrain before choosing a picnic area or campsite. When a poisonous plant is in a garden or cannot be avoided, it should be chemically destroyed or physically removed. The U.S. Department of Agriculture has literature on specific chemicals used to eradicate poison-ivy or poison-oak.[21]

Treatment of poison-ivy/poison-oak

No treatment is effective unless the offending agent is removed so that continued contact is avoided. The most prevalent method of treatment for localized inflammatory reactions is topical. When the reaction is spread over the body and/or is associated with major swelling, systemic treatment is necessary. The latter treatment always involves prescription drugs such as anti-inflammatory steroids. Oral antihistamines which theoretically should be of value have proved ineffective.[11] One of the first precepts of local treatment is to avoid unnecessary, local skin irritation by cautioning against frequent bathing and scrubbing of the lesions and using irritating chemicals, cosmetics, greases, and soaps.

The initial signs and symptoms of the reaction may be alarming, and the temptation to meddle therapeutically is strong. Simplicity and safety are keynotes of treatment. Many claims for products used for self-medication take credit for natural processes; in most cases, contact dermatitis is self-resolved. The major objectives of treatment are to provide protection to the damaged tissue until the acute reaction has subsided; to prevent excessive accumulation of debris resulting from oozing, scaling, and crusting, without disturbing normal tissue; and to relieve itching and prevent excoriation.

Generally, the local treatment should be adapted to the stage or severity of the lesions. During the acute weeping and oozing stage, aluminum acetate, saline, or sodium bicarbonate solution should be used either as soothing or astringent soaks, baths, or wet dressings for 30 minutes, three or four times a day. Shake lotions (calamine, zinc oxide, starch) are used at night or when wet dressings are not desirable. Greasy ointments should not be used during active vesiculation and oozing. Creams and ointments should be reserved for subacute and chronic dermatitis.

Large bullae should be drained to reduce itching. Aseptic techniques should be used and the blister punctured at the edge. The tops of the lesions should be kept intact because they protect the underlying, denuded epidermis of the lesions as they dry. The patient should be reassured that the fluid from the lesions will not lead to spreading of the dermatitis nor will touching someone with the dermatitis produce the disease. During the healing phase, application of a neutral soothing cream, e.g., cold cream, helps prevent crusting, scaling, and lichenification of the lesions.

Ingredients in OTC products

Four major types of pharmacologic agents—local anesthetics, antipruritics, antiseptics, and astringents—are used in topical OTC products for poison-ivy and poison-oak dermatitis.

Local anesthetics. Local anesthetics affect sensation by interfering with the transmission of the action potential along the nerve fiber. Many nerve fibers, specialized endings or receptors, and free nerve endings are in the epidermis. The superficially applied anesthetic acts very near the site of application. However, it is questionable whether the agent can reach the nerve endings when applied to unbroken skin. The most commonly used anesthetic in poison-ivy and poison-oak products is benzocaine. Other products contain diperodon hydrochloride, pramoxine hydrochloride, and tetracaine. Systemic, toxic effects attributed to local anesthetics occur at relatively high serum concentrations. Fortunately, these high levels are difficult to obtain by applying topical products now

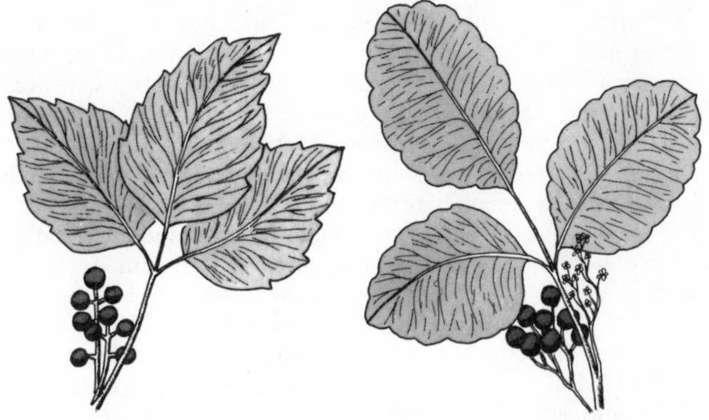

Figure 1.
Poison-ivy leaves. Poison-oak leaves.

available. A more likely, undesirable effect is an allergic one characterized by cutaneous lesions, urticaria, edema, and anaphylactoid reactions. Topically applied "caine" anesthetics are strong sensitizers in susceptible individuals.

Antipruritics. Antipruritics, which include antihistamines and counterirritants, are agents which alleviate itching. Antihistamines (diphenhydramine, pyrilamine, methapyrilene) are used essentially as local anesthetics, but, like the "caine" anesthetics, they can also be sensitizers. Counterirritants, such as menthol, phenol, and camphor, produce a feeling of coolness and reduce the irritation of the dermatitis. The sensation is difficult to explain because these chemicals produce local hyperemia. However, the counterirritants have a local anesthetic effect.

Antiseptics. Antiseptics in poison-ivy and poison-oak products are probably intended for prophylaxis against secondary infections, but their effectiveness is questionable. Of the available antiseptics (phenols, alcohols, oxidizing agents) and quaternary ammonium compounds such as benzalkonium chloride, the quaternary ammonium agents seem more effective. Unfortunately, their action is antagonized by anionic compounds such as soap.

Astringents. Astringents are mild protein precipitants that form a thick coagulum on the surface of lesions or they coagulate and remove overlying debris. They include aluminum acetate, tannic acid, zinc, iron and zirconium oxides, and potassium permanganate. These substances are used to stop oozing, reduce inflammation, and promote healing. Astringents are also antiseptic. Potassium permanganate may not be desirable because it leaves an objectionable stain.

Guidelines for product selection

Selection of products depends on the severity of the dermatitis. Mild to moderately severe cases of poison-ivy or poison-oak dermatitis can usually be treated with local or topical products. Preparations that contain benzocaine or zirconium oxide should be avoided because they can act as sensitizers. Products containing iron salts should also be avoided because they can leave a permanent tattoo. A physician should be consulted in severe cases of poison-ivy dermatitis.

Individuals who are sensitive to Toxicodendron plants should be informed of certain cosmetics, hair dyes, bleaches, and other commercial products that contain compounds related to 3-PDC which could exhibit cross-allergenicity. Shake lotions (which may contain phenol or menthol) provide immediate relief due to the cooling effect of water evaporation. Phenol and menthol lengthen the antipruritic activity. However, consultation should include cautioning against the frequent use of shake lotions, which pile masses of plasterlike material on the skin that are difficult and painful to remove. Men with facial dermatitis should shave, because shaving is less uncomfortable and irritating than accumulating crust and debris in the beard. In more severe cases, potassium permanganate baths (1 tsp potassium permanganate crystals per tub of lukewarm water, for 15 to 20 minutes) should be recommended for their drying effect and the prevention of secondary infection after the vesicles and bullae are open. Colloid baths (oatmeal colloid or a protein complex) also clean and soothe, but they make the tub slippery. If a soap is used, it should be bland.

Summary

Poison-ivy and poison-oak cause a contact dermatitis in many people every year. Prophylaxis and therapy of this allergy are still in the early stages of study, although much research is being done and progress is being made. Better understanding of the mechanism of allergic reaction, or cross-sensitivity, and of hyposensitization will help in the design of better products which alleviate and possibly eradicate this annoying and often serious disorder.

References

1. A. A. Fisher, "Contact Dermatitis," 2d ed., Lea and Febiger, Philadelphia, Pa., 1973, p. 1.
2. M. A. Lesser, *Drug Cosmet. Ind.*, **70,** 610(1952).
3. C. R. Dawson, *Trans. N.Y. Acad. Sci., Section of Physics and Chemistry,* **18,** 427(1956).
4. A. A. Fisher, "Contact Dermatitis," 2d ed., Lea and Febiger, Philadelphia, Pa., 1973, p. 260.
5. J. H. Doyle, *Pediatr. Clin. North Am.*, **8,** 259(1961).
6. S. V. Sunthankar and C. R. Dawson, *J. Am. Chem. Soc.*, **76,** 5070(1954).
7. W. E. Symes and C. R. Dawson, *J. Am. Chem. Soc.*, **76,** 2959(1954).
8. B. Loev and C. R. Dawson, *J. Am. Chem. Soc.*, **78,** 1180(1956).
9. A. M. Kligman, *Arch. Dermatol.*, **77,** 149(1958).
10. F. A. Stevens, *J. Am. Med. Assoc.*, **127,** 912(1945).
11. A. L. de Weck, in "Dermatology in General Medicine," T. B. Fitzpatrick *et al.*, Eds., McGraw-Hill, New York, N.Y., 1971, p. 669.
12. P. M. Selfon, *Mil. Med.*, **128,** 895(1963).
13. B. Shelmire, *J. Am. Med. Assoc.*, **113,** 1085(1939).
14. O. Grisvold, *J. Am. Pharm. Assoc. (Sci. Ed.),* **30,** 17(1941).
15. J. B. Howell, *Arch. Dermatol. Syphilol.*, **48,** 373(1943).
16. P. J. LoPresti and G. W. Hambrick, Jr., *Arch. Dermatol.*, **92,** 188(1965).
17. W. L. Epstein and J. R. Allen, *J. Am. Med. Assoc.*, **190,** 940(1964).
18. N. A. Hall, *J. Am. Pharm. Assoc.*, **NS12,** 576(1972).
19. A. M. Kligman, *Arch. Dermatol.*, **78,** 47(1958).
20. A. M. Kligman, *Arch. Dermatol.*, **78,** 359(1958).
21. D. M. Crooks and L. W. Kephart, *U.S. Farmers' Bull.*, No. 1972, Washington, D. C., U.S. Dept. of Agriculture, 1951, 30 pp.

Product (manufacturer)	Application form	Anesthetic	Antipruritic/ Antihistamine	Antiseptic	Astringent	Other
Caladryl (Parke-Davis)	cream lotion spray	—	diphenhydramine hydrochloride, 1% camphor, 0.1%	—	calamine	isopropyl alcohol, 10% (spray) alcohol, 2% (lotion)
Calamatum (Blair)	ointment lotion spray	benzocaine, 3%	phenol camphor	—	zinc oxide calamine	—
CZO (Elder)	lotion	—	—	—	calamine, 1.95 g/30 ml zinc oxide, 1.95 g/30 ml	glycerin aromatics
Dalicote (Dalin)	lotion	diperodon hydrochloride, 0.25%	pyrilamine maleate camphor	—	zinc oxide	dimethyl polysiloxane silicone greaseless base
Dermapax (Recsei)	lotion	—	pyrilamine maleate, 0.22% methapyrilene hydrochloride, 0.22% chlorpheniramine maleate, 0.06%	chlorobutanol, 1% benzyl alcohol, 1%	—	isopropyl alcohol, 40%
Didelamine (Commerce)	gel	—	tripelennamine hydrochloride methapyrilene hydrochloride menthol	benzalkonium chloride	—	clear gel
Dri Toxen (Walker Corp)	cream	—	methapyrilene hydrochloride, 1% phenol, 1% menthol, 0.5%	—	zinc oxide, 10% zinc sulfate, 0.5%	washable greaseless base
Hist-A-Balm Medicated Lotion (Columbia Medical)	lotion	diperodon hydrochloride, 0.25%	phenyltoloxamine dihydrogen citrate, 0.75% menthol camphor	benzalkonium chloride, 0.1%	—	—
Hista-Calma Lotion (Rexall)	lotion	benzocaine, 1%	phenyltoloxamine dihydrogen citrate, 1%	—	calamine	—
Ivarest (Carbisulphoil)	cream lotion	benzocaine, 1%	pyrilamine maleate, 1.5% menthol, 0.7% camphor, 0.3%	—	calamine, 10% zirconium oxide, 4%	—
Ivy Dry Cream (Ivy)	cream	benzocaine	menthol camphor	—	tannic acid, 8%	methylparaben propylparaben isopropyl alcohol, 7.5%
Neoxyn (Rorer)	solution	—	—	hydrogen peroxide, 2.85% benzethonium chloride, 0.26%	—	acetic acid, 1.15% propylparaben, 0.02% acetanilide, 0.0169%

Product (manufacturer)	Application form	Anesthetic	Antipruritic/ Antihistamine	Antiseptic	Astringent	Other
Nupercainal Cream (Ciba)	cream	dibucaine, 0.5%	—	—	—	acetone sodium bisulfite, 0.37% water-washable base
Nupercainal Ointment (Ciba)	ointment	dibucaine, 1%	—	—	—	acetone sodium bisulfite, 0.5%
Nupercainal Spray (Ciba)	spray	dibucaine, 0.25%	—	—	—	alcohol, 46%
Obtundia Calamine Cream (Otis Clapp)	cream	—	cresol–camphor complex	—	calamine zinc oxide	—
Peterson's Ointment (Peterson's Ointment Co.)	ointment	—	camphor, 3.88% phenol, 2.50%	—	zinc oxide, 6.60% tannic acid, 2.20%	beeswax, 4% lavender oil petrolatum
Poison Ivy Cream (McKesson)	cream	benzocaine, 2.5%	pyrilamine maleate	povidone	zirconium oxide, 4% (as carbonated hydrous zirconia)	—
Poison Ivy Spray (McKesson)	aerosol	benzocaine, 0.5%	menthol camphor	—	calamine, 2% zinc oxide, 1%	isopropyl alcohol, 9.44%
Pontocaine (Winthrop)	cream ointment	tetracaine hydrochloride, (equivalent to 1% base) (cream) base, 0.5% (ointment)	menthol, 0.5% (ointment)	—	—	methylparaben (cream) sodium bisulfite (cream) white petrolatum (ointment) white wax (ointment)
Pyribenzamine (Ciba)	cream ointment	—	tripelennamine, 2%	—	—	water-washable base (cream) petrolatum base (ointment)
Rhuli Cream (Lederle)	cream	benzocaine, 1%	menthol, 0.7% camphor, 0.3%	—	zirconium oxide, 1%	isopropyl alcohol, 8.8%
Rhuligel (Lederle)	gel	—	menthol, 0.3% camphor, 0.3%	benzyl alcohol, 2%	—	alcohol, 31%
Rhulihist (Lederle)	lotion	benzocaine, 1%	tripelennamine hydrochloride, 1% camphor, 0.1% menthol, 0.1%	—	calamine, 3% zirconium oxide, 1%	methylparaben, 0.08% propylparaben, 0.02%
Rhuli Spray (Lederle)	spray	benzocaine, 0.98%	camphor, 0.098% menthol, 0.009%	—	zirconium oxide, 1% calamine, 0.98%	isopropyl alcohol, 9.5%
Surfadil (Lilly)	cream lotion	cyclomethycaine, 0.5%	methapyrilene hydrochloride, 2%	—	—	titanium dioxide, 5% (lotion)
Topic (Ingram)	gel	—	camphor menthol	benzyl alcohol, 9%	—	isopropyl alcohol, 30% greaseless base
Tronothane Hydrochloride (Abbott)	cream jelly	pramoxine hydrochloride, 1%	—	—	—	water-miscible base

Product (manufacturer)	Application form	Anesthetic	Antipruritic/ Antihistamine	Antiseptic	Astringent	Other
Tyrohist Cream (Columbia Medical)	cream	benzocaine	pyrilamine maleate camphor menthol	benzalkonium chloride	neocalamine	—
Ziradryl (Parke-Davis)	lotion	—	diphenhydramine hydrochloride, 2% camphor, 0.1%	—	zinc oxide, 2%	alcohol, 2%
Zotox (Commerce)	spray	benzocaine	menthol camphor	—	calamine zinc oxide	isopropyl alcohol

Diaper Rash and Prickly Heat Products

Gary H. Smith

Questions to ask the patient

Is the rash confined to the diaper area?
How long has the rash been present?
Can you relate the rash to a change of diet?
What types of laundry soaps do you use for diapers?
Do you use a disinfectant rinse for the diapers?
Are any products or procedures currently being used for the condition? Which ones?

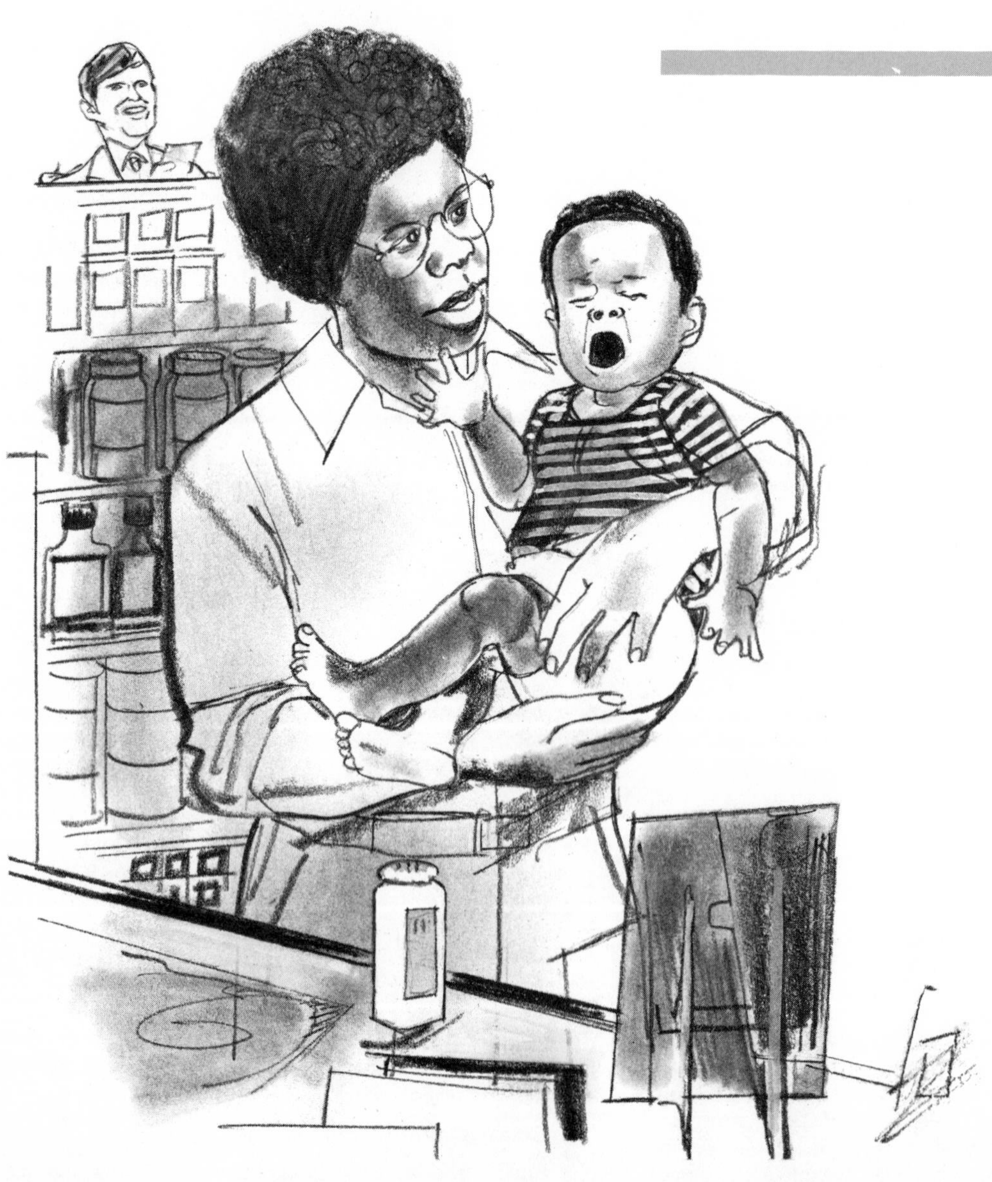

CHAPTER 31

Diaper rash and prickly heat (miliaria rubra) are acute, transient, inflammatory skin conditions which occur in nearly all infants and young children. Both conditions are unpleasant to the child. They cause burning and itching which result in restlessness, irritability, and interruption of the sleep cycle. Prevention is the best treatment, but most cases can be easily reversed by simple home remedies.

The skin of most adults is about 2 mm thick, but the infant's is considerably thinner—about 1 mm. Because the epidermis (the outermost layer of the skin) is about one-twentieth the thickness of the skin, the external barrier that protects the infant from the environment is very thin.[1] (See Chapter 27 for a discussion of skin anatomy.) The main functions of the skin are to retard the loss of body fluids to the external environment, to retard the exchange of fluids between the body and the environment, and to protect the body from external factors, such as heat, bacteria, fungi, and chemical toxins. For the skin to function most efficiently, it should remain dry, smooth, and at a low pH.

Diaper rash

Diaper rash, or diaper dermatitis, is one of the most common dermatitides in infants, occurring during the diaper-wearing period. It is an acute, inflammatory reaction of the skin in the diaper area caused by one or more factors (Table 1). A recent report indicated a 17-percent incidence the first week of life.[2]

Etiology and signs and symptoms

The histopathological changes vary with the causative factors and the severity of the dermatitis. Several predisposing factors that should also be considered include: inherited skin anomalies, such as hypersensitive skin and seborrheic diathesis and systemic diseases such as syphilis, acrodermatitis, chronica enteropathica, and Letterer-Siwe disease, all of which may produce a lowering of skin resistance.[3]

Normal newborns begin urinating within 24 hours after birth. They urinate from 1 to 20 times a day until 2 months of age and as many as eight times a day from 2 months to 8 years of age. Defecation also occurs several times a day.[4] Breast-fed infants tend to urinate less frequently and have a lower incidence of dermatitis than infants who are bottle fed because of the lower alkalinity of the urine and feces.[5,6]

Diaper rash begins between folds of skin, e.g., between the buttocks or between the scrotum and the thighs. It can spread to the entire diaper area depending on the time therapy begins and the nature of the cause. The diaper area is vulnerable to inflammation because the skin is often warm and moist and is exposed to irritants and bacteria. Diaper rash may range from mild erythema with maceration and chafing to nodular, infiltrated lesions that may become vesicular, pustular, and bullous, depending on the primary cause of the dermatitis. The causative factors of diaper rash include: ammonia, sweat retention, mechanical and chemical irritants, and secondary infections and complications.

Ammonia. The most widely accepted theory of the etiology of diaper rash is the presence of ammonia and other end products of the enzymatic breakdown of the urine. Ammoniacal dermatitis was first described by Jacquet[7] in 1886, followed by others in the early part of the 20th century.[8,9] In 1921, Cooke[10] determined that the production of ammonia in the diaper area was caused by urea-splitting bacteria found in the stool. He isolated the causative organism, which he named *Bacillus ammoniagenes,* from all the stool samples of 31 children with diaper rash. The organism is an aerobic, nonmotile, gram-positive bacillus. It is a saprophyte which has the ability to ferment urea to produce ammonia as follows:

$$CO(NH_2)_2 + 2H_2O \rightleftharpoons (NH_4)_2CO_3 \rightleftharpoons 2NH_3 + H_2O + CO_2$$

Ammonia was shown to be the cause of the diaper rash because it raises the pH and forms soaps with some of the constituents of the natural oils of the skin.

In 1955, Rapp[11] observed that a close correlation existed between the odor of urine and its ability to produce erythema, regardless of the pH of the urine. This extensive study showed that malodorous putrescent materials, in the absence of ammonia and high pH, can cause erythema. These materials are also produced by enzymatic degradation in the urine. Urine can cause diaper dermatitis that is characterized by the pungent odor of ammonia and erythematous papules on the buttocks, the inner surface of the thighs, and other sites in the diaper area.

Sweat retention. If a soiled diaper is not promptly changed, the stratum corneum in the diaper area becomes waterlogged. This causes keratotic plugging of the sweat glands (plugging with loose protein material on the skin) which results in sweat retention and may cause erythematous papules.[12]

Mechanical and chemical irritants. Tightly fitting diapers covered with plastic pants increase the humidity and temperature in the diaper area and keep air away from the skin, producing an environment conducive to irritation.[13] If diapers are changed frequently, irritation may be prevented. Irritation can result from the diaper constantly rubbing against the skin. Feces remaining in contact with the skin can cause irritation, especially if the infant's diet promotes the elimination of irritating substances. Preparations that are commonly applied to the diaper area, such as proprietary antiseptic agents and harsh soaps containing mercury, phenol, tars, salicylic acid, or sulfur, may also cause diaper rash. Diapers which are inadequately rinsed after washing may irritate the diaper area or cause an allergic reaction. Improper rinsing of the diaper area after bathing may leave a residue of soap that can cause irritation. Therefore, precautions should be taken to avoid exposing the sensitive skin of infants and young children to these irritating substances.[12]

Complications of diaper rash

Fungal and bacterial infections are the most common complications of diaper rash. They are cutaneous infec-

Table 1. Diaper Rash and Prickly Heat

Predisposing factors	Causes	Secondary infections	Prophylactic measures
Diaper rash			
Acrodermatitis	Ammonia produced by fecal bacteria	Bacterial; *Staphylococcus aureus*, Streptococcus	Avoid harsh detergents in laundering.
Chronica enteropathica	Antiseptic agents	Fungal: *Candida albicans*	Avoid plastic pants.
Congenital syphilis	Fecal and urinary irritants		Change diapers frequently.
Hypersensitive skin	Scratchy diapers		Rinse diapers well to remove soap and detergent residue and use chlorinated compound in first rinse water to remove bacteria.
Letterer-Siwe disease	Soap and detergent residue		Soak soiled diapers in disinfectant solution prior to laundering.
Seborrheic diathesis	Sweat retention caused by occlusion of pores by diaper		Use mild, protective ointments (zinc oxide paste, white petrolatum) between changes to keep the skin dry.
	Topical medicaments		Use soft, loosely fitting diapers.
Prickly heat	Sweat retention		Bathe the infant frequently to prevent sweat retention during hot weather.
	Heavy clothing		Do not overclothe the infant.
	Hot, humid environment		Keep the infant's environment cool during hot weather (air conditioner).

tions which usually result from untreated or improperly treated diaper dermatitis. The moist, warm, alkaline environment created by unchanged diapers is conducive to the development and multiplication of many pathogenic bacteria and fungi.[14] Most bacteria and fungi do not produce lesions on normal skin. However, if the skin is broken or macerated or the normal balance of the skin's bacterial flora is disturbed in some way, these organisms may become pathogenic and cause a serious infection in the diaper area.[6]

Fungal infections are most commonly caused by *Candida albicans*, an organism which is part of the normal flora of the colon. The stool, therefore, is the most common source of this organism.[13] Because monilial infections of the diaper area are usually a complication of ammoniacal diaper dermatitis, the clinical picture is often obscure and the only precise method of diagnosis is by demonstration of *C. albicans* in scrapings and cultures from the skin lesions.[15] In newborns who are less than 2 weeks old, monilial diaper dermatitis usually is accompanied by oral thrush. Both conditions are probably a result of the mother having had a *Candida* vaginal infection prior to and during delivery. Monilial dermatitis is characterized by lesions in the groin, intergluteal fold, and lower abdomen. The lesions are usually eroded and weeping and are surrounded by satellite pustules. When a parent gives this description of an infant's diaper rash, a physician should be consulted for appropriate treatment.

Bacterial infection of the diaper area is most commonly caused by *Staphylococcus* and is often a form of folliculitis. The lesions are pinhead-sized or slightly larger pustules surrounded by a narrow area of erythema. They may coalesce to form an area of infectious eczematoid dermatitis. Occasionally, bullous impetigo (also staphylococcal in origin) may occur. In some cases, Group A *Streptococcus* may be the pathogen and glomerulonephritis may be a sequela. As with monilia, if a bacterial infection in the diaper area is suspected, a physician should be consulted for appropriate diagnosis and therapy.[16]

Ulceration of the penal meatus may be a painful complication of diaper rash in circumsized babies. The pain associated with this condition leads to reflex inhibition of micturition and secondary distention of the bladder.[17 18]

Diaper rash may also accompany other dermatologic conditions, such as eczema, seborrheic dermatitis, or systemic disease.

Prickly heat: an acute dermatitis

The lesions associated with this condition result from obstruction of the ducts of the sweat glands. Sweat that is retained behind the obstruction causes the dilation and rupture of the epidermal part of the sweat duct, which produces swelling and inflammation. The term "prickly heat" was coined because the lesions usually produce itching and stinging. Prickly heat occurs mostly during hot, humid weather or during a febrile illness with heavy sweating. It may also occur as a result of overclothing and overcovering at night in warm rooms.

The lesions appear in areas of maceration and under plastic pants, diapers, adhesive tape, or anything that occludes the duct of the sweat gland. The lesions, which are erythematous and papulovesicular, occur most frequently on the cheeks, neck, trunk, and in the diaper area.[3 19]

Diaper rash vs. prickly heat

In general, if the diaper dermatitis is confined to the diaper area and does not present signs or symptoms of fungal or bacterial infection, the pharmacist can recommend OTC therapy.

If the infant has had diaper rash for only a few days, the diapers smell of ammonia, and the diapers have not been changed frequently, self-treatment can be recommended. The pharmacist can determine if parents are using laundry detergents that contain irritants. If diaper rash persists for 1 week or more after the infant has been treated with protectants and has been changed frequently, the rash may be caused by a problem other than the diaper and a physician should be consulted. If the infant has had consistent diarrhea, has awakened frequently, and is resistant to OTC treatment, a physician should be consulted because the problem may be more serious than simple diaper rash.

If the rash is more widespread than the diaper area (groin, intergluteal fold, lower abdomen), the infant may be hypersensitive to food in the diet, and the cause of the allergy should be ascertained by a physician. Eroded, weeping lesions surrounded by satellite pustules may be secondary to *Candida* infection; a definitive diagnosis should be made by a physician. If the lesions are of the pinhead kind, bullous, or look like impetigo, a staphylococcal or bacterial infection may be the cause.

The pharmacist may be able to recognize the cause of many conditions by questioning the parents. In addition to explaining the steps that must be taken to prevent diaper rash and prickly heat, the pharmacist can recommend several products suited to the child's condition. If the pharmacist ascertains that the dermatitis has persisted and appears to be complicated by infection or other process, it should be suggested that the child be taken to a physician.

Methods of prevention

Diaper rash and prickly heat are good examples of where "an ounce of prevention is worth a pound of cure." Good prophylactic practices depend on parental cooperation and responsibility (Table 1). Common sense is perhaps the best guide for preventive therapy.

A diaper should be changed as soon as it is soiled; leaving a wet diaper on for several hours increases the chances of diaper rash. Diapers should be made of soft material and fastened loosely to prevent rubbing. Plastic pants should be used as seldom as possible. They impede the passage of air through the diaper, and their use at night should be discouraged.

Infants often urinate soon after they are put to bed for the night. Parents can reduce the time a child is exposed to a wet diaper and the amount of urine accumulated at night by changing the diaper several hours after putting the child to bed.

The diaper area should be cleaned at each diaper change. A mild ointment or dusting powder (such as white petrolatum or talcum powder) may be recommended after washing. Mild soaps, Oilatum, or one of the various kinds of baby soaps should be used for cleaning the diaper area and for bathing. It is important that skin folds that entrap sweat and feces be cleaned thoroughly and rinsed well with clean water. The diaper area should be completely dry before a clean diaper is put on. Exposing the diaper area to warm, dry air for a few minutes between changes helps to keep the skin dry.

To prevent ammoniacal diaper rash, it is important to keep urea-splitting bacteria at a minimum. Several reports have dealt with the use of antibacterial compounds in laundering diapers. If home-laundered diapers are used, they should be soaked in a solution of Borax (0.5-cup Borax/gallon of water) prior to washing.[20] Other antibacterial compounds that can be used for presoaking, to reduce odor, and to disinfect diapers are quaternary ammonium compounds or a diluted sodium hypochlorite solution. Diapers should be washed with mild soap. The use of harsh detergents and water softeners should be avoided. After they are washed, the diapers should be rinsed thoroughly and, if possible, dried in the sun.

If an antibacterial presoak is not used, a disinfectant should be used during the washing process. A 5.25-percent sodium hypochlorite bleach (Clorox) properly diluted has been shown to reduce the number of organisms from 277/in ^{2} to 2 organisms/in ^{2}.[21] The use of chlorophene [(*o*-benzyl-*p*-chloro)phenol] in the first rinse of diapers in a concentration of 1 part chlorophene to 2,500 parts water has also been shown to be effective in treating and preventing ammoniacal diaper dermatitis.[22]

Grant *et al.*[23] showed that diapers cleaned by a diaper service were associated with the lowest incidence of diaper rash (24.4 percent), disposable diapers showed a similar low incidence (25 percent), and home-laundered diapers were associated with the greatest incidence of diaper rash (35.6 percent). The home-laundered diapers were not rinsed with a bacteriostatic agent. These reports show the necessity of using a bacteriostatic agent either in the rinse water or diaper pail. Diapers containing fecal material should be rinsed well in the toilet prior to placing in the diaper pail. Commercial diaper services provide essentially sterile diapers. Although disposable diapers were comparable in this study, their routine use should be discouraged because they have a plastic covering that reduces the amount of air available to the skin under the diaper.

The prevention of prickly heat consists of eliminating the cause—overheating. Overclothing and overcovering of infants should be avoided. Light clothing and covering is recommended to allow air to reach the skin. In hot weather, frequent removal of clothes for relatively short periods helps to keep the skin dry. Air conditioning the environment helps lower humidity and temperature. Perspiration can be reduced by frequent bathing or sponge baths and the use of bland dusting powder. Oatmeal (1 cup of Aveeno colloidal oatmeal/tub of warm water) and soyprotein (1 packet of protein colloidal bath powder/tub of warm water) may also help in the treatment of prickly heat.

Few infants escape diaper rash. The pharmacist can be helpful in teaching parents the proper procedures for preventing diaper rash and prickly heat. Parents should understand that the indiscriminate use of medication is not the proper way of treating either condition and is ill advised. Drugs alone cannot stop or prevent diaper rash or prickly heat. Many newborns, infants, and young children may be hypersensitive to various medicaments, and more harm than good can result from their use. Diaper dermatitis may be inadvertently induced by the overuse of medications (especially those containing sulfonamides, neomycin, and other sensitizing antibacterial agents). Fontana[24] refers to this as "dermatitis medicamentosa."

Treatment

The treatments for diaper rash and prickly heat may be considered together. The active treatment of diaper rash involves removing the source of irritation, reducing the immediate skin reaction, relieving discomfort, and preventing secondary infection and other complications. The treatment plan should be individualized for both diaper rash and prickly heat. Products which have been shown to be helpful in treatment include protectants, agents to promote healing, antiseptics, and antifungal and anti-inflammatory agents. The pharmacist is in a good position to advise parents as to which of the many products should be used for a particular kind of dermatitis. It should be noted that as with most forms of therapy, the simplest regimen is the one most likely to be followed by parents. As mentioned, babies' skin is sensitive, and many babies may be allergic to some of the available products.

In the treatment of mild forms of diaper rash, the best remedy is changing diapers frequently and leaving diapers off during naps, thus exposing the buttocks to the air. An incandescent lamp has also been recommended as a source of heat which may speed the healing process.[20 25] A lamp with a 25-watt bulb should be placed about 12 inches from the buttocks. The condition of infants with ammoniacal dermatitis improved when they were exposed to light for 20 minutes every 4 hours.[25] Parents should be warned not to hold the bulb too close to the buttocks because of the danger of burning the skin.

Corticosteroid creams and ointments are also used in the treatment of severe diaper dermatitis and prickly heat. They are prescription-only items. Several studies have shown systemic effects resulting from percutaneous absorption of steroids after topical application.[26-28] It has also been shown that occlusive dressings facilitate the absorption of topically applied steroids through normal (not inflamed) skin.[26] When steroid creams are applied topically to inflamed or abraded skin, systemic levels may be higher than when applied to normal skin.[27] Due to the large absorptive area of diaper rash and the covering of the area with a diaper, infants treated with topical steroids may experience systemic steroid effects resulting from adrenal suppression. The use of topical steroids for the treatment of diaper dermatitis should be discouraged and only used for the most severe cases, and then for only short periods.

Removal of irritants

When irritants cause diaper rash, the best treatment is their removal. The theory that various foods cause a higher incidence of diaper rash has not been substantiated in the literature. Grant *et al.*,[29] in a study of 1,184 infants, failed to show a significant difference in diaper rash between infants who were fed an iron-fortified formula and those who were fed formulas without iron. If an infant displays hypersensitivity to a particular food, a rash may appear, but it is not confined to the diaper area.

Treatment of secondary complications

Secondary complications of diaper dermatitis require special treatment. In the case of secondary infections caused by bacteria or fungi, the condition should be diagnosed and treated by a physician. Various antiseptic agents have been used to treat *Staphylococcus-* and *Streptococcus-*induced infections. These infections usually respond to local treatment with neomycin, bacitracin, and polymyxin B sulfate. Quaternary ammonium chloride compounds are often used as a component of dermatological preparations for the treatment of diaper rash and prickly heat. However, their antibacterial action has been questioned and they may not be effective. In addition, these compounds may act as irritants in some cases, resulting in a worsening of the inflammation.[30]

Burow's solution is also used for its astringent action. All of these agents may be irritating to an infant's skin, causing discomfort when applied. Antibiotic ointments, especially neomycin, should be used only when clearly indicated because they may cause hypersensitivity reactions.[31]

In *Candida*-induced diaper rash, the use of antifungal agents may be necessary, and physicians as well as patients may need to know which agents are effective. Burow's-solution soaks may be used for severe dermatitis followed by the application of nystatin dusting powder or ointment at a concentration of 100,000 units/g.[15 32] A 2-percent amphotericin B ointment has also been shown to be effective.[33] Hydroxyquinoline is applied topically for its antibacterial and antifungal activity. Calcium undecylenate is used for its antifungal activity. Nystatin, amphotericin B, and hydroxyquinoline are prescription-only products; Burow's solution and calcium undecylenate are OTC.

Ingredients in OTC products

Protectants. Prior to putting on a dry diaper, a thin layer of petroleum jelly or zinc oxide paste (Lassar's paste) serves as a protectant. Zinc oxide is found in many products used to treat diaper rash and prickly heat. It is a mild astringent that has weak antiseptic properties and is an excellent protectant. Zinc oxide paste has the highest concentration of zinc oxide of any available preparation. Ointments that contain vitamins A and D alone or in combination with other ingredients (Desitin, Balmex) are very popular for the treatment of diaper rash. They are promoted for healing purposes, but their efficacy beyond that of the ointment base has not been substantiated. All medication must be thoroughly removed at each diaper changing.

Ammoniacal diaper dermatitis, which involves abraded skin, requires a more complex treatment. In a study of 10 infants with ammoniacal diaper dermatitis, the inflammation was completely reversed in an average of 66 hours with continuous exposure of the infant to air and light.[25] It is important in this severe diaper dermatitis that the buttocks be exposed to air as often as possible. In other respects, treatment is the same as for mild cases and includes the use of a good protective agent such as zinc oxide paste.

Powders. Powdered agents are used in the treatment of diaper rash and prickly heat. Talc is a natural hydrous magnesium silicate which allays irritation, prevents chafing, and can adsorb sweat. Talc is similar to ointments and creams in that it adheres well to the skin.[13] Magnesium stearate is included in some dusting powders promoted for infant use because of its ability to adhere to the skin and to serve as a mechanical barrier to irritants. When applied after each changing, these products serve primarily to keep the diaper area dry. They should be used cautiously because inhalation of the dust by the infant may be harmful and could lead to chemical pneumonia.

Antiseptics. Boric acid has been used extensively in

the past for the treatment of diaper dermatitis and prickly heat. It has been incorporated into ointments in concentrations of as much as 3 percent and into dusting powders. It was used for its bacteriostatic and fungistatic activity. There have been reports of toxicity and, in two instances, death associated with the use of boric acid.[34 35] In one quantitative study of 16 infants, boron levels were significantly high in patients treated with 3-percent boric acid/borate ointments.[36] Concern about boron toxicity has prompted the American Academy of Pediatrics Committee on Drugs to recommend to the Food and Drug Administration that products containing boric acid be reformulated, eliminating boric acid as an ingredient.

Pharmacists should advise parents about the correct use of any product recommended. Some general precautions should be mentioned such as expiration dates on antimicrobial ointments and the possibility of stinging and irritation upon application of the ointment. If powders are recommended, parents should be instructed to apply them carefully to prevent inhalation of the powder by the infant which could lead to chemical pneumonia. When soaks and solution (such as Burow's solution) are used, the unused portion should be discarded after each use, i.e., only fresh preparations should be used each time. Above all, pharmacists should caution parents about the general use of any medicament for a baby's skin. The best therapy for diaper dermatitis is keeping the skin clean and dry.

Summary

Pharmacists should be prepared to offer sound advice on a good prophylactic program and to recommend therapy for uncomplicated, uninfected cases. They should also be prepared to assess severity of the rash and be able to recommend appropriate action—either referral to a physician or a treatment plan. Diaper dermatitis and prickly heat are the two most common afflictions of newborns, infants, and young children. The cure is toilet training, but the incidence and severity can be reduced by following the procedures outlined in this chapter. If the dermatitis does not respond to frequent diaper changes, frequent exposure to air, and application of a good protectant, such as zinc oxide paste, within 1 week, a physician should be consulted.

References

1. M. Lieder, "Practical Pediatric Dermatology," Mosby, St. Louis, Mo., 1961, p. 220.
2. G. Weipple, *Klin. Paediatr.*, **186,** 259(1974).
3. W. E. Nelson *et al.*, "Textbook of Pediatrics," 9th ed., Saunders, Philadelphia, Pa., 1969, p. 1398.
4. K. S. Shepard, "Care of the Well Baby," Lippincott, Philadelphia, Pa., 1968, p. 2310.
5. D. R. Marlow, "Textbook of Pediatric Nursing," Saunders, Philadelphia, Pa., 1973, pp. 136-137.
6. P. J. Koblenzer, *Clin. Pediatr.*, **12,** 386-392(1973).
7. L. Jacquet, *Rev. Mens. de Mal de L'enf.*, **4,** 208(1886).
8. T. S. Southworth, *Arch. Pediatr.*, **30,** 730(1913).
9. J. Zahorsky, *Am. J. Dis. Child.*, **10,** 436(1915).
10. J. V. Cooke, *Am. J. Dis. Child.*, **22,** 481(1921).
11. G. W. Rapp, *Arch. Pediatr.*, **72,** 113-118(1955).
12. L. M. Solomon and N. E. Easterly, "Neonatal Dermatology: Major Problem in Clinical Pediatrics," vol. 9, Saunders, Philadelphia, Pa., 1973.
13. F. Sadik, "Handbook of Non-Prescription Drugs," G. Griffenhagen and L. Hawkins, Eds., American Pharmaceutical Association, Washington, D. C., 1973, pp. 184-189.
14. R. F. Pittillo, *J. Dermatol.*, **12,** 245-249(1973).
15. P. J. Kozinn, *Antibiot. Annu.*, 910-913(1958-59).
16. L. F. Montes *et al.*, *Arch. Dermatol.*, **103,** 400-406(1971).
17. S. Swift, *Pediatr. Clin. North Am.*, **3,** 759-769(1956).
18. J. Brennemann, *Am. J. Dis. Child.*, **21,** 38(1921).
19. H. L. Barnett, "Pediatrics," Appleton-Century-Crofts, New York, N.Y., 1968, pp. 1808-1089.
20. M. M. Alexander and M. S. Brown, "Pediatric Physical Diagnosis for Nurses," McGraw-Hill, New York, N.Y., 1974, pp. 22-23.
21. H. S. Whitehouse and N. W. Ryan, *Am. J. Dis. Child.*, **112,** 225-228(1967).
22. W. Friend, *Calif. Med.*, **97,** 56-57(1962).
23. W. W. Grant *et al.*, *Clin. Pediatr.*, **12,** 714-716(1973).
24. V. J. Fontana, *J. Med. Soc. N. J.*, **70,** 819-825(1973).
25. D. A. Humphries, Master of Nursing Thesis, University of Washington, Seattle, Wash., 1966.
26. R. B. Scoggins and B. Kliman, *N. Engl. J. Med.*, **273,** 831-840(Oct. 14, 1965).
27. R. J. Feldman and H. I. Maibach, *Arch. Dermatol.*, **91,** 661-666(June 1965).
28. R. D. Carr and W. M. Tarnowski, *Acta Derm. Venereol.*, **48,** 417-428(1968).
29. W. W. Grant *et al.*, *J. Pediatr.*, **81,** 973-974(1972).
30. E. Shmunes and E. J. Levy, *Arch. Dermatol.*, **105,** 91(Jan. 1972).
31. J. Patrick *et al.*, *Arch. Dermatol.*, **102,** 532-535(Nov. 1970).
32. P. J. Kozinn, *J. Pediatr.*, **59,** 76-80(1961).
33. P. Kozinn, *Antibiot. Annu.*, 128-134(1956-1957).
34. W. T. Maxon, *J. Ky. Med. Assoc.*, **52,** 423-424(1954).
35. Correspondence, *Br. Med. J.*, **2,** 603(1970).
36. P. Jensen, *Nord. Med.*, **86,** 1425-1429(1971).

Products 31 DIAPER RASH/PRICKLY HEAT

Product (manufacturer)	Application form	Protectant	Powdered agent	Antimicrobial	Other
A and D Ointment (Schering)	ointment	—	—	—	petrolatum–lanolin base fish liver oil
Ammens Medicated Powder (Bristol-Myers)	powder	zinc oxide, 9.10%	talc, 45.06% starch, 41%	boric acid, 4.55% 8-hydroxyquinoline, 0.1% 8-hydroxyquinoline sulfate, 0.05%	aromatic oils, 0.14%
Ammorid Dermatologic Ointment (Kinney)	ointment	zinc oxide	—	benzethonium chloride	lanolin
Ammorid Diaper Rinse (Kinney)	powder	—	—	methylbenzethonium chloride	edetate disodium
Aveeno Bar (Cooper)	cleanser	—	—	—	colloidal oatmeal, 50% mild sudsing agent (soap free) lanolin
Aveeno Colloidal Oatmeal (Cooper)	powder	—	—	—	oatmeal derivatives
Aveeno Oilated (Cooper)	liquid	—	—	—	colloidal oatmeal, 43% lanolin fraction liquid petrolatum
Bab-Eze Diaper Rash Cream (A.V.P.)	cream	zinc oxide	starch	—	cod liver oil diperodon hydrochloride, 0.25% aluminum acetate balsam Peru
Baby Magic Lotion (Mennen)	lotion	—	—	benzalkonium chloride	lanolin refined sterols
Baby Magic Oil (Mennen)	oil	—	—	—	mineral oil lanolin
Baby Magic Powder (Mennen)	powder	—	—	methylbenzethonium chloride	—
Baby Ointment (Beecham Labs)	ointment	zinc oxide benzoin	—	boric acid	aluminum hydroxide balsam tolu phenol lanolin–petrolatum base
Balmex Baby Powder (Macsil)	powder	zinc oxide	talc starch	—	balsam Peru, purified calcium carbonate
Balmex Medicated Lotion (Macsil)	lotion	—	—	—	allantoin balsam Peru, purified silicone lanolin fraction
Balmex Ointment (Macsil)	ointment	zinc oxide	—	—	vitamins A and D balsam Peru, purified bismuth subnitrate base containing silicone

Product (manufacturer)	Application form	Protectant	Powdered agent	Antimicrobial	Other
B-Balm Baby Ointment (North American)	ointment	zinc oxide, 10% compound benzoin tincture, 0.155 ml/30 g	—	—	phenol, 65 mg/30 g methyl salicylate, 20 mg/30 g
Biotres (Central)	ointment	—	—	polymyxin B sulfate, 10,000 units/g bacitracin zinc, 500 units/g	—
Borofax (Burroughs Wellcome)	ointment	—	—	boric acid, 5%	lanolin
Caldesene Medicated Ointment (Pharmacraft)	ointment	zinc oxide	talc	—	cod liver oil lanolin petrolatum
Caldesene Medicated Powder (Pharmacraft)	powder	—	talc	calcium undecylenate, 10%	—
Codanol A & D (Amer. Pharm.)	ointment	—	—	—	vitamin A, 1500 units/g vitamin D, 200 units/g white petrolatum lanolin
Comfortine (Dermik)	ointment	zinc oxide, 2%	—	boric acid, 2%	lanolin vitamins A and D
Comfortine Ointment (Dermik)	ointment	zinc oxide	—	—	vitamins A and D lanolin
Cruex (Pharmacraft)	aerosol powder powder	—	talc	calcium undecylenate, 10%	—
Dalicreme (Dalin)	cream	—	—	methylbenzethonium chloride, 0.1%	vitamins A and D diperodon hydrochloride, 0.25% scented greaseless base
Dalisept (Dalin)	ointment	—	—	methylbenzethonium chloride, 0.1% hexachlorophene, 1%	vitamin A, 750 units/g vitamin D, 75 units/g diperodon hydrochloride, 1% petrolatum–lanolin base
Desitin Baby Powder (Leeming)	powder	—	talc	benzethonium chloride	—
Desitin Ointment (Leeming)	ointment	zinc oxide	talc	—	cod liver oil petrolatum lanolin
Diapakare Baby Powder (Canfield)	powder	—	corn starch	benzethonium chloride	sodium bicarbonate

Product (manufacturer)	Application form	Protectant	Powdered agent	Antimicrobial	Other
Diaparene Baby Powder (Breon)	powder	—	corn starch	methylbenzethonium chloride, 1:1800	magnesium carbonate
Diaparene Ointment (Breon)	ointment	—	—	methylbenzethonium chloride, 1:1000	petrolatum glycerin
Diaparene Peri-Anal Creme (Breon)	cream	—	—	methylbenzethonium chloride, 1:1000	cod liver oil water-repellent base
Diaprex (Moss, Belle)	ointment	zinc oxide	zinc stearate	boric acid	balsam Peru water-resistant base
Johnson & Johnson Medicated Powder (Johnson & Johnson)	powder	zinc oxide	talc	—	menthol fragrance
Johnson's Baby Cream (Johnson & Johnson)	cream	—	—	—	mineral oil paraffin lanolin white beeswax ceresin
Johnson's Baby Powder (Johnson & Johnson)	powder	—	talc	—	—
Mediconet (Medicone)	cloth wipe	—	—	benzalkonium chloride, 0.02%	hamamelis water, 50% glycerin, 10% ethoxylated lanolin, 0.5% methylparaben, 0.15% perfume
Methakote Pediatric Cream (Syntex)	cream	—	talc	benzethonium chloride	protein hydrolysate
Mexsana Medicated Powder (Plough)	powder	zinc oxide	corn starch	triclosan	kaolin camphor eucalyptus oil
Moruguent (Beecham Labs)	ointment	—	—	—	cod liver oil concentrate lanolin–petrolatum base
Oilatum Soap (Stiefel)	cleanser	—	—	—	polyunsaturated vegetable oil, 7.5%
Panthoderm (USV)	cream	—	—	—	dexpanthenol, 2% water-miscible base
Rexall Baby Powder (Rexall)	powder	—	talc	—	fragrance
Silicote (Arnar-Stone)	cream ointment	dimethicone, 30% (cream) 33.3% (ointment) titanium dioxide, 1% (cream)	—	—	—

Product (manufacturer)	Application form	Protectant	Powdered agent	Antimicrobial	Other
Spectro-Jel (Recsei)	gel	—	—	cetylpyridinium chloride, 0.1%	glycol–polysiloxane, 1% isopropyl alcohol, 15% methylcellulose, 1.5%
Taloin (Warren-Teed)	ointment	zinc oxide calamine	—	methylbenzethonium chloride	eucalyptol silicone base
Vaseline Pure Petroleum Jelly (Chesebrough-Pond)	gel	—	—	—	white petrolatum, 100%
ZBT Baby Powder (Glenbrook)	powder	—	talc, 95.148% magnesium stearate, 1.9%	—	mineral oil, 2%
Zincofax Cream (Burroughs Wellcome)	cream	zinc oxide, 15%	—	—	petrolatum–lanolin base

Foot Care Products

Nicholas G. Popovich

Questions to ask the patient

What characterizes the condition—inflammation, blisters, oozing lesions, scaling, or bleeding?

Where is the lesion located—on top or between the toes or on the sole?

Is the condition painful?

How long has the condition existed?

Are other members of your family affected?

Do your feet sweat excessively?

Do you have any allergies?

Can you relate the onset of the condition to the use of new shoes, socks, or soaps?

Have you consulted a physician about this problem?

Are you under the care of a physician for other diseases such as diabetes or asthma?

What medicines are you taking?

Have you attempted any self-treatment? If so, which medication was used and for how long? Was the treatment effective?

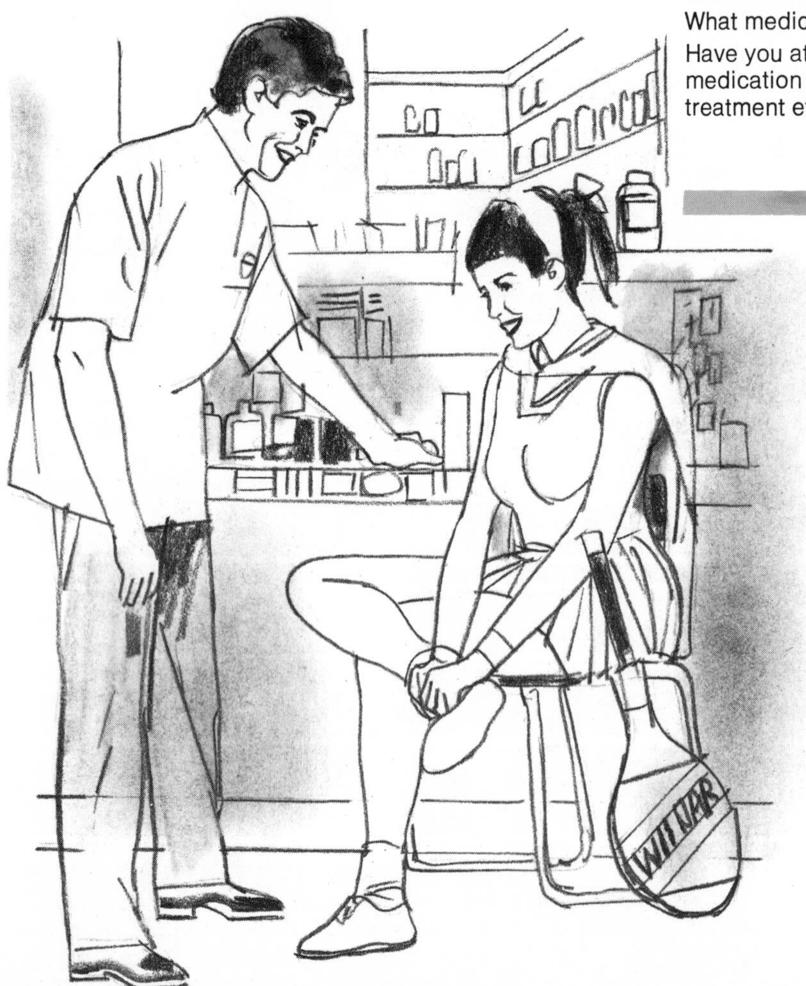

CHAPTER 32

Although foot conditions are seldom life-threatening, they can cause impaired mobility—from a limitation of activity to a serious disease condition.[1] Corns and calluses, for example, are common and widespread and can contribute to impairment.

Corns and calluses

Corns and calluses usually are confined to the feet, but calluses can appear on other sites, e.g., the palms of the hands. Corns and calluses are caused by pressure or friction against the skin for long periods. The affected areas respond by a thickening of the skin. Corns and calluses can be painless. It is usually when they are painful that advice and consultation are sought.

Pressure (tightly fitting shoes) is the most frequent cause of the pain of corns. Friction (loosely fitting shoes), walking barefooted, and orthopedic problems contribute to the development of calluses. Orthopedic problems include improper weight distribution, pressure, and the development of bunions with age.[2] Improperly fitting hosiery and nonlubricated friction in hosiery can cause blisters, calluses, and corns.

A corn and callus are strikingly similar in one aspect: each has a marked hyperkeratosis of the stratum corneum. (See Chapter 27 for a discussion of skin anatomy.) Beyond this, however, there are marked differences.

A corn (clavus) is a small, sharply demarcated, hyperkeratotic lesion having a central core (Fig. 1).[3] It is raised and yellowish gray and ranges from a few millimeters to one or more centimeters in diameter. The base of the corn is on the surface of the skin; the apex points inwardly and presses nerve endings in the dermis, causing pain.[4]

Corns are hard or soft. Hard corns occur on the surfaces of the toes and are shiny and polished. Soft corns are whitish thickenings of the skin that are usually found on the webs between the fourth and fifth toes. They are continually macerated by accumulated sweat.[5]

Soft and hard corns usually are caused by underlying bony prominences. A bony spur, or exostosis (a bony tumor in the form of an ossified muscular attachment to the surface of the bone), nearly always exists beneath long-lasting hard and soft corns. A lesion located over non-weight-bearing bony prominences or joints, such as metatarsal heads, the bulb of the large toe, the dorsum of the fifth toe, or the tips of the middle toes, is usually a corn.[5]

A callus differs from a corn in that it has no central core and has more diffuse thickening of the skin (Fig. 2).[2,3] It has indefinite borders and ranges from a few millimeters to several centimeters in diameter. It is usually raised, yellow, and has a normal pattern of skin ridges on its surface. Calluses form on weight-bearing areas other than joints (e.g., on the palms of the hands, the sides and soles of the feet).

During corn or callus development, the cells in the basal cell skin layer undergo mitotic division which leads to the migration of maturing cells through the prickle cell (stratum spinosum) and the granular (stratum granulosum) layers of skin. The rate is equal to the continual surface cellular desquamation. Normal mitotic activity and subsequent desquamation lead to complete replacement of the epidermis in about 1 month.[6] In the case of a callus, friction and pressure cause faster mitotic activity of the basal cell layer.[6] This activity produces a thicker stratum corneum as more cells reach the outer surface of the skin. When the friction or pressure is relieved, mitotic activity returns to normal causing remission and disappearance of the callus.

Bunions

Bunions are swellings of the bursae caused by various conditions. Pressure from a tightly fitting shoe is generally attributed as a cause of this condition, but pressure can result from the way a person sits, walks, or stands. When a bunion appears on the lateral side of the fifth metatarsal head, for example, it is called a "tailors" bunion, or "bunionette." The term "bunionette" was coined many years ago from the observation of people, like tailors, who predominantly sat cross-legged. By crossing the legs for long periods, an abnormal amount of pressure was applied to the fifth metatarsal head of the foot. The result of this friction and pressure caused an inflammatory swelling, or bunion formation, on the side of the fifth toe.[7]

The hallux, or great toe, along with the inner side of the foot provide the elasticity and mobility needed to propel oneself. The hallux is, therefore, a dynamic organ.[8] However, this mobility causes a number of anatomic disorders associated with the foot. Among the anatomical disorders of the great toe is hallux valgus [deviation of the great toe toward the lateral (outer) side of the foot].[9] Prolonged pressure caused by hallux valgus may result in pressure over the angulation of the metatarsophalangeal joint of the great toe. This may lead to inflammatory swelling of the bursa over the metatarsophalangeal joint and resultant bunion formation (Fig. 3).[10]

Bunions can result from pressure or friction on the toes caused by malformations of the bones of the toes (e.g., wide heads, lateral bending) or tightly fitting shoes.

Corrective steps to alleviate the condition often depend on the degree of discomfort. Bunions may be asymptomatic but usually become quite painful, swollen, and tender. The bunion area itself is usually covered by an extensive overgrowth of the horny layer of the skin.

Warts (verrucae)

Warts (intraepidermal tumors of the skin) are the most common viral infection of the skin; they are caused by a human wart virus (human papilloma virus).[11] Although there are several kinds of warts, it is presumed that the human papilloma virus is responsible for a majority of them. Human papilloma virus belongs biologically to the papovavirus group (*pa*pilloma, *po*lyoma, *va*cuolating viruses).[12] This virus has not been grown in tissue culture or laboratory animals. Thus, little information is known about its growth pattern, immunology, or metabolism. Information is based on various observations of infections in humans.

Warts begin as minute, smooth-surfaced, skin-colored lesions that enlarge over time. Repeated irritation causes the wart to continue enlarging. Plantar warts (on the soles of the feet) are usually asymptomatic and may not be noticed. However, if the plantar warts are large, the pain can be bothersome to the point of seeking professional advice.

Three criteria must be met for an individual to develop a wart. The papovavirus must be in the area, there must be an open avenue for the virus to enter through the skin, and the patient must be susceptible to the virus (probably the key factor as to why certain individuals develop warts and others do not).

Warts are most common in children and young adults and usually appear on exposed areas of the fingers, hands, face, and soles of the feet. They can spread by contact or autoinoculation. The incubation period after inoculation ranges from 1 to 20 months, with an average of 4 months.[13] Pegum[14] suggests that an increase in plantar warts in England was due to an increase in the number and use of swimming pools. The hypothesis was that swimming, especially in warm water with a pH greater than 5, produced swelling and softening of the cells of the horny layer of the skin on the sole of the foot. The surrounding surface area of the pool and diving board is abrasive enough to contribute to tissue debridement, and inoculation in an area of heavy foot traffic around the pool (e.g., the diving board) is likely, especially when running and springing contribute to stress on the soles of the feet. Scrapings of the horny layer of plantar warts contain virus particles, and therefore, it is conceivable that an area of heavy traffic of a pool can easily be contaminated by one person with a plantar wart.

Warts are not necessarily permanent—30 percent clear spontaneously in 6 months; 65 percent in 2 years.[15,16] Acquired immunity may account for the remission.[17] The wart virus stimulates the production of two immunoglobulins (IgM and IgG).[18] However, there has been no evidence that the increase in immunoglobulin titer was responsible for the disappearance of warts or the prevention of subsequent infections. Bunney *et al.*,[19] in a study involving the topical treatment of plantar warts, reported that 65 percent of the subjects cured in a 12-week treatment period had wart antibody; of those who were not cured, 23 percent had wart antibody. The results show

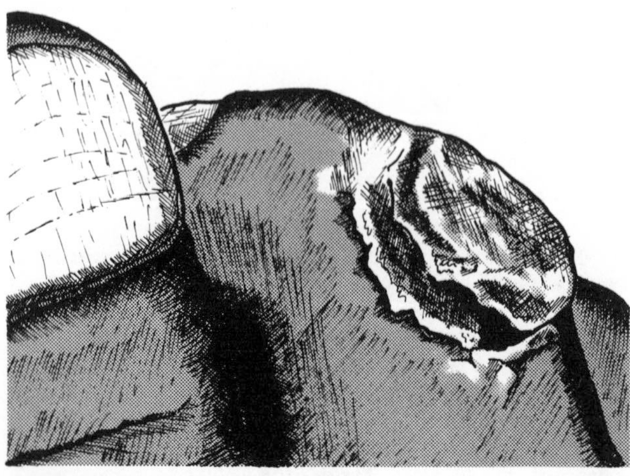

Figure 1. Toe with corns.

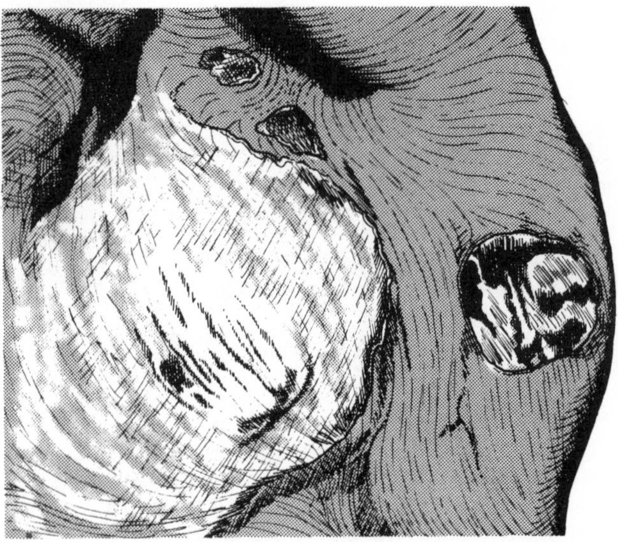

Figure 2. Sole of foot with plantar heloma (callus).

that topical therapy allows for the formation of protective antibodies as does the removal of the antigenic stimulus by early curettage of the wart. Destroying a wart too early by curettage can lead to reinfection because protective immunity seems to develop in about 6 months. Immunity can be correlated with the "not exceptionally high" rate of cure of electrodestruction and curettage.[15] Electron microscopic counting procedures demonstrate that warts contain their highest concentration of virus particles when they are about 6 months old. It is in the period between 6 and 12 months after inoculation that peak antibody titers in the body are reached.[12] In light of this, it is questionable whether warts should be treated at all. The determination can only be made after making appropriate differential diagnosis and weighing the advantages and disadvantages of therapy predicated on patient circumstance. Many practitioners believe that because of the contagious nature of plantar warts, early and vigorous treatment provides the best results. Prolonged treatment with OTC products may make the lesions more resistive to future treatment.

Common virogenic warts are defined depending on their location. Common warts (verruca vulgaris) are located on the hands and fingers, although they can occur on the face. Juvenile, or flat, warts (verruca plana) usually occur in groups on the face, neck, dorsa of the hands, wrists, and knees. Venereal warts (condylomatum latum) occur near the genitalia and anus. Plantar warts (verruca plantaris) are common on the soles of the feet.[20]

Plantar warts are more common in older children and adolescents, but they also occur in adults.[21] They are hyperkeratotic lesions that result from pressure. They may be confined to the weight-bearing areas of the foot (the sole of the heel, the big toe, the areas below the heads of the metatarsal bones, and the ball), or they may occur in non-weight-bearing areas of the sole of the foot (Fig. 4). Because calluses are also more commonly found under weight-bearing areas of the foot, a differential diagnosis must be made by a podiatrist.

Plantar warts demonstrate marked hypertrophy of the horny layer of skin, thickening of the prickle cell layer (acanthosis), formation of minute spaces (vacuolization) in the granular layer, and the development of many papillomas (circumscribed overgrowth of a small nipplelike process).[17] The causative virus stimulates mitosis in the prickle cell layer, resulting in the formation of the warty lesion.[22] The warts are circumscribed undurated lesions under constant pressure and are usually not raised above the surface of the skin unless they are on non-weight-bearing surfaces. In the center of the lesion is the wart itself. It is roughly circular and is 0.5 to 1 cm wide. The surface is grayish and friable. The skin surrounding the wart is thick and heaped. The entire area forms a uniform, slight swelling.[21 23] The surface of the plantar wart may contain small black points which are the result of hypertrophied papillae that contain highly distended blood vessels. Rupture of the vessels allows coagulated blood into the epidermis and is eventually carried to the outer surface of the epidermis.[11]

Plantar warts occur in clusters, or several contiguous warts are fused, giving the appearance of one wart (mosaic wart).[16] They are often confused with corns and calluses which are mainly thickened areas of the corneous layer.[21] Plantar warts can grow under a callus.[11]

Signs and symptoms

Pain is usually associated with corns and warts. In corns, it can be severe and sharp (when downward pressure is applied) or dull and discomforting. Calluses usually are asymptomatic, causing pain only when pressure is applied.[24] Individuals who suffer from calluses on the sole of the foot frequently draw a parallel of their discomfort to that of a person walking with a pebble in the shoe. Another important sign with foot problems is the hardening of the skin. The hardening is a sign that there is a biochemical problem that is causing abnormal weight distribution in that particular area of the foot. This hardening can physically be identified by the attending physician and the patient. Hardening of the skin is an objective sign as opposed to pain, which is subjective. A podiatric examination is warranted to determine whether an imbalance is present.

A physician [either a doctor of medicine (MD) or podiatrist (DPM)] should be consulted if:

- ☐ A peripheral circulatory disease, diabetes, or a condition that is already under a physician's care exists.
- ☐ Hemorrhaging or oozing of purulent material occurs.
- ☐ Corns and calluses indicate an anatomical defect or faulty weight distribution.
- ☐ Corns or calluses are extensive on the foot and are painful and debilitating.
- ☐ Warts are not confined to the foot, are extensive on one site, or are in the perianal and genital areas.
- ☐ Proper self-medication for warts has been tried for an adequate period with no beneficial results.

Self-treatment is appropriate if:

- ☐ The directions for use of the products can be followed with no difficulty.
- ☐ Chronic, debilitating diseases do not contraindicate the use of these products.
- ☐ Predisposing factors (ill-fitting footwear and hosiery) of corns and calluses are removed.
- ☐ Corns and calluses are minor.
- ☐ Neither an anatomical defect nor faulty weight distribution is indicated by corns and calluses.
- ☐ Plantar warts are not spread extensively over the sole of the foot.
- ☐ No medication (e.g., immunosuppressives) is being taken for another condition that contraindicates the use of these products.

Treatment

The success of treatment of corns and calluses with OTC products depends on eliminating the causes—pressure and friction. This entails the use of well-fitting, nonbinding footwear that distributes body weight evenly; for anatomical foot deformities, orthopedic corrections must be made. These measures relieve pressure and friction to allow for efficacious use of topical products used for corns and calluses, the resumption of normal mitosis of the basal cell layer, and the normalization of the stratum corneum after total desquamation of the hyperkeratotic tissue.

Many foot conditions require the attention of a physician, especially in cases of accompanying chronic, debilitating diseases (e.g., diabetes mellitus or arteriosclerosis). Without proper supervision, OTC products can induce more ulceration and possibly gangrene, especially in cases of vascular insufficiency in the foot.[1] In addition, simple lesions can mask more serious abscesses or ulcerations. If exostoses associated with corns are not excised by a physician, the corns will persist. Sites with many corns and calluses and lesions that ooze purulent material (a sign of secondary infection) should be examined by a physician.

An OTC product may be unnecessary for warts because some warts disappear spontaneously. Because it cannot be predicted whether an existing plantar wart will grow larger or how many more will develop if left untreated, self-treatment must be viewed with caution.

Warts are a result of infection by a virus. No specific effective medication is available, but topical agents and procedures help in their removal and relief of pain. Treatment is extremely difficult. Warts can reappear as long as several months after they have been supposedly "cured."

Simple, not widespread warts can be helped by self-medication depending on how the products are used (administration, dosage) and the use of ancillary procedures (foot baths, debridement with emery board) that help make the treatment effective. When warts are widespread in a specific area, especially the perianal or genital area, medical attention and supervision are necessary.

Ingredients in OTC products

There are a few drugs that have enough keratolytic activity for use in products intended for the treatment of corns, calluses, and warts. Among these drugs are salicylic acid, glacial acetic acid, lactic acid, zinc chloride, castor oil, calcium pantothenate, ascorbic acid, and podophyllum resin. Certain drugs, such as castor oil, are included in proprietary drug products for their emollient properties. Several topical products contain a local anesthetic, e.g., diperodon hydrochloride, to help alleviate the pain of corns or calluses. Salicylic acid is the most common ingredient in OTC drug products intended for corns, calluses, and warts. It usually appears in these products alone but may appear with other agents as well.

Salicylic acid. Salicylic acid, in concentrations of 5 to 10 percent and higher, softens and destroys the stratum corneum by increasing endogenous hydration, probably the result of lowering the pH which causes the cornified epithelium to swell, soften, macerate, and then desquamate.[25] This concentration is advantageous in hyperkeratotic conditions such as corns and calluses. However, on normal skin tissue, damage and necrosis are associated with the overuse (six times daily) or long-term use of salicylic acid in concentrations as low as 3 to 6 percent.[26 27]

The presence of moisture is important for therapeutic efficacy of salicylic acid in corn and callus therapy. If there is no moisture, tolerable amounts of salicylic acid will not soften cornified epithelium. Thus, salicylic acid usually is incorporated in dosage forms (plasters, flexible collodions, occlusive ointments) that occlude the area and promote moisture buildup, causing maceration and sloughing of tissue.[28] These occlusive dosage forms may cause percutaneous absorption of salicylic acid.[27] If enough salicylic acid is absorbed, salicylism could result. However, this condition develops only when the salicylic acid preparation is used over an extensive area of the foot. Absorbed salicylic acid is metabolized to a degree and excreted in urine; patients with impaired liver and/or kidney function are predisposed to systemic salicylate buildup. These patients cannot tolerate absorbed salicylate because toxic serum levels may develop.[26 29]

In concentrations of 3 to 6 percent, salicylic acid is keratolytic and will slough tissue. In acne and dandruff preparations, salicylic acid in concentrations below 3 percent, in combination with other keratolytics (e.g., sulfur, resorcinol), is used to facilitate keratin removal from "normal skin." For the treatment of hyperkeratotic conditions, such as corns and calluses, salicylic acid preparations of 10 to 40 percent, in appropriate dosage forms, applied only to the affected area are needed. Thus, large amounts of salicylic acid preparations should be applied carefully to avoid destruction of skin, particularly on adjacent healthy skin. Salicylic acid preparations must be used cautiously by patients with diabetes mellitus or peripheral vascular disease, where acute inflammation or ulcer formation from topical salicylic acid would be difficult to treat. Products containing salicylic acid are contraindicated in these individuals unless the products are used under the direct supervision of a physician.

Salicylic acid plaster (USP XIX) is a uniform mixture of salicylic acid in a suitable base, spread on appropriate backing material.[30] The usual concentration of salicylic acid in the base is 40 percent.

Salicylic acid is used most often in conjunction with lactic acid or glacial acetic acid in the following classic prescription for corns and warts: [2] one part each of salicylic and lactic acids to up to 10 parts flexible collodion. Apply every day to corn.

There are no clear-cut guidelines for how much salicylic acid or other keratolytic in an appropriate vehicle is needed before the product is considered a prescription-only item.

Glacial acetic acid and lactic acid. Glacial acetic acid and lactic acid are organic acids which are included in OTC formulations for corns, calluses, and warts because of their corrosive properties.[31] Both are extremely corrosive and must be applied only on the affected area, not on surrounding healthy skin. Either of these acids is usually included in low concentration (less than 10 percent) in formulations that also contain salicylic acid.

These acids are contraindicated in cases involving debilitating diseases. Overuse can cause skin irritation and ulceration. Used appropriately, these agents are safe for adults and children.

Zinc chloride. Zinc chloride is included in several formulations of topical OTC products for corns and calluses. Because it is irritating and caustic, its concentration is low, usually less than 3 percent. Zinc chloride is very water soluble and ether soluble and can be used in either drug delivery system. It owes its activity to zinc ion which precipitates protein.[32] Because zinc chloride is extremely corrosive and irritating, it should not come in contact with mucous membranes or healthy skin.[33] It also should not be used for long periods.

Castor oil. Castor oil is included in several proprietary products for corns and calluses for its emollient properties; it can also be used by itself.[34] It keeps the keratinous tissue soft by forming an occlusive film. The film prevents water loss and sweat evaporation from the surface of the corn or callus, and the tissue remains soft and pliable.

The oil usually is applied at bedtime, and the foot is covered by a sock. The sock serves a dual purpose in that it prevents oil stains on bed linens and helps occlude the affected area for better penetration of the medication.

Pantothenic acid and derivatives. Calcium pantothenate is used for warts. Application of the alcohol derivative, pantothenol, in various ulcerative and pyogenic dermatoses stimulates epithelialization and allays itching. There have been no reports of sensitization or allergic reaction to topical therapy with pantothenic acid or its derivatives.[35] The use of these drugs in adults and children seems safe. Topical formulations have a 2- to 5-percent concentration of the active pantothenic acid derivative.

Ascorbic acid. Ascorbic acid is included in one topical product for wart therapy. Although ascorbic acid is essential in the development of supporting tissue (collagen, intracellular ground substance) and healing, there are no clinical reports to substantiate or refute its efficacy in topical wart therapy.[35] Because ascorbic acid is a polar molecule, it is unlikely that percutaneous absorption will occur with its topical use. However, even if it is absorbed percutaneously, the minimal amount absorbed would not create problems.

Collodions. Topical keratolytics used in treatment of corns, calluses, and warts usually are formulated in flexible collodion drug delivery systems. These systems usually contain pyroxylin, volatile solvents (ether, alcohol), and a plasticizer, usually castor oil. Pyroxylin is a nitrocellulose derivative that, after evaporation of the volatile solvents, remains on the skin as a water-repellent film.[36] Collodion drug delivery systems are advantageous because they form an adherent, flexible or rigid film.[37] They also prevent moisture evaporation which facilitates penetration of the active ingredient into the affected tissue, resulting in sustained local action of the drug. The systems are water insoluble, as are a majority of the active ingredients they contain, e.g., salicylic acid. They are less apt to run than aqueous solutions.

The disadvantages of collodions are that they are extremely flammable and volatile and they can be mechanically irritating by occluding normal water transport through the skin. In addition, the collodions can favor systemic absorption of some drugs by their occlusive nature, and aromatic odors of the collodion make it a vehicle which children or adults might abuse by sniffing its contents.[38]

A plaster, e.g., salicylic acid, provides direct and prolonged contact of drugs with corns, calluses, and warts. It is a solid or semisolid, adhesive mass which is spread onto an appropriate backing (felt, moleskin, cotton, plastic) and applied to the affected area. Plasters are adhesive at body temperature, and the backing can be cut to conform to the size of the affected area. They are occlusive and prevent the dissipation of moisture.[39]

Local anesthetics. To ease the pain of a corn or

callus, several topical products contain a local anesthetic used with the keratolytic agents. Diperodon hydrochloride is usually incorporated into preparations at a concentration of 1 percent.[40] It is as potent as cocaine and has a longer duration of action.[41] It should not be applied to abraded or denuded areas where systemic absorption is possible. Diperodon hydrochloride is contraindicated in patients who are hypersensitive to other local anesthetic agents, e.g., benzocaine.

Menthol or camphor is included in several OTC products for wart removal as a counterirritant and mild, local anesthetic.

Prescription drugs

The pharmacist should be cognizant that there are several prescription products that might better serve the patient. At times, injection of a small amount of a corticosteroid (Aristocort, Celestone, Kenalog) beneath a painful corn will result in a dramatic relief of symptoms for the patient.[24]

Podophyllum. Podophyllum resin (20 percent) dispersed in compound benzoin tincture or as a solution in alcohol is effective in the treatment of condyloma acuminatum (genital warts).[4] It is a caustic and powerful skin irritant. In 24 to 48 hours after application, lesions become necrotic. In the following days, these lesions begin to slough off and gradually disappear.

The primary toxicological problem associated with the use of podophyllum resin, aside from its topical irritant qualities, is peripheral neuropathy when it is percutaneously absorbed into the systemic circulation. In fact, Chamberlain *et al.*[42] reported the development of peripheral neuropathy and intrauterine death that occurred in a young woman in the 32d week of pregnancy after the application of podophyllum resin to vulvar warts. There are other examples that can be found in the literature of peripheral neuropathy associated with the oral ingestion of podophyllum or its application to anal warts.[43 44]

Podophyllum should be applied only by a physician and then, only in small amounts. In all cases of its application (i.e., to genital warts or plantar warts), the patient should be instructed to wash off the podophyllum preparation with water within 8 to 12 hours from the time of application.

The dosage form in which podophyllum is delivered may present problems from the standpoint of delivery of the drug solely to the wart. Because the usual delivery system is a suspension (compound tincture of benzoin) or tincture (alcohol), the system does not have much viscosity. Thus, there is a tendency for the solution to run onto adjacent tissue and cause damage. This risk can be minimized by applying white petrolatum to healthy surrounding skin before applying the podophyllum preparation to the wart.[45]

Podophyllum resin for vulvar warts in pregnant women should be used cautiously, if at all. Similarly, the drug should not be used in conditions where there is hemorrhaging or an extensive skin surface area involved. These conditions increase the possibility of percutaneous absorption. Because podophyllum is such a potent corrosive, it should not be used in conjunction with other keratolytic agents (e.g., salicylic acid). The result could be a supereffect with extensive damage to the skin.

Based on the potent topical effects of podophyllum as well as its unfortunate systemic effects once absorbed, podophyllum should not be used over a long period. In fact, if used properly, it is applied only by a physician and

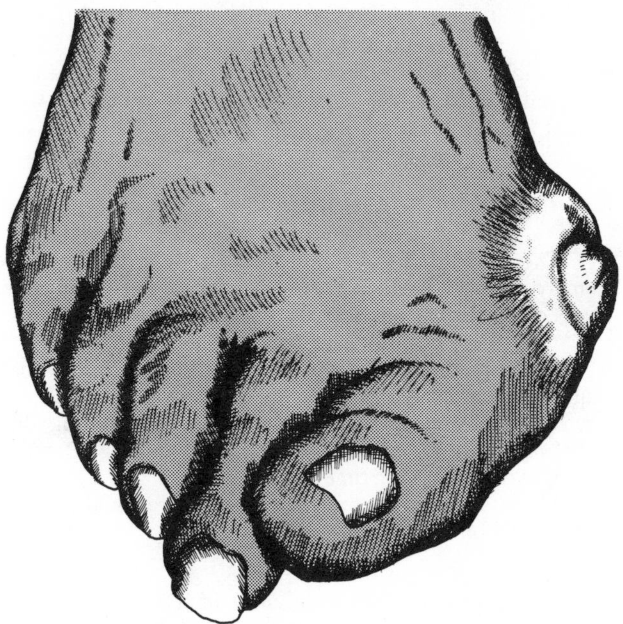

Figure 3. Foot with typical hallux valgus (bunion).

washed away after several hours of contact with the lesion. Thus, it should not be used for self-medication in adults or children.

Product evaluation

To date, there have been no definite clinical trials to indicate whether prescription-only products (e.g., cantharidin) are superior to OTC products. Conclusions can be based only on subjective physician evaluation reports infrequently found in the literature.[5 24] In light of the literature, salicylic acid in the form of a plaster or collodion dosage form is the most effective treatment for corns and calluses. Some studies advocate the use of a 50-percent solution of silver nitrate, applied by the physician, followed by weekly applications of 40 percent salicylic acid plasters for corns.[2 5]

There are many opinions about the best treatment for warts. The opinions vary from Tutunji's [46] recommendations to use nitric acid for plantar warts to other physicians' recommendations of cantharidin preparations for common warts.[17 47] Although the main use of tretinoin is in the treatment of acne vulgaris, it has been reported to be useful in the treatment of warts.[48 49]

Bunney *et al.*[19] evaluated four plantar wart products. In this study, a benzyldimethylammonium dibromide solution (Callusolve paint) was less effective than either a preparation of 50 percent podophyllum resin/liquid paraffin preparation or an established salicylic acid/lactic acid/collodion preparation (1 part:1 part:4 parts). A flexible collodion was used as the control preparation. The study also showed that the basic treatment time for simple plantar warts was about 6 weeks and that the rate of cure was fastest with salicylic acid paint. The conclusion stated that the treatment of plantar warts with salicylic acid/lactic acid/flexible collodion mixture was enhanced when the method of application of the product was understood and was carried out under the supervision of a physician.

The salicylic acid/lactic acid/flexible collodion preparation used in this study was safe and effective in children and adults; no incidences of hypersensitivity or systemic involvement were reported. Podophyllum was also used with no acute reactions, but it was used under the direct supervision of a physician, and the therapy was for plantar, not genital, warts. Podophyllum toxicity is associated with genital warts.[43 44]

Patient considerations

The medical history and medication profile are extremely valuable, particularly in cases where self-medication has been tried. Lesions such as warts or calluses and corns can mask more serious abscesses and ulcerations, and, if left medically unattended, they may lead to conditions that require hospitalization, such as osteomyelitis. Because circulation is impaired in these chronic, debilitating diseases, injury to normal skin treated with these OTC products may require a long time to heal.

Medical history and medication profile should include information on:

- ☐ Duration of the condition. Did it appear recently, with a new pair of shoes or with all footwear?
- ☐ Corns, calluses, and warts or corrective footwear in other members of the family.
- ☐ Present medical treatment of the problems.
- ☐ Present medical treatment and medication for other problems (e.g., immunosuppressive therapy).
- ☐ Characteristics of the foot problem—pain on walking, continual pain, pain when shoes are worn, or pain when pressure is applied (warts).
- ☐ Which self-medication products have been tried and for how long. Other preventive measures, e.g., new footwear.
- ☐ Allergy or allergic conditions and the kind of substances or drugs that cause them.
- ☐ Oozing or bleeding of the wart.

The seriousness of the problem must be evaluated before a helpful OTC product is recommended. However, the product cannot treat corns and calluses successfully if ill-fitting footwear, anatomical malfunctions, or faulty weight distribution is not corrected. Another factor in product selection is the ability to distinguish between corns, calluses, and warts. The pharmacist will probably not see the lesion and must be assured that the person has properly distinguished the lesion as a corn, callus, wart, or bunion.

Bunions are not amenable to topical drug therapy. The patient should correct the condition by wearing properly fitting shoes or seeing a podiatrist. If the condition is not severe, shielding the bunion with protective pads (e.g., moleskin) may be all that is necessary. However, if the manifestation is severe or particularly unsightly, surgical correction is usually indicated. If the pharmacist recommends the use of topical, adhesive cushioning to alleviate the pressure on the bunion, this should be accompanied with instructions on proper use. Before the protective pad is applied, the foot should be bathed and dried thoroughly. The pad is then cut into a shape that conforms to the bunion. If the intent is to relieve the pressure from the center of the bunion area, the pad can be cut in such a way that it surrounds the bunion. The pressure is then transferred to the surrounding pad instead of to the bunion. Precut pads are available for immediate patient use.

Larger footwear may be necessary in order to compensate for the space taken up by the pad; not increasing shoe size may cause pressure in other areas. Also, protective pads should not be used on bunions when the skin is broken or blistered. In these cases, palliative treatment should first involve treatment of the abraded skin before pads are applied. If these conditions persist (e.g., in diabetic patients), the pharmacist should recommend that the patient see a podiatrist. Surgical treatment may be necessary to save the patient from further suffering and expense.

Remission of corns, calluses, and warts does not happen quickly; it can take from several days to several months (in cases of persistent warts). Usually, treatment lasts from 3 to 7 days for corns and calluses, and 6 to 7 days for warts and is repeated, if necessary. (If the wart remains, a physician should be consulted.) Bunney *et al.*[19] showed that plantar wart therapy, in the majority of cases, took at least 6 weeks. Adherence to the dosage regimen and selection of a convenient time to apply the product are important during the course of therapy. The lack of mobility and pain associated with corns, calluses, or warts usually is a strict reminder to adhere to the medication. Topical products are to be applied daily—in the morning and at bedtime are the most convenient times.

The pharmacist should explain how to use the medication. The information that the pharmacist transmits to the patient should be clear. Because many products contain corrosive materials, it should be understood that the product is applied only to the corn, callus, or wart. If a plaster or pad is used, the process of trimming it to follow the contours of the corn or callus should be explained.

If a solution is used, it is applied, one drop at a time, directly to the corn, callus, or wart and is allowed to dry and harden to avoid running; the procedure continues until the entire affected area is covered. Adjacent areas of normal healthy skin should not come in contact with the product. If the solution does touch healthy skin, it should be washed off immediately with soap and water. If the solution is intended for a soft corn between the toes, the toes should be held apart comfortably until the solution is applied and is allowed to dry. This procedure should be followed for 3 to 6 days. The solution should solidify before applying a dressing.

A plaster should be cut to the size of the lesion, applied

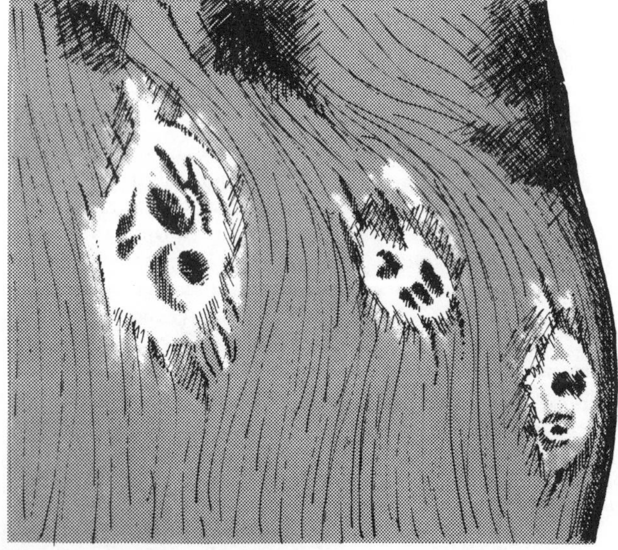

Figure 4. Sole of foot with multiple verrucae (plantar warts).

to the skin, and covered with adhesive, occlusive tape. The next day the dressing is removed and the foot is soaked in warm water. The macerated, soft white skin of the corn or callus is then removed with gentle scrubbing using a rough towel, pumice stone, or callus file, and the plaster is reapplied. Patients must be careful not to debride "healthy" skin when using a pumice stone or callus file.

Creams should be applied after the wart has been washed with soap and water. Then, an occlusive dressing generally is placed over the wart.

Because OTC preparations contain volatile and irritating ingredients, precautions should be taken in using them. After use, the container should be tightly capped, avoiding evaporation and preventing the active ingredients from assuming a greater concentration. The volatile delivery systems are quite flammable, and the product should be stored away from direct sunlight or heat in amber or light-resistant containers.

The products that contain collodions are poisonous when they are taken orally, and they should be stored out of the reach of children. They have an odor similar to that of airplane glue and can be abused by inhaling the vapors.[39]

Nonprescription products are not recommended for patients with diabetes or circulatory problems. Contraindications should be pointed out to all patients to avoid the possibility of other family members who have such conditions inadvertently using such products.

These products are keratolytic and cause skin tissue to slough off, leaving an unsightly, slightly pinkish tinge to the skin; nevertheless, they should continue being used. They should be discontinued only when a severe inflammatory response (swelling, reddening) or irritation occurs.

In addition to OTC products, self-therapy measures include:

- ☐ Daily soaking of the affected area throughout the treatment period in very warm (not hot) water to remove dead tissue.
- ☐ Gentle removal of dead tissue after normal washing. Skin should not be forcibly removed because further damage could result. Sharp knives or razor blades should not be used to cut dead tissue because they are not sterile and can cause bacterial infections. A rough towel, callus file, or pumice stone effectively removes dead tissue of corns and calluses.
- ☐ Application of petroleum jelly on the healthy skin surrounding the affected area to avoid accidental application of corrosive products. This is especially important in cases where poor eyesight increases the chances of misapplication.
- ☐ Correction of footwear involved with corns and calluses.
- ☐ Procedures to avoid the spread of warts, which are contagious: washing hands before and after treating or touching wart tissue, using a specific towel only for drying the affected area after cleaning, not picking at the wart, wearing footwear or stockings in the case of plantar warts.

Summary

The OTC drug of choice in the treatment of corns, calluses, and warts is salicylic acid. Salicylic acid may be delivered to the affected area in the form of a flexible collodion (10 percent) or a plaster (40 percent), whichever is more convenient. However, it is ineffective if predisposing factors responsible for corns and calluses are not corrected. (Surgical excision of corns associated with exostoses prevents development of corns only in that area.) The effectiveness of salicylic acid in warts is increased if the wart is pared to the point of bleeding or pain. This procedure should be performed only by a physician. Plantar warts should be treated with a higher concentration (20 to 40 percent of salicylic acid); warts on thin epidermis require a lower concentration (10 to 20 percent). Because warts are usually self-limiting, treatment should be conservative; vigorous therapy with salicylic acid can scar tissue.

Before recommending OTC treatment for corns, calluses, and warts, a patient's medical history should be studied for chronic, debilitating diseases that warrant medical treatment. Lower extremities affected by vascular insufficiency are extremely susceptible to the irritating agents in OTC products. In these areas, corns and calluses can mask deeper ulcerations and abscesses, and, if they are left medically unattended, the lesions can lead to more serious consequences.

Finally, when the pharmacist recommends a product for the patient, instructions on the use, amount, duration, and storage of medication should be understood by the patient. Extended use or misuse of these products can irritate otherwise healthy skin. Other self-therapy procedures, e.g., foot baths and tissue debridement, should be recommended when appropriate.

These instructions will help the patient better understand the condition. The patient can then understand the rationale of the treatment and the need to comply appropriately with the chosen product. Beyond this, the patient should be cautioned to consult a physician if the lesions do not respond to treatment.

Athlete's foot

Fungal infections of the skin are divided into two classes—deep systemic mycosis and superficial fungal infections. Of the two, it is usually the superficial type that warrants the pharmacist's advice and counsel.

The most prevalent superficial fungal infection in humans is athlete's foot (dermatophytosis of the foot, tinea pedis). This disease is classified symptomatically either as acute (characterized by weeping and inflammatory lesions) or subacute/chronic (characterized by dry, scaly skin).[50] In both cases, itching, burning, and stinging sensations of the feet are the primary complaints.

Etiology and predisposing factors

Species of the genera *Trichophyton, Microsporum,* and *Epidermophyton* are the most common pathogens in fungal infections of the nails, hair, and skin. The most common pathogens of tinea pedis are *Trichophyton* sp., specifically *T. mentagrophytes* and *T. rubrum*.[51]

Tinea pedis may occur at all ages but is more commonly restricted to adults. The infection is probably most often acquired by walking barefoot on infected floors, such as those in hotel bathrooms and locker rooms of clubs, schools, and camps of the armed forces. Tinea pedis may be present among several members of a family, presumably due to the spread of the fungi via the bathroom floor, bath mats, or rugs. Pathogenic fungi are also found in contaminated shoes and socks.

Among the predisposing factors contributing to the development of superficial fungal infections such as tinea pedis are poor nutrition; poor hygiene; a mild, humid climate; and debilitating diseases (e.g., diabetes). Occlusive footwear can also be included as a strong predisposing factor. Tinea pedis is not transmitted simply by exposure to fungal infections. Trauma to the skin, especially blister-producing trauma (e.g., wearing ill-fitting footwear), may contribute significantly to the occurrence of human fungal infections.[52]

Susceptibility. Although there are many pathogenic fungi in the environment, the overall incidence of actual superficial fungal infections is remarkably low. Many degrees of susceptibility produce a clinical infection —from instantaneous "takes" by as little as one spore to severe trauma by massive exposure.[53] One of the most important determinants of susceptibility to clinical fungal infection may be undefined, host-resistant factors.[54] Acquired protective immunity occurs in the majority of infected patients. Reinfection in such patients requires a greater exposure to fungi, and lesions appear to heal more rapidly. About 20 percent of those afflicted with an acute superficial fungal infection will develop a chronic fungal infection. An adequate immune response is not acquired by these patients.[55]

Pathophysiology

Superficial fungi, such as dermatophytes, attach to, proliferate, and live in the horny layer of the skin. These fungi produce keratinase, an enzyme that enables them to digest keratin, causing the outermost skin layer to disintegrate and scale.[56 57] The more severe reactions characterized by vesicles, erythema, and infiltration are presumably due to the fungi releasing an exotoxin or metabolic product.[58] Dermatophytic fungi grow only in keratinous tissue because there is a potent serum antifungal factor present that protects living tissue against deep penetration of fungal elements.[59]

The primary lesions of tinea pedis often consist of macerated tissues, slight scaling, occasional vesiculation, and fissuring between and under the toes. Any or all of the interdigital webs of the foot may be affected, although usually the skin beneath the fourth and fifth toes of each foot is involved. A relapse of the disease process often is the result of an infected toenail.[60]

There are two main clinical types of tinea pedis—vesicular and intertriginous.

Vesicular. In this form, the fungus causes a vesicular or blisterlike eruption in the epidermis beneath the surface. *T. mentagrophytes,* which causes a majority of the cases, produces this acute inflammatory condition.[51] The vesicles are about 2 to 3 mm wide and may be few in number and isolated or closely grouped into areas 2.5 to 5 cm wide. These vesicles or blisters may appear on the soles or sides of the feet or between the toes. The erythema, or skin-reddening, varies widely between patients afflicted with vesicular tinea pedis. It may be extensive or absent altogether.

After a few days, these vesicles may become yellowish and purulent. They may rupture, causing a weeping surface which may eventually become infected secondarily with pyrogenic cocci. On the other hand, the vesicles may not rupture spontaneously and may dry up as the acute stage subsides, leaving yellowish-brown crusts.

Hyperhidrosis (excessive sweating) is frequently present in this type of dermatophytosis. The sweat between the toes and on the soles of the feet has a high pH (between 6 and 7), which serves as a good culture medium for the fungi to proliferate. Burning and itching accompany the formation of the vesicles in most cases and cause discomfort.

Intertriginous. *T. rubrum* is the primary pathogenic fungus responsible for this type of "chronic dermatophytosis." In intertriginous dermatophytosis, the horny layer of the skin becomes white and macerated and usually peels off in large, friable scales. Beneath the scales, the epidermis appears dull and red. Some weeping may occur.

This type of tinea pedis may be restricted to a small patch adjacent to a fungus-infected toenail (usually caused by *T. rubrum*) or to a patch between or under the toes.[59] The absence of vesiculation is characteristic of this type of superficial fungal infection.

Signs and symptoms

The most common complaint of patients suffering from tinea pedis is pruritus. However, if fissures are present, particularly between the toes, the patient may also complain of painful burning and stinging sensations. If the foot area is abraded, denuded, or inflamed, weeping or oozing may occur in addition to frank pain. Some patients may merely remark on the bothersome scaling of dry skin, particularly if it has progressed around and to the soles of the feet. Small vesicular lesions may combine to form a larger bullous eruption marked by pain and irritation. The only symptoms may be brittleness and discoloration of a hypertrophied toenail.

The only true determinant of a fungal infection of the foot is clinical laboratory evaluation of tissue scrapings from the foot. This involves a potassium hydroxide mount preparation of the scrapings and cuttings on special growth media to show the actual presence of fungi and the specific type.[61] This procedure, however, can only be ordered and performed at the direction of a physician.

When consulted for advice, the pharmacist must question the patient thoroughly as to the condition and its characteristics. The pharmacist should try to obtain information from the patient with regard to: the acuity and description of the condition; the extent of the disease process; mitigating circumstances (e.g., diabetes, obesity) that would render the patient susceptible to the disease process; and previous patient compliance with medications.

The pharmacist must differentiate between tinea pedis and:

☐ Hyperhidrosis (excessive sweating). In this instance, tender vesicles cover the sole of the foot and toes and may be quite painful. The skin generally turns white, erodes, and becomes macerated. This condition is accompanied by a foul foot odor.

☐ Allergic contact dermatitis. This condition is characterized by a reddening of the skin and vesiculation that involves the dorsum of the foot and toes. The dermatitis may result from contact with leather, dyes, or ointments. It may be caused by new shoes, new socks, or even a topical foot powder.

☐ Atopic dermatitis. This is characterized by dry, itchy scaling of the skin and dorsum of the foot. This condition may be a reaction to a new oral medication or contact with external factors such as soaps, wool, or heat.[53]

The pharmacist should recommend that the patient consult a physician for a foot condition if:

☐ The toenail is involved. In these cases, topical treatment is ineffective and does not allay the condition until the primary focus of the disease is treated with oral griseofulvin or other preventive measures are instituted (e.g., surgical avulsion of the nail).

□ Vesicular eruptions are oozing. This includes purulent material that could be indicative of a secondary bacterial infection. In this case, topical astringent therapy and/or appropriate antibiotic therapy might be appropriate.

□ The foot is seriously inflamed and/or swollen and involves a major portion of the foot. Supportive therapy must be instituted before an antifungal agent may be applied.

□ The patient is under a physician's supervision for a disease process (e.g., diabetes, asthma) where the normal defense mechanism may be deficient.

□ The disease process is not confined to a minor portion of the foot area.

□ The patient has used an OTC product appropriately for several weeks without relief. This may be indicative of a disease other than tinea pedis.

□ The patient is suffering from hyperhidrosis, allergic contact dermatitis, or atopic dermatitis.

Treatment

Before self-medication can be effective, the correct stage of tinea pedis as well as correct treatment must be evaluated. Treatment of an actual superficial tinea infection of the foot can be effective if certain conditions are met. In acute, inflammatory tinea pedis, characterized by reddened, oozing, vesicular eruptions, the inflammatory process must be counteracted before antifungal therapy can be instituted. This is especially important if the eruptions are caused by a secondary bacterial infection.[53]

The role of self-treatment in the eradication of the disease process is effective only if the patient understands the importance of compliance with all facets of the treatment plan. Specific antifungal products must be used appropriately in conjunction with other treatment objectives (e.g., general hygienic measures).

The role of physician-directed medical treatment is implicit if the condition is in the acute, inflammatory stage. In addition, if the toenail is involved, therapy can be effective only if the nail is treated with oral griseofulvin or is surgically excised. Griseofulvin has had only moderate success in curing onychomycosis (tinea of the nail). Patient noncompliance is no doubt a contributing factor to therapeutic failures.

Ingredients in OTC products

Organic fatty acids. Sodium and calcium propionates have been used extensively in the preparation of bakery products as nontoxic mold inhibitors. Peck and Rosenfeld[62] studied the antifungal effect of various fatty acids and their salts on dermatophytes and reported encouraging clinical results with sodium propionate, a constituent of sweat. Keeney *et al.*[63] reported that the sodium salt of caprylic acid (C_8 fatty acid) was more effective than sodium undecylenate in the treatment of dermatophytosis of the foot. However, both propionic and undecylenic acids are weakly fungistatic.[64]

Whether organic fatty acids are more effective than sulfur and/or iodine preparations in the treatment of superficial fungal infections is questionable. Organic acid preparations should be used, if at all, only for very mild or for chronic forms of tinea pedis.

The concentration of the organic fatty acids and/or their salt forms is usually too low to be irritating to the skin. Although these products are nonsensitizing, if irritation or sensitivity develops with their use, treatment should be discontinued.

These organic fatty acids and/or their salts are available in a variety of dosage forms. The cream or ointment forms are usually used at bedtime, and solutions should be used for their soothing effects after a footbath. The powder is usually sprinkled into the socks and shoes in the morning. The efficacy of the powder forms of these weak organic acids must be questioned from the standpoint of drug delivery. Most powder dosage forms of these organic fatty acids contain the salts of the acids. If the vehicle of the powder contains "inert" ingredients which are either adsorbent or absorbent, such as talc, corn starch, magnesium carbonate, etc., it is questionable whether the salt can convert to the fungistatic acid with minimal moisture. For example, it may be that the efficacy of the product is attributable to the absorbent "inert" ingredients preventing moisture buildup. So far, no clinical study has compared the salt of the organic acid in its powder form with the powder vehicle itself.

Undecylenic acid–zinc undecylenate. This combination is widely used for various superficial fungal infections exclusive of those involving nails and/or hairy parts of the body. It is fungistatic and is effective in mild, chronic cases of tinea pedis. Compound undecylenic acid ointment (USP XIX) contains undecylenic acid and 20 percent zinc undecylenate in a polyethylene glycol vehicle.[65] It is believed that zinc undecylenate liberates undecylenic acid (the active antifungal entity) when it comes in contact with moisture (e.g., perspiration). In addition, zinc undecylenate has astringent properties due to the presence of zinc ion.[58] This astringent activity decreases the irritation and inflammation of the infection.

When applied to the skin in the form of an ointment, diluted solution, or dusting powder, the combination (undecylenic acid–zinc undecylenate) is relatively nonirritating, and hypersensitivity reactions associated with its use are uncommon. The undiluted solution, however, can cause transient stinging when applied to broken skin due to its alcoholic content. Caution must be exercised by the patient to ensure that these ingredients do not come in contact with the eye or that the powder is not inhaled.

The vehicle in compound undecylenic acid ointment has a water-miscible base, which would make it nonocclusive, water-removable, and easy to apply. The powder uses talc as its vehicle and adsorbent. The aerosol contains menthol, which serves as a counterirritant and antipruritic. The solution contains 10 percent undecylenic acid in a vehicle solution of propanol, propylene glycol, and water. The product is applied twice daily after cleansing the affected area. The usual period for therapeutic results is dependent upon the patient. However, improvement should occur in 2 to 4 weeks, after which the condition should be reevaluated and an alternative medication tried.

To avoid contamination of the product, a small amount of solution is poured from the stock solution into a smaller glass container. With an applicator or cotton swab, the solution is then applied from the smaller container. Another precaution is to allow the solution to air-dry after it has been applied. If this is not done, the water will accumulate, resulting in further maceration of tissue. A problem associated with the use of products that have undecylenic acid as their main ingredient is that undecylenic acid has a rancid odor. This may be objectionable to some patients and may promote ultimate patient noncompliance.

The combination is beneficial to patients with mild, chronic forms of tinea pedis. In a controlled drug efficacy study involving guinea pigs, various Desenex products (undecylenic acid–zinc undecylenate liquid, ointment, and aerosol powder) were evaluated in the treatment of *T. mentagrophytes* superficial fungal infections.[66] None of the products was capable of effecting a complete cure of the infection. However, each tested preparation controlled the severity of the infection in a majority of the animals after several daily applications. Control of the disease was measured by the reduction of erythema, swelling, and scaliness of the infected zone. However, once therapy ceased, the disease process in several guinea pigs returned to a more severe lesion response within 48 hours.

The efficacy and use of undecylenic acid–zinc undecylenate combinations must be questioned when the condition is complicated by an infected toenail. In these cases, the combination is useless and cannot eradicate the primary foci of the disease.

Other preparations, e.g., ointments, powders, and tinctures, incorporate undecylenic acid (10 percent) by itself in the vehicle. This concentration of undecylenic acid has minor irritative effects on the skin. However, undecylenic acid should not be applied directly to mucous membranes in concentrations of more than 1 percent.

Acetic acid. In addition to caprylic, propionic, and undecylenic acids, acetic acid is used in treating tinea pedis. In OTC products, acetic acid is delivered to the infected area as triacetin (glyceryl triacetate). The fungistatic activity of triacetin is based on the fact that at the neutral or alkaline pH of infected skin, fungal esterase enzymes cleave triacetin into acetic acid and glycerin.[67] The acetic acid then effects antifungal activity by lowering the pH at the site of infection. As the pH increases after the initial release of acetic acid, more acetic acid is generated by the enzymes and the process is repeated. The efficacy of products containing triacetin has not been proved by controlled clinical trials.[68]

In the concentrations used, the small amount of acetic acid liberated is probably nonirritating to the skin in a majority of cases. The corresponding incidence of sensitization would also be low. However, there are some precautions that must be taken with the use of triacetin. The acetic acid formed can damage rayon fabrics, so the treated areas should be covered with a clean bandage to prevent contact. Triacetin must not come in contact with the eyes.

Triacetin [topical aerosol (15 percent), cream (25 percent), or powder pack (33.3 percent)] should be applied every evening after thorough cleansing. The aerosol and powder may be used adjunctively to the cream form. The product should be used until the infection is cleared entirely. Then, it is suggested that it be used once a week as a preventive measure.

Triacetin is relatively odorless and colorless when used topically. Odor emanating from the formation of acetic acid is dependent on the amount of acetic acid formed.

Phenolic compounds and derivatives. These aromatic compounds are included in topical OTC athlete's foot products for their keratolytic or fungicidal effects.

Salicylic acid. In high concentrations, salicylic acid is a keratolytic agent, causing a shedding of the keratin layer of the skin and facilitating penetration of other drugs. Lower concentrations (less than 2 percent) are keratoplastic; they aid normal keratinization. Salicylic acid (5 to 10 percent) softens the stratum corneum by increasing the endogenous hydration of this layer. This is probably the result of a lowering of the pH which causes the cornified epithelium to swell, soften, macerate, and then desquamate.[69] If no moisture is present, cornified epithelium will not be significantly softened by tolerable amounts of salicylic acid. Because salicylic acid accelerates exfoliation of the infected keratin tissue, its use in conjunction with topical antifungals in appropriate conditions can be very beneficial.[68]

Salicylic acid alone has little or no antifungal activity. It usually is applied to the skin as a combination of 3 percent salicylic acid and 6 percent benzoic acid in a polyethylene glycol base.[70] Benzoic acid alone is alleged to have some fungistatic activity, but this is debatable at best. This ointment is available in double strength and half strength. The half-strength formula (1.5 percent salicylic acid) does not have the keratolytic properties of the regular or double strength and should, therefore, never be used when keratolytic activity is necessary. The basic criterion for evaluating the efficacy of salicylic acid products as keratolytic agents is the concentration of salicylic acid. Thus, based on current literature, these products should contain concentrations of more than 2 percent salicylic acid.

The pharmacist should be aware of the irritant properties of topically applied salicylic acid. No doubt many skin irritations have been reported following unsupervised self-medication.

Phenol and substituted phenols. Phenol and substituted phenols (e.g., resorcinol) are included in many topical antifungal products. Phenol is fungicidal at a concentration of 1.3 percent. Resorcinol is also fungicidal, but its potency is about one-third that of phenol. Phenol is reported to be more effective in aqueous solutions than in glycerin or fats; it is relatively ineffective when incorporated into fats.[71]

When applied to unabraded skin in low concentrations, phenol causes warmth and a tingling sensation. Its irritant qualities usually restrict phenol's effectiveness in athlete's foot remedies. In order to be fungicidal in these preparations, concentrations that are irritating to human skin generally must be used.

Resorcinol, in concentrations usually applied topically (less than 10 percent), is nonirritating; higher concentrations can be irritating. Although resorcinol has the potential to produce allergic reactions, they rarely occur.

Phenol and resorcinol resemble each other with regard to systemic action, particularly on the CNS. Thus, preparations containing either of these should never be applied to large areas or to irritated or denuded skin because of possible absorption and systemic toxicity.

Chloroxylenol, a substituted phenol, is a nonirritating antiseptic agent. Chloroxylenol (0.5-percent solution) was reported to be effective in treating and preventing athlete's foot.[72] Observations were that the chloroxylenol solution was nonirritating to the skin, relieved itching in a majority of cases, seemed to increase evaporation of perspiration, and controlled hyperhidrosis. The solution appeared more effective against new, acute conditions than against chronic cases of athlete's foot. Therapy with the solution averaged between 1 and 4 weeks.

Chloroxylenol is included in some topical preparations. It is used in liquid, cream, and powder forms. Because chloroxylenol has limited water solubility, its efficacy is questionable in powder drug delivery systems. If the inert agents of the vehicle are effective in adsorbing moisture, the effect of the chloroxylenol would be diminished.

Chloroxylenol causes no cutaneous irritation at a concentration of 5 percent.[73] It is less toxic than phenol, but eczematous reactions have followed its use.[74]

Carbol-fuchsin solution. Basic fuchsin (NF XIII) dye is a mixture of rosaniline and pararosaniline hydrochlorides. It is used only in superficial fungal infections of the foot in the form of carbol-fuchsin solution (NF XIII), or Castellani's paint.[75] The solution is dark purple but appears red when painted onto the affected area in a fine film. It has local anesthetic and fungicidal properties.

The indications for the use of carbol-fuchsin solution in tinea pedis are in the subacute or chronic stages of infection, when there is little or no inflammation. The solution should not be applied to inflamed or denuded skin. Carbol-fuchsin solution in tinea pedis is not as effective as other agents.[69]

The staining property of basic fuchsin and the poisonous nature of the solution limit the usefulness of carbol-fuchsin solution. Several precautions should be taken:

☐ The solution must not be applied to an extensive area of the foot. No more than 10 percent of the foot should be treated with the solution at one time.

☐ The area to which the solution has been applied must be allowed to dry thoroughly.

☐ The solution must not come in contact with inanimate objects, including clothing, due to its staining properties.

☐ Because the alcohol and acetone in the solution are volatile the container must be tightly covered. When not in use, this solution should be kept out of the reach of children.

☐ If the solution is ingested accidentally, a physician should be consulted immediately.

Before the solution is applied, the affected area should be thoroughly cleaned with soap and water and dried. The solution is then applied to the area with an applicator and reapplied once or twice daily for one week. After this time, if the condition has not improved, choice of medication as well as assessment of the actual condition should be reevaluated.

The efficacy of carbol-fuchsin solution must be questioned, especially if an infected toenail is involved. Use of the applicator tip back and forth into the stock solution may cause contamination. Because the preparation contains several volatile components, the patient should securely tighten the cap to avoid evaporation. Otherwise, volatile ingredients escape and other nonvolatile components become more concentrated (e.g., resorcinol), and irritation can result with subsequent applications.

The effectiveness of the product is limited because it can only be applied to 10 percent of the foot area. This limitation, its staining properites, and the fact that a patient could be sensitive to ingredients in the product limit the usefulness of carbol-fuchsin solution for tinea pedis.

Naphthol derivatives. The most notable naphthol derivative synthesized for antifungal activity is tolnaftate.[76] Its spectrum of action encompasses typical fungi responsible for tinea pedis, including *T. mentagrophytes* and *T. rubrum.* In addition, it is effective against *E. floccosum* and *Microsporum* sp. Although the exact mechanism of action of tolnaftate has not been reported, it is believed that it distorts the hyphae and stunts the mycelial growth of the fungi species. Tolnaftate is more effective in tinea pedis than in onychomycosis or tinea capitis. For onychomycosis and tinea capitis, concomitant administration of oral griseofulvin is necessary, unless the condition is superficial.

Tolnaftate is tolerated well when applied to intact or broken skin in either exposed or intertriginous areas. Tolnaftate usually causes a slight stinging sensation when applied. Although there has been one report of a developed delayed hypersensitivity reaction to tolnaftate, there have been no references to hypersensitivity associated with its use.[77] As with all topical medicaments, irritation, sensitization, or worsening of the skin condition warrants discontinuance of the product.

Tolnaftate (1-percent solution or 1-percent cream) is applied sparingly twice daily after thoroughly cleansing the affected area. The usual period for effective therapy is 2 to 4 weeks, although treatment from 4 to 6 weeks may be necessary for some individuals, e.g., patients with lesions between the toes or on pressure areas of the foot. When medication is applied to pressure areas of the foot, where the horny layer of skin is thicker than normal, concomitant use of a keratolytic agent might be advisable. Neither keratolytic agents nor wet compresses, such as aluminum acetate (Burow's) solution, which promote the healing of oozing lesions, interfere with the efficacy of tolnaftate. If weeping lesions are present, the inflammation should be treated before tolnaftate is applied.

The cream dosage form of tolnaftate is formulated in a polyethylene glycol 400/propylene glycol vehicle, the solution in polyethylene glycol 400. These vehicles are particularly advantageous in superficial antifungal therapy because they are nonocclusive, nontoxic, nonsensitizing, water-miscible, anhydrous, easy to apply, and efficient in delivering the drug to the affected area.

High molecular weight polyethylene glycol bases have been reported to form associated complexes with some medicaments, e.g., benzoic and salicylic acids. Although diffusion of the medicament to the skin is adequate with polyethylene glycol bases, little percutaneous absorption occurs.[78,79] In regard to topical antifungal therapy, however, complex formation seems inconsequential because the role of the vehicle in this instance is to supply the drug to the horny layer of the skin.

Tolnaftate solution solidifies when exposed to cold. However, if the preparation is allowed to warm, it will liquefy with no loss in potency.

The topical powder formulation of tolnaftate uses corn starch–talc as its vehicle. This vehicle is not only an effective drug delivery system but also offers therapeutic advantage due to the water-retaining nature of the two agents. Tolnaftate powder was shown to be more effective than its vehicle in reducing the incidence of tinea pedis in patients who, upon initial examination, demonstrated laboratory-confirmed dermatophytosis of the foot.[80] The topical aerosol formulation of tolnaftate includes talc in addition to the propellant vehicle.

Tolnaftate has demonstrated marked clinical efficacy since its commercial introduction in the U.S. in 1965, and, since then, it has become the standard, ethical, topical antifungal medicament.[81] In addition, there has been a consistent absence of signs of irritation or hypersensitivity to tolnaftate, in the form of a cream, solution, or powder.

In a drug efficacy study involving guinea pigs infected with *T. mentagrophytes,* Wolin[82] reported that tolnaftate solution was capable of controlling the infection with several daily applications. Desenex solution, however, was found to be ineffective in the treatment of *T. mentagrophytes* infection in guinea pigs in that same study. From this small scale study, it would appear that the tolnaftate (i.e., Tinactin) solution was superior to Desenex solution in the control of *T. mentagrophytes* in guinea pigs.

There have been implications in the literature of superficial fungal infection relapse after tolnaftate therapy has been discontinued.[68] However, this relapse may be caused by an inadequate time for treatment, patient noncompliance with the medication, or the use of tolnaftate where oral griseofulvin therapy should have been instituted.

Quinoline derivatives. Oster and Golden [83] examined 24 derivatives of quinoline in *in vitro* testing for fungistatic or fungicidal activity. Of the series of compounds investigated, only benzoxiquine (8-hydroxyquinoline benzoate) was found to be active in fungistatic and fungicidal testing. Zentmyer [84] postulated that the activity of 8-hydroxyquinoline was due to chemical inactivation via chelation of trace metals, essential for the growth of fungi, either in the nutritive media or the cell of the fungus. Three percent benzoxiquine in a vanishing cream base was shown to be fungicidal in *in vitro* testing when compared to other antifungal ointments.[64] Subsequently, an antifungal preparation containing 2.5 percent benzoxiquine was used successfully in the treatment of dermatophytosis.[85]

Several proprietary powder antifungals use 8-hydroxyquinoline sulfate in their formulations. This compound is fungicidal. Because the sulfate salt is fairly water soluble and forms an acidic solution in the pressure of moisture, it may lend more efficacy to the antifungal effect of the 8-hydroxyquinoline. However, there is no clinical evidence to substantiate or refute this assumption.

Quaternary ammonium compounds. Quaternary ammonium compounds (e.g., benzethonium chloride, methylbenzethonium chloride) are used in several antifungal aids for their skin antiseptic and detergent properties. Solutions of these agents have emulsifying properties, all of which favor wetting and penetration of surfaces to which they are applied. These compounds are germicidal to most pathogenic fungi.

The disinfectant action of these compounds may not be as great as expected. These compounds are cationic and have a chemical incompatibility with anionic compounds such as soaps. Thus, if there is any residual soap or soap film on the skin, it will inactivate their usefulness.[86] In athlete's foot, where patients are told to clean their feet thoroughly on a daily basis, patients must also be instructed to rinse the affected area thoroughly before drying it. Otherwise, if the product used contains one of these quaternary ammonium compounds, any beneficial effects may be negated. Price [87] reported that a tincture delivery system of these cationic compounds is more effective as a skin disinfectant and is less affected by soap than an aqueous solution. Accordingly, tincture forms of these agents are used in more dilute concentrations than aqueous solutions.

Therefore, in a liquid form, especially a tincture, these quaternary compounds should be effective if appropriate concentrations are used. However, when applied topically in powder form with adsorbent agents included in the formulation, their efficacy may be in doubt. If all moisture is removed effectively by the adsorbing material, the quaternary compound will not be able to dissolve and exert its germicidal activity, but these compounds will dissolve in a minimal amount of water.

Quaternary ammonium compounds generally are safe when applied topically. However, each compound has its own sensitization index and its own ability to produce contact dermatitis as a result of widespread usage and multiple sources of patient exposure to these chemicals.

Salts of aluminum. The foremost astringent used in the acute inflammatory stage of tinea pedis probably is aluminum acetate. Aluminum acetate is usually applied as a wet dressing to the affected area as a 5-percent solution.

The action of aluminum acetate and all external astringents is as a protein precipitant which, when applied to cell surfaces, will limit secretions of glands by contracting and hardening tissue. The astringent will decrease edema, exudation, and inflammation by reducing the permeability of the cell membrane and hardening the cement substance of the capillary epithelium.[88]

Aluminum acetate solution for use in tinea pedis generally is diluted with about 10 to 40 parts of water. Depending on the situation, the patient will either immerse the whole foot for 20 minutes up to three times daily into the solution or merely apply the solution in the form of a wet dressing to the area.

When topical aluminum acetate solution dressings are indicated, an appropriate product can be selected depending on the involvement of the acute, inflammatory lesion. Where lesions cover a limited area of the foot, Burowets, a disposable dressing saturated with 1:20 aluminum acetate solution, would be convenient. If the lesions are extensive and a foot soak is desired, Buro-Sol powder can be made into a solution. Similarly, the use of Domeboro (powder or tablets) or Bluboro powder diluted with appropriate amounts of water will form a modified aluminum acetate solution. These latter products use aluminum sulfate and calcium acetate to form the solution.

These products are convenient to use. They are intended for external use and are not to be ingested and should be kept away from contact with the eyes. Prolonged or continuous use of aluminum acetate solution for extended periods can produce necrosis.[89] However, in the acute, inflammatory stage of tinea pedis, this solution should only be used for less than one week. The pharmacist should instruct the patient to discontinue use of the solution if extensive inflammatory lesions appear to worsen or if irritation becomes more apparent.

If used appropriately, aluminum acetate solution is valuable in the acute, inflammatory stage of tinea pedis. However, its potential for misuse (e.g., ingesting the solution or tablets by children) is real, and precautions must be taken to prevent this.

Other ingredients and dosage forms

The primary drug delivery systems used for treatment of tinea pedis are creams, solutions, and powders. Powders, including those in aerosol dosage forms, are generally indicated for adjunctive use with solutions and creams. In very mild conditions, powders may suffice as the sole therapy.

These delivery systems play an integral and vital role in the treatment of tinea pedis. The basic premise of these specialized dosage forms is ease of administration as well as efficacy in presenting the active medicament to the affected area of the skin.

The vehicle of the solution or cream forms should be:

- ☐ Nonocclusive. The vehicle should not retain moisture or sweat which exacerbates the condition.
- ☐ Water-miscible or water-washable. The patient should be able to remove the vehicle with minimal cleansing effort. Hard scrubbing of the affected area further abrades the skin.
- ☐ Anhydrous. Inclusion of water into the formulation introduces a variable that is one of the primary causes of the condition.
- ☐ Spreadable. The vehicle should be applicable with minimal effort and without waste.
- ☐ Capable of efficient drug delivery. The vehicle must not interact with the active ingredient, but allow it to penetrate to the seat of the fungal infection.
- ☐ Nonsensitizing and nontoxic when applied to in-

tact or denuded skin. If the vehicle is absorbed into the systemic circulation, it should be nontoxic.

Most vehicles used to deliver topical solutions and creams are essentially polyethylene glycol bases with variable amounts of propylene glycol and alcohols. These vehicles meet the above criteria. Polyethylene glycol bases are very efficient in delivering water-insoluble drugs topically as compared to delivering water-soluble agents. This is an added advantage because most topical antifungal drugs are basically water insoluble (e.g., tolnaftate).

The criteria for the powder dosage form (normal or under pressure) are basically the same as those for creams or solutions. Certain agents in powder dosage forms are therapeutic and also serve as vehicles, e.g., talc and/or corn starch. Some OTC powder formulations state that the active ingredient is contained in a moisture-absorbent base (i.e., Enzactin). Powder dosage forms inhibit the propagation of fungi by absorbing moisture and preventing skin maceration. Thus, powder forms actually alter the ecological conditions of the fungi, but the actual effective agent in these powder formulations is unknown.[80] For example, the adsorbing material within the powder, rather than the active ingredients, might be responsible for the remission of the disease.

Product evaluation

Methods

Current clinical trials used to evaluate the efficacy of topical antifungal products usually are well controlled. In general, the studies are randomized, double-blind investigations involving human subjects with tinea pedis. All patients in these experiments are diagnosed subjectively (physical examination) and objectively (microscopic evaluation) to determine if dermatophytosis is present. Approximately one-half of the sample patients are then given the active medicament in its intended vehicle for use; the rest are given a placebo. The subjects are periodically examined subjectively and objectively, and the efficacy of the product is determined using the two criteria together. Most studies try to follow patients beyond the normal treatment time. Although this is limited and difficult, the followup helps ascertain the extended effectiveness of the products in eradicating the disease and preventing remission.

The current trend toward evaluation of topical antifungals involves newer prescription-only drugs (clotrimazole, haloprogin, miconazole nitrate). Tolnaftate is used as the standard for comparison because it is tolnaftate that appears to be the most effective OTC topical antifungal agent.

Effectiveness and safety

Unlike other ringworm infections, tinea pedis generally occurs only in adults; the infection is rare in children. Efficacy and safety of drugs are based on clinical reports involving human subjects affected with tinea pedis. Clinical evaluation methods such as microscopic analysis of tissue scrapings have helped confirm dermatophytosis prior to the study as well as determine drug efficacy after the termination of the study.

Laboratory test methods have included toxicity and efficacy studies in animals. Usually, these have involved guinea pigs inoculated with *Trichophyton* sp. and treated with the active medicament under investigation.[66 82] Because tinea pedis afflicts many people and is amenable to topical therapy, clinical efficacy studies usually involve human subject panels. This is extremely beneficial because the effects of species, animals vs. humans, is obviated and effectiveness of the medications can be judged in those for whom the medication is intended.

The effectiveness of products for superficial fungal infections (e.g., tinea pedis) is not predicated only on the action of the drug itself but also on predisposing factors. In general, these products are nonsensitizing and nonirritating when applied topically. Although they appear to be safe for application in children if the situation warranted, the poison potential from misuse of some products should be noted. If accidentally ingested, particularly by young children, some preparations can be toxic. Ingredients that are classified as extremely dangerous in this regard include phenols, salicylic acid, and carbol-fuchsin. These products must be kept out of the reach of children, especially those dosage forms that appear drinkable (solutions) or are capable of being accidentally inhaled (powders). In addition, adequate preventive measures must ensure that products that are potential irritants (e.g., salicylic acid, phenols) do not come in contact with the eyes.

Guidelines for product selection

Once the pharmacist is convinced that the patient's condition is amenable to topical OTC therapy, patient acceptance and compliance with the product recommended must be dealt with. The pharmacist must discern from interacting with the patient whether the patient is an "at risk" patient or not. An "at risk" patient is one who usually cannot be bothered to take the time to adhere to a prescribed or recommended dosage regimen. Thus, any merit that can be gained from therapy is usually lost by noncompliance. In all cases, however, the pharmacist is charged with the responsibility of choosing the appropriate product, in an appropriate form, in such a way that the product will cause the least interference with daily habits and activities and yet be efficacious.

The pharmacist should consider the patient's current mental and physical status in the selection of a product. The foremost concern is that the patient understand the directions for use in order to comply with them. The pharmacist should choose the product which is as simple as possible to use but which, at the same time, is most effective. Product selection must also be geared to the particular patient. For example, if the patient is elderly, the pharmacist may need to recommend a product which is easier than normal to use; if the patient is obese, excessive sweating may contribute significantly to the disease process, and the pharmacist may consider recommending topical talcum powders as an adjunctive measure.

The pharmacist must clearly understand for whom the product is intended. Although children rarely suffer from tinea pedis, parents often ask the pharmacist to recommend a product, without stating that the product is for a child.

The medical history of the patient is invaluable in assessing patient response to suggested therapy. If the patient is diabetic, an overabundance of glucose (a normal constituent of sweat) is secreted.[72] Glucose is an excellent growth medium for fungi. In order for topical therapy to be effective, the diabetes must be under control. The medical history is also important for patients who suffer from allergic dermatitides because these individuals are extremely sensitive to most agents, oral and topical.

An atopic individual will usually have a history of asthma, hay fever, or atopic dermatitis. The medication profile should list these conditions, and the medications indicated for treatment will be apparent. It is extremely important that atopic dermatitis not be confused with a tinea infection. Selection of the wrong topical product might result in skin irritation and an allergic reaction. An up-to-date medication profile will show if the patient is on immunosuppressive therapy (e.g., corticosteroids). If so, this therapy may not only impede the healing process of a tinea infection but may also be a predisposing factor to the infection. In order to ascertain a patient's compliance record, the pharmacist can check the medication record for chronic medications on which the patient is maintained and the patient's timing of refill requests.

The pharmacist must bear in mind that prescription-only drugs available for tinea pedis might be more beneficial. Haloprogin (Halotex), miconazole nitrate (Mica-Tin), and clotrimazole (Lotrimin) have demonstrated efficacy in the treatment of cutaneous candidiasis in addition to the treatment of dermatophytoses. Thus, their spectrum of activity appears broader than that of tolnaftate.

Pharmacist advice to the patient

Patients should be advised by the pharmacist not to expect dramatic remission of the condition initially. The onset of relief of the symptoms may take several days because healing generally is a gradual process. Patients should be advised that, depending on certain factors (e.g., extent of the affected area, patient variability to medication), the medication may have to be used for a minimum of 2 to 4 weeks. The patient should be told of the necessity to adhere to the dosage regimen prescribed by the physician or the suggested directions contained on the OTC product label. This is especially appropriate for the use of the OTC topical products because they probably will be used by the patient for a minimum of 2 weeks. Although patient noncompliance is not documented in the literature, it probably contributes to the failure of topical products in the treatment of tinea pedis. Assuming topical therapy will be successful the pharmacist should ask the patient to continue the medication for a few days after the recommended time period to help prevent the possibility of a relapse of the infection.

All topical antifungal products can induce various hypersensitivity reactions. Although the incidence is small, patients should be advised to discontinue the product if itching, swelling, or further exacerbations of the disease occur.

Because topical antifungal products are intended for topical use, patients should avoid contact of these products with their eyes. After applying the product, patients should wash their hands thoroughly with soap and water.

General recommendations

Before effective drug therapy for athlete's foot can be instituted, the pharmacist should emphasize the need for proper hygiene.

☐ The feet should be cleaned and dried thoroughly each day. Even though transmission of the disease to other individuals is rare, patients should have their own washcloths and towels for cleansing and washing. The affected area should be thoroughly patted dry. After bathing, the feet should be dried last so as not to spread the infection with the towel to other sites.

☐ General measures should be taken to eliminate the predisposing factors—heat and perspiration. Shoes and light cotton socks that allow ventilation should be worn. Wool and some newer synthetic fabrics interfere with the dissipation of moisture originating from the foot. Occlusive footwear, including canvas, rubber-soled, athletic shoes should not be worn. Shoes should be alternated as often as possible to permit adequate drying of the inside of the shoes. Socks should be changed daily and washed thoroughly after use. Shoes should be dusted with drying powders.

☐ Clothing and towels should be changed frequently and well laundered in hot water.

☐ The feet, particularly the area between the toes, should be dusted with a drying powder at every change of socks. Whenever possible, the feet should be aired to prevent moisture buildup.

☐ Nonocclusive, protective footwear (e.g., rubber or wooden sandals) should be worn in areas of family or public use such as the home bathroom, community showers, or bathing areas.

The pharmacist should inform the patient of the need for protective measures which aid the topical antifungal product in eradicating the fungal infection. However, patients should be cautioned against overzealous cleansing with soap and water and vigorous drying between the toes; this can further irritate the area.

Summary

The pharmacological OTC drug of choice, from the standpoint of proven efficacy, in the treatment of tinea pedis, is tolnaftate. However, other predisposing factors to tinea pedis must be eliminated by the patient in order that tolnaftate be effective. In this regard, recommendations from the pharmacist are important and should be emphasized.

Tolnaftate is effective in all its drug delivery systems. However, the powder form should be reserved only for extremely mild conditions or as adjunctive therapy.

When it is recommended for suspected or actual dermatophytosis of the foot, tolnaftate should be used twice a day, morning and night. Because the vehicle forms of the solution and cream are spreadable, they should be used sparingly. Treatment should be continued for 2 to 4 weeks, depending on the symptoms. After this time, effectiveness should be evaluated by the patient and pharmacist. It may be that therapy should be continued or a physician should be consulted if the condition persists or if there is a possibility of another disease process. Depending on the severity, when the condition is characterized by oozing or acute lesions, soaks and compresses may be suggested. After the initial inflammatory response has subsided, topical therapy with tolnaftate can be instituted. Alleviation of the symptoms does not occur overnight. Patients should be aware of this to avoid noncompliance associated with a product which they believe to be ineffective.

References

1. S. Rosen, *J. Med. Assoc. State Ala.*, **43,** 617(1974).
2. A. N. Domonkos, "Andrews' Diseases of the Skin," 6th ed., Saunders, Philadelphia, Pa., 1971, pp. 54-58.
3. G. K. Potter, *J. Am. Podiatr. Assoc.*, **63,** 57(1973).

4. F. Sadik, "Handbook of Non-Prescription Drugs," American Pharmaceutical Association, Washington, D. C., 1973, pp. 180-184.
5. "Current Dermatologic Management," S. Maddin and T. H. Brown, Eds., Mosby, St. Louis, Mo., 1970, pp. 114-116.
6. W. D. Stewart, *et al.*, "Dermatology: Diagnosis and Treatment of Cutaneous Disorders," 3d ed., Mosby, St. Louis, Mo., 1974, pp. 3-21.
7. N. J. Giannestras, "Foot Disorders: Medical and Surgical Management," 2d ed., Lea and Febiger, Philadelphia, Pa., 1973, pp. 420-421.
8. N. J. Giannestras, "Foot Disorders: Medical and Surgical Management," 2d ed., Lea and Febiger, Philadelphia, Pa., 1973, pp. 24-26.
9. I. Yale, "Podiatric Medicine," Williams and Wilkins, Baltimore, Md., 1974, pp. 244-246.
10. "DuVries' Surgery of the Foot," 3d ed., V. T. Inman, Ed., Mosby, St. Louis, Mo., 1973, pp. 206-223.
11. A. N. Domonkos, "Andrews' Diseases of the Skin," 6th ed., Saunders, Philadelphia, Pa., 1971, pp. 548-553.
12. E. Jawetz *et al.*, "Review of Medical Microbiology," 11th ed., Lange Medical Publications, Los Altos, Calif., 1974, pp. 449-450.
13. "Harrison's Principles of Internal Medicine," M. M. Wintrobe *et al.*, Eds., 7th ed., McGraw-Hill, New York, N.Y., 1974, p. 977.
14. J. S. Pegum, *Practitioner,* **209,** 453(1972).
15. F. A. Ive, *Br. Med. J.,* **4,** 475(1973).
16. K. A. Arndt, "Manual of Dermatological Therapeutics," Little, Brown, Boston, Mass., 1974, pp. 167-173.
17. W. D. Stewart *et al.*, "Dermatology: Diagnosis and Treatment of Cutaneous Disorders," 3d ed., Mosby, St. Louis, Mo., 1974, pp. 281-285.
18. A. P. Goffe *et al., Lancet,* **2,** 607(1966).
19. M. H. Bunney *et al., Practitioner,* **207,** 197(1971).
20. J. H. Graham *et al.*, Eds., "Dermal Pathology," Harper and Row, Hagerstown, Md., 1972, pp. 533-535.
21. F. R. Bettley, "Skin Diseases in General Practice," Charles C Thomas, Springfield, Ill., 1965, pp. 243-253.
22. N. Tobias, "Essentials of Dermatology," 6th ed., Lippincott, Philadelphia, Pa., 1963, p. 210.
23. H. T. Behrman *et al.*, "Common Skin Diseases: Diagnosis and Treatment," 2d ed., Grune and Stratton, New York, N.Y., 1971, pp. 139-142.
24. K. A. Arndt, "Manual of Dermatological Therapeutics," Little, Brown, Boston, Mass., 1974, pp. 23-25.
25. "Drug Design," vol. 4, E. J. Ariens, Ed., Academic Press, New York, N.Y., 1973, p. 134.
26. J. F. vonWeiss and W. F. Lever, *Arch. Dermatol.,* **90,** 614(1964).
27. M. E. Stolar *et al., J. Am. Pharm. Assoc. (Sci. Ed.),* **49,** 144(1960).
28. "Drug Design," vol. 4, E. J. Ariens, Ed., Academic Press, New York, N.Y., 1973, p. 178.
29. J. A. Mills, *N. Engl. J. Med.,* **290,** 781(1974).
30. "The United States Pharmacopoeia," 19th rev., Mack Publishing Easton, Pa., 1975, p. 446.
31. N. W. Blacow, "Martindale: The Extra Pharmacopoeia," 26th ed., Pharmaceutical Press, London, England, 1972, pp. 879-882.
32. "The Pharmacological Basis of Therapeutics," 5th ed., L. S. Goodman and A. Gilman, Eds., Macmillan, New York, N.Y., 1975, p. 1000.
33. M. N. Gleason *et al.*, "Clinical Toxicology of Commercial Products, Acute Poisoning," 3d ed., Williams and Wilkins, Baltimore, Md., 1969, Section 2, p. 154.
34. N. W. Blacow, "Martindale: The Extra Pharmacopoeia," 26th ed., Pharmaceutical Press, London, England, 1972, pp. 1256-1257.
35. "AMA Drug Evaluations," 2d ed., Publishing Sciences Group, Acton, Mass., 1973, pp. 153-170.
36. "Sprowls' American Pharmacy," 7th ed., L. W. Dittert, Ed., Lippincott, Philadelphia, Pa., 1974, p. 167.
37. H. C. Ansel, "Introduction to Pharmaceutical Dosage Forms," Lea and Febiger, Philadelphia, Pa., 1969, p. 260.
38. E. M. Brecher and Editors of Consumer Reports, "Licit and Illicit Drugs," Little, Brown, Boston, Mass., 1972, pp. 309-320.
39. H. C. Ansel, "Introduction to Pharmaceutical Dosage Forms," Lea Febiger, Philadelphia, Pa., 1969, p. 339.
40. "Remington's Pharmaceutical Sciences," 14th ed., A. Osol *et al.*, Eds., Mack Publishing, Easton, Pa., 1970, p. 1076.
41. "AMA Drug Evaluations," 2d ed., Publishing Sciences Group, Acton, Mass., 1973, p. 214.
42. M. J. Chamberlain *et al., Br. Med. J.,* **3,** 391(1972).
43. A. N. G. Clark and M. J. Parsonage, *Br. Med. J.,* **2,** 1155(1957).
44. C. G. Schirren, Sr., *Hautarzt,* **17,** 321(1966).
45. A. S. Wigfield, *Br. Med. J.,* **3,** 585(1972).
46. D. F. Tutunji, *Br. Med. J.,* **4,** 241(1972).
47. W. L. Epstein and A. M. Kligman, *Arch. Dermatol.,* **77,** 508(1958).
48. R. R. M. McLaughlin, *Arch. Dermatol.,* **106,** 129(1972).
49. R. Lester and D. Rosenthal, *Arch. Dermatol.,* **104,** 330(1971).
50. "Current Diagnosis and Treatment," M. A. Krupp and M. J. Chatton, Eds., Lange Medical Publications, Los Altos, Calif., 1973, pp. 56-57.
51. G. C. Sauer, "Manual of Skin Diseases," 3d ed., Lippincott, Philadelphia, Pa., 1973, pp. 159-181.
52. R. L. Baer and S. A. Rosenthal, *J. Am. Med. Assoc.,* **197,** 187(1966).
53. W. D. Stewart *et al.*, "Dermatology: Diagnosis and Treatment of Cutaneous Disorders," 3d ed., Mosby, St. Louis, Mo., 1974, pp. 234-259.
54. "An Introduction to the Biology of the Skin," R. H. Champion *et al.*, Eds., Davis, Philadelphia, Pa., 1970, pp. 206-221.
55. K. A. Arndt, "Manual of Dermatologic Therapeutics," Little, Brown, Boston, Mass., 1974, pp. 61-77.
56. A. Jarrett, "The Physiology and Pathophysiology of the Skin: The Epidermis," vol. 1, Academic Press, London, England, 1973, p. 155.
57. R. J. Yu *et al., J. Bacteriol.,* **96,** 1435(1968).
58. F. Sadik, *PharmIndex,* **15(7A),** 5(1973).
59. "Dermal Pathology," J. H. Graham *et al.*, Eds., Harper and Row, Hagerstown, Md., 1972, pp. 137-253.
60. H. T. Behrman *et al.*, "Common Skin Diseases: Diagnosis and Treatment," 2d ed., Grune and Stratton, New York, N.Y., 1971, p. 39.
61. "Current Therapy, 1972," H. F. Conn, Ed., Saunders, Philadelphia, Pa., 1972, p. 585.
62. S. M. Peck and H. Rosenfeld, *J. Invest. Dermatol.,* **1,** 237(1938).
63. E. L. Keeney *et al., Bull. Johns Hopkins Hosp.,* **77,** 422(1945).
64. M. J. Golden and K. A. Oster, *J. Am. Pharm. Assoc. (Sci. Ed.),* **39,** 47(1950).
65. "The United States Pharmacopeia," 19th rev., Mack Publishing, Easton, Pa., 1975, p. 532.
66. H. L. Wolin, "The Effectiveness of Various Desenex Preparations Against *Trichophyton mentagrophytes* Infected Guinea Pigs," Research Laboratories, The Brookdale Hospital Center, Brooklyn, N.Y., July 19, 1966, unpublished.
67. W. C. Cutting, "Handbook of Pharmacology," 5th ed., Meredith Corp., New York, N.Y., 1972, p. 56.
68. "AMA Drug Evaluations," 2d ed., Publishing Sciences Group, Acton, Mass., 1973, pp. 595-606.
69. "The United States Dispensatory and Physician's Pharmacology," 26th ed., A. Osol *et al.*, Eds., Lippincott, Philadelphia, Pa., 1024(1967).
70. "The United States Pharmacopeia," 19th rev., Mack Publishing, Easton, Pa., 1975, p. 49.
71. "The Pharmacological Basis of Therapeutics," 4th ed., L. S. Goodman and A. Gilman, Eds., Macmillan, New York, N.Y., 1970, p. 1036.
72. M. H. Walker, *J. Am. Podiatr. Assoc.,* **52,** 737(1962).
73. M. N. Gleason *et al.*, "Clinical Toxicology of Commercial Products, Acute Poisoning," 3d ed., Williams and Wilkins, Baltimore, Md., 1969, p. 37.
74. J. K. Morgan, *Br. J. Clin. Prac.,* **22,** 261(1968).
75. "The National Formulary," 13th ed., Mack Publishing, Easton, Pa., 1970, p. 139.
76. T. Noguchi *et al.*, "Antitrichophyton Activity of Naphthiomates in Antimicrobial Agents and Chemotherapy," American Society for Microbiology, Ann Arbor, Mich. 1962, p. 259.
77. G. A. Gellin *et al., Arch. Dermatol.,* **106,** 715(1972).
78. J. B. Shelmire, Jr., *J. Invest. Dermatol.,* **26,** 105(1956).
79. K. H. Kaidbey and A. M. Kligman, *Arch. Dermatol.,* **110,** 868(1974)
80. E. B. Smith *et al., South. Med. J.,* **67,** 776(1974).
81. A. H. Gould, *Dermatol. Trop.,* **3,** 255(1964).
82. H. L. Wolin, "A Comparison of Tinactin Liquid and Desenex Liquid Preparations Against *Trichophyton mentagrophytes* Infected Guinea Pigs," Research Laboratories, The Brookdale Hospital Center, Brooklyn, N.Y., August 24, 1966, unpublished.
83. K. A. Oster and M. J. Golden, *J. Am. Pharm. Assoc. (Sci. Ed.),* **37,** 429(1948).
84. G. A. Zentmyer, *Science,* **100,** 294(1944).
85. K. A. Oster and M. J. Golden, *Exp. Med. Surg.,* **1,** 37(1949).
86. "Sprowls' American Pharmacy," 7th ed., L. W. Dittert, Ed., Lippincott, Philadelphia, Pa., 1974, p. 49.
87. P. B. Price, *Arch. Surg.,* **61,** 23(1950).
88. "Remington's Pharmaceutical Sciences," 14th ed., A. Osol *et al.*, Eds., Mack Publishing, Easton, Pa., 1970, p. 768.
89. M. N. Gleason *et al.*, "Clinical Toxicology of Commercial Products, Acute Poisoning," 3d ed., Williams and Wilkins, Baltimore, Md., 1969, p. 27.

Products 32 ATHLETE'S FOOT

Product (manufacturer)	Application form	Antifungal	Keratolytic	Other
Aftate (Plough)	spray liquid spray powder powder gel	tolnaftate, 1%	—	—
Bevill's Lotion (Bevill)	lotion	—	salicylic acid	alcohol, 68% ether, 8% methyl salicylate, 1%
Blis-To-Sol (Chattem)	liquid gel aerosol powder powder	undecylenic acid, 5% (gel) 50 mg/g (liquid) zinc stearate, 10 mg/g (aerosol, powder)	salicylic acid, 90 mg/g (liquid) 10 mg/g (aerosol) 19 mg/g (powder) benzoic acid, 10 mg/g (aerosol) 19 mg/g (powder)	—
Bluboro (Derm-Arts)	powder	—	—	aluminum sulfate calcium acetate boric acid
Buro-Sol (Doak)	powder cream	—	—	aluminum acetate
Campho-Phenique (Glenbrook)	liquid powder	phenol, 4.75% (liquid) 2% (powder)	—	camphor, 10.86% (liquid) 4.38% (powder)
Daliderm (Dalin)	powder	zinc undecylenate sodium propionate	salicylic acid	methylbenzethonium chloride corn starch magnesium carbonate boric acid bentonite zinc oxide talc aromatic oils
Desenex (Pharmacraft)	ointment powder aerosol powder soap	zinc undecylenate, 20% (not in soap) undecylenic acid, 5% (ointment) 2% (powder, soap)	—	—
Desenex Liquid (Pharmacraft)	solution	undecylenic acid, 10%	—	isopropyl alcohol, 40% propylene glycol triethanolamine
Deso-Creme (Columbia Medical)	cream	zinc undecylenate, 20% caprylic acid, 5% sodium propionate, 2%	—	—
Domeboro (Dome)	liquid	—	—	aluminum sulfate calcium acetate
Enzactin (Ayerst)	cream spray powder	triacetin, 250 mg (cream) 15% (spray) 33.3% (powder)	—	—
Fungacetin (Blair)	liquid ointment powder	triacetin, 30% (liquid) 25% (ointment) 33.3% (powder)	—	—
Jim Wade Deodorant Foot Powder (Wade)	powder	8-hydroxyquinoline, 0.01%	—	aluminum sulfate, 15% menthol, 1% corn starch boric acid talc
Jim Wade Foot Medicine (Wade)	liquid	—	salicylic acid	sucrose octaacetate acetone
NP 27 Aerosol Powder (Norwich)	aerosol powder	zinc undecylenate	salicylic acid	dichlorophene

Product (manufacturer)	Application form	Antifungal	Keratolytic	Other
NP 27 Cream (Norwich)	cream	8-hydroxyquinoline	salicylic acid	benzoic acid propylparaben methylparaben
NP 27 Liquid (Norwich)	liquid	—	salicylic acid	benzoic acid isopropyl alcohol, 50% propylparaben benzyl alcohol chlorothymol
NP 27 Powder (Norwich)	powder	—	salicylic acid	benzoic acid eucalyptol menthol
Podiaspray (Dalin)	spray	undecylenic acid	salicylic acid	cetyltrimethylammonium bromide chloroxylenol aromatic base
Quinsana Foot Powder (Mennen)	powder	zinc undecylenate, 20% undecylenic acid, 2%	—	—
Rid-Itch Cream (Thomas & Thompson)	cream	zinc undecylenate, 20% undecylenic acid, 5%	—	emulsion base
Rid-Itch Liquid (Thomas & Thompson)	liquid	resorcinol, 1%	salicylic acid, 7%	boric acid, 5% benzoic acid, 2% chlorothymol, 1% alcohol glycerin
Salicresen (Upjohn)	liquid	—	salicylic acid, 2%	acetone, 10% benzoic acid, 2% secondary amyltricresols, 0.1% *o*-hydroxyphenylmercuric chloride, 0.1% alcohol, 50%
Solvex Ointment (Scholl)	ointment	—	salicylic acid	thymol benzoic acid
Solvex Powder (Scholl)	powder	8-hydroxyquinoline sulfate	colloidal sulfur salicylic acid	chlorothymol
Solvex Spray (Scholl)	spray	undecylenic acid	—	dichlorophene chlorothymol benzocaine propylene glycol alcohol
Sopronol (Wyeth)	liquid ointment powder	sodium propionate, 12.3% (liquid & ointment) 5% (powder) sodium caprylate, 10% zinc caprylate, 5% (ointment) zinc propionate, 5% (powder)	—	—
Tinactin Cream and Liquid (Schering)	cream solution	tolnaftate, 1%	—	polyethylene glycol 400 propylene glycol (cream) butylated hydroxytoluene titanium dioxide (cream)
Tinactin Powder (Schering)	powder aerosol powder	tolnaftate, 1%	—	corn starch (powder) talc propellants (aerosol) butylated hydroxytoluene (aerosol)
Ting (Pharmacraft)	cream powder	zinc stearate	—	benzoic acid boric acid zinc oxide alcohol, 16% (cream)

Products 32 ATHLETE'S FOOT

Product (manufacturer)	Application form	Antifungal	Keratolytic	Other
Verdefam Cream (Texas Pharmacal)	cream	propionic acid, 3% undecylenic acid, 2% sodium propionate, 1% sodium caprylate, 1% copper undecylenate, 0.5%	salicylic acid, 3%	—
Verdefam Solution (Texas Pharmacal)	solution	undecylenic acid, 5% propionic acid, 3% sodium propionate, 2% sodium caprylate, 2% copper undecylenate, 0.5%	salicylic acid, 5%	—

Products 32 CALLUS/CORN/WART

Product (manufacturer)	Application form	Active ingredients	Other
Bevill's Corn Remedy (Bevill)	lotion	salicylic acid ferric chloride tincture	alcohol, 70% ether methyl salicylate
Blis-To-Sol Corn and Callus Remover (Chattem)	liquid	salicylic acid, 18% diperodon hydrochloride, 1% zinc chloride	collodion
Blue Jay Callus Pads and Discs (Colgate-Palmolive)	unmedicated pads and medicated discs	phenoxyethanoic acid	—
Blue Jay Callus Plaster (Colgate-Palmolive)	plaster	phenoxyethanoic acid	—
Blue Jay Corn Pads (Colgate-Palmolive)	medicated and unmedicated pads	phenoxyethanoic acid	—
Blue Jay Corn Pad Treatment (Colgate-Palmolive)	unmedicated pads ointment	phenoxyethanoic acid benzocaine chlorobutanol thymol benzoxiquine zinc oxide	—
Blue Jay Corn Plaster (Colgate-Palmolive)	plaster	phenoxyethanoic acid	—
Blue Jay Liquid Corn-Callus Remover (Colgate-Palmolive)	liquid	phenoxyethanoic acid	pyroxylin acetone
Compound W Wart Remover (Whitehall)	liquid	salicylic acid, 14% glacial acetic acid, 11% menthol, 2% camphor, 1.5% castor oil	alcohol ether acetone
Derma-Soft Creme (Creighton)	cream	salicylic acid, 2.5%	cream base
Dr. Scholl's Corn/Callous Salve (Scholl)	ointment	salicylic acid	eucalyptus oil petrolatum lanolin mineral oil
Dr. Scholl's "2" Drop Corn-Callous Remover (Scholl)	liquid	salicylic acid camphor	alcohol, 15% ether, 9.65 g/30 ml
Dr. Scholl's Fixo Corn Plaster (Scholl)	plaster	salicylic acid	—
Dr. Scholl's Waterproof Corn Pads (Scholl)	unmedicated pads and medicated discs	salicylic acid	—
Dr. Scholl's Zino-Pads (Scholl)	unmedicated pads and medicated discs	salicylic acid	—

Product (manufacturer)	Application form	Active ingredients	Other
Freezone Corn and Callus Remover (Whitehall)	liquid	salicylic acid zinc chloride hypophosphorous acid	alcohol Oregon balsam fir collodion
Solvex Liquid (Scholl)	liquid	benzoic acid salicylic acid benzocaine chlorothymol	alcohol, 45%
Vergo (Daywell)	ointment	calcium pantothenate ascorbic acid	starch
Wart Fix (Alvin Last)	liquid	castor oil	—

PRODUCT INDEX

A

B

C

PRODUCT INDEX

D

E

PRODUCT INDEX

J

K

L

M

N

O

P

Q

R

S

T

U

V

W

X

Y

Z